Treatment of Psychiatric Disorders Among Older Adults

Rajesh R. Tampi • Deena J. Tampi
Editors

Treatment of Psychiatric Disorders Among Older Adults

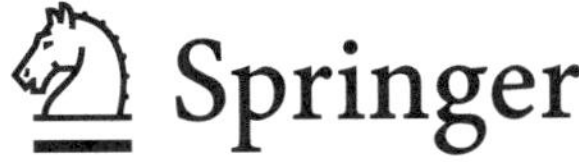
Springer

Editors
Rajesh R. Tampi
Department of Psychiatry
Creighton University
Omaha, NE, USA

Deena J. Tampi
Co-Founder & Managing Principal
Behavioral Health Advisory Group
Princeton, NJ, USA

ISBN 978-3-031-55713-2   ISBN 978-3-031-55711-8   (eBook)
https://doi.org/10.1007/978-3-031-55711-8

This Springer imprint is published by the registered company Springer Nature Switzerland AG
The registered company address is: Gewerbestrasse 11, 6330 Cham, Switzerland

If disposing of this product, please recycle the paper.

Contents

Contributors

Esther Akinyemi Department of Psychiatry, Henry Ford Health, Detroit, MI, USA

Ali Abbas Asghar-Ali Department of Psychiatry, Baylor College of Medicine, Houston, TX, USA

Mack Bozman UAB Heersink School of Medicine, Birmingham, AL, USA

Amanda L. Campbell Department of Psychiatry, St. Luke's University Health Network, Easton, PA, USA

Adiel Carlo Department of Psychiatry, University of Arizona School of Medicine, Tucson, AZ, USA

Hadley Cameron-Carter Department of Psychiatry, Henry Ford Health, Detroit, MI, USA

Seetha Chandrasekhara Department of Psychiatry, Lewis Katz School of Medicine at Temple University, Philadelphia, PA, USA

Rosalyn Chi Department of Internal Medicine, Division of Pulmonary, Critical Care, Sleep, and Occupational Medicine, Indiana University School of Medicine, Indianapolis, IN, USA

Michael Duerden Department of Psychiatry, University of Arizona School of Medicine, Tucson, AZ, USA

Mathew Erisman Department of Psychiatry, University of Arizona School of Medicine, Tucson, AZ, USA

Marisa Fallone Department of Psychiatry, Henry Ford Health, Detroit, MI, USA

Gibson George St. Luke's Penn Foundation, Department of Psychiatry, St. Luke's University Health Network, Easton, PA, USA

Ganesh Gopalakrishna Department of Psychiatry, University of Arizona-COMP, Phoenix, AZ, USA

Banner Alzheimer's Institute, Phoenix, AZ, USA

Darlon Jan Department of Psychiatry, Carilion Clinic-Virginia Tech Carilion School of Medicine, Roanoke, VA, USA

Melvin Joseph Department of Psychiatry, Henry Ford Health, Detroit, MI, USA

Pallavi Joshi Department of Psychiatry, University of Arizona-COMP, Phoenix, AZ, USA

Banner Alzheimer's Institute, Phoenix, AZ, USA

Amber Khan, MD Department of Psychiatry, Yale School of Medicine, New Haven, CT, USA

Babar Khan Department of Internal Medicine, Division of Pulmonary, Critical Care, Sleep, and Occupational Medicine, Indiana University School of Medicine, Indianapolis, IN, USA

Siddharth Khasnavis Department of Psychiatry, Yale University School of Medicine, New Haven, CT, USA

Marianne Klugheit Department of Psychiatry, University of Arizona School of Medicine, Tucson, AZ, USA

Michael G. Li Department of Psychiatry, University of Texas at Southwestern Medical Center, Dallas, TX, USA

North Texas Veterans Health Administration, Dallas Veterans Affairs Medical Center, Dallas, TX, USA

Alison Liss Temple University Hospital, Philadelphia, PA, USA

Padmapriya Marpuri Department of Psychiatry, St. Luke's University Health Network, Easton, PA, USA

Megan Mazzella Department of Psychiatry, Henry Ford Health, Detroit, MI, USA

Ali M. Molaie Department of Mental Health/Psychiatry, VA Greater Los Angeles Healthcare System, Los Angeles, CA, USA

Ty Owens Department of Neurology, Indiana University School of Medicine, Indianapolis, IN, USA

Nisha Patel Department of Psychiatry, University of Arizona-COMP, Phoenix, AZ, USA

Manju Pillai Temple University Hospital, Philadelphia, PA, USA

Senthil Vel Rajan Rajaram Manoharan Department of Psychiatry, Huntsville Hospital, Huntsville, AL, USA

UAB Heersink School of Medicine, Birmingham, AL, USA Laureen Raelly-Muze Long School of Medicine, University of Texas Health Science Center at San Antonio, San Antonia, TX, USA

Badr Ratnakaran Department of Psychiatry, Carilion Clinic-Virginia Tech Carilion School of Medicine, Roanoke, VA, USA

Ashish Sarangi Department of Psychiatry, University of Missouri-Columbia, Columbia, MO, USA

Christina Spoleti Department of Psychiatry, St. Luke's University Health Network, Easton, PA, USA

Deena J. Tampi Behavioral Health Advisory Group, Princeton, NJ, USA

Rajesh R. Tampi Department of Psychiatry, Creighton University School of Medicine, Omaha, NE, USA

Department of Psychiatry, Yale School of Medicine, New Haven, CT, USA

Hans F. von Walter Department of Mental Health/Psychiatry, VA Greater Los Angeles Healthcare System, Los Angeles, CA, USA

Department of Psychiatry and Biobehavioral Sciences, David Geffen School of Medicine at University of California, Los Angeles (UCLA), Los Angeles, CA, USA

Jessy Walia Huntsville Hospital, Huntsville, AL, USA

Sophia Wang Department of Psychiatry, Indiana University School of Medicine, Indianapolis, IN, USA

Department of Psychiatry, Indiana Alzheimer's Disease Research Center, Indiana University School of Medicine, Indianapolis, IN, USA

Demetrius Woodard Department of Psychiatry, University of Pennsylvania Health System, Philadelphia, PA, USA

Brandon C. Yarns Department of Mental Health/Psychiatry, VA Greater Los Angeles Healthcare System, Los Angeles, CA, USA

Department of Psychiatry and Biobehavioral Sciences, David Geffen School of Medicine at University of California, Los Angeles (UCLA), Los Angeles, CA, USA

Part I

Neurocognitive Disorders

Pallavi Joshi, Nisha Patel,
and Ganesh Gopalakrishna

Epidemiology

Alzheimer's disease (AD) is the most common type of dementia in the United States. It is the sixth leading cause of death in adults in the United States and the fifth leading cause of death in adults over the age of 65 years [1, 2]. The most important risk factor is age [3]. The risk of AD is 5% in those aged 65–74, 13.1% in those aged 75–84, and 33.2% in those over age 85 [4]. This increased risk with age is critical to note when looking at the population trends overall. In America, it is estimated that the population of people aged 65 and older will be 88 million by 2050 [5]. In 2022, from a global perspective, the total world population over the age of 65 is 10% of the total population, and it is expected to grow to 16% by 2050, which is twice the population of children aged 5 or younger [6, 7]. In 2022, 6.5 million Americans 65 years and older are estimated to have AD, and the number is predicted to increase to 12.7 million by 2050 [5]. Worldwide, it is estimated that 131 million will live with dementia by 2050 [8, 9].

The increase in the population of adults aged 65 and older compared to younger people is termed population aging, which is a result of decline in fertility, a rise in life expectancy, and decrease in mortality [5, 9]. The life expectancy increases with the advance in management and treatment of chronic health conditions such as cardiovascular disease and diabetes, both of which are associated with dementia.

The incidence of AD appears to be declining since the early 2000s. This is attributed to better management of chronic health conditions and increase in life expectancy, which in turn reduces the risk of developing AD [5, 10]. However, given the current increase in the number of people aging over 65, the annual incidence rate is expected to grow. It is important to note that epidemiological studies often have mixed results due to multiple factors. This includes data gathered from limited regions versus global populations, race, sex, genetics, differences in diagnostic categories, and finally screening with clinical symptoms rather than objective findings such as structural changes or biomarkers [10–12]. Often, misdiagnosis, overdiagnosis, lack of recognizing mild cognitive impairment versus dementia, and lack of use of biomarkers present as limitations in global reviews and meta-analyses [10, 12, 13]. Recently, the COVID-19 pandemic has impacted the life expectancy of individuals with AD, who are more vulnerable to death from COVID. In fact, one in ten death certificates with the initial cause of death as COVID-19 had listed the secondary cause as AD [14, 15].

P. Joshi (✉) · N. Patel · G. Gopalakrishna
Department of Psychiatry, University of Arizona-COMP, Phoenix, AZ, USA
e-mail: Pallavi.joshi@bannerhealth.com;
nisha.patel1@va.gov;
ganesh.gopalakrishna@bannerhealth.com

Prevalence of AD varies with biological sex, genetics, and race or ethnicity. Older Hispanic and Black Americans are more likely to have AD than older White Americans [10]. Many studies have shown that Blacks are twice as likely, and Hispanics are one and one-half times more likely to have any dementia compared to Whites [10, 16–18]. This may be associated with the marginalization of people of color in the United States, which leads to socioeconomic disparities such as suboptimal living environments and exposure to toxins, pollutants, and violence [5]. Reduced access to good education can reduce the cognitive reserve. These factors, in addition to disparities in the medical health system, predispose minorities to develop chronic conditions, which increases the risk of dementia [19–22].

Two-thirds or 4 million of Americans with AD over 65 are women [4, 23–25]. Women have a longer life span, which in turn may lead to a higher prevalence of dementia than men. It is postulated that estrogen regulates neurotransmission, neural development, protection against oxidative stress, reduction in amyloid beta-peptides, and reduction in effects of tau hyperphosphorylation [26]. With aging and menopause, ovarian function declines and the reduction in estrogen is associated with dementia. Some studies have also noted that the APOE-e4 genotype, the gene that increases the risk of developing AD, has a stronger association in women when specifically looking at ages 55–70 years [27–29].

Risk Factors

This section consists of an overview of the different risk factors and protective factors. The main risk factors include age, genetics, and family history. Other risk factors include gender; cerebrovascular disease; diabetes; dyslipidemia; obesity; diet; education; physical, social, and cognitive activity levels; sleep; smoking; and low vitamin D levels. Risk factors can be categorized into non-modifiable and modifiable or acquired [8, 30, 31]. The non-modifiable factors include age, gender, race, ethnicity, and genetics. The rest are modifiable or combination of both modifiable

and non-modifiable. In fact, from a pathological perspective, mixed dementia is a very common cause with the combination of non-modifiable and modifiable factors being AD and cardiovascular disease, respectively [8, 31, 32]. Addressing these factors may decrease the risk of developing AD, but it does not necessarily prevent cognitive decline altogether.

Age is the greatest risk factor, and the risk of AD increases with age. Late-onset AD (LOAD), which is diagnosed after the age of 65, is the most common type. Early-onset Alzheimer's disease (EOAD) starts before age 65 and is rare, accounting for only 6% of cases of AD [26, 32]. Genetics and family history play a strong role in the development of this disease. Family history of AD in a first-degree relative(s) increases the risk of developing AD. Early-onset cases involve inherited autosomal dominant patterns and mutations in dominant genes such as amyloid precursor protein (APP), presenilin-1 (PSEN-1), and presenilin-2 (PSEN-2). The autosomal dominant pattern and mutations in the three dominant genes only account for less than 1% of all AD cases; however, these mutations increase the beta-amyloid plaque burden and rate of development [26, 33, 34].

Apolipoprotein E (APOE) is involved in intercellular and interstitial transport of lipid metabolism [35, 36]. Every individual has one of the three APOE genes, e2, e3, and e4. These are inherited from each parent, and with this, there are a total of six different pairs with the possible combination of the gene type [5, 36]. Just having one copy of e4 form may lead to three times the risk of developing AD, and having two copies of the e4 will increase the risk 12-fold [5, 37]. A meta-analysis by Farrer studied the frequency of APOE and odds ratio of developing Alzheimer's disease [38]. The data showed that different ethnicities have variable risk. African and Hispanic e4 carriers have a lower APOE Alzheimer's risk compared to Caucasians and Japanese e4 carriers. This data did show an APOE e4 frequency that is inversely associated with e4-related risk [36, 38]. Other studies supported this by revealing a lower increase in AD incidence in Africans despite African Americans having the higher baseline incidence [35, 39]. Mutations in APP lead to pathological accumulation of beta-amyloid fragments. This is seen in trisomy 21 (Down syndrome) and may explain the early onset of Alzheimer's disease in Down syndrome [5, 40]. The mutations in presenilin gene 1 come from genes in chromosome 14, and mutations of presenilin gene 2 come from genes in chromosome 1. Both of these contribute to beta-amyloid pathology [23].

As mentioned, there are many modifiable factors outside of age, genetics, and family history. Cerebrovascular disease includes ischemia or hemorrhagic strokes, vasculopathy, and damage to white matter [31]. Suboptimal functioning of heart and blood vessels can lead to hypoxia, accumulation of neurotoxins, and neuronal damage by amyloidogenic pathways [5, 31, 41]. These events can increase the risk of AD. Postmortem pathological studies in those diagnosed with Alzheimer's have revealed concurrent cerebrovascular disease [30, 42].

Cardiovascular disease is an acquired but modifiable risk factor. Cardiovascular injury or disease occurs from smoking, diabetes, midlife obesity, hypertension, prehypertension, high cholesterol, and reduced physical activity [5, 26, 43]. Hypertension can damage or thicken the vascular wall leading to the cerebrovascular events mentioned previously along with peripheral vascular disease and atherosclerosis, which in turn can lead to neuronal damage and accumulation of beta amyloid. Hypercholesterolemia causes atherosclerosis and damage to the blood–brain barrier, which is a potential mechanism contributing to increased risk of dementia. In animal models, beta-amyloid peptide deposition and neurofibrillary tangles were noted to increase with elevated cholesterol [26, 44, 45]. Smoking increases oxidative stress, free radicals and inflammation, and cardiovascular disease, all of which are associated with dementia [31]. The Finnish Geriatric (FINGER) Intervention Study to Prevent Cognitive Impairment and Disability is a multidomain intervention study, which showed a slowing of cognitive decline with multidomain interventions such as physical exercise, management of metabolic and vascular risk factors, cognitive training, social stimulation, and dietary modifications [26, 46].

Obesity is associated with increased adipose tissue, which releases pro-inflammatory cytokines, which in turn can lead to systemic and brain inflammation. Obesity can also cause hyperglycemia and diabetes, both of which can cause oxidative stress, neuroinflammation, and insulin resistance or deficiency. Diabetes mellitus type 2 has been implicated in increasing the risk of AD by possible mechanism of reduction in beta-amyloid clearance and tau hyperphosphorylation [26, 44, 47].

Other modifiable risk factors contributing to Alzheimer's include poor sleep, early adult depression, smoking and alcohol, environment and pollution, trauma, and infection and delirium. Sleep disorders such as insomnia and sleep disordered breathing increase the risk for all dementias; however, it is important to note that sleep disorders might develop at the onset of dementia [30, 48].

Protective factors include physical activity, education, social engagement, cognitively stimulating jobs, and healthy diets. These factors allow for access to healthy and safe environments free from pollution, violence, and toxic metals such as lead and aluminum. Education is a protective factor and reduces the risk of Alzheimer's. Education supports cognitive agility, flexibility, and efficiency [5, 49, 50]. Cognitive training and engagement such as mind games as well as music and art therapy can help maintain functioning and improve quality of life [5, 26]. Incorporating a heart-healthy diet such as the Mediterranean diet which consists of vegetables, whole grains, healthy fats, chicken, nuts, fish, leafy greens, and legumes can provide antioxidant activity and reduce the risk of cardiovascular disease. Ensure that vitamin D is supplemented because deficiency can cause oxidation, inflammation, and amyloidogenic disease. Vitamin D regulates neurotrophic factors and reduces inflammation, which can reduce the risk of dementia. Physical exercise also reduces blood pressure, obesity, and inflammatory activity and can activate neurogenetic and synaptic plasticity [5, 51].

Assessment

Clinical Presentation

The initial clinical evaluation for an older adult presenting with cognitive impairment (outlined in Fig. 1.1) should consist of a thorough clinical interview with a collateral historian including a functional assessment; a physical examination including a focused neurological examination and mental status examination; a brief objective cognitive examination tool; selected laboratory tests to assess for reversible causes of cognitive impairment; and structural brain imaging [52, 53].

Evaluation of cognitive impairment requires thorough history taking from the patient as well as LoL from collateral, usually a close family member or friend. Collateral information is key since some patients may have difficulty recalling pertinent details or lack insight into their condition. In cases of more advanced cognitive impairment, a collateral informant may be the only source of information available.

The typical presentation of AD consists of slowly progressive memory decline with an insidious onset. However, less common non-amnestic forms of AD have a different presentation. Early on, individuals with AD typically present with impairment in memory and thinking that often manifests as subtle forgetfulness, occasional repetition of stories, and, of special importance, difficulty recalling the details of recent events. In contrast, memories of the distant past, immediate recollection of a recently learned address or phone number, or memory for vocabulary or concepts is not commonly affected early in the disease. As the disease progresses, other cognitive domains become affected, with executive function and problem-solving typically being the first to deteriorate [54, 55].

Although the extent and rate of progression vary between individuals, disease staging (mild, moderate, and severe) is based on the extent of functional impairment defined by instrumental activities of daily living (IADLs) and basic activities of daily living (ADLs). IADLs are activities which allow for independent living in the community such as shopping, food preparation, housekeeping, and finances; ADLs encompass basic activities such as feeding, dressing, bathing, toileting, and ambulation. Available instruments to assess functioning include the Functional Assessment Staging Tool (FAST Scale), the Lawton Instrumental Activities of Daily Living (IADL) Scale, and Katz Index of Independence in Activities of Daily Living (ADL). In the milder stages, individuals are relatively independent in many IADLs but require assistance in more complex activities (e.g., managing finances). Functioning in ADLs is preserved in the milder stages. Moderate stages are characterized by difficulties in some of the ADLs, while individuals in the severe stage consistently need assistance with almost all ADLs.

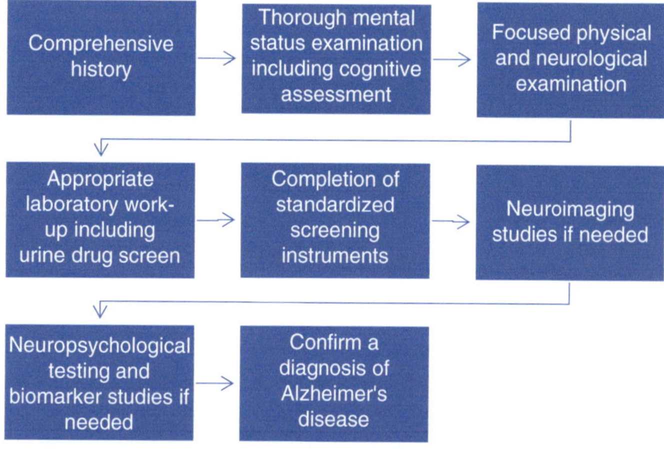

Fig. 1.1 Workup for Alzheimer's disease (adapted from [52, 53])

An office-based standardized cognitive test is essential to quantify the cognitive deficits. The most commonly used assessments are the Montreal Cognitive Assessment (MoCA), Mini Mental Status Examination (MMSE), and Saint Louis University Mental Status (SLUMS) Exam. The MoCA is more sensitive and comprehensive in identifying cognitive decline compared to the MMSE [56]. Both the SLUMS and MoCA have been found to be more sensitive than the MMSE in detecting MCI [57]. Several comparative studies have found the MoCA and SLUMS to be similarly effective at detecting MCI and dementia [57, 58]. In contrast to the MMSE and MoCA which are both copyrighted, the SLUMS can be used without incurring a charge. Formal neuropsychological testing, which provides a comprehensive profile of each cognitive domain, may be pursued if the cognitive deficits are either borderline or for highly educated and highly functioning patients [56, 59].

Physical/Neurological Examination

The physical/neurological examination, including a mental status examination, is an indispensable part of the initial evaluation. Physical and neurological examination in early AD is essentially normal unless a comorbid medical or neurological condition is present. The use of "smell cards" can help identify olfactory dysfunction, seen in early AD [60, 61]. The presence of focal neurological signs such as aphasia, apraxia, hemineglect, motor weakness, hyperreflexia, visual field deficits, and somatosensory loss can suggest an additional vascular etiology and may prompt a referral to a specialist for further assessment [62].

Diagnostic Criteria

The *Diagnostic and Statistical Manual of Mental Disorders, Fifth Edition (DSM-5)*, specifies the following criteria for the diagnosis of major neurocognitive disorder due to Alzheimer's disease [63]:

(a) The diagnostic criteria for major or mild neurocognitive disorder are fulfilled.
(b) Insidious onset and gradual decline of cognitive function in one or more areas for mild neurocognitive disorder, or two or more areas for major neurocognitive disorder.
(c) The diagnostic criteria for either possible or probable Alzheimer's dementia are fulfilled, as defined by the following:

Presence of causal Alzheimer's dementia genetic mutation based on family history or genetic testing.

The following three indicators are present:

1. Decline in memory or learning, and one other cognitive area, based on history or trials of neuropsychological testing
2. Steady cognitive decline, without periods of stability
3. No indicators of other psychological, neurological, or medical problems responsible for cognitive decline

Blood Tests and Imaging

Blood tests are useful in excluding some reversible comorbidities. These include vitamin B12, folate, thyroid-stimulating hormone (TSH), calcium, glucose, complete blood cell count, renal and liver function, rapid plasma reagin test, and HIV [63, 64]. Structural neuroimaging is useful in identifying potentially treatable causes of cognitive impairment such as an operable tumor or normal pressure hydrocephalus (NPH) and in identifying specific patterns observed in different neurocognitive disorders. Although computer tomography (CT) and magnetic resonance imaging (MRI) are both routinely used to rule out reversible causes of cognitive impairment, MRI is more sensitive in identifying patterns of neurodegeneration in AD [65]. Photon emission tomography (PET) scan can show beta-amyloid or tau deposition, and fluorodeoxyglucose (FDG) PET hypometabolism can be used to differentiate atypical presentations of AD from other neurodegenerative conditions such as frontotemporal dementia [66]. Structural MRI is the only widely available neuroimaging modality. Amyloid PET has limited clinical utilization outside of research. Amyloid PET can be appropriately used by a dementia expert as a single piece of information to support or oppose a clinical diagnosis of AD in an individual in whom cognitive impairment has been objectively verified, in whom there is substantial uncertainty as to the underlying pathology, and for whom greater diagnostic certainty would change management [65]. However, coverage by commercial health insurance or Medicare is limited. It is approved for coverage in the Veterans Health Administration system only when ordered by a dementia expert.

The National Institute on Aging and Alzheimer's Association (NIA-AA) guidelines recommend that MRI, PET, or CSF biomarkers be used as optional clinical tools for use where available and when deemed appropriate by the clinician to enhance the certainty of AD pathophysiology [66]. A low cerebrospinal fluid (CSF) AB42/AB40 ratio points to beta-amyloid deposition and is suggestive of AD pathology. Overall, AD biomarkers are used as a supportive diagnostic tool in clinical practice only when the clinician deems that their use will change the management, not as a routine test.

Biomarker evidence of neurodegeneration is the least specific finding in AD but is useful in staging the disease. The A/T/N classification of clinical criteria for probable AD is based on AB deposition (A), tau deposition (T), and neurodegeneration (N). Of note, individuals with cognitive impairment concomitant with biomarker evidence of AB deposition and a second biomarker (T or N) have a significantly increased rate of cognitive decline compared to individuals who have neither or only AB deposition [67]. Several blood biomarkers are being developed for AB deposition, tau deposition, and neurodegeneration. Biomarkers for tau deposition and neurodegeneration include CSF phosphorylated tau (P-tau) and elevated CSF total tau, respectively. Although these blood biomarkers are currently used for research purposes, there is great promise that they will eventually be used in clinical practice given their similar efficiency in detecting biomarker abnormalities when compared to more expensive imaging biomarkers and more invasive CSF biomarkers.

Treatments

The management of nonreversible neurocognitive disorders focuses on reducing the burden of the disease on patients and their caregivers by delaying the progression of cognitive decline and loss of functionality and treating neuropsychiatric symptoms when present. Both non-pharmacological and pharmacological treatments are available and are often used in conjunction. Treatment should be tailored based on the etiology and severity of the neurocognitive disorder; nevertheless, some non-pharmacological treatments are often useful in any kind of neurocognitive disorder. Atri proposes the treatment paradigm outlined in Fig. 1.2 [54].

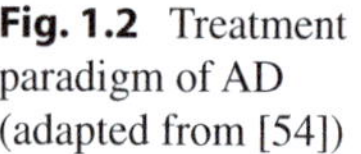

Fig. 1.2 Treatment paradigm of AD (adapted from [54])

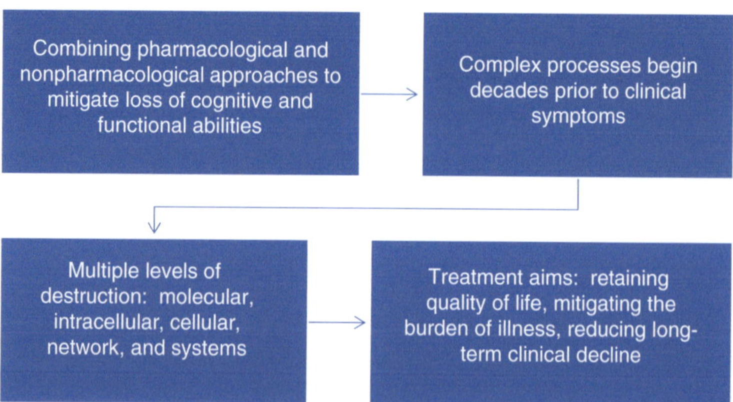

Non-pharmacological

Management of AD focuses on lifestyle modifications to try to slow the progression of cognitive impairment. Diet, exercise, and cognitive stimulation have shown to be effective, albeit modestly, in this regard. The Mediterranean-Dietary Approaches to Stop Hypertension (DASH) diet Intervention for Neurological Delay (MIND) diet, a hybrid of the Dietary Approaches to Stop Hypertension (DASH) and the Mediterranean diet, was developed specifically for dementia prevention by emphasizing the dietary components and servings linked to neuroprotection [68]. The MIND diet has been shown to be superior to other plant diets, including the Mediterranean Lol diet, in decreasing the risk of some types of neurocognitive disorder, slowing the progression of cognitive decline, and has even been found to improve cognition [68–70]. Table 1.1 gives a brief overview of the MIND diet. When possible, consulting a nutritionist to assist with implementing the MIND diet may be helpful.

Physical exercise has been shown to slow cognitive decline and promote independent functioning in mild cognitive impairment (MCI) as well as in dementia [71]. Although most of the studies have focused on aerobic exercise as an intervention, the ideal type or amount of physical activity needed to maximize its benefits on cognition is still not well understood.

Cognitively stimulating leisure activities may also be effective in delaying cognitive decline [72–74]. Cognitively stimulating activities should be carefully chosen based on the individual's cognitive abilities so as to avoid undue frustration and stress. Reminiscence therapy, music therapy, art therapy, and CST have shown to be of potential benefit to people with dementia by improving the quality of life and some even improving cognition [75–77].

Due to the complexity of neurocognitive disorders and its global effect on functionality and health, a collaborative approach with social workers, clinician managers, occupational therapists, nutritionists, speech therapists, physical therapists, palliative care, and others is helpful. Direct collaboration with caregivers is key, and support and education for them should be readily available due to the high caregiver burden of caring for someone with dementia [78, 79]. Table 1.2 lists online resources for patients and caregivers. Close attention to potential safety

Table 1.1 No brief overview of the Mediterranean-DASH diet Intervention for Neurological Delay (MIND) diet [66]

Food groups	Servings
Whole grains	3 or more per day
Green leafy vegetables	2 or more per day
Other vegetables	1 or more a day
Berries	2 or more per week
Fish	1 or more per week
Poultry	2 or more per week
Beans	3 or more per week
Nuts	5 or more per week
Olive oil	Primary oil
Butter, margarine	Less than 1 tablespoon per day
Red meats and products	Less than 4 per week
Fast and fried food	Less than 1 per week
Cheese	Less than 1 per week
Pastries and sweets	Less than 5 per week
Wine	Less than 1 glass per day

Table 1.2 Selected online resources for dementia care

Alzheimer's Association (alz.org)	Offers extensive information, a 24/7 helpline and services for patients with AD and their caregivers. Patient and caregivers can also connect with local chapters
National Institute on Aging (NIA) Information Center (nia.nih.gov/health)	Offers free publications in English and Spanish about aging
Eldercare Locator (eldercare.acl.gov)	A public service of the US administration on aging that aims to connect patient and caregivers to local support resources such as meals, home care, or transportation
National Institute on Aging (NIA) Alzheimer's and Related Dementias Education and Referral (ADEAR) Center	Offers information of diagnosis, treatment, patient care, caregiver needs, long-term care, and research and clinical trials related to AD

issues (i.e., driving, proper use of kitchen appliances and furnaces, medication management, access to firearms, elderly abuse), finances, long-term healthcare planning, medical and advanced care directives, and personal hygiene is essential [8, 80–82]. In cases where caregiver support is either not available or insufficient to meet the needs of individuals with dementia, home care, meal services, adult day care programs, respite services, and/or placement in assisted living facilities or skilled nursing facilities should be considered.

available, and their efficacy is similar [84]. However, their adverse effect profile varies. Table 1.3 lists the different acetylcholinesterase inhibitors and their indications, dosage titration, and common adverse effects. Overall, a slow titration over 4–8 weeks is recommended. If adverse effects arise, the dosage may be lowered temporarily before re-titrating more slowly and monitoring for recurrence of adverse effect. Alternatively, the medication can be discontinued, and a different one in the same class can be trialed.

Pharmacological

Cholinesterase Inhibitors

Acetylcholinesterase inhibitors were the first drugs approved in the United States for AD. These drugs inhibit the enzyme acetylcholinesterase, resulting in relative increase in available acetylcholine at the synaptic cleft. In a meta-analysis review of ten randomized, double-blind, placebo-controlled trials, each with a 6-month duration of drug exposure, acetylcholinesterase inhibitors were associated with 2.4 points slower decline (95% CI, −2.7 to −2.0; $P < 0.001$) for a cognitive outcome with a range of 0–70.9 [83]. Modest improvements were also seen in activities of daily living and behaviors. Three acetylcholinesterase inhibitors—donepezil, rivastigmine, and galantamine—are

NMDA Receptor Agonist

Memantine is an N-methyl-D-aspartate receptor antagonist which is FDA approved for moderate to severe AD, and it can be used as monotherapy or in combination with an acetylcholinesterase inhibitor. There is evidence that combination therapy with an acetylcholinesterase inhibitor and memantine is more beneficial for cognitive and functional function in patients with moderate to severe AD when compared with monotherapy with a ChEI [85, 86]. The clinical guideline is to start with an acetylcholinesterase inhibitor in the mild stage of AD and then to add memantine once the disease progresses to the moderate stage. Memantine monotherapy is usually reserved for individuals who cannot tolerate an acetylcholinesterase inhibitor [8]. Table 1.4 lists

Table 1.3 Cholinesterase inhibitors: FDA-approved indications, dosage titration, and common adverse effects [54]

Cholinesterase inhibitors	FDA-approved indication	Dosage titration	Adverse effects
Donepezil	Mild to severe stages of AD	*Mild to moderate stages (tablet or orally disintegrating tablet):* 5 mg once daily initially; may increase to 10 mg once daily after 4–6 weeks *Moderate to severe stages (tablet or orally disintegrating tablet):* 5 mg once daily initially; may increase to 10 mg once daily after 4–6 weeks; may increase further to 23 mg once daily if stable on 10 mg once daily for more than 3 months	Nausea, vomiting, diarrhea, loss of appetite, decrease in weight, abnormal dreams, insomnia; caution in patients with bradycardia, respiratory disease, seizure disorder, peptic ulcer disease, and urinary tract obstruction

Table 1.3 (continued)

Cholinesterase inhibitors	FDA-approved indication	Dosage titration	Adverse effects
Rivastigmine	Oral: Mild to severe stages of AD Transdermal: all stages of AD	*Capsule:* 1.5 mg twice daily initially; increase by 3 mg daily in every 2 weeks up to 6 mg twice daily *Transdermal patch in mild to moderate stages:* 4.6 mg per 24 h initially; increase as tolerated to 9.5 mg per 24 h after 4 weeks; may increase to a maximum dose of 13.3 mg per 24 h after 4 weeks if needed (9.5–13.3 mg recommended effective dose) *Transdermal patch in severe stage:* Same as in mild to moderate stages but target dose is 13.3 mg per 24 h	Nausea, vomiting, diarrhea, loss of appetite, decrease in weight, abnormal dreams, insomnia; caution in patients with bradycardia, respiratory disease, seizure disorder, peptic ulcer disease, and urinary tract obstruction Transdermal patch can cause local skin irritation and reactions (change patch location with each placement to minimize the risk); has less risk of GI adverse events compared to oral preparation
Galantamine	Mild to moderate stages of AD	*Extended-release capsule:* 8 mg once daily for 4 weeks; if tolerated, increase to 16 mg once daily for 4 more than 4 weeks; if tolerated, increase to 24 mg once daily (recommended target dose range, 16–24 mg once daily) *Immediate-release tablet or solution:* 4 mg twice daily for 4 weeks initially; if tolerated, increase to 8 mg twice daily for 4 or more weeks; if tolerated, increase to 12 mg twice daily (recommended target dose range, 16–24 mg daily in two divided doses)	Nausea, vomiting, diarrhea, loss of appetite, decrease in weight, abnormal dreams, insomnia; caution in patients with bradycardia, respiratory disease, seizure disorder, peptic ulcer disease, and urinary tract obstruction

Table 1.4 Memantine: FDA-approved indications, dosage titration, and common adverse effects [54]

Drug	FDA-approved indication	Dosing	Adverse effects
Memantine	Moderate to severe stages of AD	Starting dose: 5 mg/d; increase dose in 5 mg increments minimum 1 week apart Max dose: 20 mg/d divided	Dizziness, confusion, headache, constipation
Memantine XR	Moderate to severe stages of AD	Starting dose: 7 mg/d Target dose: 28 mg/d, increase in 7 mg increments every seventh day	Dizziness, confusion, headache, constipation

the indication, dosage titration, and common adverse effects of memantine. A fixed-dose combination drug of memantine and donepezil (brand name Namzaric) is also available and can be used to improve adherence and decrease pill burden [87].

Anti-Amyloid Monoclonal Antibodies

Aducanumab

Aducanumab is a human IgG1 anti-Aβ monoclonal antibody selective for Aβ aggregates [88]. On June 7, 2021, aducanumab became the first anti-amyloid monoclonal antibody to receive accelerated FDA approval, which was subsequently updated to clarify mild cognitive impairment and mild AD as approved indications. Evidence for the efficacy and tolerability of aducanumab comes from two randomized, double-blind, placebo-controlled, parallel-group studies (EMERGE and ENGAGE) conducted by its manufacturer, Biogen. On post hoc analysis in the EMERGE trial, high-dose aducanumab was shown to be better than placebo on the following scales: −0.39 points on the CDR-SB, 0.6 points on the MMSE, −1.4 points on the ADAS-Cog13, and 1.7 points on the ADCS-ADL-MCI [87]. The ENGAGE trial did not show any benefit for aducanumab on any of the outcomes when compared to placebo.

Adverse Events

Aducanumab was associated with dose-related amyloid-related imaging abnormalities related to cerebral edema (ARIA-E) and to intracerebral hemorrhage (ARIA-H) [88]. The risk for these events was greater in ApoE ε4 carriers and tended to occur early (12–32 weeks) during treatment [89]. The risk for intracranial hemorrhage with aducanumab was low and similar to the placebo group.

Expert panel recommendations for the use of aducanumab include titrating aducanumab to the highest dose (10 mg/kg); dose interruption or treatment discontinuation for symptomatic ARIA and moderate to severe ARIA; and brain MRIs prior to initiating therapy, during the titration of the drug, and at any time that the patient has symptoms suggestive of ARIA [90]. There remains substantial uncertainty to the clinical benefit and ongoing dosing considerations of aducanumab. At the writing of this chapter, aducanumab is only covered by Medicare under coverage with evidence development (CED), such as enrollment in an FDA or National Institutes of Health (NIH)-approved clinical trials [91].

Lecanemab

Lecanemab is a humanized monoclonal antibody with high affinity for soluble Aβ protofibrils [92]. On January 6, 2023, lecanemab received accelerated FDA approval for the treatment of AD [93]. Evidence for the efficacy and tolerability of lecanemab comes from Clarity AD, an 18-month, multicenter, double-blind, placebo-controlled, parallel-group trial involving participants with early Alzheimer's disease. A phase 3 trial with 1795 participants showed that lecanemab was better than placebo in modifying the primary endpoint, the CDR-SB (−0.45 points on the CDR-SB, 95% CI, −0.67 to −0.23). A substudy with 698 participants showed greater reductions in brain amyloid burden with lecanemab than with placebo (−59.1 centiloids, 95% CI, −62.6 to −55.6), −1.44 points on the ADAS-Cog14 and 2.0 points on the ADCS-ADL-MCI [94].

Adverse Events

Similar to aducanumab, lecanemab was associated with dose-related ARIA-E and ARIA-H [94]. In the Clarity AD trial, the most common adverse events in the lecanemab group were ARIA-H (lecanemab: 17.3%, placebo: 9.0%), ARIA-E (lecanemab: 12.6%, placebo: 1.7%), headache (lecanemab: 11.1%, placebo: 8.1%), and falls (lecanemab: 10.4%, placebo: 9.6%). The risk for these events was greater in ApoE ε4 carriers [94]. Longer trials are needed to determine the efficacy and safety of lecanemab in early AD and to establish clinical guidelines.

Additional therapies such as gantenerumab and donanemab are in various stages of development.

A Note on Behavioral and Psychological Symptoms of Dementia (BPSD)

Behavioral and neuropsychiatric symptoms are common in dementia. Detailed assessment and management of BPSD are covered in Chap. 6 of this book.

Conclusions

Alzheimer's disease (AD) is the most common cause of dementia and the sixth leading cause of death in the United States. It carries significant burden to society, increases healthcare costs, and causes significant distress to patients and caregivers. In addition to history taking, cognitive and physical examination, and laboratory workup, neuroimaging and fluid biomarkers can help with the diagnosis of AD in clinically challenging cases. Management includes non-pharmacological and pharmacological treatments tailored to the etiology and to the individual. The first-line pharmacological treatment for AD is an acetylcholinesterase inhibitor. Memantine can be added in the moderate to severe stages of the disease. Anti-amyloid monoclonal antibodies are emerging therapies that hold promise in modifying the treatment paradigm. A collaborative approach is key due to the complexity of neurocognitive disorders and its global effect on functionality and health.

References

1. Centers for Disease Control and Prevention (CDC). Health, United States, 2015: With special feature on racial and ethnic health disparities. CDC website. https://www.cdc.gov/nchs/data/hus/hus15.pdf. Published 2016. Accessed 23 Dec 2022.
2. GBD 2015 Mortality and Causes of Death Collaborators. Global, regional, and national life expectancy, all-cause mortality, and cause-specific mortality for 249 causes of death, 1980–2015: a systematic analysis for the Global Burden of Disease Study 2015. Lancet. 2016;388(10053):1459–544. https://doi.org/10.1016/S0140-6736(16)31012-1.
3. Guerreiro R, Bras J. The age factor in Alzheimer's disease. Genome Med. 2015;7:106.
4. Rajan KB, Weuve J, Barnes LL, McAninch EA, Wilson RS, Evans DA. Population estimate of people with clinical AD and mild cognitive impairment in the United States (2020-2060). Alzheimers Dement. 2021;17:1966. https://doi.org/10.1002/alz.12362.
5. Alzheimer's Association. Alzheimer's disease facts and figures. Alzheimers Dement. 2022;2022:18.
6. He W, Goodkind D, Paul Kowal US, Bureau C. International population reports, P95/16–1, an aging world: 2015, U.S. Washington, DC: Government Publishing Office; 2016.
7. United Nations Department of Economic and Social Affairs, Population Division (2022). World Population Prospects 2022: Summary of Results. UN DESA/POP/2022/TR/NO.
8. Arvanitakis Z, Shah RC, Bennett DA. Diagnosis and management of dementia: review. JAMA. 2019;322(16):1589–99. https://doi.org/10.1001/jama.2019.4782.
9. Wimo A, Ali GC, Guerchet M, Prince M, Prina M, Wu YT. World Alzheimer report 2015. He global impact of dementia: an analysis of prevalence, incidence, cost and trends. Alzheimer's Disease International; 2015. https://www.alzint.org/resource/world-alzheimer-report-2015/Arvanitakis.
10. Rajan KB, Weuve J, Barnes LL, Wilson RS, Evans DA. Prevalence and incidence of clinically diagnosed Alzheimer's disease dementia from 1994 to 2012 in a population study. Alzheimers Dement. 2019;15(1):1–7.
11. Tahami Monfared AA, Byrnes MJ, White LA, Zhang Q. Alzheimer's disease: epidemiology and clinical progression. Neurol Ther. 2022;11(2):553–69. https://doi.org/10.1007/s40120-022-00338-8. Epub 2022 Mar 14
12. Hudomiet P, Hurd M, Rohwedder S. Dementia prevalence in the United States in 2000 and 2012: estimates based on a nationally representative study. J Gerontol B Psychol Sci Soc Sci. 2018;73(Suppl 1):S10–9.
13. Fiest KM, Roberts JI, Maxwell CJ, et al. The prevalence and incidence of dementia due to Alzheimer's disease: a systematic review and meta-analysis. Can J Neurol Sci. 2016;43(Suppl 1):S51–82.
14. Centers for Disease Control and Prevention. National Center for Health Statistics. Excess deaths associated with COVID-19. https://www.cdc.gov/nchs/nvss/vsrr/covid19/excess_deaths.htm
15. U.S. Department of Health and Human Services. Centers for Disease Control and Prevention. National Center for Health Statistics. CDC WONDER online database: about provisional mortality statistics, 2018 through last month. https://wonder.cdc.gov/mcd-icd10-provisional.html
16. Potter GG, Plassman BL, Burke JR, Kabeto MU, Langa KM, Llewellyn DJ, et al. Cognitive performance and informant reports in the diagnosis of cog-

nitive impairment and dementia in African Americans and whites. Alzheimers Dement. 2009;5(6):445–53.

17. Gurland BJ, Wilder DE, Lantigua R, Stern Y, Chen J, Killeffer EH, et al. Rates of dementia in three ethnoracial groups. Int J Geriatr Psychiatry. 1999;14(6):481–93.

18. Mehta KM, Yeo GW. Systematic review of dementia prevalence and incidence in United States race/ethnic populations. Alzheimers Dement. 2017;13(1):72–83.

19. Bailey ZD, Feldman JM, Bassett MT. How structural racism works—racist policies as a root cause of U.S. racial health inequities. N Engl J Med. 2021;384(8):768–73.

20. Bailey ZD, Krieger N, Agenor M, Graves J, Linos N, Bassett MT. Structural racism and health inequities in the USA: evidence and interventions. Lancet. 2017;389(10077):1453–63.

21. Zhang Z, Hayward MD, Yu YL. Life course pathways to racial disparities in cognitive impairment among older Americans. J Health Soc Behav. 2016;57(2):184–99.

22. Lines LM, Sherif NA, Wiener JM. Racial and ethnic disparities among individuals with Alzheimer's disease in the United States: a literature review. Research Triangle Park, NC: RTI Press; 2014.

23. U.S. Census Bureau. 2014 National population projections: downloadable files. https://www.census.gov/data/datasets/2014/demo/popproj/2014-popproj.html. Accessed 24 Dec 2022.

24. Seshadri S, Wolf PA, Beiser A, Au R, McNulty K, White R, et al. Lifetime risk of dementia and Alzheimer's disease. The impact of mortality on risk estimates in the Framingham study. Neurology. 1997;49(6):1498–504. 265.

25. Hebert LE, Scherr PA, McCann JJ, Beckett LA, Evans DA. Is the risk of developing Alzheimer's disease greater for women than for men? Am J Epidemiol. 2001;153(2):132–6.

26. Van Cauwenberghe C, Van Broeckhoven C, Sleegers K. The genetic landscape of Alzheimer disease: clinical implications and perspectives. Genet Med Off J Am Coll Med Genet. 2016;18:421–30.

27. Altmann A, Greicius MD. Apolipoprotein E, gender, and Alzheimer's disease: an overlooked, but potent and promising interaction. Brain Imaging Behav. 2014;8(2):262–73.

28. Ungar L, Altmann A, Gericius MD. Apolipoprotein E, gender, and Alzheimer's disease: an overlooked, but potent and promising interaction. Brain Imaging Behav. 2014;8(2):262–73.

29. Neu SC, Pa J, Kukull W, Beekly D, Kuzma A, Gangadharan P, et al. Apolipoprotein E genotype and sex risk factors for Alzheimer disease: a meta-analysis. JAMA Neurol. 2017;74(10):1178–89.

30. Silva MVF, Loures CMG, Alves LCV, de Souza LC, Borges KBG, Carvalho MDG. Alzheimer's disease: risk factors and potentially protective measures. J Biomed Sci. 2019;26(1):33. https://doi.org/10.1186/s12929-019-0524-y.

31. Schneider JA, Arvanitakis Z, Leurgans SE, Bennett DA. The neuropathology of probable Alzheimer disease and mild cognitive impairment. Ann Neurol. 2009;66(2):200–8. https://doi.org/10.1002/ana.21706.

32. Breijyeh Z, Karaman R. Comprehensive review on Alzheimer's disease: causes and treatment. Molecules. 2020;25(24):5789. https://doi.org/10.3390/molecules25245789.

33. Khanahmadi M, Farhud DD, Malmir M. Genetic of Alzheimer's disease: a narrative review article. Iran J Public Health. 2015;44:892–901.

34. Ward A, Crean S, Mercaldi CJ, Collins JM, Boyd D, Cook MN, et al. Prevalence of apolipoprotein e4 genotype and homozygotes (APOE e4/4) among patients diagnosed with Alzheimer's disease: a systematic review and meta-analysis. Neuroepidemiology. 2012;38:1–17.

35. Zhang R, Xu X, Yu H, Xu X, Wang M, Le W. Factors influencing Alzheimer's disease risk: whether and how they are related to the APOE genotype. Neurosci Bull. 2022;38(7):809–19.

36. Farrer LA, Cupples LA, Haines JL, Hyman B, Kukull WA, Mayeux R. Effects of age, sex, and ethnicity on the association between apolipoprotein E genotype and Alzheimer disease. A meta-analysis. APOE and Alzheimer Disease Meta Analysis Consortium. JAMA. 1997;278:1349–56.

37. National Down Syndrome Society. Alzheimer's disease and down syndrome. https://www.ndss.org/resources/alzheimers/.

38. Mayeda ER, Glymour MM, Quesenberry CP, Whitmer RA. Inequalities in dementia incidence between six racial and ethnic groups over 14 years. Alzheimers Dement. 2016;12:216–24.

39. Samieri C, Perier MC, Gaye B, Proust-Lima C, Helmer C, Dartigues JF, et al. Association of cardiovascular health level in older age with cognitive decline and incident dementia. JAMA. 2018;320(7):657–64.

40. Hauser PS, Narayanaswami V, Ryan RO. Apolipoprotein E: from lipid transport to neurobiology. Prog Lipid Res. 2011;50:62–74.

41. Fitzpatrick A, Kuller LH, Lopez OL, Diehr P, O'Meara ES, Longstreth WT, et al. Mid- and late-life obesity: risk of dementia in the Cardiovascular Health Cognition Study. Arch Neurol. 2009;66(336–42):122.

42. Anjum I, Fayyaz M, Wajid A, Sohail W, Ali A. Does obesity increase the risk of dementia: a literature review. Cureus. 2018;10:e2660.

43. Corrada MM, Hayden KM, Paganini-Hill A, Bullain SS, DeMoss J, Aguirre C, et al. Age of onset of hypertension and risk of dementia in the oldest-old: the 90+ study. Alzheimer Dement. 2017;13:103–10.

44. Nordestgaard LT, Tybjaerg-Hansen A, Nordestgaard BG, Frikke-Schmidt R. Loss-of-function mutation in ABCA1 and risk of Alzheimer's disease and cerebrovascular disease. Alzheimer's Dement J Alzheimer's Assoc. 2015;11:1430–8.

45. Proserpio P, Arnaldi D, Nobili F, Nobili L. Integrating sleep and Alzheimer's disease pathophysiology: hints

for sleep disorders management. J Alzheimers Dis. 2018;63(3):871–86.

46. Ballarini T, Melo van Lent D, Brunner J, Schroder A, Wolfsgruber S, Altenstein S, et al. Mediterranean diet, Alzheimer disease biomarkers and brain atrophy in old age. Neurology. 2021;96(24):e2920–32.

47. Pegueroles J, Jimenez A, Vilaplana E, Montal V, Carmona-Iragui M, Pane A, Alcolea D, Videla L, Casajoana A, Clarimon J, et al. Obesity and Alzheimer's disease, does the obesity paradox really exist? A magnetic resonance imaging study. Oncotarget. 2018;9:34,691–8.

48. Shi L, Chen SJ, Ma MY, Bao YP, Han Y, Wang YM, et al. Sleep disturbances increase the risk of dementia: a systematic review and meta-analysis. Sleep Med Rev. 2018;40:4–16.

49. Stern Y, Arenaza-Urquijo EM, Bartres-Faz D, Belleville S, Cantilon M, Chetelat G, et al. Whitepaper: defining and investigating cognitive reserve, brain reserve, and brain maintenance. Alzheimers Dement. 2018;pii:S1552-5260(18):33,491–5.

50. Love S, Miners JS. Cerebrovascular disease in ageing and Alzheimer's disease. Acta Neuropathol. 2016;131(5):645–58.

51. Najar J, Ostling S, Gudmundsson P, Sundh V, Johansson L, Kern S, et al. Cognitive and physical activity and dementia: a 44-year longitudinal population study of women. Neurology. 2019;92(12):e1322–30.

52. Pérez Palmer N, Trejo Ortega B, Joshi P. Cognitive impairment in older adults: epidemiology, diagnosis, and treatment. Psychiatr Clin North Am. 2022;45(4):639–61. https://doi.org/10.1016/j.psc.2022.07.010. Epub 2022 Oct 14.

53. McKhann GM, Knopman DS, Chertkow H, et al. The diagnosis of dementia due to Alzheimer's disease: recommendations from the National Institute on Aging-Alzheimer's Association workgroups on diagnostic guidelines for Alzheimer's disease. Alzheimers Dement J Alzheimers Assoc. 2011;7(3):263–9. https://doi.org/10.1016/j.jalz.2011.03.005.

54. Atri A. Current and future treatments in Alzheimer's disease. Semin Neurol. 2019;39(2):227–40.

55. Dubois B, Feldman HH, Jacova C, et al. Revising the definition of Alzheimer's disease: a new lexicon. Lancet Neurol. 2010;9(11):1118–27. https://doi.org/10.1016/S1474-4422(10)70223-4. Epub 2010 Oct 9.

56. Elkana O, Tal N, Oren N, Soffer S, Ash EL. Is the cutoff of the MoCA too high? Longitudinal data from highly educated older adults. J Geriatr Psychiatry Neurol. 2020;33(3):155–60. https://doi.org/10.1177/0891988719874121.

57. Sanford AM. Mild cognitive impairment. Clin Geriatr Med. 2017;33(3):325–37. https://doi.org/10.1016/j.cger.2017.02.005.

58. Cao L, Hai S, Lin X, et al. Comparison of the Saint Louis university mental status examination, the mini-mental state examination, and the Montreal cognitive assessment in detection of cognitive impairment in Chinese elderly from the geriatric department. J Am Med Dir Assoc. 2012;13(7):626–9. https://doi.org/10.1016/j.jamda.2012.05.003.

59. Cummings-Vaughn LA, Chavakula NN, Malmstrom TK, Tumosa N, Morley JE, Cruz-Oliver DM. Veterans affairs Saint Louis University mental status examination compared with the Montreal cognitive assessment and the short test of mental status. J Am Geriatr Soc. 2014;62(7):1341–6. https://doi.org/10.1111/jgs.12874.

60. de Moraes e Silva M, Mercer PBS, Witt MCZ, Pessoa RR. Olfactory dysfunction in Alzheimer's disease systematic review and meta-analysis. Dement Neuropsychol. 2018;12(2):123–32. https://doi.org/10.1590/1980-57642018dn12-020004.

61. Carnemolla SE, Hsieh JW, Sipione R, et al. Olfactory dysfunction in frontotemporal dementia and psychiatric disorders: a systematic review. Neurosci Biobehav Rev. 2020;118:588–611. https://doi.org/10.1016/j.neubiorev.2020.08.002.

62. Seraji-Bzorgzad N, Paulson H, Heidebrink J. Neurologic examination in the elderly. Handb Clin Neurol. 2019;167:73–88. https://doi.org/10.1016/B978-0-12-804766-8.00005-4.

63. American Psychiatric Association. Diagnostic and statistical manual of mental disorders. 5th ed. Washington, DC: American Psychiatric Publishing; 2013.

64. Albert MS, DeKosky ST, Dickson D, et al. The diagnosis of mild cognitive impairment due to Alzheimer's disease: recommendations from the National Institute on Aging-Alzheimer's Association workgroups on diagnostic guidelines for Alzheimer's disease. Alzheimers Dement J Alzheimers Assoc. 2011;7(3):270–9. https://doi.org/10.1016/j.jalz.2011.03.008.

65. Staffaroni AM, Elahi FM, McDermott D, et al. Neuroimaging in dementia. Semin Neurol. 2017;37(5):510–37. https://doi.org/10.1055/s-0037-1608808.

66. Johnson KA, Minoshima S, Bohnen NI, et al. Appropriate use criteria for amyloid PET: a report of the amyloid imaging task force, the Society of Nuclear Medicine and Molecular Imaging, and the Alzheimer's Association. Alzheimers Dement J Alzheimers Assoc. 2013;9(1):e-1–16. https://doi.org/10.1016/j.jalz.2013.01.002.

67. Jack CR, Bennett DA, Blennow K, et al. NIA-AA research framework: toward a biological definition of Alzheimer's disease. Alzheimers Dement J Alzheimers Assoc. 2018;14(4):535–62. https://doi.org/10.1016/j.jalz.2018.02.018.

68. Morris MC, Tangney CC, Wang Y, Sacks FM, Bennett DA, Aggarwal NT. MIND diet associated with reduced incidence of Alzheimer's disease. Alzheimers Dement J Alzheimers Assoc. 2015;11(9):1007–14. https://doi.org/10.1016/j.jalz.2014.11.009.

69. Kheirouri S, Alizadeh M. MIND diet and cognitive performance in older adults: a systematic review. Crit

Rev Food Sci Nutr. Published online May 14, 2021:. 2022;62:8059–77. https://doi.org/10.1080/10408398. 2021.1925220.

70. Hosking DE, Eramudugolla R, Cherbuin N, Anstey KJ. MIND not Mediterranean diet related to 12-year incidence of cognitive impairment in an Australian longitudinal cohort study. Alzheimers Dement J Alzheimers Assoc. 2019;15(4):581–9. https://doi.org/10.1016/j.jalz.2018.12.011.

71. Nuzum H, Stickel A, Corona M, Zeller M, Melrose RJ, Wilkins SS. Potential benefits of physical activity in MCI and dementia. Behav Neurol. 2020;2020:7807856. https://doi.org/10.1155/2020/7807856.

72. Butler M, McCreedy E, Nelson VA, et al. Does cognitive training prevent cognitive decline?: a systematic review. Ann Intern Med. 2018;168(1):63–8. https://doi.org/10.7326/M17-1531.

73. Hall CB, Lipton RB, Sliwinski M, Katz MJ, Derby CA, Verghese J. Cognitive activities delay onset of memory decline in persons who develop dementia. Neurology. 2009;73(5):356–61. https://doi.org/10.1212/WNL.0b013e3181b04ae3.

74. Altschul DM, Deary IJ. Playing analog games is associated with reduced declines in cognitive function: a 68-year longitudinal cohort study. J Gerontol Ser B. 2020;75(3):474–82. https://doi.org/10.1093/geronb/gbz149.

75. Wang JJ. Group reminiscence therapy for cognitive and affective function of demented elderly in Taiwan. Int J Geriatr Psychiatry. 2007;22(12):1235–40. https://doi.org/10.1002/gps.1821.

76. Lam HL, Li WTV, Laher I, Wong RY. Effects of music therapy on patients with dementia-a systematic review. Geriatr Basel Switz. 2020;5(4):E62. https://doi.org/10.3390/geriatrics5040062.

77. Emblad SYM, Mukaetova-Ladinska EB. Creative art therapy as a non-pharmacological intervention for dementia: a systematic review. J Alzheimers Dis Rep. 2021;5(1):353–64. https://doi.org/10.3233/ADR-201002.

78. Connors MH, Seeher K, Teixeira-Pinto A, Woodward M, Ames D, Brodaty H. Dementia and caregiver burden: a three-year longitudinal study. Int J Geriatr Psychiatry. 2020;35(2):250–8. https://doi.org/10.1002/gps.5244.

79. Adelman RD, Tmanova LL, Delgado D, Dion S, Lachs MS. Caregiver burden: a clinical review. JAMA. 2014;311(10):1052–60. https://doi.org/10.1001/jama.2014.304.

80. Thyrian JR, Hertel J, Wucherer D, et al. Effectiveness and safety of dementia care management in primary care: a randomized clinical trial. JAMA Psychiatry. 2017;74(10):996–1004. https://doi.org/10.1001/jamapsychiatry.2017.2124.

81. Laakkonen ML, Kautiainen H, Hölttä E, et al. Effects of self-management groups for people with dementia and their spouses—randomized controlled trial. J Am Geriatr Soc. 2016;64(4):752–60. https://doi.org/10.1111/jgs.14055.

82. Widera E, Steenpass V, Marson D, Sudore R. Finances in the older patient with cognitive impairment: "He didn't want me to take over.". JAMA. 2011;305(7):698–706. https://doi.org/10.1001/jama.2011.164.

83. Birks J. Cholinesterase inhibitors for Alzheimer's disease. Cochrane Database Syst Rev. 2006;(1):CD005593.

84. Chodosh J, Colaiaco BA, Connor KI, et al. Dementia care management in an underserved community: the comparative effectiveness of two different approaches. J Aging Health. 2015;27(5):864–93. https://doi.org/10.1177/0898264315569454.

85. Schmidt R, Hofer E, Bouwman FH, et al. EFNS-ENS/EAN guideline on concomitant use of cholinesterase inhibitors and memantine in moderate to severe Alzheimer's disease. Eur J Neurol. 2015;22(6):889–98. https://doi.org/10.1111/ene.12707.

86. Matsunaga S, Kishi T, Iwata N. Combination therapy with cholinesterase inhibitors and memantine for Alzheimer's disease: a systematic review and meta-analysis. Int J Neuropsychopharmacol. 2015;18(5):pyu115. https://doi.org/10.1093/ijnp/pyu115.

87. Cummings JL, Tong G, Ballard C. Treatment combinations for Alzheimer's disease: current and future pharmacotherapy options. J Alzheimers Dis JAD. 2019;67(3):779–94. https://doi.org/10.3233/JAD-180766.

88. Food and Drug Administration. Aducanumab (Marketed as Aduhelm) Information. https://www.accessdata.fda.gov/drugsatfda_docs/label/2021/761178s003lbl.pdf. Accessed 22 Dec 2022.

89. Liu KY, Schneider LS, Howard R. The need to show minimum clinically important differences in Alzheimer's disease trials. Lancet Psychiatry. 2021;8:1013. https://doi.org/10.1016/S2215-0366(21)00197-8.

90. Cummings J, Salloway S. Aducanumab: appropriate use recommendations. Alzheimers Dement. 2021;18:531. https://doi.org/10.1002/alz.12444.

91. Centers for Medicare & Medicaid Services. Monoclonal antibodies directed against amyloid for the treatment of Alzheimer's disease. https://www.cms.gov/medicare-coverage-database/view/ncacal-decision-memo.aspx?proposed=N&ncaid=305. Accessed 22 Dec 2022.

92. Tucker S, Möller C, Tegerstedt K, et al. The murine version of BAN2401 (mAb158) selectively reduces amyloid-β protofibrils in brain and cerebrospinal fluid of tg-ArcSwe mice. J Alzheimers Dis. 2015;43:575–88.

93. Food and Drug Administration. FDA Grants Accelerated Approval for Alzheimer's Disease Treatment. https://www.fda.gov/news-events/press-announcements/fda-grants-accelerated-approval-alzheimers-disease-treatment. Accessed 25 Jan 2023.

94. van Dyck CH, Swanson CJ, Aisen P, et al. Lecanemab in early Alzheimer's disease. N Engl J Med. 2023;388(1):9–21. https://doi.org/10.1056/NEJMoa2212948. Epub 2022 Nov 29.

Major Neurocognitive Disorder Due to Vascular Disease

2

Melvin Joseph, Hadley Cameron-Carter, and Esther Akinyemi

Epidemiology

Vascular dementia is a form of dementia caused by impaired blood flow to the brain, leading to cell damage and/or death. This can be caused by a myriad of cerebrovascular pathologies. Vascular dementia is widely known to be the second most common type of dementia after Alzheimer's disease [1–3], accounting for 15–20% of dementias [3, 4]. The incidence of vascular dementia increases with age, and risk doubles approximately every 5 years after the age of 65 [5, 6]. A meta-analysis published in 2020 found that the prevalence of vascular dementia was 40 per 10,000 in people aged 60–69, 105 per 10,000 in people aged 70–79, 235 per 10,000 in people aged 80–89, and 548 per 10,000 in people over the age of 90 [6]. A meta-analysis published in 2021 found that the average age of onset was 67.5, the average age of diagnosis was 73.5, and the average age of death was 77 [7]. However, studying the epidemiological aspects of vascular dementia is limited due to lack of a standard diagnostic definition, variation in different populations, and high rates of dementias with multiple etiologies [8].

Risk Factors Including Neurobiology

Vascular dementia has many similarities with Alzheimer's disease; however, there are some changes that have been found in the neurobiology of vascular dementias that are different from Alzheimer's disease and other types of dementias. Vinciguerra et al. reviewed the evidence on the neurobiology of vascular cognitive impairment (VCI). They found that oxidative stress, neuroinflammation, endothelial dysfunction, hypoperfusion, blood–brain barrier (BBB) disruption, cortical hyperexcitability, and neurotransmitter imbalance all play a role in VCI. They found changes in the serum biomarkers, cerebrospinal fluid (CSF) analysis, neuroimaging, as well as histopathology [9].

Changes described in the serum markers include increases in inflammatory markers such as cytokines (including IL-1β, TNF-α, IFN-γ, IL-4, IL-5, IL-8, G-CSF, and MIP-1b) and markers of endothelial dysfunction including homocysteine in patients with vascular dementia. They also found that reduction in antioxidant enzymes, such as the activity of arylesterase and paraoxonase, was associated with the risk of developing dementia. CSF albumin levels were found to be higher than in patients with Alzheimer's disease and was thought to be due to disruption in the BBB. They noted that mitochondrial DNA mutations may have a cumulative effect by increasing

M. Joseph (✉) · H. Cameron-Carter · E. Akinyemi
Department of Psychiatry, Henry Ford Health, Detroit, MI, USA
e-mail: mjoseph5@hfhs.org; hcamero3@hfhs.org; eakinye2@hfhs.org

© The Author(s), under exclusive license to Springer Nature Switzerland AG 2024
R. R. Tampi, D. J. Tampi (eds.), *Treatment of Psychiatric Disorders Among Older Adults*,
https://doi.org/10.1007/978-3-031-55711-8_2

the probability of developing an energy failure and possibly lowering the age of onset of vascular dementia. Histopathologic changes revealed loss of glutaminergic synapse and that the preservation of glutamatergic synapses supports cognition and protects against dementia after a cerebrovascular accident (CVA) or a stroke. Vesicular glutamate transporter 1 upregulation seems to correlate with preserved cognitive function in subjects with cerebrovascular disease. A mechanism likely related to the promotion of brain-derived neurotrophic factor (BDNF) expression and subsequent restoration of cholinergic system activity in the hippocampus was also observed [9].

Risk factors for vascular dementia include risk factors for vascular pathology. Age is one of the strongest non-modifiable risk factors for vascular dementia and is associated with arterial stiffness, endothelial changes, and BBB dysfunction [10, 11]. Moreover, age is a risk factor for CVAs [12], which have been found to increase the risk for all-cause dementia [13]. In a longitudinal study of 355 stroke patients over 75 years of age, 10% of participants developed poststroke dementia within 3–15 months after a stroke and 24% developed delayed post-stroke dementia during a mean follow-up time of 3.79 years [14]. In a meta-analysis including 7511 patients, it was found that the prevalence of poststroke dementia was 10% shortly after their first stroke and 30% after recurrent strokes [15].

Hypertension is a strong modifiable risk factor for CVAs [12] and vascular dementia. A meta-analysis of 20 studies found that higher blood pressure and blood pressure variability were associated with dementia and cognitive impairment [16]. Analysis stratified by subgroups found that the association between blood pressure and dementia was strongest for vascular dementia [16]. A meta-analysis of six longitudinal studies found that hypertension is significantly associated with the risk of vascular dementia [17]. In addition, a 2022 study showed that a midlife high blood pressure at a single time point predicts all-

cause dementia and more than doubles the risk for vascular dementia later in life [18].

Diabetes has also been found to be a strong modifiable risk factor for vascular dementia in multiple studies. A meta-analysis of 26 observational studies found that there is a 126% increased risk of vascular dementia in diabetic patients [19]. Another meta-analysis including 122 studies found that diabetes increased the risk by 1.25–1.91-fold for all-cause dementias, including vascular dementia [20]. Moreover, studies have shown that type 2 diabetic patients with hypoglycemic episodes are at significantly increased risk of developing dementia than diabetic patients without significant hypoglycemic episodes [21, 22].

Decreased levels of physical and cognitive activity may also be a risk factor for vascular dementia. A study showed that cognitive and physical activity in midlife was protective against dementia, which suggests that being sedentary in midlife increases the risk of dementia later in life [23].

There is conflicting evidence on whether smoking is a risk factor for vascular dementia. Multiple studies have shown that smoking increases the risk of vascular dementia [24, 25], and heavy smoking in midlife was shown to increase the risk of both Alzheimer's dementia and vascular dementia after two decades in a meta-analysis including 37 studies [26]. However, a more recent study suggests that smoking may not increase the risk of dementia, including vascular dementia [27].

There are also multiple genetic risk factors for developing vascular dementia, including hereditary disorders, such as cerebral autosomal dominant arteriopathy with subcortical infarcts and leukoencephalopathy (CADASIL) and cerebral autosomal recessive arteriopathy with subcortical infarcts and leukoencephalopathy (CARASIL), which are small-vessel diseases that lead to vascular dementia [28]. Furthermore, there are multiple polymorphisms associated with vascular dementia, including APOE E2/E3/E4, MTHFR C677T, PON1 L55M, TGF-B1 +29C/T, and TNF-a-850 C/T [29].

Assessment

The diagnostic criteria for vascular dementia vary between different organizations, including the Diagnostic and Statistical Manual (DSM); the International Classification of Diseases, tenth Revision (ICD-10); the Ischemic Scale of Rosen; the State of California Alzheimer's Disease Diagnostic and Treatment Centers (ADDTC); and the National Institute of Neurological Disorders and Stroke/Association Internationale Pour La Recherche Et L'Enseignement En Neurosciences (NINDS-AIREN) [30, 31]. Similarities include establishment of cognitive impairment; identification of cerebrovascular disease, especially stroke; and cerebrovascular disease/event considered to be the cause of cognitive impairment [30, 31].

When assessing individuals with vascular dementia, it is important to take a thorough history and to elucidate timing of cognitive decline relative to vascular disease, especially strokes. Assessment should include a cognitive screen, such as the Montreal Cognitive Assessment (MoCA). The Hachinski Ischemic Score (HIS) can be used to predict the likelihood of vascular contribution to dementia by assigning points for features of abrupt onset, fluctuating course, history of stroke, focal neurologic symptoms, focal neurologic signs, stepwise deterioration, nocturnal confusion, preservation of personality, depression, somatic complaints, emotional incontinence, hypertension, and associated atherosclerosis [32]. HIS can accurately discern Alzheimer's disease from vascular dementia [32]. Neuropsychological testing is important if the etiology of cognitive impairment is not clear [3].

Physical examination is essential for patients with vascular dementia and can reveal signs suggestive of strokes. Laboratory tests, including complete blood count, comprehensive metabolic panel, vitamin B12, folate, human immunodeficiency virus testing, rapid plasma reagin test, and thyroid screen, are necessary to look for reversible causes of cognitive impairment or other contributing disorders. It is also important to assess for modifiable risk factors, including diet, hypertension, diabetes, and smoking [3].

Neuroimaging can be used to evaluate for evidence of cerebrovascular disease including previous strokes. Magnetic resonance imaging (MRI) is typically more sensitive than computed tomography (CT) for assessing small-vessel disease, while CT scans are useful for assessing acute hemorrhagic events [3].

Treatment

There is currently no cure for vascular dementia similar to most other types of major neurocognitive disorders. However, there are certain modalities used to address the symptoms or behavioral concerns caused by the illness. Treatment of vascular dementia symptoms can be accomplished by both non-pharmacological and pharmacological modalities. The importance of non-pharmacological management of vascular dementia should not be underscored when compared to medication management as to decrease the exposure of medication side effects.

Non-pharmacological

In a 2-year randomized control trial, Ngandu et al. investigated a multidomain intervention of diet, exercise, cognitive training, and vascular risk monitoring versus control to determine its effects on cognitive decline in at-risk elderly people (Finnish Geriatric Intervention Study to Prevent Cognitive Impairment and Disability). Diet was monitored for protein, fats, carbohydrates, fiber, salt, and alcohol intake [33]. Exercise regimens were guided by trainers and focused on aerobics, strength training, and exercise to improve postural balance. Cognitive training was conducted through computers and focused specifically on executive processes, working memory, episodic memory, and mental speed. Vascular risk factors were monitored including blood pressure, weight, body mass index (BMI), hip and waist circumference, and physical examinations, and recommendations for lifestyle management were made. The control group was given general health advice. Estimated mean change in neuropsychological test battery (NTB) total Z score at 2 years was 0.20 (SE 0.01, SD 0.51) in the intervention group and 0.16 (0.01, 0.51) in the control group. The mean difference between groups (group × time interaction) in change of NTB total score per year was 0.022 (95% CI 0.002–0.042, P = 0.030). Improvement in NTB total score after 24 months was 25% higher in the intervention group than in the control group.

Physical activity has been shown to have a positive effect on cognition, even when this begins later in life [34]. A trial in 2008 demonstrated the benefit of physical activity on cognitive function in older adults with subjective and objective mild cognitive impairment. It was thought that physical activity improves cognition, possibly by improving cerebral vascular function and brain perfusion [35]. In the review by Elizabeth et al., they discuss how exercise may be an effective strategy for reducing the risk of cognitive decline, promoting brain health by increasing the bioavailability of neurotrophins, reducing vessel damage by targeting endothelial function, and controlling vascular risk factors [36].

Smoking has been previously identified to increase the risk of dementia, although the evidence is mixed. Choi et al. explored the effects of smoking cessation and the risk for developing dementia. They compared continual smokers, short-term quitters (less than 4 years), long-term quitters (4 years or more), and never smokers over a period of 8 years to determine the risk of Alzheimer's and vascular dementia [24]. They found that long-term quitters and never smokers had decreased incidence of developing dementia compared to their counterparts. Hence, every effort should be made to help patients quit smoking.

In the Delphi Consensus, researchers found that the DICE (describe, investigate, create, and evaluate) process was the best non-pharmacologic treatment option for behavioral and psychological symptom management of dementia [37]. They also found that the use of music was beneficial as a treatment option. Prioritized factors included caregiver training, environmental adaptations, person-centered care, and tailored activities as primary approaches in addressing behavioral and symptom care.

Pharmacological

A mainstay of pharmacologic management of vascular dementia is prevention. This is primarily by adequate control of treatable underlying risk factors including high blood pressure and diabetes, among others. Hence, a number of medications to treat vascular dementia will be to address underlying disorders.

Antihypertensives

Hypertension is known to be a risk factor for the development of strokes and subsequent vascular dementia. There is evidence that the use of antihypertensives [angiotensin-converting enzyme (ACE) inhibitors or diuretics] can prevent future strokes, but there is insufficient evidence to verify if its usage decreases the risk of developing vascular dementia [38]. However, the TRIUMPH Trial, which studied cognitive changes in individuals with resistant hypertension, showed that lifestyle modification improved cognition. This appeared to be associated with reduced ambulatory systolic blood pressure changes through weight loss and was accompanied by parallel improvements in endothelial and microvascular function [39].

Acetylcholinesterase Inhibitors

Acetylcholinesterase inhibitors have some benefits in vascular dementia. In a network meta-analysis by Battle et al., authors reviewed donepezil, rivastigmine, and galantamine against placebo on its safety, effects on cognition, and adverse events in patients diagnosed with vascular dementia. They included 8 randomized controlled studies with 4373 participants. They found that donepezil 10 mg/d and galantamine had slight improvements in cognition and memory; however, this was not clinically significant. There did not appear to be a difference in outcome with the use of rivastigmine and placebo. Of note, they only utilized the oral formulation and not the patch. Regarding adverse outcomes, donepezil 10 mg/d and galantamine 16–24 mg/d were associated with more side effects including vomiting, diarrhea, dizziness, headache, and hypertension, while rivastigmine did not demonstrate significant adverse effects against placebo [40]. Another study looked at the effects of donepezil specifically on cognition and global functioning in patients with vascular dementia and found significant improvements. They also noted low rates of withdrawal from the study due to adverse effects of donepezil [41].

Another meta-analysis by Kim et al. reviewed the differences in Mini-Mental State Examination (MMSE) and Alzheimer's Disease Assessment Scale-Cognitive subscale (ADAS-Cog) scores, prior to and after administration of cholinesterase inhibitors (donepezil, rivastigmine, and galantamine) [42]. Mean differences (MD) of MMSE score in poststroke cognitive impairment and vascular dementia with the use of cholinergic augmentation were significantly increased throughout the 24 weeks: 3.000 (95% confidence interval [CI] 2.135–3.865) at 4 weeks, 1.732 (95% CI 0.555–2.910) at 4–8 weeks, 1.578 (95% CI 1.308–1.848) at 8–12 weeks, 1.516 (95% CI 1.203–1.829) at 12–18 weeks, and 1.222 (95% CI 0.727–1.718) at 18–24 weeks. Only minimal change of MMSE score was observed compared to placebo in poststroke cognitive impairment and vascular dementia after 4 weeks. The changes in ADAS-Cog scores were analyzed in vascular dementia patients treated with cholinergic medications, which showed decreases by MD of −2.333 (95% CI −2.778 to −1.889) at 6 weeks, MD of −2.913 (95% CI −3.490 to −2.335) at 12 weeks, MD of −2.416 (95% CI −3.009 to −1.824) at 18 weeks, and MD of −1.859 (95% CI −2.514 to −1.204) at 24 weeks, and this decreased pattern was maintained for 24 weeks. In patients with vascular dementia treated with placebo, no changes in ADAS-Cog scores were noted at 6, 18, and 24 weeks (MD −0.763, 95% CI −2.104 to 0.578; MD 0.148, 95% CI −0.365 to 0.133; and MD −0.204, 95% CI −0.541 to 0.133, respectively); however, a reduction in score was observed at 12 weeks (MD −0.699, 95% CI −1.092 to −0.307).

Antidepressants

Liu et al. worked to identify the effects of fluoxetine on brain-derived neurotropic factor (BDNF) and its effect of increasing cognitive functioning in patients diagnosed with vascular dementia. Fifty patients with vascular dementia were given fluoxetine 20 mg/d versus a control group who did not and monitored over 12 weeks. Serum BDNF level, MMSE score, Ten-Point Clock Drawing score, and Digit Span Test and Verbal Fluency Test scores were measured at baseline and at week 12 for both groups. In the group given fluoxetine, serum BDNF level, MMSE score, and Ten-Point Clock Drawing score all increased. These increases were not seen in the control group [43].

Stimulants

In a small study, Leijenaar et al. investigated methylphenidate's ability to improve executive functioning through increasing dopamine and norepinephrine at the synaptic cleft in those with vascular cognitive impairment. They also looked at the acetylcholinesterase inhibitor galantamine's ability to improve memory. They found that by administering 10 mg/d of methylphenidate, participants improved in cognitive abilities when compared against placebo (estimated difference in mean performance (%) compared to baseline, 1.40% (95% confidence interval [CI] 0.56–2.25), $P = 0.002$). There was no difference with the use of galantamine on memory [44].

Antipsychotics

Agitation, aggression, and behavioral issues are common concerns for patients diagnosed with vascular dementia. In the review by Muhlbauer et al., the authors discuss the effectiveness of typical and atypical antipsychotics in addressing agitation and psychosis in patients diagnosed with Alzheimer's disease and vascular dementia. They found that haloperidol and thiothixene likely improved aggression in patients and did slightly improve psychosis. Typical antipsychotics did increase the risk of extrapyramidal symptoms. Atypical antipsychotics such as risperidone, olanzapine, aripiprazole, and quetiapine did improve agitation slightly, but had negligible effects towards psychosis. These drugs increased the incidence of somnolence and were also found to cause a slight increase in the risk of extrapyramidal symptoms [45].

Pimavanserin, an antipsychotic with a novel mechanism of action, primarily used for the treatment of Parkinson's disease psychosis was found to be effective in the management of dementia-related psychosis, and maintenance with the medication was helpful in preventing relapse in patients who had a positive response [46].

Antipsychotics have been known to increase all-cause mortality in patients with dementia; hence, they have an FDA black box warning for their use in patients with dementia. Most patients who died had causes related to cardiac issues or infections [47].

Evidence-Based Treatment Algorithm

When treating a vulnerable population such as individuals with vascular dementia, it is important to identify specifically the goals of treatment. As stated before, there is no cure for vascular dementia; however, there are strategies to prevent the illness and to address the symptoms associated with the illness. Firstly, clinicians should use non-pharmacological treatment options for this population, as it does not add to the medication burden which many older patients may struggle with. Strength training, aerobic exercise, diet, and movement in general have been shown to improve cognition including memory [33].

Although there is no robust data on the effects of medications in improving overall cognition, memory, or executive functioning in patients with vascular dementia, there is some modest evidence for acetylcholinesterase inhibitors assisting with the improvement of cognition [40–42]. There is no significant evidence that any specific acetylcholinesterase inhibitor is better than others; however, studies show that donepezil and galantamine may be better as first-line options when compared to rivastigmine [40]. Other medications such as antidepressants and stimulants have been shown to produce some mild improvements in cognition including memory [43, 44]. However, there are yet to be any definitive recommendations regarding their use among individuals with vascular dementia.

When addressing behavioral concerns with agitation and aggression in patients with vascular dementia, antipsychotics are commonly used. However, these medications should be used with caution as they have a risk of causing life-threatening side effects [47]. In addition, they have a risk of causing extrapyramidal side effects including tardive dyskinesia after chronic use. These drugs should be used only after non-pharmacological options have failed. When using them, these drugs should only be used at their lowest effective doses and for the shortest time possible (Fig. 2.1).

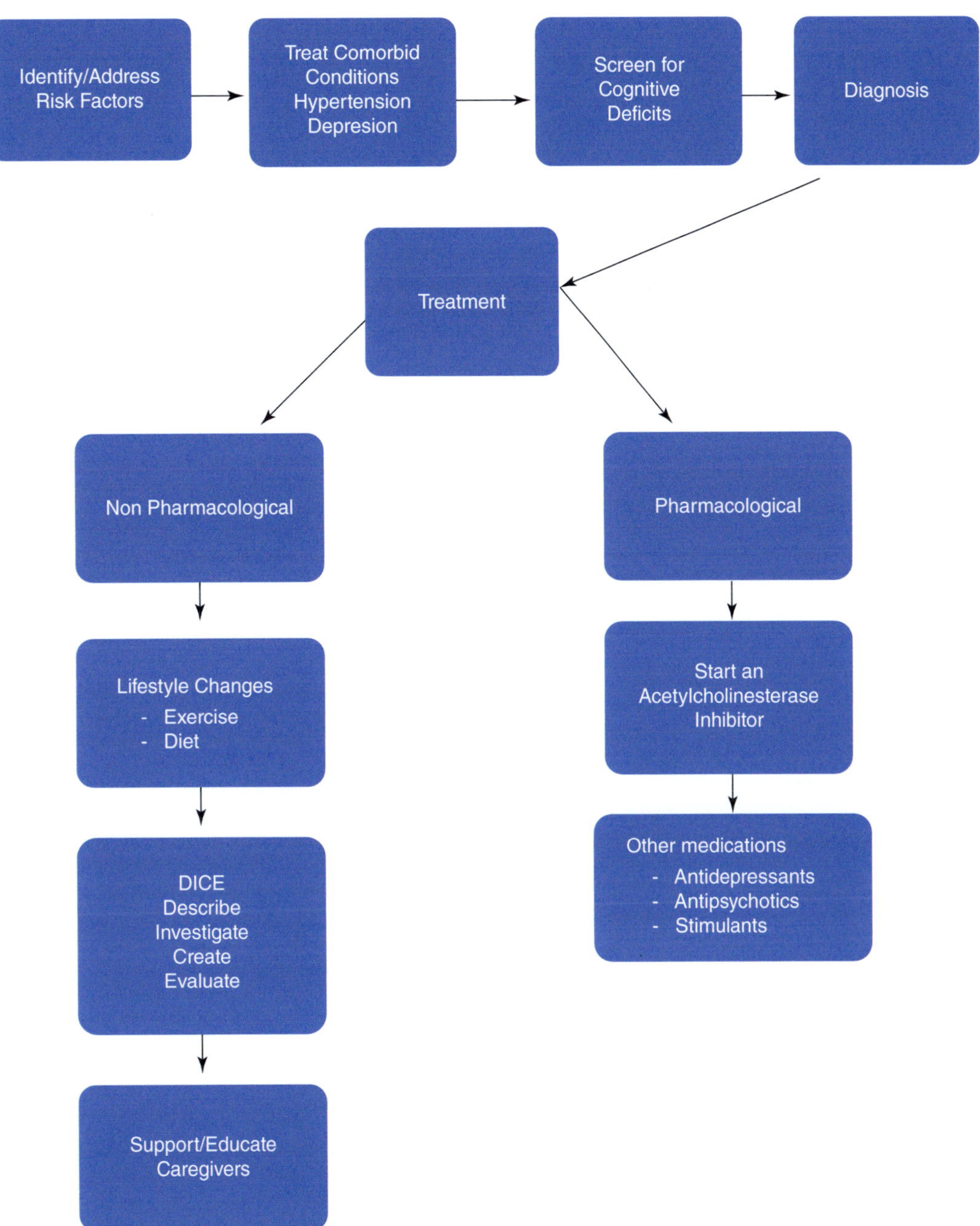

Fig. 2.1 Management of major neurocognitive disorder due to vascular disease

Conclusion

Vascular dementia is very common in the aging population. This condition can negatively impact the quality of life for the patient as well as their caregivers. The best intervention is prevention, which can be achieved by lifestyle changes and aggressively addressing health conditions that increase the risk of vascular dementia. As there are no curative treatments for vascular dementia, symptom management and treatment of behavioral concerns are the mainstay for care. When evaluating treatment options, one should use non-pharmacological options first before using medications, if possible. Medication management, primarily the use of acetylcholinesterase inhibitors, can be somewhat helpful in addressing cognitive decline. While antipsychotics are used for the management of behavioral and psychological symptoms of dementia, there should be caution with their use given their significant adverse effects. Other medications such as antidepressants and stimulants may provide some benefit to individuals with vascular dementia. More research is needed to identify other potential treatment options for vascular dementia.

References

1. Chan KY, Wang W, Wu JJ, et al. Global Health Epidemiology Reference Group (GHERG). Epidemiology of Alzheimer's disease and other forms of dementia in China, 1990–2010: a systematic review and analysis. Lancet. 2013;381(9882):2016–23.
2. Lobo A, Launer LJ, Fratiglioni L, et al. Prevalence of dementia and major subtypes in Europe: a collaboratory study of population-based cohorts. Neurologic Diseases in the Elderly Research Group. Neurology. 2000;54(11 Suppl 5):S4–9.
3. Uwagbai O, Kalish VB. Vascular dementia. [Updated 2022 Jan 14]. In: StatPearls [Internet]. Treasure Island (FL): StatPearls Publishing; 2022.
4. Rizzi L, Rosset I, Roriz-Cruz M. Global epidemiology of dementia: Alzheimer's and vascular types. Biomed Res Int. 2014;2014:908915.
5. Jorm AF, Jolley D. The incidence of dementia: a meta-analysis. Neurology. 1998;51(3):728–33.
6. Cao Q, Tan CC, Xu W, et al. The prevalence of dementia: a systematic review and meta-analysis. J Alzheimer Dis. 2020;73(3):1157–66.
7. Liang CS, Li DJ, Yang FC, et al. Mortality rates in Alzheimer's disease and non-Alzheimer's dementias: a systematic review and meta-analysis. Lancet Healthy Longev. 2021;2(8):e479–88.
8. Schneider JA, Arvanitakis A, Bang W, et al. Mixed brain pathologies account for most dementia cases in community-dwelling older persons. Neurology. 2007;69:2197.
9. Vinciguerra L, Lanza G, Puglisi V, et al. Update on the neurobiology of vascular cognitive impairment: from lab to clinic. Int J Mol Sci. 2020;21(8):2977.
10. Akinyemi RO, Mukaetova-Ladinska EB, Attems J, et al. Vascular risk factors and neurodegeneration in ageing related dementias: Alzheimer's disease and vascular dementia. Curr Alzheimer Res. 2013;10(6):642–53.
11. Day S, Roberts S, Launder NH, et al. Age of symptom onset and longitudinal course of sporadic Alzheimer's disease, frontotemporal dementia, and vascular dementia: a systematic review and meta-analysis. J Alzheimers Dis. 2022;85(4):1819–33.
12. Boehme AK, Esenwa C, Elkind MS. Stroke risk factors, genetics, and prevention. Circ Res. 2017;120(3):472–95.
13. Kuźma E, Lourida I, Moore SF, et al. Stroke and dementia risk: a systematic review and meta-analysis. Alzheimers Dement. 2018;14(11):1416–26.
14. Allan LM, Rowan EN, Firbank MJ, et al. Long term incidence of dementia, predictors of mortality and pathological diagnosis in older stroke survivors. Brain. 2011;134(Pt 12):3716–27.
15. Pendlebury ST, Rothwell PM. Prevalence, incidence, and factors associated with pre-stroke and post-stroke dementia: a systematic review and meta-analysis. Lancet Neurol. 2009;8(11):1006–18.
16. de Heus RAA, Tzourio C, Lee EJL, et al. Association between blood pressure variability with dementia and cognitive impairment: a systematic review and meta-analysis. Hypertension. 2021;78(5):1478–89.
17. Sharp SI, Aarsland D, Day S, et al. Hypertension is a potential risk factor for vascular dementia: systematic review. Int J Geriatr Psychiatry. 2011;26(7):661–9.
18. Moberg L, Leppert J, Liljeström S, et al. Blood pressure screening in midlife aids in prediction of dementia later in life. Ups J Med Sci. 2022;127
19. Gudala K, Bansal D, Schifano F, et al. Diabetes mellitus and risk of dementia: a meta-analysis of prospective observational studies. J Diabetes Investig. 2013;4(6):640–50.
20. Xue M, Xu W, Ou YN, et al. Diabetes mellitus and risks of cognitive impairment and dementia: a systematic review and meta-analysis of 144 prospective studies. Ageing Res Rev. 2019;55:100944.
21. Kim YG, Park DG, Moon SY, et al. Hypoglycemia and dementia risk in older patients with type 2 diabetes mellitus: a propensity-score matched analysis of a population-based cohort study. Diabetes Metab J. 2020;44(1):125–33.
22. Huang L, Zhu M, Ji J. Association between hypoglycemia and dementia in patients with diabetes: a systematic review and meta-analysis of 1.4 million patients. Diabetol Metab Syndr. 2022;14(1):31.
23. Najar J, Östling S, Gudmundsson P, et al. Cognitive and physical activity and dementia: a 44-year longitudinal population study of women. Neurology. 2019;92(12):e1322–30.
24. Choi D, Choi S, Park SM. Effect of smoking cessation on the risk of dementia: a longitudinal study. Ann Clin Transl Neurol. 2018;5(10):1192–9.
25. Rusanen M, Kivipelto M, Quesenberry CP Jr, et al. Heavy smoking in midlife and long-term risk of

Alzheimer disease and vascular dementia. Arch Intern Med. 2011;171(4):333–9.

26. Zhong G, Wang Y, Zhang Y, et al. Smoking is associated with an increased risk of dementia: a meta-analysis of prospective cohort studies with investigation of potential effect modifiers. PLoS One. 2015;10(3):e0118333.

27. Otuyama LJ, Oliveira D, Locatelli D, et al. Tobacco smoking and risk for dementia: evidence from the 10/66 population-based longitudinal study. Aging Ment Health. 2020;24(11):1796–806.

28. Tikka S, Baumann M, Siitonen M, et al. CADASIL and CARASIL. Brain Pathol. 2014;24(5):525–44.

29. Sun JH, Tan L, Wang HF, et al. Genetics of vascular dementia: systematic review and meta-analysis. J Alzheimers Dis. 2015;46(3):611–29.

30. Wiederkehr S, Simard M, Fortin C, et al. Comparability of the clinical diagnostic criteria for vascular dementia: a critical review. Part I. J Neuropsychiatry Clin Neurosci. 2008;20(2):150–61.

31. Sachdev P, Kalaria R, O'Brien J, et al. Diagnostic criteria for vascular cognitive disorders: a VASCOG statement. Alzheimer Dis Assoc Disord. 2014;28(3):206–18.

32. Moroney JT, Bagiella E, Desmond DW, et al. Meta-analysis of the Hachinski Ischemic Score in pathologically verified dementias. Neurology. 1997;49(4):1096–105.

33. Ngandu T, Lehtisalo J, Solomon A, et al. A 2 year multidomain intervention of diet, exercise, cognitive training, and vascular risk monitoring versus control to prevent cognitive decline in at-risk elderly people (FINGER): a randomised controlled trial. Lancet. 2015;385(9984):2255–63.

34. Morovic S, Budincevic H, Govori V, et al. Possibilities of dementia prevention—it is never too early to start. J Med Life. 2019;12(4):332–7.

35. Lautenschlager NT, Cox KL, Flicker L, et al. Effect of physical activity on cognitive function in older adults at risk for Alzheimer disease: a randomized trial. JAMA. 2008;300(9):1027–37. [published correction appears in JAMA].

36. Dao E, Hsiung GR, Liu-Ambrose T. The role of exercise in mitigating subcortical ischemic vascular cognitive impairment. J Neurochem. 2018;144(5):582–94.

37. Kales HC, Lyketsos CG, Miller EM, et al. Management of behavioral and psychological symptoms in people with Alzheimer's disease: an international Delphi consensus. Int Psychogeriatr. 2019;31(1):83–90.

38. Zonneveld TP, Richard E, Vergouwen MD, et al. Blood pressure-lowering treatment for preventing recurrent stroke, major vascular events, and dementia in patients with a history of stroke or transient ischaemic attack. Cochrane Database Syst Rev. 2018;7(7):CD007858.

39. Smith PJ, Sherwood A, Hinderliter AL, et al. Lifestyle modification and cognitive function among individuals with resistant hypertension: cognitive outcomes from the TRIUMPH trial. J Hypertens. 2022;40(7):1359–68.

40. Battle CE, Abdul-Rahim AH, Shenkin SD, et al. Cholinesterase inhibitors for vascular dementia and other vascular cognitive impairments: a network meta-analysis. Cochrane Database Syst Rev. 2021;2(2):CD013306.

41. Wilkinson D, Doody R, Helme R, et al. Donepezil in vascular dementia: a randomized, placebo-controlled study. Neurology. 2003;61(4):479–86.

42. Kim JO, Lee SJ, Pyo JS. Effect of acetylcholinesterase inhibitors on post-stroke cognitive impairment and vascular dementia: a meta-analysis. PLoS One. 2020;15(2):e0227820.

43. Liu X, Zhang J, Sun D, et al. Effects of fluoxetine on brain-derived neurotrophic factor serum concentration and cognition in patients with vascular dementia. Clin Interv Aging. 2014;9:411–8.

44. Leijenaar JF, Groeneveld GJ, Klaassen ES, et al. Methylphenidate and galantamine in patients with vascular cognitive impairment-the proof-of-principle study STREAM-VCI. Alzheimers Res Ther. 2020;12(1):10.

45. Mühlbauer V, Möhler R, Dichter MN, et al. Antipsychotics for agitation and psychosis in people with Alzheimer's disease and vascular dementia. Cochrane Database Syst Rev. 2021;12(12):CD013304.

46. Tariot PN, Cummings JL, Soto-Martin ME, et al. Trial of pimavanserin in dementia-related psychosis. N Engl J Med. 2021;385(4):309–19.

47. Rubino A, Sanon M, Ganz ML, et al. Association of the US Food and Drug Administration antipsychotic drug boxed warning with medication use and health outcomes in elderly patients with dementia. JAMA Netw Open. 2020;3(4):e203630.

Michael G. Li

Epidemiology

Historically, dementia with Lewy bodies (DLB) was once considered a rare disease. The true prevalence was challenging to determine, due in part to the variation in diagnostic criteria and terminology used to define this phenomenon. Early studies analyzed patients with a dementia diagnosis who were referred to inpatient hospitals for treatment, which may not have been a generalizable population [1]. Following the consensus guidelines from the First International Workshop of the Consortium on Dementia with Lewy Bodies in 1996, which armed clinicians with a more standardized diagnostic approach, and the revised International Consensus Criteria in 2005, there was a dramatic increase in diagnosing DLB cases [2–4]. Currently, the most recent systematic reviews between 2014 and 2018 indicate that there is roughly a 5–7% prevalence of DLB in the general population, with an incidence of 3.8% in all new dementia cases [5, 6]. However, these studies examined groups that were isolated in specific treatment settings, with a relatively weak statistical power, which likely gave rise to the common quote of DLB's prevalence ranging from 5 to 30% in all cases of dementia. Despite this controversy, DLB is widely considered to be a leading cause of major neurocognitive disorder behind Alzheimer's disease (AD).

Risk Factors

DLB was historically considered a sporadic and late-onset disease [5]. However, the strong hereditary component in related conditions like Parkinson's disease (PD) and AD suggests that genetics may play a significant role in DLB [7, 8]. The current list of suspected culprits within the genome includes also established risk factors for PD and AD, and there has not been a gene specific for DLB. This deficit might be due to the phenotypic variability of DLB, which poses challenges to study designs that attempt to identify a genetic correlate and complicates the firm conclusions that could be drawn from published studies [7]. Accurate identification of genetic risk factors requires a firm understanding of the pathophysiology and pathogenesis of DLB, which revolves primarily around the hypothesis of abnormal expression and accumulation of alpha-synuclein [9]. Naturally, the genes associated with alpha-synuclein expression and maintenance have been the front-running genetic risk factors for DLB. In 2018, a comprehensive, well-powered genome-wide

M. G. Li (✉)
Department of Psychiatry, University of Texas at Southwestern Medical Center, Dallas, TX, USA

North Texas Veterans Health Administration, Dallas Veterans Affairs Medical Center, Dallas, TX, USA
e-mail: Michael.li2@utsouthwestern.edu;
michael.li@va.gov

© The Author(s), under exclusive license to Springer Nature Switzerland AG 2024
R. R. Tampi, D. J. Tampi (eds.), *Treatment of Psychiatric Disorders Among Older Adults*,
https://doi.org/10.1007/978-3-031-55711-8_3

Table 3.1 Summary of genetic risk factors for DLB

Gene	Significance
Synuclein alpha *(SNCA)*	Encodes the alpha-synuclein protein and is implicated in both DLB and PD. Mutations are suspected to increase the propensity for aggregation of alpha-synuclein
Apolipoprotein E (APOE)	The APOEε2 and ε4 alleles, classically related to AD pathogenesis, have been identified as protective and risk factors for DLB, respectively
Glucocerebrosidase (GBA)	Encodes glucocerebrosidase. Mutations resulted in decreased activity of beta-glucocerebrosidase and leads to impaired degradation of alpha-synuclein. Frequency of mutations ranges from 4 to 28% in patients with DLB. Mutations also carry a threefold higher phenoconversion rate from RBD to dementia and/or parkinsonism
Amyloid precursor protein (APP)	53% of autopsies in individuals with the APP717 mutation revealed presence of Lewy bodies
Presenilin 1 *(PSEN1)*, **presenilin 2** *(PSEN2)*	Key components of the gamma-secretase complex that process amyloid. Mutations result in increased levels of beta-amyloid, creating an intracellular environment that is hypothesized to enable Lewy body formation
Contactin-1 *(CNTN1)*	A novel locus identified in 2018 which encodes for the contactin-1 protein, a neuronal membrane protein that functions as a cell adhesion molecule significant for axonal function
Leucine-rich repeat kinase 2 (**LRRK2**)	A common gene associated with Lewy body deposition in both familial and sporadic disease
Chromosome 2q35–q36 region	Strong association with familial Lewy body disease

association study estimated the hereditary component of DLB to be 36% [7]. In addition, recent studies have independently highlighted the association between DLB with mutations in the *SNCA, APOE,* and *GBA* genes and other chromosomal regions highlighted in Table 3.1 [7, 8, 10–17]. While there seems to be promise in the reproducibility of these studies, it is important to take note that single nucleotide polymorphisms (SNPs) often explain only a small proportion of the total estimated heritability [18]. Indeed, there are puzzling findings such as the generally discordant incidence of DLB observed among monozygotic twins, which suggests the likelihood that environmental and epigenetic factors could also play significant roles in disease progression [19]. Therefore, further studies are needed to clarify the risk factors that are specific to DLB.

The phenomenon of rapid eye movement (REM) sleep behaviors has emerged as a powerful clinical indicator of neurodegenerative synucleinopathies including multiple system atrophy (MSA), PD, and DLB [20]. In 2019, a study that included the largest group of polysomnographically diagnosed RBD (REM behavioral disorder) identified a conversion rate from idiopathic RBD to a neurodegenerative syndrome at 6.3% per year [20]. Attempts of identifying a genetic correlate for RBD have pointed to the *GBA* gene as a likely culprit, which in turn raised interest in *GBA*'s role in LBD. Mutations in *GBA* were associated with a 3.2 higher rate of conversion from RBD to parkinsonism and/or dementia [21].

Assessment

The diagnostic process for DLB can be challenging, due to the heterogenous and often nonspecific clinical manifestations. In addition, the primary criticism of previous iterations of the DLB diagnostic criteria was its low sensitivity, despite having high specificity according to autopsy-confirmed studies, which likely contributed to the prior misconception that it was a rare disease [22–25]. However, the fundamental principles remain the same as any other major neurocognitive disorder, which is to first rule out any reversible causes and assess for functional deficits in basic and instrumental activities of daily living:

1. Cognitive screen (e.g., Montreal Cognitive Assessment, neuropsychology evaluation)
2. Neuroimaging study (e.g., MRI brain)
3. Laboratory tests (e.g., thyroid function, infection, vitamin B12 level)
4. Psychiatric evaluation

Clinicians may refer to the most recent set of diagnostic guidelines that was updated in 2017 in the fourth consensus report by the DLB Consortium summarized in Table 3.2 [26].

The 2017 criteria were designed to increase the sensitivity in diagnosis, although the degree of improvement currently remains to be validated. From a quick glance, clinicians might be puzzled by how to accurately screen and assess some of the core clinical features that mimic delirium or hyperarousal-nocturnal states in post-traumatic stress disorder. The following section will expand on the core features, advise basic strategies for assessment, and review the sensitivity and specificity of the indicative biomarkers as well as other possibilities on the horizon:

Fluctuations in Cognition

The cardinal feature in DLB is the profound disturbance of attention and alertness. When DLB diagnostic criteria were first described, this phe-

Table 3.2 Criteria for the clinical diagnosis of probable and possible DLB

Essential for a diagnosis of DLB is dementia, defined as a progressive cognitive decline of sufficient magnitude to interfere with normal social or occupational functions, or with usual daily activities:
- Prominent or persistent memory impairment may not necessarily occur in the early stages but is usually evident with progression.
- Deficits on tests of attention, executive function, and visuo-perceptual ability may be especially prominent and occur early.

Core clinical features	*Indicative biomarkers*
• Fluctuating cognition with pronounced variations in attention and alertness • Recurrent visual hallucinations that are typically well formed and detailed • REM sleep behavior disorder (RBD), which may precede cognitive decline • One or more spontaneous cardinal features of parkinsonism	• Reduced dopamine transporter (DaT) uptake in basal ganglia demonstrated by SPECT or PET • Abnormal (low uptake) 123-iodine-metaiodobenzylguanidine scintigraphy (MIBG) myocardial scintigraphy • Polysomnographic confirmation of REM sleep without atonia
Supportive clinical features	*Supportive biomarkers*
• Severe sensitivity to antipsychotics • Postural instability • Repeated falls • Syncope or other transient episodes of unresponsiveness • Severe autonomic dysfunction (e.g., orthostatic hypotension, constipation) • Apathy, anxiety, or depression	• Relative preservation of medial temporal lobes on computer tomography (CT)/magnetic resonance imaging (MRI) scan • Generalized low uptake on single-photon emission computerized tomography (SPECT)/positron emission tomography (PET) perfusion/metabolism scan with reduced occipital activity +/− cingulate island sign on *fluorodeoxyglucose* (FDG-PET) imaging • Prominent posterior slow-wave activity on electroencephalogram (EEG) with periodic fluctuations in the pre-alpha/theta range

- *Probable DLB* = "2 or more core clinical features" or "1 core clinical feature with 1 or more indicative biomarkers"
- *Possible DLB* = "1 core clinical feature" or "no core clinical features with 1 or more indicative biomarkers"

A diagnosis of DLB is less likely:
- In the presence of cerebrovascular disease evident as focal neurologic signs or on brain imaging
- In the presence of any other physical illness or brain disorder sufficient to account in part or in total for the clinical picture
- If parkinsonism is the only core feature and appears for the first time at a stage of severe dementia

nomenon was even considered mandatory for diagnosis. However, the substantial difficulties for clinicians to define and quantify this feature ultimately led to its softening from mandatory to core criteria. The challenge with this symptom stems from its ephemeral and heterogenous nature, as patients will most likely be unable to describe their experiences accurately. The terms "confusion" and "fluctuating" are often used by caregivers to describe patients, but these are generally vague and nonspecific and offer no additional value to the clinician who may be considering other neurocognitive disorders in the differential. Prior, albeit few, attempts of distinguishing the qualitative characteristics from Alzheimer's disease have been made [27]. Data regarding the prevalence of fluctuating cognition in probable DLB are mixed, with rates between 45 and 90%. In possible DLB, the rates are generally reported to be lower at around 29% [28]. It is unclear whether there is a correlation between this feature's presence and prognosis [29]. Several cross-sectional studies have determined that fluctuating cognition does not lead to a poorer outcome or greater rates of cognitive decline [30–32].

Currently, there are a handful of clinical scales with fair interrater reliability, sensitivity, and specificity, and they are listed in Table 3.3 [27, 33–35]. They generally take between 5 and 10 min to administer, but may be limited by clinician experience and accuracy of report by the caregiver.

Recurrent Visual Hallucinations

There are currently a variety of proposed mechanisms for visual hallucinations in DLB, but the consensus points to a combination of neurobio-

Table 3.3 Clinical scales to assess fluctuating cognition

Name	Year	Description	Strengths	Weaknesses
Dementia Cognitive Fluctuation Scale	2014	17-item questionnaire, adapted from previous scales to improve sensitivity and specificity of DLB over other forms of dementia	– Directly compared DLB against Alzheimer's and vascular dementia – Decent sensitivity (78.6–80.3%) and specificity (73.9–79.3%) to detect DLB over other dementias	– May need larger studies to repeat and validate findings
Mayo Fluctuation Scale	2004	19-item questionnaire for symptoms 1 month before the assessment	– Differentiates between sleep/arousal and cognitive causes of fluctuation – Positive predictive value of 83% to diagnose DLB over AD	– Does not distinguish DLB from non-AD subtypes of dementia
Clinician Assessment of Fluctuation	2000	2 questions that evaluate symptoms 1 month before assessment. Rated by the presence, duration, and frequency of symptoms	– Fair interrater reliability – Good sensitivity (~81%) and specificity (~82%) to differentiate DLB from AD – Good sensitivity (81%) and specificity (92%) to differentiate DLB from vascular dementia	– Relies on a clinician with greater experience with the scale and pathophysiology
One Day Fluctuation Assessment Scale	2000	7-item clinician-rated scale to evaluate 24 h before assessment	– Allows for a tighter window for snapshot assessment	Low sensitivity in detecting fluctuating cognition in DLB

logical, environmental, social, and psychological factors [36]. Prior reviews that have surveyed visual hallucinations in the setting of DLB have characterized the hallucinations as complex, vivid, binocular, and occurring throughout the entire visual field [26, 37]. They may also occur earlier in the disease course, before the onset of parkinsonism features. Depending on the level of cognitive impairment, patients may have varying abilities to characterize the visual disturbances. In addition, there may be different levels of insight and distress towards the hallucinations. Clinicians may orient their questions to clarify these qualitative and temporal traits, but the sensitivity and specificity to distinguish from other neuropsychiatric disorders remain undetermined. A proposed set of questions to characterize visual hallucinations are listed in Table 3.4 [26, 36, 37].

Rapid Eye Movement (REM) Sleep Behavioral Disorder

RBD has been classically considered to be a strong clinical predictor for neurodegenerative synucleinopathies. Usually, patients would experience violent dream enactment behaviors that their spouses might witness in the middle of the night but may have poor recollection of those events. The gold standard according to the International Classification of Sleep Disorders third Edition requires a polysomnography (PSG) study [38]. But if access to a sleep study is not readily available, clinicians may refer to the first question of the Mayo Sleep Questionnaire, which has a sensitivity of 100% and specificity of 95% in diagnosing RBD, confirmed in PSG-verified subjects [39].

Table 3.4 Proposed clinical questions to assess visual hallucinations in DLB

Are the visions well-formed?	Y/N
Are they visible through both eyes?	Y/N
Do the visions cause distress?	Y/N
Did the visions begin before parkinsonism traits?	Y/N

Parkinsonism

Parkinsonism is an essential criterion of PD and requires the presence of bradykinesia and either a resting tremor or rigidity. The resting tremor is described as 4–6 Hz at rest that is suppressed with movement initiation. Clinicians should first exclude any other organic or drug-induced etiologies and should consider diagnoses other than DLB if the onset of parkinsonism occurs in the setting of severe dementia without other clinical features of DLB [26].

Indicative Biomarkers

Dopamine transporter (DAT) imaging by single-photon emission computed tomography (SPECT) and positron emission tomography (PET) has an impressive sensitivity and specificity range [26, 40]. A large multicentered study in 2007 showed a sensitivity of 78% and specificity of 90% in distinguishing probable DLB from non-DLB pathology [40]. A smaller study in 2017 analyzed autopsy validated samples with DAT imaging and found a sensitivity of 80% and specificity of 92% for differentiating DLB from AD [41].

Iodine-123 metaiodobenzylguanidine (MIBG) cardiac scintigraphy holds a rather high sensitivity and specificity with differentiating DLB from AD [26, 42]. While there had been multiple studies looking into the diagnostic utility of MIBG scintigraphy since the turn of the century, it was in 2015 that the first multicentered study compared accuracy between an automated calculation of the heart-to-mediastinum (H/M) ratio and visual assessment by readers who were blind to the subjects' diagnosis [42]. Both groups had a remarkably similar sensitivity (68.9%) and specificity (87–89.1%) in differentiating probable DLB from probable AD. There was a 3-year follow-up to this study in 2018 that tracked MIBG scintigraphy's diagnostic accuracy by using an independent consensus panel who reassessed the subjects' diagnoses matched with the baseline scintigraphy data [43]. Here, it was determined

Table 3.5 Indicative biomarkers of DLB

Biomarker	Strengths	Limitations
DAT imaging by SPECT or PET	Great sensitivity (78–80%) and specificity (90–92%) for distinguishing DLB from non-DLB and AD pathology	Does not distinguish between synucleinopathies like MSA, PD, and PDD
MIBG cardiac scintigraphy	Decent sensitivity (70–100%) and specificity (87–94%) in distinguishing DLB from AD. May offer good utility in detecting earlier signs of disease	Studies have used different H/M ratio cutoffs, which may be confusing to interpret for clinicians, and explain the variance in sensitivity data
Polysomnography showing REM stage without muscle atonia	Identifies RBD with high diagnostic sensitivity (84%) and specificity (98%) for neurodegenerative synucleinopathies	Does not distinguish between other related Lewy body disorders like PD, PDD, and MSA

that there was a sensitivity and specificity of 77% and 94%, respectively, with differentiating DLB from AD. However, clinicians should be cognizant of the H/M cutoff ratio used to distinguish DLB from other dementia subtypes, as the sensitivity and specificity may change depending on the H/M ratio cutoffs used [44]. Table 3.5 summarizes the biomarkers' strengths and weaknesses [40–45].

Treatments

Non-pharmacological

In general, evidence for non-pharmacologic management of DLB has been limited to case reports and case series, which leads to inadequately powered studies with limited generalizability [46, 47]. Primary outcome measures have mostly pointed towards overall quality of life, caregiver burden, and neuropsychiatric symptoms like depression and anxiety. The low number of high-quality studies dedicated to DLB has consequently forced clinicians to extrapolate the findings for other dementia subtypes, like AD, and there is a significant need for adequately powered comparison studies. The non-pharmacologic interventions with the most available data for DLB are summarized below:

Exercise

One randomized controlled trial in 2015 with 170 subjects with dementia was assessed, but it only included 4 patients with DLB, which showed a significant level of improvement in apathy within the exercise groups [48]. However, the small number of DLB participants prevented quality statistical comparisons with the other dementia groups. Other case series have generally demonstrated improvements in gait speed, attention, and quality of life but primarily recruited patients with PD and PDD [49, 50].

Environmental Modifications

Two case studies with a combined total of two DLB subjects reported decreased anxiety distress around visual hallucinations and improved caregiver burden [51, 52].

Music Therapy

One cluster randomized controlled trial of 17 subjects (1 with DLB) showed significant improvement in quality of life and symptom burden as indicated by feedback from semi-structured interviews and program evaluations [53].

Electroconvulsive Therapy (ECT)

There are several case series that aimed to treat neuropsychiatric symptoms like depression and hallucinations, and most were made up of 4–8 DLB subjects. In general, there is modest improvement of depressive symptoms by interview, although the primary outcome measures were not standardized between studies from 2003 to 2016 as some chose to analyze various combinations of the Mini-Mental State Examination (MMSE), Neuropsychiatric Inventory (npi), and Hamilton Depression Rating Scale (HDRS) [54–57]. Study designs were also complicated by the different lengths of treatment (6–15 sessions), varying settings of electrode placement (unilateral vs. bilateral), and a non-standardized inclusion criteria with different degrees of concurrent psychopharmacologic treatment.

Transcranial Magnetic Stimulation (TMS)

Two case series in 2009 and 2016 recruited DLB subjects to examine the effects of TMS on depression and cognitive deficits [56, 58]. Both showed significant improvements in their primary outcome measures on the HAM-D rating and reaction speed in attention testing, although these effects were not sustained. The studies differed in the number of TMS treatments received and coil placement; therefore, additional studies are needed to construct a standardized treatment protocol.

Pharmacological

Pharmacologic management of DLB poses a complex set of challenges, ranging from the wide constellation of neuropsychiatric symptoms to the adverse effects of medications. The pathophysiology and clinical manifestations of DLB present a fundamental dilemma that clinicians must balance when deciding on a treatment approach. For example, treating the parkinsonian symptoms with antiparkinsonian medications may exacerbate psychotic features, but addressing the neuropsychiatric symptoms like psychosis may worsen parkinsonism [59]. Furthermore, there are no disease-modifying drugs available currently, although research in targeting alpha-synuclein aggregates has gained more traction in recent years [60–62]. Due to the lack of high-quality studies concerning pharmacologic treatment of DLB, the general approach to treatment is focused on identifying the target symptom that causes most distress to the patient and caregivers [59].

Out of the available classes of medications to address DLB, cholinesterase inhibitors (ChEIs) may have the most evidence that can address both the cognitive impairment and neuropsychiatric symptoms in DLB [59]. Rivastigmine was the first to be tested in a randomized, double-blind, placebo-controlled international study for DLB, where nearly twice as many patients on rivastigmine showed an improvement of 30% on a computerized cognitive examination and experienced less anxiety and hallucinations [63]. Galantamine has also been shown to improve the fluctuations in cognition, sleep disturbances, and psychosis in a retrospective comparison study, where the results were then replicated in a 24-week, open-label study with 50 test subjects [64, 65]. Donepezil was first examined in 2012 within a large group of 140 subjects with DLB over the course of 12 weeks, after which there were significant improvements in the MMSE, caregiver burden, and behavioral symptoms [66]. Subsequent safety data demonstrated sustained improvement in MMSE scores with higher plasma concentrations of donepezil, without significantly worsened side effect burden [67]. Furthermore, a meta-analysis and systematic review investigating the safety and efficacy of donepezil, rivastigmine, and galantamine showed significant benefits in cognitive function, and overall improvement in the clinical global impression of change (CGIC) without worsening of parkinsonism [68]. Memantine, an N-methyl D-aspartate (NMDA) receptor antagonist, has also demonstrated significant improvements in the CGIC scores in two separate randomized, double-blinded, placebo-controlled studies [69, 70]. However, meta-analyses have suggested that high doses of donepezil and galantamine were superior in improving cognitive functioning and behavioral symptoms when compared with memantine alone in patients with DLB [68]. Authors have reported significant heterogeneity in study designs, which may impact the overall generalizability of the data.

Hallucinations in DLB generally cause significant distress for patients and caregivers. Antipsychotics are typically avoided in elderly patients due to the increased risk of mortality and sensitivity of worsening parkinsonism. In a recent systematic review, all second-generation antipsychotics had equivocal results in managing visual hallucinations, except for clozapine which significantly reduced psychotic symptoms [71].

However, there are no studies of clozapine specifically for DLB, as the adverse effects of constipation, orthostatic hypotension, and risk of agranulocytosis are strong deterrents for many clinicians. A review of five double-blinded RCTs and two open-label RCTs for quetiapine at 100 mg daily dose indicated very modest efficacy in reducing psychosis while at a tolerable dose that did not worsen motor symptoms [72]. Only one RCT for olanzapine at 5 mg daily dose has been conducted, which showed improvements of hallucinations and delusions [73]. Again, there was significant heterogeneity of study designs, with some including a greater sample of PD and PDD patients rather than DLB. In addition, visual hallucinations often get clustered with other psychotic symptoms in the study outcomes, thus further limiting the generalizability of the data. Novel antipsychotics like pimavanserin, a 5-HT2a inverse agonist, have shown early, though modest, benefits in dementia-related psychosis. However, most studies analyze subjects primarily with PD, and those that include DLB have a rather modest sample size and therefore are insufficient for adequate statistical comparison with the other dementia subtypes [74]. In addition, the safety profile of pimavanserin compared with atypical antipsychotics requires additional investigation. A recent observational study in 2022 showed no differences in mortality rates between pimavanserin and atypical antipsychotics after 180 days of treatment in nursing home patients [75].

Despite the frequency of other neuropsychiatric symptoms like depression and apathy in DLB which might initiate the start of an antidepressant, there is a significant lack of studies to support this decision [59]. A randomized trial in 2010 analyzing citalopram to treat depression in DLB showed poor tolerance and high dropout rate, though there was a positive response noted for PDD [76]. Further standardized studies of antidepressants in DLB patients are desperately needed.

Parkinsonism in DLB can be treated with the dopamine precursor, levodopa, although its benefits are less effective than in patients with PD

[77, 78]. The evidence is severely limited by small sample sizes for DLB, and mean doses are generally low around 303 mg/day. Zonisamide, a sodium and T-type calcium channel blocker, has promising early evidence as an adjunct treatment of parkinsonism over levodopa. A Phase 2 trial that enrolled 158 patients with DLB showed significant improvement in motor signs without worsening of caregiver burden, cognitive function, and behavioral symptoms [79].

Sleep disturbances are common in DLB, with RBD and insomnia being the primary presentations. Judicious use of low-dose clonazepam at 0.5–1 mg has been shown to reduce injuries in patients and their sleep partners [80]. However, more recent recommendations encourage modification of the sleep environment over benzodiazepines [81]. Systematic reviews for melatonin indicate fair effectiveness in reducing the severity and frequency of RBD signs at doses of 3–9 mg/day, and a safer risk profile when compared to clonazepam [82, 83]. Other sleep disturbances like restless leg syndrome may be treated with iron supplementation, dopamine agonists (though caution for worsening psychosis), and gabapentin, but studies are lacking to support their use specifically in DLB.

While there is currently no available disease-modifying treatment for DLB, several potentially promising options focused on the alpha-synuclein pathway are in their early phases of development. An alpha-synuclein misfolding inhibitor, NPT200–11, has been shown to reduce the accumulation of Lewy bodies in mice [60]. E2027, a phosphodiesterase-I inhibitor (PDE-I) is currently in a 12-week phase 2 clinical trial, under the premise that the PDE-I inhibitor may rescue alpha-synuclein toxicity through increasing levels of cyclic guanosine monophosphate (cGMP) [61]. Ambroxol, a medication for respiratory distress, can increase glucocerebrosidase activity, thus lowering alpha-synuclein levels, but there are only trials for PDD, and none for DLB at this time [62].

Table 3.6 summarizes the report listed above, for only the medications with evidence in DLB

Table 3.6 Pharmacologic management in DLB

Drug name	Drug class	Daily target dose	Dose schedule	Target symptom	Adverse effects
Donepezil	Acetylcholinesterase inhibitor	5–10 mg (oral)	Start 5 mg at bedtime for 4 weeks, then may increase to 10 mg	Cognitive impairment Neuropsychiatric symptoms	Bradycardia Diarrhea Nausea Weight loss
Rivastigmine	Acetylcholinesterase inhibitor	12 mg (oral) 13.3 mg (patch)	Oral—start 1.5 mg twice a day, then increase by 1.5 mg dose increments every 4 weeks as tolerated Patch—start 4.6 mg daily for 4 weeks, then may increase to 9.5 mg daily for 4 weeks, then may increase to 13.3 mg daily	Cognitive impairment Neuropsychiatric symptoms	Bradycardia Diarrhea Nausea Weight loss
Galantamine	Acetylcholinesterase inhibitor	24 mg (immediate-release oral) 24 mg (extended-release oral)	IR—start 4 mg BID, increase by 4 mg BID every 4-week increments as tolerated ER—start 8 mg daily, then increase by 8 mg increments every 4 weeks as tolerated	Cognitive impairment Neuropsychiatric symptoms	Bradycardia Diarrhea Nausea Weight loss
Memantine	NMDA receptor antagonist	20 mg (oral)	Start 5 mg daily, then increase by 5 mg increments every week as tolerated. Doses greater than 5 mg daily should be divided into twice-a-day dosing	Cognitive impairment Behavioral symptoms	Agitation Constipation Dizziness Headache
Quetiapine	Atypical antipsychotic	100 mg	Start at 50 mg at bedtime, may increase as tolerated up to 100 mg split in twice-a-day dosing	Hallucinations	Orthostatic hypotension Sedation
Olanzapine	Atypical antipsychotic	5 mg	Start at 2.5 mg at bedtime, may increase as tolerated and consider twice-a-day dosing	Hallucinations	Orthostatic hypotension Constipation Sedation
Levodopa	Dopamine precursor	303 mg (mean dose of response in trials)	Depending on formulation, start at lowest dose split in 3×/day or 4×/day dosing. Increase as tolerated every 2 days for response	Parkinsonism	Psychosis Nausea Hypotension Irritability
Zonisamide	Anticonvulsant	25–50 mg (mean dose of response in trials)	Start at 25 mg daily, and increase to 50 mg daily based on tolerability	Parkinsonism	Decreased appetite Weight loss
Melatonin	Melatonin receptor 1 agonist	3–12 mg	Start at 3 mg at bedtime and increase as tolerated for response	Sleep disturbances (RBD) Neuropsychiatric symptoms	Sedation
Clonazepam	Benzodiazepine	0.5–1 mg	Start judiciously at bedtime and may increase as tolerated for response	Sleep disturbances (RBD)	Dizziness Falls Sedation

[59, 63–70, 72, 73, 77–80, 82, 83]. Medications that had either poor response, poor tolerability, or no trials are not included.

In general, management of the adverse effects should begin with an open discussion about the patient's and caregiver's concern. Clinicians should conduct a robust medication reconciliation, monitor the time onset of symptoms, and consider other physiologic causes. If the culprit happens to be the medication prescribed for DLB, clinicians may ask patients about their desire to continue, reduce the dose, or consider alternatives.

Due to the significant lack of standardized trials for multiple medication classes, there is no consensus algorithm available for the treatment of DLB. Clinicians should start by identifying the key symptom that causes the most distress for the patient and caregiver. Non-pharmacologic interventions should be considered first line whenever possible. Acetylcholinesterase inhibitors appear to have the most robust data in addressing both the cognitive impairment and neuropsychiatric symptoms of DLB. Management should strongly weigh polypharmacy risks when deciding on a treatment approach, and thus being able to address multiple symptom clusters with the least number of medications is ideal.

Conclusions

Dementia due to Lewy bodies is a common neurodegenerative disorder with a complex array of clinical manifestations and diagnostic and treatment challenges. The phenotypic heterogeneity of this disease has posed challenges for standardizing study designs, thus limiting the quality of the available data and treatment protocols. The most recent consensus report for the diagnostic criteria was designed to increase diagnostic sensitivity, which in turn may facilitate study recruitment. However, these benefits remain to be determined. The future of research development lies within improving the accuracy of diagnostic biogenetic markers and creating disease-modifying drugs.

References

1. Shergill SS, Mullan E, D'Ath PJ, Katona C. What is the clinical prevalence of Lewy body dementia? Int J Geriatr Psychiatry. 1994;9:907.
2. Zaccai J, McCracken C, Brayne C. A systematic review of prevalence and incidence studies of dementia with Lewy bodies. Age Ageing. 2005;34(6):561–6.
3. Chan SS, Chiu HF, Lam LC, Leung VP. Prevalence of dementia with Lewy bodies in an inpatient psychogeriatric population in Hong Kong Chinese. Int J Geriatr Psychiatry. 2002;17(9):847–50.
4. Heidebrink JL. Is dementia with Lewy bodies the second most common cause of dementia? J Geriatr Psychiatry Neurol. 2002;15(4):182–7.
5. Vann Jones SA, O'Brien JT. The prevalence and incidence of dementia with Lewy bodies: a systematic review of population and clinical studies. Psychol Med. 2014;44(4):673–83.
6. Kane JPM, Surendranathan A, Bentley A, Barker SAH, Taylor JP, Thomas AJ, Allan LM, McNally RJ, James PW, McKeith IG, Burn DJ, O'Brien JT. Clinical prevalence of Lewy body dementia. Alzheimers Res Ther. 2018;10(1):19.
7. Guerreiro R, Ross OA, Kun-Rodrigues C, Hernandez DG, Orme T, Eicher JD, Shepherd CE, Parkkinen L, Darwent L, Heckman MG, Scholz SW, Troncoso JC, Pletnikova O, Ansorge O, Clarimon J, Lleo A, Morenas-Rodriguez E, Clark L, Honig LS, Marder K, et al. Investigating the genetic architecture of dementia with Lewy bodies: a two-stage genome-wide association study. Lancet Neurol. 2018;17(1):64–74.
8. Bras J, Guerreiro R, Darwent L, Parkkinen L, Ansorge O, Escott-Price V, Hernandez DG, Nalls MA, Clark LN, Honig LS, Marder K, Van Der Flier WM, Lemstra A, Scheltens P, Rogaeva E, St George-Hyslop P, Londos E, Zetterberg H, Ortega-Cubero S, Pastor P, et al. Genetic analysis implicates APOE, SNCA and suggests lysosomal dysfunction in the etiology of dementia with Lewy bodies. Hum Mol Genet. 2014;23(23):6139–46.
9. Spillantini MG, Schmidt ML, Lee VM, Trojanowski JQ, Jakes R, Goedert M. Alpha-synuclein in Lewy bodies. Nature. 1997;388(6645):839–40.
10. Nalls MA, Duran R, Lopez G, Kurzawa-Akanbi M, McKeith IG, Chinnery PF, Morris CM, Theuns J, Crosiers D, Cras P, Engelborghs S, De Deyn PP, Van Broeckhoven C, Mann DM, Snowden J, Pickering-Brown S, Halliwell N, Davidson Y, Gibbons L, Harris J, et al. A multicenter study of glucocerebrosidase mutations in dementia with Lewy bodies. JAMA Neurol. 2013;70(6):727–35.
11. Tolea MI, Galvin JE. The genetics of dementia with Lewy bodies. Handb Clin Neurol. 2018;148:431–40.
12. Mata IF, Samii A, Schneer SH, Roberts JW, Griffith A, Leis BC, Schellenberg GD, Sidransky E, Bird TD, Leverenz JB, Tsuang D, Zabetian CP. Glucocerebrosidase gene mutations: a risk

factor for Lewy body disorders. Arch Neurol. 2008;65(3):379–82.

13. Clark LN, Kartsaklis LA, Wolf Gilbert R, Dorado B, Ross BM, Kisselev S, Verbitsky M, Mejia-Santana H, Cote LJ, Andrews H, Vonsattel JP, Fahn S, Mayeux R, Honig LS, Marder K. Association of glucocerebrosidase mutations with dementia with Lewy bodies. Arch Neurol. 2009;66(5):578–83.

14. Gegg ME, Schapira AHV. The role of glucocerebrosidase in Parkinson disease pathogenesis. FEBS J. 2018;285(19):3591–603.

15. Rosenberg CK, Pericak-Vance MA, Saunders AM, Gilbert JR, Gaskell PC, Hulette CM. Lewy body and Alzheimer pathology in a family with the amyloid-beta precursor protein APP717 gene mutation. Acta Neuropathol. 2000;100(2):145–52.

16. Meeus B, Theuns J, Van Broeckhoven C. The genetics of dementia with Lewy bodies: what are we missing? Arch Neurol. 2012;69(9):1113–8.

17. Castro-Chavira SA, Fernandez T, Nicolini H, Diaz-Cintra S, Prado-Alcala RA. Genetic markers in biological fluids for aging-related major neurocognitive disorder. Curr Alzheimer Res. 2015;12(3):200–9.

18. Manolio TA, Collins FS, Cox NJ, Goldstein DB, Hindorff LA, Hunter DJ, McCarthy MI, Ramos EM, Cardon LR, Chakravarti A, Cho JH, Guttmacher AE, Kong A, Kruglyak L, Mardis E, Rotimi CN, Slatkin M, Valle D, Whittemore AS, Boehnke M, et al. Finding the missing heritability of complex diseases. Nature. 2009;461(7265):747–53.

19. Wang CS, Burke JR, Steffens DC, Hulette CM, Breitner JC, Plassman BL. Twin pairs discordant for neuropathologically confirmed Lewy body dementia. J Neurol Neurosurg Psychiatry. 2009;80(5):562–5.

20. Postuma RB, Iranzo A, Hu M, Högl B, Boeve BF, Manni R, Oertel WH, Arnulf I, Ferini-Strambi L, Puligheddu M, Antelmi E, Cochen De Cock V, Arnaldi D, Mollenhauer B, Videnovic A, Sonka K, Jung KY, Kunz D, Dauvilliers Y, Provini F, et al. Risk and predictors of dementia and parkinsonism in idiopathic REM sleep behaviour disorder: a multicentre study. Brain. 2019;142(3):744–59.

21. Honeycutt L, Montplaisir JY, Gagnon JF, Ruskey J, Pelletier A, Gan-Or Z, Postuma RB. Glucocerebrosidase mutations and phenoconversion of REM sleep behavior disorder to parkinsonism and dementia. Parkinsonism Relat Disord. 2019;65:230–3.

22. Mega MS, Masterman DL, Benson DF, Vinters HV, Tomiyasu U, Craig AH, Foti DJ, Kaufer D, Scharre DW, Fairbanks L, Cummings JL. Dementia with Lewy bodies: reliability and validity of clinical and pathologic criteria. Neurology. 1996;47(6):1403–9.

23. Luis CA, Barker WW, Gajaraj K, Harwood D, Petersen R, Kashuba A, Waters C, Jimison P, Pearl G, Petito C, Dickson D, Duara R. Sensitivity and specificity of three clinical criteria for dementia with Lewy bodies in an autopsy-verified sample. Int J Geriatr Psychiatry. 1999;14(7):526–33.

24. Hohl U, Tiraboschi P, Hansen LA, Thal LJ, Corey-Bloom J. Diagnostic accuracy of dementia with Lewy bodies. Arch Neurol. 2000;57(3):347–51.

25. Verghese J, Crystal HA, Dickson DW, Lipton RB. Validity of clinical criteria for the diagnosis of dementia with Lewy bodies. Neurology. 1999;53(9):1974–82.

26. McKeith IG, Boeve BF, Dickson DW, Halliday G, Taylor JP, Weintraub D, Aarsland D, Galvin J, Attems J, Ballard CG, Bayston A, Beach TG, Blanc F, Bohnen N, Bonanni L, Bras J, Brundin P, Burn D, Chen-Plotkin A, Duda JE, et al. Diagnosis and management of dementia with Lewy bodies: fourth consensus report of the DLB Consortium. Neurology. 2017;89(1):88–100.

27. Bradshaw J, Saling M, Hopwood M, Anderson V, Brodtmann A. Fluctuating cognition in dementia with Lewy bodies and Alzheimer's disease is qualitatively distinct. J Neurol Neurosurg Psychiatry. 2004;75(3):382–7.

28. Walker Z, Moreno E, Thomas A, Inglis F, Tabet N, Stevens T, Whitfield T, Aarsland D, Rainer M, Padovani A, DaTSCAN DLB Phase 4 Study Group. Evolution of clinical features in possible DLB depending on FP-CIT SPECT result. Neurology. 2016;87(10):1045–51.

29. Cagnin A, Gnoato F, Jelcic N, Favaretto S, Zarantonello G, Ermani M, Dam M. Clinical and cognitive correlates of visual hallucinations in dementia with Lewy bodies. J Neurol Neurosurg Psychiatry. 2013;84(5):505–10.

30. Graff-Radford J, Aakre J, Savica R, Boeve B, Kremers WK, Ferman TJ, Jones DT, Kantarci K, Knopman DS, Dickson DW, Kukull WA, Petersen RC. Duration and pathologic correlates of Lewy body disease. JAMA Neurol. 2017;74(3):310–5.

31. Kramberger MG, Auestad B, Garcia-Ptacek S, Abdelnour C, Olmo JG, Walker Z, Lemstra AW, Londos E, Blanc F, Bonanni L, McKeith I, Winblad B, de Jong FJ, Nobili F, Stefanova E, Petrova M, Falup-Pecurariu C, Rektorova I, Bostantjopoulou S, Biundo R, et al. Long-term cognitive decline in dementia with Lewy bodies in a large multicenter, international cohort. J Alzheimer's Dis. 2017;57(3):787–95.

32. O'Dowd S, Schumacher J, Burn DJ, Bonanni L, Onofrj M, Thomas A, Taylor JP. Fluctuating cognition in the Lewy body dementias. Brain. 2019;142(11):3338–50.

33. Lee DR, McKeith I, Mosimann U, Ghosh-Nodial A, Grayson L, Wilson B, Thomas AJ. The dementia cognitive fluctuation scale, a new psychometric test for clinicians to identify cognitive fluctuations in people with dementia. Am J Geriatr Psychiatry. 2014;22(9):926–35.

34. Ferman TJ, Smith GE, Boeve BF, Ivnik RJ, Petersen RC, Knopman D, Graff-Radford N, Parisi J, Dickson DW. DLB fluctuations: specific features that reliably differentiate DLB from AD and normal aging. Neurology. 2004;62(2):181–7.

35. Walker MP, Ayre GA, Cummings JL, Wesnes K, McKeith IG, O'Brien JT, Ballard CG. The clini-

cian assessment of fluctuation and the one day fluctuation assessment scale. Two methods to assess fluctuating confusion in dementia. Br J Psychiatry. 2000;177:252–6.

36. Aarsland D. Epidemiology and pathophysiology of dementia-related psychosis. J Clin Psychiatry. 2020;81(5):AD19038BR1C.

37. Barnes J, David AS. Visual hallucinations in Parkinson's disease: a review and phenomenological survey. J Neurol Neurosurg Psychiatry. 2001;70(6):727–33.

38. Hu MT. REM sleep behavior disorder (RBD). Neurobiol Dis. 2020;143:104996.

39. Boeve BF, Molano JR, Ferman TJ, Lin SC, Bieniek K, Tippmann-Peikert M, Boot B, St Louis EK, Knopman DS, Petersen RC, Silber MH. Validation of the Mayo Sleep Questionnaire to screen for REM sleep behavior disorder in a community-based sample. J Clin Sleep Med. 2013;9(5):475–80.

40. McKeith I, O'Brien J, Walker Z, Tatsch K, Booij J, Darcourt J, Padovani A, Giubbini R, Bonuccelli U, Volterrani D, Holmes C, Kemp P, Tabet N, Meyer I, Reininger C, DLB Study Group. Sensitivity and specificity of dopamine transporter imaging with 123I-FP-CIT SPECT in dementia with Lewy bodies: a phase III, multicentre study. Lancet Neurol. 2007;6(4):305–13.

41. Thomas AJ, Attems J, Colloby SJ, O'Brien JT, McKeith I, Walker R, Lee L, Burn D, Lett DJ, Walker Z. Autopsy validation of 123I-FP-CIT dopaminergic neuroimaging for the diagnosis of DLB. Neurology. 2017;88(3):276–83.

42. Yoshita M, Arai H, Arai H, Arai T, Asada T, Fujishiro H, Hanyu H, Iizuka O, Iseki E, Kashihara K, Kosaka K, Maruno H, Mizukami K, Mizuno Y, Mori E, Nakajima K, Nakamura H, Nakano S, Nakashima K, Nishio Y, et al. Diagnostic accuracy of 123I-meta-iodobenzylguanidine myocardial scintigraphy in dementia with Lewy bodies: a multicenter study. PLoS One. 2015;10(3):e0120540.

43. Komatsu J, Samuraki M, Nakajima K, Arai H, Arai H, Arai T, Asada T, Fujishiro H, Hanyu H, Iizuka O, Iseki E, Kashihara K, Kosaka K, Maruno H, Mizukami K, Mizuno Y, Mori E, Nakamura H, Nakano S, Nakashima K, et al. 123I-MIBG myocardial scintigraphy for the diagnosis of DLB: a multicentre 3-year follow-up study. J Neurol Neurosurg Psychiatry. 2018;89(11):1167–73.

44. Slaets S, Van Acker F, Versijpt J, Hauth L, Goeman J, Martin JJ, De Deyn PP, Engelborghs S. Diagnostic value of MIBG cardiac scintigraphy for differential dementia diagnosis. Int J Geriatr Psychiatry. 2015;30(8):864–9.

45. Boeve BF, Silber MH, Ferman TJ, Lin SC, Benarroch EE, Schmeichel AM, Ahlskog JE, Caselli RJ, Jacobson S, Sabbagh M, Adler C, Woodruff B, Beach TG, Iranzo A, Gelpi E, Santamaria J, Tolosa E, Singer C, Mash DC, Luca C, et al. Clinicopathologic correlations in 172 cases of rapid eye movement sleep behavior disorder with or without a coexisting neurologic disorder. Sleep Med. 2013;14(8):754–62.

46. Connors MH, Quinto L, McKeith I, Brodaty H, Allan L, Bamford C, Thomas A, Taylor JP, O'Brien JT. Non-pharmacological interventions for Lewy body dementia: a systematic review. Psychol Med. 2018;48(11):1749–58.

47. Morrin H, Fang T, Servant D, Aarsland D, Rajkumar AP. Systematic review of the efficacy of non-pharmacological interventions in people with Lewy body dementia. Int Psychogeriatr. 2018;30(3):395–407.

48. Telenius EW, Engedal K, Bergland A. Effect of a high-intensity exercise program on physical function and mental health in nursing home residents with dementia: an assessor blinded randomized controlled trial. PLoS One. 2015;10(5):e0126102.

49. Tabak R, Aquije G, Fisher BE. Aerobic exercise to improve executive function in Parkinson disease: a case series. J Neurol Phys Ther. 2013;37(2):58–64.

50. Rochester L, Burn DJ, Woods G, Godwin J, Nieuwboer A. Does auditory rhythmical cueing improve gait in people with Parkinson's disease and cognitive impairment? A feasibility study. Movement Disorders. 2009;24(6):839–45.

51. Huh TJ, Areán PA, Bornfeld H, Elite-Marcandonatou A. The effectiveness of an environmental and behavioral approach to treat behavior problems in a patient with dementia with Lewy bodies: a case study. Ann Long-Term Care. 2008;16(11):17–21.

52. Gil-Ruiz N, Osorio RS, Cruz I, Agüera-Ortiz L, Olazarán J, Sacks H, Álvarez-Linera J, Martínez-Martín P, Alzheimer Center of The Queen Sofia Foundation Multidisciplinary Therapy Group. An effective environmental intervention for management of the 'mirror sign' in a case of probable Lewy body dementia. Neurocase. 2013;19(1):1–13.

53. Hsu MH, Flowerdew R, Parker M, Fachner J, Odell-Miller H. Individual music therapy for managing neuropsychiatric symptoms for people with dementia and their carers: a cluster randomised controlled feasibility study. BMC Geriatr. 2015;15:84.

54. Kung S, O'Connor MK. ECT in Lewy body dementia: a case report. Primary Care Companion J Clin Psychiatry. 2002;4(4)

55. Rasmussen KG Jr, Russell JC, Kung S, Rummans TA, Rae-Stuart E, O'Connor MK. Electroconvulsive therapy for patients with major depression and probable Lewy body dementia. J ECT. 2003;19(2):103–9.

56. Takahashi S, Mizukami K, Yasuno F, Asada T. Depression associated with dementia with Lewy bodies (DLB) and the effect of somatotherapy. Psychogeriatrics. 2009;9(2):56–61.

57. Yamaguchi Y, Matsuoka K, Ueda J, Takada R, Takahashi M, Kiuchi K, et al. The effect of electroconvulsive therapy on psychiatric symptoms of dementia with Lewy bodies. J Neuropsychiatry Clin Neurosci. 2016;28:e66.

58. Elder GJ, Firbank MJ, Kumar H, Chatterjee P, Chakraborty T, Dutt A, Taylor JP. Effects of transcranial direct current stimulation upon attention and visuoperceptual function in Lewy body dementia: a preliminary study. Int Psychogeriatr. 2016;28(2):341–7.

59. Stinton C, McKeith I, Taylor JP, Lafortune L, Mioshi E, Mak E, Cambridge V, Mason J, Thomas A, O'Brien JT. Pharmacological management of lewy body dementia: a systematic review and meta-analysis. Am J Psychiatry. 2015;172(8):731–42.

60. Price DL, Koike MA, Khan A, Wrasidlo W, Rockenstein E, Masliah E, Bonhaus D. The small molecule alpha-synuclein misfolding inhibitor, NPT200-11, produces multiple benefits in an animal model of Parkinson's disease. Sci Rep. 2018;8(1):16165.

61. Höllerhage M, Moebius C, Melms J, Chiu WH, Goebel JN, Chakroun T, Koeglsperger T, Oertel WH, Rösler TW, Bickle M, Höglinger GU. Protective efficacy of phosphodiesterase-1 inhibition against alpha-synuclein toxicity revealed by compound screening in LUHMES cells. Sci Rep. 2017;7(1):11469.

62. McNeill A, Magalhaes J, Shen C, Chau KY, Hughes D, Mehta A, Foltynie T, Cooper JM, Abramov AY, Gegg M, Schapira AH. Ambroxol improves lysosomal biochemistry in glucocerebrosidase mutation-linked Parkinson disease cells. Brain. 2014;137(Pt 5):1481–95.

63. McKeith I, Del Ser T, Spano P, Emre M, Wesnes K, Anand R, Cicin-Sain A, Ferrara R, Spiegel R. Efficacy of rivastigmine in dementia with Lewy bodies: a randomised, double-blind, placebo-controlled international study. Lancet (London, England). 2000;356(9247):2031–6.

64. Bhasin M, Rowan E, Edwards K, McKeith I. Cholinesterase inhibitors in dementia with Lewy bodies: a comparative analysis. Int J Geriatr Psychiatry. 2007;22(9):890–5.

65. Edwards K, Royall D, Hershey L, Lichter D, Hake A, Farlow M, Pasquier F, Johnson S. Efficacy and safety of galantamine in patients with dementia with Lewy bodies: a 24-week open-label study. Dement Geriatr Cogn Disord. 2007;23(6):401–5.

66. Mori E, Ikeda M, Kosaka K, Donepezil-DLB Study Investigators. Donepezil for dementia with Lewy bodies: a randomized, placebo-controlled trial. Ann Neurol. 2012;72(1):41–52.

67. Mori E, Ikeda M, Nakai K, Miyagishi H, Nakagawa M, Kosaka K. Increased plasma donepezil concentration improves cognitive function in patients with dementia with Lewy bodies: an exploratory pharmacokinetic/pharmacodynamic analysis in a phase 3 randomized controlled trial. J Neurol Sci. 2016;366:184–90.

68. Wang HF, Yu JT, Tang SW, Jiang T, Tan CC, Meng XF, Wang C, Tan MS, Tan L. Efficacy and safety of cholinesterase inhibitors and memantine in cognitive impairment in Parkinson's disease, Parkinson's disease dementia, and dementia with Lewy bodies: systematic review with meta-analysis and trial sequential analysis. J Neurol Neurosurg Psychiatry. 2015;86(2):135–43.

69. Aarsland D, Ballard C, Walker Z, Bostrom F, Alves G, Kossakowski K, Leroi I, Pozo-Rodriguez F, Minthon L, Londos E. Memantine in patients with Parkinson's disease dementia or dementia with Lewy bodies: a double-blind, placebo-controlled, multicentre trial. Lancet Neurol. 2009;8(7):613–8.

70. Emre M, Tsolaki M, Bonuccelli U, Destée A, Tolosa E, Kutzelnigg A, Ceballos-Baumann A, Zdravkovic S, Bladström A, Jones R, 11018 Study Investigators. Memantine for patients with Parkinson's disease dementia or dementia with Lewy bodies: a randomised, double-blind, placebo-controlled trial. Lancet Neurol. 2010;9(10):969–77.

71. Swann P, O'Brien JT. Management of visual hallucinations in dementia and Parkinson's disease. Int Psychogeriatr. 2019;31(6):815–36.

72. Desmarais P, Massoud F, Filion J, Nguyen QD, Bajsarowicz P. Quetiapine for psychosis in Parkinson disease and neurodegenerative parkinsonian disorders: a systematic review. J Geriatr Psychiatry Neurol. 2016;29(4):227–36.

73. Cummings JL, Street J, Masterman D, Clark WS. Efficacy of olanzapine in the treatment of psychosis in dementia with Lewy bodies. Dement Geriatr Cogn Disord. 2002;13(2):67–73.

74. Tariot PN, Cummings JL, Soto-Martin ME, Ballard C, Erten-Lyons D, Sultzer DL, Devanand DP, Weintraub D, McEvoy B, Youakim JM, Stankovic S, Foff EP. Trial of pimavanserin in dementia-related psychosis. N Engl J Med. 2021;385(4):309–19.

75. Mosholder AD, Ma Y, Akhtar S, Podskalny GD, Feng Y, Lyu H, Liao J, Wei Y, Wernecke M, Leishear K, Nelson LM, MaCurdy TE, Kelman JA, Graham DJ. Mortality among Parkinson's disease patients treated with Pimavanserin or atypical antipsychotics: an observational study in medicare beneficiaries. Am J Psychiatry. 2022;179(8):553–61.

76. Culo S, Mulsant BH, Rosen J, Mazumdar S, Blakesley RE, Houck PR, Pollock BG. Treating neuropsychiatric symptoms in dementia with Lewy bodies: a randomized controlled-trial. Alzheimer Dis Assoc Disord. 2010;24(4):360–4.

77. Goldman JG, Goetz CG, Brandabur M, Sanfilippo M, Stebbins GT. Effects of dopaminergic medications on psychosis and motor function in dementia with Lewy bodies. Movement Disorders. 2008;23(15):2248–50.

78. Drach LM. Pharmakotherapie bei Demenz mit Lewy-Körperchen und Parkinson-Demenz. Gemeinsamkeiten und Unterschiede [Drug treatment of dementia with Lewy bodies and Parkinson's disease dementia--common features and differences]. Medizinische Monatsschrift fur Pharmazeuten. 2011;34(2):47–54.

79. Murata M, Odawara T, Hasegawa K, Iiyama S, Nakamura M, Tagawa M, Kosaka K. Adjunct zonisamide to levodopa for DLB parkinsonism: a randomized double-blind phase 2 study. Neurology. 2018;90(8):e664–72.

80. Massironi G, Galluzzi S, Frisoni GB. Drug treatment of REM sleep behavior disorders in dementia with Lewy bodies. Int Psychogeriatr. 2003;15(4):377–83.
81. Aurora RN, Zak RS, Maganti RK, Auerbach SH, Casey KR, Chowdhuri S, Karippot A, Ramar K, Kristo DA, Morgenthaler TI, Standards of Practice Committee, & American Academy of Sleep Medicine. Best practice guide for the treatment of REM sleep behavior disorder (RBD). J Clin Sleep Med. 2010;6(1):85–95.
82. McGrane IR, Leung JG, St Louis EK, Boeve BF. Melatonin therapy for REM sleep behavior disorder: a critical review of evidence. Sleep Med. 2015;16(1):19–26.
83. Boeve BF, Silber MH, Ferman TJ. Melatonin for treatment of REM sleep behavior disorder in neurologic disorders: results in 14 patients. Sleep Med. 2003;4(4):281–4.

Major Neurocognitive Disorders Due to Frontotemporal Disease

4

Ganesh Gopalakrishna, Ashish Sarangi, and Pallavi Joshi

Introduction

Major neurocognitive disorder or dementia due to frontotemporal disease is a syndromal term that includes multiple neurodegenerative diseases characterized by gradual deterioration of frontal and temporal lobe functions and is associated with problems in behavior, language, and executive functioning [1]. It primarily encompasses three distinct clinical subtypes: behavioral variant of FTD (bvFTD), semantic variant primary progressive aphasia (PPA), and nonfluent agrammatic variant PPA (nfPPA). The latter two are subtypes of primary progressive aphasia (PPA), a neurodegenerative disease characterized by early and prominent language impairment with little to no memory impairment, behavioral symptoms, or motor dysfunction [2]. Logopenic variant of PPA is frequently caused by Alzheimer's disease (AD) [3] and hence will not be discussed here. Diagnostic criteria for PPA are noted in Table 4.1 as described by Mesulam [4]. FTD motor neuron disease, pro-

Table 4.1 Inclusion and exclusion criteria for PPA based on the criteria by Mesulam [2, 4]

Criteria for the diagnosis of primary progressive aphasia: Based on the criteria by Mesulam
Inclusion criteria 1–3 must be present: 1. Most prominent clinical feature is difficulty with language 2. These deficits are the principal cause of impaired daily living activities 3. Aphasia should be the most prominent deficit at the symptom onset and for the initial phases of the disease
Exclusion criteria: One to four must be absent for a diagnosis of PPA 1. Pattern of deficits is better accounted for by other neurodegenerative or medical disorders 2. Cognitive disturbance is better accounted for by a psychiatric diagnosis 3. Prominent initial episodic memory, visual memory, and visuoperceptual impairment 4. Prominent initial behavioral disturbance

gressive supranuclear palsy syndrome, and corticobasal syndrome are also often considered part of FTD by some clinical researchers [5].

Epidemiology

Frontotemporal dementia (FTD) is one of the most common types of dementia among patients under the age of 65, also known as early-onset dementia (EOD) [6]. Among the clinical subtypes, the behavioral variant accounts for about 50% of all FTD [7]. FTD can affect people anywhere between the fourth and eighth decades of

G. Gopalakrishna (✉) · P. Joshi
Banner Alzheimer's Institute, Phoenix, AZ, USA
e-mail: Ganesh.gopalakrishna@bannerhealth.com;
Pallavi.joshi@bannerhealth.com

A. Sarangi
Department of Psychiatry, University of Missouri-Columbia, Columbia, MO, USA
e-mail: aks5dg@health.missouri.edu

life but commonly affects people in their 50s and 60s [8]. Behavioral variant FTD (bvFTD) is most common among patients between ages 45 and 65. Other variants of FTD like PPA may have a later peak age at diagnosis [9]. Due to its predilection for younger patients, the loss of productivity and overall costs per patient are estimated to be higher among individuals with FTD when compared to individuals with AD [10]. Prevalence and incidence of FTD are often difficult to determine due to the rarity of the disorders among a large at-risk population, especially when compared to Alzheimer's dementia. Also, FTD is frequently missed or misdiagnosed as a psychiatric disorder or other types of dementia [1]. The prevalence estimates for FTD range from 15 to 22 per 1,000,000 person-years, while the incidence is estimated to be about 2–4 per 100,000 person-years [11]. FTD affects both genders nearly equally, but females have a higher prevalence of granulin-related FTD [12, 13].

Risk Factors

FTD is a strongly familial disorder with genetic heterogeneity, despite a large number of cases being sporadic. About 40% of patients with FTD have a family history of a similar disorder, highlighting the major role genetic factors play in its etiology. Approximately 10% of patients have an autosomal dominant pattern of inheritance [14]. Heritability is also known to vary between the different clinical syndromes, with the highest heritability noted in bvFTD and the lowest in semantic PPA [14, 15]. More than 80% of the hereditable FTD is attributed to mutations of three genes—chromosome 9 open reading frame 72 (C9ORF72), progranulin (GRN), and microtubule-associated protein tau (MAPT) [12]. Other factors associated with higher risk of sporadic FTD include head trauma and thyroid disease [16]. Histopathologically, FTD is predominantly related to the abnormal accumulation of three types of protein—microtubule-binding protein tau, TAR DNA-binding protein (TDP-43), and fused in sarcoma protein (FUS) (Fig. 4.1). Neuro-inflammation and autoimmune processes can also contribute towards the pathogenesis of FTD, as seen with other neurodegenerative diseases [17, 18]. People with a history of traumatic brain injury appear to be at a higher risk of developing FTD in some studies [19, 20]. Table 4.2 enumerates the genetic mutations associated with the subtypes of FTD.

Clinical syndromes	Major genetic mutations	Most common pathology
• Behavioral Variant • Semantic variant PPA • Non fluent variant PPA	• C9ORF72 • GRN • MAPT	• Microtubule-binding protein tau • TDP-43 • FUS

Fig. 4.1 FTD considered as a syndrome of threes that has three distinct clinical syndromes, three major gene mutations, and three predominant pathologies

Assessment

A comprehensive history from the patient, and more importantly from the family, is vital to the assessment of FTD. Like the genetic and pathological heterogeneity, FTD also has heterogeneity in clinical presentation. Behavioral variant FTD is characterized by behavioral changes early in the course of the disease. These include social disinhibition, apathy, loss of sympathy and empathy for others, and loss of insight. Repetitive, obsessive, and stereotyped behaviors, and hyperorality or dietary changes, are also commonly noted [7, 21]. The clinical features of possible FTD are summarized in Table 4.2. A diagnosis of probable FTD indicates significant functional decline and imaging results consistent with bvFTD, in addition to the criteria listed for possible FTD. A definitive diagnosis of bvFTD is confirmed only with histopathological evidence on biopsy or autopsy [22]. Psychosis may be present in about 10% of patients with FTD, with higher prevalence among patients with genetic mutations of C9ORF72 and GRN [23]. PPA is characterized by a gradual, progressive decline in language over many months or years affecting the ability of the individual to understand, create, and deliver messages [24]. It is important to apply the diagnostic criteria for PPA before identifying the subtype to avoid conflating the diagnosis with speech apraxia [25].

nfvPPA often presents with slow, effortful speech with hesitancies, mispronunciations, and distortions. Patients tend to be frustrated with their inability to communicate and comprehend conversations or complex instructions [24]. On the other hand, patients with semantic PPA are able to produce well-articulated sentences, but the speech content lacks substance. Speech problems start with word-finding difficulty and progress to circumlocutory and empty speech. Family may provide a history of the patient forgetting the meaning of previously familiar words and an erosion of vocabulary. The anomia that is characteristic of semantic variant PPA is due to failure of recognition or comprehension of words and

Table 4.2 Clinical criteria for possible behavioral variant of frontotemporal dementia [22]

Diagnostic criteria for possible behavioral variant FTD

Three of the following behavioral/cognitive symptoms (A–F) must be present to meet the criteria. Ascertainment requires that symptoms be persistent or recurrent, rather than single or rare events.

    A. Early behavioral disinhibition [one of the following symptoms (A.1–A.3) must be present]:
        A.1. Socially inappropriate behavior
        A.2. Loss of manners or decorum
        A.3. Impulsive, rash, or careless actions
    B. Early apathy or inertia [one of the following symptoms (B.1–B.2) must be present]:
        B.1. Apathy
        B.2. Inertia
    C. Early loss of sympathy or empathy [one of the following symptoms (C.1–C.2) must be present]:
        C.1. Diminished response to other people's needs and feelings
        C.2. Diminished social interest, interrelatedness, or personal warmth
    D. Early perseverative, stereotyped, or compulsive/ritualistic behavior [one of the following symptoms (D.1–D.3) must be present]:
        D.1. Simple repetitive movements
        D.2. Complex, compulsive, or ritualistic behaviors
        D.3. Stereotypy of speech
    E. Hyperorality and dietary changes [one of the following symptoms (E.1–E.3) must be present]:
        E.1. Altered food preferences
        E.2. Binge eating, increased consumption of alcohol or cigarettes
        E.3. Oral exploration or consumption of inedible objects
    F. Neuropsychological profile: Executive/generation deficits with relative sparing of memory and visuospatial functions [all of the following symptoms (F.1–F.3) must be present]:
        F.1. Deficits in executive tasks
        F.2. Relative sparing of episodic memory
        F.3. Relative sparing of visuospatial skills

Table 4.3 Clinical criteria for nfv variant and semantic variant PPA adapted from Gorno-Tempini, M.L. et al. [28]

Clinical diagnostic criteria for agrammatic variant and semantic variant PPA	
Nonfluent/agrammatic variant PA	**Semantic variant**
At least one of the following core features must be present: 1. Agrammatism in language production 2. Effortful, halting speech with inconsistent speed sound errors and distortions (apraxia of speech)	Both of the following core features must be present: 1. Impaired confrontation naming 2. Impaired single-word comprehension
At least two of the three following other features must be present: 1. Impaired comprehension of syntactically complex sentences 2. Spared single-word comprehension 3. Spared object knowledge	At least two of the four following features must be present: 1. Impaired object knowledge, particularly for low-frequency or low-familiarity items 2. Surface dyslexia or dysgraphia 3. Spare repetition 4. Spared speech production (grammar and motor speech)

objects [24]. The diagnostic criteria for nonfluent/agrammatic variant and semantic variant PPA are presented in Table 4.3 [2].

A thorough neurological examination should be completed to identify any frontal release signs, to rule out other pathologies, and to identify any comorbidity such as motor neuron disease or parkinsonism. A formal neuropsychological evaluation can be very useful in diagnosing FTD and identifying the correct subtype. Frontal dysfunction is evident as impaired executive functioning which is characterized by impairments in attention, abstraction, planning, and problem-solving. Patients with bvFTD may demonstrate deficits in memory, albeit with better performance when compared to individuals with AD [26]. Social cognition is significantly impaired in FTD, which may distinguish it from AD [27]. Multiple neuropsychological assessments are available to aid in the diagnosis of PPA and further identify the subtype accurately. The Repeat and Point Test is a brief measure which can differentiate semantic and nonfluent variants with 100% accuracy. The Sydney Language Battery (SydBat) can also differentiate among the PPA subtypes. Clinical Dementia Rating (CDR) scale also includes a language domain offering additional sensitivity to detect and track symptoms consistent with PPA [28].

Imaging

MRI brain is a structural scan intended to exclude pathologies (like masses, infarcts) as part of a standard assessment for suspected neurodegenerative disorders. Focal atrophy, symmetric or asymmetric, in the frontal or temporal lobes can support a diagnosis of FTD. However, the absence of such atrophic pattern does not rule out a diagnosis of FTD [22].

A functional imaging modality like PET-*fluorodeoxyglucose* (FDG) could enhance the sensitivity for diagnosis of FTD by demonstrating the decreased uptake of FDG in the fronto-temporal distribution [29]. Similarly, single-photon emission computerized tomography (SPECT) or arterial spin labelling can identify hypoperfusion aiding the diagnosis [30]. It is important to be aware of the possibility of false-positive FDG-PET scans in individuals with primary psychiatric disorders [31]. Imaging abnormalities in the left posterior fronto-insular region, such as predominant atrophy on MRI brain or hypometabolism on the PET-FDG, support the clinical diagnosis of nfvPPA [32]. Likewise, similar changes in the anterior temporal lobe support the diagnosis of semantic variant of PPA [2, 33].

An amyloid PET scan can identify amyloid deposition in the brain suggesting an AD pathology, but this may not be the causative etiology [34]. On the other hand, a negative amyloid scan may help exclude AD. Similarly, Tau PET scan with currently available ligands is not specific enough to accurately diagnose FTD [34].

Fluid-Based Biomarkers

Blood-based biomarkers and cerebrospinal fluid (CSF) markers have an increasingly important role in the assessment of FTD. Neurofilament light (NfL) is a nonspecific marker of neuronal injury and degeneration with good correlation between CSF and plasma concentrations [35]. It can predict progression of illness in patients with FTD [36, 37]. NfL is not a diagnostic biomarker for FTD, but could be useful in differentiating it from primary psychiatric disorders like bipolar disorder [38].

Phosphorylated Tau (p-Tau) subtypes like p-Tau 181 and p-Tau 217, along with biomarkers of amyloid deposition like Aβ42 and Aβ40, have demonstrated high sensitivity and specificity in diagnosing patients with AD [39, 40]. P-Tau has also demonstrated efficacy in differentiating FTD from AD, another key clinical distinction with therapeutic implications [41].

TDP-43 is a cytoplasmic inclusion protein found in a large number of FTD patients across various subtypes [42]. Despite some studies showing elevated TDP-43 levels, both in CSF and in plasma, it has limited utility due to significant overlap with controls and other tauopathies [43]. Dipeptide repeat proteins (DPRs), resulting from the repeat expansions in the noncoding regions of the C9orf72 gene, can be measured in the CSF, thus helping detect patients in the asymptomatic stage of the disease [44]. But like TDP43, it has limited clinical use due to significant overlap with controls. Improved testing with more sensitive techniques could improve the accuracy of this test for future clinical use [43].

Pathogenic variants in granulin gene (GRN) cause haploinsufficiency leading to reduced progranulin levels [45]. Progranulin, measured in CSF or plasma, can separate GRN carriers from controls. The diagnostic utility of this biomarkers is limited by possible effects of other confounding variables on the progranulin levels [46]. Biomarkers are increasingly used in clinical trials during screening to enrich sample and to measure therapeutic response. Routine use of these biomarkers in clinical care would need further research.

Genetic Testing

Genetic testing may be considered for individuals presenting with symptoms of FTD and have a family history of dementia or other neurodegenerative diseases like ALS. The three major gene mutations in FTD-C9ORF72, GRN, and MAPT can be tested. Testing for other less common genetic mutations is also available. Testing patients with no family history of FTD should be based on individual cases as some mutations like the C9ORF72 have significant heterogeneity in clinical presentation [34]. It is also vital to provide pretest and posttest counselling for genetic testing given the tremendous psychosocial impact the results have on patients and their families.

Treatments

Non-pharmacological

With lack of effective pharmacological interventions, supportive therapy is the mainstay of treatment for FTDs. The role of a multidisciplinary team comprised of clinicians, speech therapists, and social workers, which incorporates the family's input into treatment planning that cannot be overstated. Psychoeducation is an important part of management and can provide key insights to the caregivers, family members, and other healthcare providers. Following the diagnosis, it is important to address safety-related issues including driving and supervision with both the patients and their caregivers. The risk of road traffic accidents is often increased even in the mild disease stage and is related to inattention, impulsivity, and poor emotion regulation [8]. It is also vital to educate the family about advance directives and financial planning. Financial planning in FTD has the added challenge of lost income with dependent children at home, due to earlier age at onset of symptoms [47]. Poor judgement and executive functioning can lead to bad financial decisions and severe financial problems [48].

Very few randomized controlled trials have been reported on non-pharmacological management interventions for FTD [49]. Cognitive training or rehabilitation has limited effectiveness in FTD. Behavioral interventions such as reintroducing old hobbies and replacing stimulus-bound behaviors with appropriate behaviors could be used to reduce disruptive behaviors in social settings. Family will need education regarding dietary restriction to avoid excessive weight gain secondary to hyperorality. Despite the lack of evidence specific to FTD, physical exercise can enhance mood and cognition among patients with dementia and should be encouraged with all patients with FTD [50].

Speech Therapy

Several studies have substantiated the benefits of speech and language therapies in the management of PPA. Targeted word retrieval interventions with individualized training sets using patient's own items promote relearning and maintenance of gains, specifically in nfvPPA [51]. Script training, an established intervention used in stroke aphasia/apraxia, has resulted in significant improvements in accurate production of trained topics among patients with nfvPPA. Many language therapists prioritize functional communication skill training aimed at improving day-to-day conversations and removing barriers of communication between the patients and their families [52].

Caregiver Support

Compared to AD, distress among caregivers is higher in FTD, particularly with bvFTD [53, 54]. Caregivers are often younger and have other socio-occupational stressors which are different from retired caregivers in late-onset dementias. Clinicians should pay close attention to caregiver burden and provide families with all the resources that are available to prevent burnout. Identifying the limits of one's capability and seeking respite care can be very effective in reducing caregiver burden [49].

Group therapy, with focus on education and support, can empower the patients and their families with problem-solving abilities, and it can also provide peer support [55]. There are multiple support groups available across the USA that can be accessed at https://www.theaftd.org/living-with-ftd/aftd-support-groups/.

Noninvasive Brain Stimulation

Transcranial magnetic stimulation (TMS) and transcranial direct current stimulation (tDCS) have shown some benefit among individuals with PPA. tDCS has shown to improve language outcomes in PPA in multiple studies. But the treatment effects can be modified by patient characteristics and methodological differences, such as intensity, frequency, combined therapy, and electrode configuration of tDCS [56]. The use of repetitive transcranial magnetic stimulation (rTMS) has also demonstrated improvement in language among individuals with PPA [57]. tDCS and TMS used in conjunction with traditional behavioral and speech therapies have been found to be beneficial in PPA [58, 59].

Pharmacological Treatment of Frontotemporal Dementia

Unfortunately, there are no current FDA-approved pharmacological treatments for frontotemporal dementia although there are several ongoing clinical trials. Due to the lack of evidence, as mentioned above, non-pharmacological

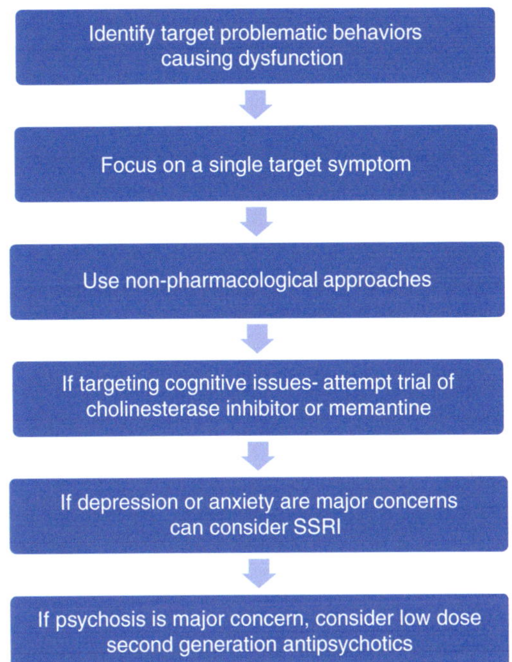

Fig. 4.2 Treatment algorithm for the management of behavioral symptoms in FTD

approaches and behavioral redirection are generally considered the preferred approach.

Currently used treatments are mostly off-label medications for symptomatic management and have minimal evidence from randomized, placebo-controlled trials to support their use on a consistent or long-term basis. These therapies rely on modulation of neurotransmitter levels and do not target the underlying pathophysiology of FTD.

Currently, there are six different classes of medications that have shown benefit among individuals with FTD (Fig. 4.2). These treatment options are outlined below:

Nootropics (Cholinesterase Inhibitors and Memantine)

Given the clinical utility of cholinesterase inhibitors in the treatment of AD, there was reasonable excitement for the use of these agents in patients with FTD. However, response rate for reduction of problematic behavioral symptoms has been less than adequate in the clinical setting. Memantine and cholinesterase inhibitors have not demonstrated clinically significant efficacy in treating FTD patients and may also hasten cognitive decline or worsen behavioral symptoms [60]. A review of such treatments has shown paradoxical agitation and increased aggressiveness in patients with FTD as well as possible exacerbation of sexual disinhibition and preexisting compulsions [61]. This is likely due to lack of significant cholinergic deficit in patients with FTD, as compared to patients with AD [62]. Conversely, at least one study reported some efficacy in improving behavioral symptoms with galantamine treatment in an aphasic subgroup of FTD patients without any reported serious adverse events, although no effect was found in the overall treatment of general FTD subjects [63]. This was based on ineffectiveness at improving scores on the Clinical Impression Severity Scale, which is a standardized severity measure. Dosages used in the treatment of patients with FTD in clinical trials are similar to those individuals with AD.

Gastrointestinal upset, insomnia, fatigue, and bradycardia are some of the common side effects that need to be considered with the use of cholinesterase inhibitors [64]. This may be counteracted by taking the medication with food, by utilizing the patch formulation, or by utilizing lower doses. Dosing the medications in the morning instead of bedtime may help with insomnia.

Antidepressants

The best evidence for effective pharmacologic intervention in FTD involves the use of antidepressants, although the clinical utility of this strategy has often been questioned. While still inconclusive, the observation of impaired serotonergic (and more broadly monoaminergic) activity in FTD again implies biologic plausibility for the use of such agents in FTD [65].

There is limited evidence that antidepressants have a role in combating irritability, impulsivity, hyperorality, and disinhibition associated with FTD [66]. Paroxetine has shown some benefit in one open-label 14-month trial in dosages up to 20 mg/day [67]. However, a follow-up study did not show any benefit, and there was concern for it potentially causing impairment in several neuropsychological tests including visual discrimination tasks, errors in paired-associate learning task, and delayed pattern recognition memory accuracy [68]. The discrepancy in efficacy may be dose related although it does suggest that higher powered studies are required in the future. Paroxetine also poses the risk of being highly anticholinergic and leading to side effects such as dry mouth and constipation, which can limit its use among older adults.

Citalopram is another selective serotonin reuptake inhibitor (SSRI) that has been recently shown to provide some improvement in behaviors among individuals with FTD. Herrmann and colleagues found improvement with a citalopram challenge at 40 mg daily dosages that led to a decrease in behavioral symptoms including irritability, depression, apathy, and disinhibition while also improving overall NPI scores among individuals with FTD [69]. Doses above 40 mg/day are still not recommended in patients above the age of 65 due to the risk of cardiac arrhythmias, which limits clinical utility and efficacy of this medication.

More recently, in a randomized double-blinded placebo-controlled crossover study, bvFTD patients who were prescribed 30 mg daily dosages of citalopram demonstrated improved disinhibition symptoms in addition to a partial restoration of serotonergic neurotransmission in dysfunctional prefrontal cortical systems as measured by magnetoencephalography and electro-encephalography [70].

Evaluation of sertraline's efficacy in treating FTD symptoms is mainly limited to observational studies. The advantage of sertraline is low drug-to-drug interactions, suggesting safety and tolerability; however, clinical efficacy has been less than desirable [71]. One study comparing stereotypical behavior in FTD and AD subjects suggested that stereotypical movements in FTD could be decreased with sertraline administration at a dosage range of 50–100 mg/day [72].

Alternatively, treatment with trazodone at dosages of at least 300 mg/day over 12 weeks has been reported to be helpful in decreasing symptoms of problematic eating, agitation, irritability, dysphoria, and depression, although adverse events were more prominent in subjects being prescribed the medication [73]. Typical emergent side effects included fatigue, dizziness, and hypotension, but the authors reported that these symptoms were mild in severity. Higher doses of trazodone also have a potential for priapism as a serious adverse effect.

One 12-week open-label trial showed a treatment response with fluvoxamine administration between dosage ranges of 50 and 150 mg/day (mean dose was 110 mg/day) in improving stereotypic behavior, eating behavior, and wandering behavior among individuals with FTD [74]. Significant drug-drug interactions limit clinical utility of fluvoxamine as many geriatric patients are on multiple medications resulting in greater risk for adverse effects.

Stimulants

Stimulants have been proposed as treatments for FTD due to their mechanism of action in elevating extracellular catecholamine concentrations that improve cognitive functioning and lessen frontostriatal and orbitofrontal dysfunction, which improves risk-taking behaviors in individuals with FTD [75]. One study found that eight patients with FTD who were prescribed methylphenidate at 40 mg/day demonstrated decreased risk-taking behavior with overall improvement in general behavior [76]. Additionally, a randomized double-blinded crossover trial comparing dextroamphetamine and quetiapine use in FTD patients found that dextroamphetamine administration decreased disinhibition and apathy symptoms while being more tolerable than quetiapine, which caused sedation in the trial population [77]. Despite these studies suggesting the safety and efficacy of stimulants in treating specific symptoms common in the FTD population, a risk-benefit analysis must be conducted prior to the use of stimulants among individuals with FTD. The data is limited due to their low power and questionable generalizability, as well as possible side effects and tolerability issues of stimulants in more elderly patients. The risk of possible psychosis and worsening anxiety with the use of stimulants should also be considered among this population. Stimulant medications pose the risk of cardiac arrhythmias and death, especially in patients with congenital cardiac anomalies or in patients with a family history of early cardiac death [78]. An electrocardiogram (EKG) at baseline and regular monitoring of pulse and blood pressures are recommended if stimulants are used among individuals with FTD.

Mood Stabilizers

Many of the behaviors noted to be problematic in FTD such as motor restlessness, agitation, irritability, and depression are commonly seen in bipolar disorder. As such, mood stabilizers might be beneficial in the treatment of such behavioral and psychiatric disturbances. There exists only a single case report in the literature on the effectiveness of topiramate, an anti-epileptic drug with potential mood-stabilizing properties among individuals with FTD [79]. Despite the lack of evidence, clinicians and researchers are intrigued by the potential of certain mood stabilizers, such as valproic acid and lithium, to inhibit glycogen synthase kinase-3β, a key enzyme responsible for the hyperphosphorylation of tau seen in degenerative diseases [80]. In a case series, when low-dose lithium was used as an add-on to antipsychotic treatment in patients with AD and FTD, several symptoms improved including auditory hallucinations, visual hallucinations, paranoia, anxiety, anger/aggression, agitation, impulsivity, and physical violence [81]. Anticonvulsants such as valproic acid may be associated with various side effects including weight gain, hair loss, and dermatological conditions among others [82]. Side effects need to be discussed thoroughly with the patient and their caregivers prior to initiation of treatment. There should also be periodic monitoring of blood levels to prevent toxicity.

Sedatives, Hypnotics, and Benzodiazepines

There are no studies of these classes of medications among individuals with FTD. Additionally, these medications can worsen cognition among individuals with FTD. The risk of paradoxical agitation with the use of these medications must also be weighed against any potential benefits. These classes of drugs are associated with risk of tolerance and dependence and can increase the risk of falls in the geriatric population [83]. These agents should generally be avoided or used as a last resort in patients with severe behavioral agitation.

Antipsychotics

Antipsychotics, especially the atypical agents, have been used in the management of severe behavioral or psychiatric symptoms among individuals with dementia. Their use has been associated with a 1.6- to 1.7-fold increased risk of death when used among older individuals with dementia [84]. Several case reports in the literature have demonstrated improvement in behavioral symptoms and even restoration of frontal glucose hypometabolism with the use of atypical antipsychotics in FTD [85, 86]. As the risk/benefit ratio may clearly be altered in individual cases, any use of antipsychotics needs to be discussed in detail with the patient and their caregivers with a full disclosure of their risks and benefits. Currently, the evidence for using antipsychotics in FTD is limited, and these medications carry the risk of extrapyramidal side effects, to which individuals with FTD are particularly vulnerable [87]. In certain situations when the behaviors associated with FTD may pose a serious risk of safety and well-being of the individual and/or their caregivers, the use of antipsychotics at their lowest possible effective doses and for the shortest period of time possible with close monitoring of their efficacy and adverse effects may be justified.

Treatment Algorithm

There are no accepted algorithms for the management of FTD due to the lack of available evidence supporting any individual treatment strategy. Hence, treating clinicians must devise an individualized treatment plan that targets the most bothersome and debilitating symptoms occurring at any given time. This plan requires a rational empiric strategy. Effective implementation of such a strategy is dependent on several key considerations for both the clinician and the caregivers. Clinical judgment is imperative on a case-by-case basis. The following strategy might be helpful in the clinical setting to dictate psychopharmacological treatment, if necessary, in patients with FTD. The strategy below is based on the presumption that non-pharmacological approaches have been attempted and have been ineffective.

Conclusions

Frontotemporal dementia is a syndrome that can have a variable constellation of symptoms and signs, especially among older adults, which is often underrecognized. It is critical to identify FTD as a separate clinical entity than AD due to the specific nature of its course and progression. There exists a dire need to accurately diagnose FTD based on biomarkers, imaging, and neuropsychological testing.

Currently, there exists a lack of disease-modifying therapies for FTD although this may be on the horizon. Psychotropic medication management is limited to ameliorating functional distress. Management of patients with FTD often entails significant collaboration between geriatric psychiatrists, geriatricians, neuropsychologists, movement disorder specialists, and speech therapists.

References

1. Bang J, Spina S, Miller BL. Frontotemporal dementia. Lancet. 2015;386(10004):1672–82.
2. Gorno-Tempini ML, Hillis AE, Weintraub S, Kertesz A, Mendez M, Cappa SF, et al. Classification of primary progressive aphasia and its variants. Neurology. 2011;76(11):1006–14.
3. Rabinovici GD, Jagust WJ, Furst AJ, Ogar JM, Racine CA, Mormino EC, et al. Abeta amyloid and glucose metabolism in three variants of primary progressive aphasia. Ann Neurol. 2008;64(4):388–401.
4. Mesulam MM. Primary progressive aphasia. Ann Neurol. 2001;49(4):425–32.
5. Younes K, Miller BL. Frontotemporal dementia: neuropathology, genetics, neuroimaging, and treatments. Psychiatr Clin North Am. 2020;43(2):331–44.
6. Vieira RT, Caixeta L, Machado S, Silva AC, Nardi AE, Arias-Carrión O, et al. Epidemiology of early-onset dementia: a review of the literature. Clin Pract Epidemiol Ment Health. 2013;9:88–95.
7. Mann DMA, Snowden JS. Frontotemporal lobar degeneration: pathogenesis, pathology and pathways to phenotype. Brain Pathol. 2017;27(6):723–36.
8. Finger EC. Frontotemporal dementias. Continuum (Minneap Minn). 2016;22(2 Dementia):464–89.
9. Coyle-Gilchrist ITS, Dick KM, Patterson K, Vázquez Rodríquez P, Wehmann E, Wilcox A, et al. Prevalence, characteristics, and survival of frontotemporal lobar degeneration syndromes. Neurology. 2016;86(18):1736–43.
10. Galvin JE, Howard DH, Denny SS, Dickinson S, Tatton N. The social and economic burden of frontotemporal degeneration. Neurology. 2017;89(20):2049–56.
11. Knopman DS, Roberts RO. Estimating the number of persons with frontotemporal lobar degeneration in the US population. J Mol Neurosci. 2011;45(3):330–5.
12. Onyike CU, Diehl-Schmid J. The epidemiology of frontotemporal dementia. Int Rev Psychiatry. 2013;25(2):130–7.
13. Curtis AF, Masellis M, Hsiung GR, Moineddin R, Zhang K, Au B, et al. Sex differences in the prevalence of genetic mutations in FTD and ALS: a meta-analysis. Neurology. 2017;89(15):1633–42.
14. Rohrer JD, Guerreiro R, Vandrovcova J, Uphill J, Reiman D, Beck J, et al. The heritability and genetics of frontotemporal lobar degeneration. Neurology. 2009;73(18):1451–6.
15. Hodges JR, Mitchell J, Dawson K, Spillantini MG, Xuereb JH, McMonagle P, et al. Semantic dementia: demography, familial factors and survival in a consecutive series of 100 cases. Brain. 2010;133(Pt 1):300–6.
16. Rosso SM, Landweer EJ, Houterman M, Donker Kaat L, van Duijn CM, van Swieten JC. Medical and environmental risk factors for sporadic frontotemporal dementia: a retrospective case-control study. J Neurol Neurosurg Psychiatry. 2003;74(11):1574–6.
17. McCauley ME, Baloh RH. Inflammation in ALS/FTD pathogenesis. Acta Neuropathol. 2019;137(5):715–30.
18. Bright F, Werry EL, Dobson-Stone C, Piguet O, Ittner LM, Halliday GM, et al. Neuroinflammation in frontotemporal dementia. Nat Rev Neurol. 2019;15(9):540–55.
19. Kalkonde YV, Jawaid A, Qureshi SU, Shirani P, Wheaton M, Pinto-Patarroyo GP, et al. Medical and environmental risk factors associated with frontotemporal dementia: a case-control study in a veteran population. Alzheimers Dement. 2012;8(3):204–10.
20. Kennedy E, Panahi S, Stewart IJ, Tate DF, Wilde EA, Kenney K, et al. Traumatic brain injury and early onset dementia in post 9-11 veterans. Brain Inj. 2022;36(5):620–7.
21. Neary D, Snowden JS, Gustafson L, Passant U, Stuss D, Black S, et al. Frontotemporal lobar degeneration:

a consensus on clinical diagnostic criteria. Neurology. 1998;51(6):1546–54.

22. Rascovsky K, Hodges JR, Knopman D, Mendez MF, Kramer JH, Neuhaus J, et al. Sensitivity of revised diagnostic criteria for the behavioural variant of frontotemporal dementia. Brain. 2011;134(9):2456–77.

23. Shinagawa S, Nakajima S, Plitman E, Graff-Guerrero A, Mimura M, Nakayama K, et al. Psychosis in frontotemporal dementia. J Alzheimer's Dis. 2014;42(2):485–99.

24. Marshall CR, Hardy CJD, Volkmer A, Russell LL, Bond RL, Fletcher PD, et al. Primary progressive aphasia: a clinical approach. J Neurol. 2018;265(6):1474–90.

25. Botha H, Josephs KA. Primary progressive aphasias and apraxia of speech. Continuum (Minneap Minn). 2019;25(1):101–27.

26. Poos JM, Jiskoot LC, Papma JM, van Swieten JC, van den Berg E. Meta-analytic review of memory impairment in behavioral variant frontotemporal dementia. J Int Neuropsychol Society. 2018;24(6):593–605.

27. Kumfor F, Honan C, McDonald S, Hazelton JL, Hodges JR, Piguet O. Assessing the "social brain" in dementia: applying TASIT-S. Cortex. 2017;93:166–77.

28. Henry ML, Grasso SM. Assessment of individuals with primary progressive aphasia. Semin Speech Lang. 2018;39(3):231–41.

29. Mendez MF, Shapira JS, McMurtray A, Licht E, Miller BL. Accuracy of the clinical evaluation for frontotemporal dementia. Arch Neurol. 2007;64(6):830–5.

30. Hu WT, Wang Z, Lee VM, Trojanowski JQ, Detre JA, Grossman M. Distinct cerebral perfusion patterns in FTLD and AD. Neurology. 2010;75(10):881–8.

31. Vijverberg EG, Wattjes MP, Dols A, Krudop WA, Möller C, Peters A, et al. Diagnostic accuracy of MRI and additional [18F]FDG-PET for behavioral variant frontotemporal dementia in patients with late onset behavioral changes. J Alzheimer's Dis. 2016;53(4):1287–97.

32. Josephs KA, Duffy JR, Strand EA, Whitwell JL, Layton KF, Parisi JE, et al. Clinicopathological and imaging correlates of progressive aphasia and apraxia of speech. Brain. 2006;129(Pt 6):1385–98.

33. Gorno-Tempini ML, Dronkers NF, Rankin KP, Ogar JM, Phengrasamy L, Rosen HJ, et al. Cognition and anatomy in three variants of primary progressive aphasia. Ann Neurol. 2004;55(3):335–46.

34. Boeve BF, Boxer AL, Kumfor F, Pijnenburg Y, Rohrer JD. Advances and controversies in frontotemporal dementia: diagnosis, biomarkers, and therapeutic considerations. Lancet Neurol. 2022;21(3):258–72.

35. Meeter LH, Dopper EG, Jiskoot LC, Sanchez-Valle R, Graff C, Benussi L, et al. Neurofilament light chain: a biomarker for genetic frontotemporal dementia. Ann Clin Transl Neurol. 2016;3(8):623–36.

36. Eratne D, Keem M, Lewis C, Kang M, Walterfang M, Farrand S, et al. Cerebrospinal fluid neurofilament light chain differentiates behavioural variant frontotemporal dementia progressors from non-progressors. J Neurol Sci. 2022;442:120439.

37. Ooi S, Patel SK, Eratne D, Kyndt C, Reidy N, Lewis C, et al. Plasma neurofilament Light chain and clinical diagnosis in frontotemporal dementia syndromes. J Alzheimer's Dis. 2022;89(4):1221–31.

38. Davy V, Dumurgier J, Fayosse A, Paquet C, Cognat E. Neurofilaments as emerging biomarkers of neuroaxonal damage to differentiate behavioral frontotemporal dementia from primary psychiatric disorders: a systematic review. Diagnostics (Basel). 2021;11(5):754.

39. Qu Y, Ma YH, Huang YY, Ou YN, Shen XN, Chen SD, et al. Blood biomarkers for the diagnosis of amnestic mild cognitive impairment and Alzheimer's disease: a systematic review and meta-analysis. Neurosci Biobehav Rev. 2021;128:479–86.

40. Olsson B, Lautner R, Andreasson U, Öhrfelt A, Portelius E, Bjerke M, et al. CSF and blood biomarkers for the diagnosis of Alzheimer's disease: a systematic review and meta-analysis. Lancet Neurol. 2016;15(7):673–84.

41. Thijssen EH, La Joie R, Strom A, Fonseca C, Iaccarino L, Wolf A, et al. Plasma phosphorylated tau 217 and phosphorylated tau 181 as biomarkers in Alzheimer's disease and frontotemporal lobar degeneration: a retrospective diagnostic performance study. Lancet Neurol. 2021;20(9):739–52.

42. Mackenzie IRA, Neumann M, Bigio EH, Cairns NJ, Alafuzoff I, Kril J, et al. Nomenclature and nosology for neuropathologic subtypes of frontotemporal lobar degeneration: an update. Acta Neuropathol. 2010;119(1):1–4.

43. Swift IJ, Sogorb-Esteve A, Heller C, Synofzik M, Otto M, Graff C, et al. Fluid biomarkers in frontotemporal dementia: past, present and future. J Neurol Neurosurg Psychiatry. 2021;92(2):204–15.

44. Lehmer C, Oeckl P, Weishaupt JH, Volk AE, Diehl-Schmid J, Schroeter ML, et al. Poly-GP in cerebrospinal fluid links C9orf72-associated dipeptide repeat expression to the asymptomatic phase of ALS/FTD. EMBO Mol Med. 2017;9(7):859–68.

45. Rhinn H, Tatton N, McCaughey S, Kurnellas M, Rosenthal A. Progranulin as a therapeutic target in neurodegenerative diseases. Trends Pharmacol Sci. 2022;43(8):641–52.

46. Ntymenou S, Tsantzali I, Kalamatianos T, Voumvourakis KI, Kapaki E, Tsivgoulis G, et al. Blood biomarkers in frontotemporal dementia: review and meta-analysis. Brain Sci. 2021;11(2)

47. Wylie MA, Shnall A, Onyike CU, Huey ED. Management of frontotemporal dementia in mental health and multidisciplinary settings. Int Rev Psychiatry. 2013;25(2):230–6.

48. Luscombe G, Brodaty H, Freeth S. Younger people with dementia: diagnostic issues, effects on carers and use of services. Int J Geriatr Psychiatry. 1998;13(5):323–30.

49. Shinagawa S, Nakajima S, Plitman E, Graff-Guerrero A, Mimura M, Nakayama K, et al. Non-

pharmacological management for patients with frontotemporal dementia: a systematic review. J Alzheimer's Dis. 2015;45(1):283–93.

50. Cheng ST, Chow PK, Song YQ, Yu EC, Chan AC, Lee TM, et al. Mental and physical activities delay cognitive decline in older persons with dementia. Am J Geriatric Psychiatry. 2014;22(1):63–74.

51. Volkmer A, Rogalski E, Henry M, Taylor-Rubin C, Ruggero L, Khayum R, et al. Speech and language therapy approaches to managing primary progressive aphasia. Pract Neurol. 2020;20(2):154–61.

52. Taylor-Rubin C, Croot K, Power E, Savage SA, Hodges JR, Togher L. Communication behaviors associated with successful conversation in semantic variant primary progressive aphasia. Int Psychogeriatr. 2017;29(10):1619–32.

53. Mioshi E, Foxe D, Leslie F, Savage S, Hsieh S, Miller L, et al. The impact of dementia severity on caregiver burden in frontotemporal dementia and Alzheimer disease. Alzheimer Dis Assoc Disord. 2013;27(1):68–73.

54. Nunnemann S, Kurz A, Leucht S, Diehl-Schmid J. Caregivers of patients with frontotemporal lobar degeneration: a review of burden, problems, needs, and interventions. Int Psychogeriatr. 2012;24(9):1368–86.

55. Jokel R, Meltzer J, D RJ, D ML, J CJ, A NE, et al. Group intervention for individuals with primary progressive aphasia and their spouses: who comes first? J Commun Disord. 2017;66:51–64.

56. Coemans S, Struys E, Vandenborre D, Wilssens I, Engelborghs S, Paquier P, et al. A systematic review of transcranial direct current stimulation in primary progressive aphasia: methodological considerations. Front Aging Neurosci. 2021;13:710818.

57. Pytel V, Cabrera-Martín MN, Delgado-Álvarez A, Ayala JL, Balugo P, Delgado-Alonso C, et al. Personalized repetitive transcranial magnetic stimulation for primary progressive aphasia. J Alzheimer's Dis. 2021;84(1):151–67.

58. Sheppard SM. Noninvasive brain stimulation to augment language therapy for primary progressive aphasia. Handb Clin Neurol. 2022;185:251–60.

59. Nissim NR, Moberg PJ, Hamilton RH. Efficacy of noninvasive brain stimulation (tDCS or TMS) paired with language therapy in the treatment of primary progressive aphasia: an exploratory meta-analysis. Brain Sci. 2020;10(9)

60. Mocellin R, Scholes A, Walterfang M, Looi JC, Velakoulis D. Clinical update on frontotemporal dementia: diagnosis and treatment. Australas Psychiatry. 2015;23(5):481–7.

61. Mendez MF, Shapira JS, McMurtray A, Licht E. Preliminary findings: behavioral worsening on donepezil in patients with frontotemporal dementia. Am J Geriatric Psychiatry. 2007;15(1):84–7.

62. Chow TW. Treatment approaches to symptoms associated with frontotemporal degeneration. Curr Psychiatry Rep. 2005;7(5):376–80.

63. Kertesz A, Morlog D, Light M, Blair M, Davidson W, Jesso S, et al. Galantamine in frontotemporal demen-

tia and primary progressive aphasia. Dement Geriatr Cogn Disord. 2008;25(2):178–85.

64. Cummings JL. Use of cholinesterase inhibitors in clinical practice: evidence-based recommendations. Am J Geriatric Psychiatry. 2003;11(2):131–45.

65. Huey ED, Putnam KT, Grafman J. A systematic review of neurotransmitter deficits and treatments in frontotemporal dementia. Neurology. 2006;66(1):17–22.

66. Swartz JR, Miller BL, Lesser IM, Darby AL. Frontotemporal dementia: treatment response to serotonin selective reuptake inhibitors. J Clin Psychiatry. 1997;58(5):212–6.

67. Moretti R, Torre P, Antonello RM, Cazzato G, Bava A. Frontotemporal dementia: paroxetine as a possible treatment of behavior symptoms. A randomized, controlled, open 14-month study. Eur Neurol. 2003;49(1):13–9.

68. Deakin JB, Rahman S, Nestor PJ, Hodges JR, Sahakian BJ. Paroxetine does not improve symptoms and impairs cognition in frontotemporal dementia: a double-blind randomized controlled trial. Psychopharmacology. 2004;172(4):400–8.

69. Herrmann N, Black SE, Chow T, Cappell J, Tang-Wai DF, Lanctot KL. Serotonergic function and treatment of behavioral and psychological symptoms of frontotemporal dementia. Am J Geriatric Psychiatry. 2012;20(9):789–97.

70. Hughes LE, Rittman T, Regenthal R, Robbins TW, Rowe JB. Improving response inhibition systems in frontotemporal dementia with citalopram. Brain. 2015;138(Pt 7):1961–75.

71. Mendez MF. Frontotemporal dementia: therapeutic interventions. Front Neurol Neurosci. 2009;24:168–78.

72. Mendez MF, Shapira JS, Miller BL. Stereotypical movements and frontotemporal dementia. Mov Disord. 2005;20(6):742–5.

73. Young JJ, Lavakumar M, Tampi D, Balachandran S, Tampi RR. Frontotemporal dementia: latest evidence and clinical implications. Ther Adv Psychopharmacol. 2018;8(1):33–48.

74. Ikeda M, Shigenobu K, Fukuhara R, Hokoishi K, Maki N, Nebu A, et al. Efficacy of fluvoxamine as a treatment for behavioral symptoms in frontotemporal lobar degeneration patients. Dement Geriatr Cogn Disord. 2004;17(3):117–21.

75. Mega MS, Cummings JL. Frontal-subcortical circuits and neuropsychiatric disorders. J Neuropsychiatry Clin Neurosci. 1994;6(4):358–70.

76. Rahman S, Robbins TW, Hodges JR, Mehta MA, Nestor PJ, Clark L, et al. Methylphenidate ('Ritalin') can ameliorate abnormal risk-taking behavior in the frontal variant of frontotemporal dementia. Neuropsychopharmacology. 2006;31(3):651–8.

77. Huey ED, Garcia C, Wassermann EM, Tierney MC, Grafman J. Stimulant treatment of frontotemporal dementia in 8 patients. J Clin Psychiatry. 2008;69(12):1981–2.

78. Martinez-Raga J, Knecht C, Szerman N, Martinez MI. Risk of serious cardiovascular problems with

medications for attention-deficit hyperactivity disorder. CNS Drugs. 2013;27(1):15–30.

79. Cruz M, Marinho V, Fontenelle LF, Engelhardt E, Laks J. Topiramate may modulate alcohol abuse but not other compulsive behaviors in frontotemporal dementia: case report. Cogn Behav Neurol. 2008;21(2):104–6.

80. Galariotis V, Bodi N, Janka Z, Kalman J. Frontotemporal dementia—part III. Clinical diagnosis and treatment. Ideggyogy Sz. 2005;58(9–10):292–7.

81. Devanand DP, Pelton GH, D'Antonio K, Strickler JG, Kreisl WC, Noble J, et al. Low-dose lithium treatment for agitation and psychosis in Alzheimer disease and frontotemporal dementia: a case series. Alzheimer Dis Assoc Disord. 2017;31(1):73–5.

82. Nanau RM, Neuman MG. Adverse drug reactions induced by valproic acid. Clin Biochem. 2013;46(15):1323–38.

83. Glass J, Lanctot KL, Herrmann N, Sproule BA, Busto UE. Sedative hypnotics in older people with insomnia: meta-analysis of risks and benefits. BMJ. 2005;331(7526):1169.

84. Salzman C, Jeste DV, Meyer RE, Cohen-Mansfield J, Cummings J, Grossberg GT, et al. Elderly patients with dementia-related symptoms of severe agitation and aggression: consensus statement on treatment options, clinical trials methodology, and policy. J Clin Psychiatry. 2008;69(6):889–98.

85. Curtis RC, Resch DS. Case of pick's central lobar atrophy with apparent stabilization of cognitive decline after treatment with risperidone. J Clin Psychopharmacol. 2000;20(3):384–5.

86. Fellgiebel A, Muller MJ, Hiemke C, Bartenstein P, Schreckenberger M. Clinical improvement in a case of frontotemporal dementia under aripiprazole treatment corresponds to partial recovery of disturbed frontal glucose metabolism. World J Biol Psychiatry. 2007;8(2):123–6.

87. Pijnenburg YA, Sampson EL, Harvey RJ, Fox NC, Rossor MN. Vulnerability to neuroleptic side effects in frontotemporal lobar degeneration. Int J Geriatr Psychiatry. 2003;18(1):67–72.

Major Neurocognitive Disorders Due to Parkinson's Disease

Senthil Vel Rajan Rajaram Manoharan, Jessy Walia, and Mack Bozman

Epidemiology

In the original description of Parkinson's disease (PD), named after James Parkinson, cognitive deficits were not described. It was not until the 1960s when patients began to survive for longer periods as a result of new treatments that dementia in PD started to become recognized [1]. The prevalence of Parkinson's disease (PD) is difficult to estimate precisely due to the variation reported, most likely due to methodological differences in studies. However, the generally accepted prevalence is 1–2 per 1000 in a given population [2]. The incidence varies widely from 5/100,000 to over 35/100,000 new cases yearly. This incidence increases five- to tenfold from the sixth to the ninth decades of life. The prevalence of this condition also increases with population age [3]. As the population's average age increases, so will the number of patients dealing with PD. PD is the fastest increasing neurological disorder; the number of people with PD doubled to over 6 million between 1990 and 2015, and by 2040, it is expected to double again to 12 million [4]. The societal and economic burdens will also parallelly rise, increasing the urgency to develop more effective methods of treatments, cures, or prevention [5]. Men are one and a half times more likely to have PD than women, and fewer African Americans or Asian Americans are affected than Whites. Rates of PD differ based on geographical location, e.g., higher rates of PD reported in the Midwest/Great Lakes region and the northeastern seaboard. This is likely due to exposure to environmental toxins or toxic chemicals such as pesticides (see Risk Factors, Table 5.1) [6].

Table 5.1 Risk factors for dementia in patients with PD [12]

Risk factor	Risk rate
Parkinsonism	Increased risk
Age	Ninefold increased risk in the
Mild cognitive	group over 80 years when
impairment	compared with the group aged
Olfactory	50–59 years [13]. Four- to
dysfunction	sixfold increased risk in the
Visual	group over 76 years of age when
hallucinations	compared with those <65 years
Rapid eye	[14]
movement sleep	Risk increased 3–3.9-fold
behavior disorder	Twenty-fold higher
Gender	Fourfold increased risk
Genetics	Twofold increased risk
Cerebrovascular	1.7-fold increased risk for men
factors	Increased cumulative risk
	Increased risk

S. V. R. Rajaram Manoharan (✉)
Department of Psychiatry, Huntsville Hospital, Huntsville, AL, USA

UAB Heersink School of Medicine, Birmingham, AL, USA

J. Walia
Huntsville Hospital, Huntsville, AL, USA

M. Bozman
UAB Heersink School of Medicine, Birmingham, AL, USA
e-mail: bozman@uab.edu

R. R. Tampi, D. J. Tampi (eds.), *Treatment of Psychiatric Disorders Among Older Adults*, https://doi.org/10.1007/978-3-031-55711-8_5

The risk of dementia in persons with PD is 4–6 times higher than in healthy individuals matched for age, sex, and education. Studies show that in PD patients who survive more than 10 years, at least 75% develop dementia (PD-D) [7]. Some longitudinal studies have shown that by the 10-year follow-up from diagnosis, 46% of individuals with Parkinson's disease had progressed to PD-D [8]. PD-related cognitive impairment can present as either Parkinson's disease mild cognitive impairment (PD-MCI) or PD-dementia (PD-D). Activities of daily living are not impaired in PD-MCI, whereas PD-D is more severe, with cognitive impairment affecting the activities of daily living (ADLs) [9]. PD-MCI and PD-D are associated with decreased quality of life and increased nursing home admissions. About 25–30% of patients with PD can have PD-MCI, and there is an increased risk of developing dementia in patients with PD-MCI as compared to PD without MCI (relative risk is 39.2 at 3 years) [10].

Risk Factors

PD dementia (PD-D) has been consistently associated with certain risk factors. These include advanced age, more severe illness (particularly rigidity, postural instability, and gait disturbance), male sex, psychiatric comorbidity, and mild cognitive impairment (MCI) [11]. MCI has also been associated consistently with the development of more severe parkinsonism [7]. Table 5.1 enumerates the risk factors for dementia in patients with PD.

There are certain constellations of symptoms that render patients more susceptible to developing dementia. Motor phenotype is strongly associated with cognitive decline. Patients with more symmetrical signs, higher disability, and bradykinesia scores, and more impairment of gait and balance, are more likely to develop dementia when compared to those who suffer from the tremor-predominant subtype of PD [15]. The prototypical form of PD-D can be described as a dysexecutive syndrome commonly associated with behavioral symptoms and a postural insta-

bility and gait disturbance (PIGD)-dominant motor phenotype [11].

The cognitive profile, severity, time course, and nature of behavioral symptoms in individual patients are also determined by the extent and topography of Lewy body (LB)-type degeneration and coexisting Alzheimer's dementia (AD) type. The cognitive characteristics of PDD might vary compared to AD. In PDD, attention, executive functions, and visuospatial abilities are often more prominently affected, while impairments in memory encoding and language abnormalities are relatively less pronounced compared to AD [16]. In a clinicopathological study, patients with a pure LB pathology had a more dysexecutive syndrome, those with pure AD pathology an amnestic syndrome, and those with both pathologies a more mixed cognitive profile [17].

There are a variety of genetic, environmental, and behavioral risk factors for the development of PD itself. Identifiable genetic mutations of known genes are noted in 5–10% of PD cases, although these mutations are notably absent in most PD patients. Moreover, the most common mutations of this disease have incomplete penetrance, indicating that other environmental or genetic factors are involved [3]. Mutations in the alpha-synuclein gene (SNCA) are associated with autosomal dominant PD [18]. There have been multiple studies over many decades assessing the risk of developing PD that is associated with toxic chemicals, notably the strong association with pesticide exposure. Farm work or rural residence has been associated with an increased risk of PD [19]. Several lifestyle factors have been associated with reduced risk of PD. A common and consistent association is the reduced risk of PD in cigarette smokers, tobacco users, and coffee and caffeine use [3, 20].

Assessment

Compared to other neurodegenerative etiologies causing dementia, the diagnosis of dementia in patients with PD can be more difficult. Several confounding factors are related to the disease itself, its treatment, and comorbid conditions, which are more frequent in this patient population. These include adverse effects of medication, acute or prolonged confusion due to systemic abnormalities or diseases, and presence of depression, all of which can mimic symptoms of dementia. At times, severe motor impairment renders it difficult to judge if the impairment in function is due to mental or motor dysfunction [21].

Assessment of Cognitive Functions

There may be cognitive changes from the early stages of PD. The impairments may be mild (mild cognitive impairment; PD-MCI) or severe enough to justify the diagnosis of PD dementia. Typically, the cognitive profile is different from that of AD, with predominant impairments in attention, executive, and visuospatial functions in PD-D, with less significant deficits in memory encoding and language abnormalities than in AD [16]. Unlike patients with AD, individuals with PDD commonly acknowledge their memory difficulties rather than denying them. They typically maintain awareness of their mental deficits and readily admit to memory issues when questioned [22]. Nevertheless, there are instances where this pattern deviates in certain patients. For instance, in the majority of cases, the memory impairment in PDD is of the retrieval type, meaning that the ability to store new information is relatively preserved. However, some individuals may develop limbic-type amnesia, a characteristic more commonly associated with AD, where the inability to store new information occurs [22]. The severity, distribution, and presence of both Lewy body (LB)-type degeneration and AD-type pathology are important factors that influence the nature, intensity, and progression of cognitive and behavioral symptoms. According to a clinicopathological study, individuals with pure LB pathology tend to exhibit a dysexecutive syndrome, while those with pure AD pathology commonly display an amnestic syndrome. In cases where both pathologies coexist, a more mixed cognitive profile is typically observed [17].

PD-D is often unrecognized and is not appropriately treated. Table 5.2 includes some of the

Table 5.2 Early signs and symptoms of preceding Parkinson's disease dementia [23]

Early signs and symptoms of preceding dementia in Parkinson's disease
Disturbances of the sleep-wake cycle
Excessive daytime sleepiness
Brief confusion on awakening
Feeling of presence of hallucinations
Disturbance in visual orientation
Increasing forgetfulness
Impaired attentiveness and concentration
Apathy

early signs and symptoms of preceding dementia in Parkinson's disease. The introduction of guidelines for the diagnosis of dementia associated with PD by the Movement Disorder Society is an important milestone in its recognition as a distinct disease entity (Fig. 5.1). A task force was created by the Movement Disorder Society (MDS) to propose clinical criteria diagnosing possible and probable PD-D [11]. Before these criteria came into existence, patients were diagnosed based on DSM-4 criteria under the label "dementia due to other general medical conditions." The proposed clinical criteria for the diagnosis of possible and probable PD-D by MDS were based on epidemiological, cognitive, and neuropsychiatric motor and other clinical features, ancillary examinations, and clinicopathological correlations. The MDS Task Force came up with two versions: one for clinicians requiring a simple, practical screening tool in the office/bedside and another, a more detailed approach for research and clinical trials [11].

A simple algorithm [24] for clinician diagnosis of PDD, as recommended by the MDS Task Force is as follows:

1. A diagnosis of PD—Queen Square Brain Bank Criteria.
2. PD precedes the onset of dementia based on patient/caregiver history or ancillary records.
3. PD associated with a decreased global cognitive efficiency—MMSE <26.
4. Cognitive deficiency severe enough to impair daily life based on caregiver interview or pill questionnaire.
5. Impairment of more than one cognitive domain as noted through impairments in at

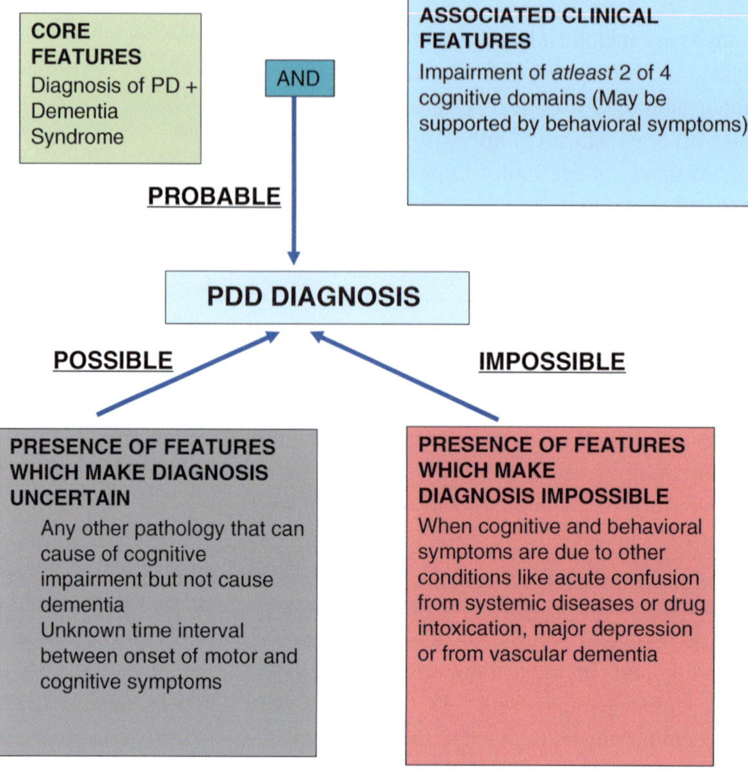

Fig. 5.1 Movement Disorder Society guidelines (2007) for diagnosis of Parkinson's disease dementia (PDD) [24]

least two of the following domains—attention, executive function, visuo-constructive ability, and memory.

The probable PDD:

Core features:

It is essential to identify idiopathic PD prior to the development of dementia, and this is the first critical step. The two core features are the following: (1) a diagnosis of PD according to the Queen Square Brain Bank Criteria [25] and (2) PD must have developed before the onset of dementia. *Dementia with Lewy bodies (DLB) is temporally distinguished using the "1-year rule." In PD, motor symptoms develop at least 1 year before, whereas in DLB, the motor symptoms occur no more than 1 year prior to or more frequently after the onset of dementia* [26].

Dementia syndrome is defined as affecting at least two cognitive domains that impair functioning, social, occupational, and personal care. This impairment must be solely caused by cognitive deficiency and must be independent of impair-ment caused by motor symptoms of Parkinson's disease. The Mini-Mental State Examination (MMSE) is a widely used screening instrument that has been recommended by the MDS task force for identifying cognitive impairment in PD-D patients. It can be quickly and easily used in a clinical setting with a score of 25 or less used as the cutoff to identify cognitive impairment [24].

Associated features of Probable PD-D:

Impairment in attention, memory, executive, and visuospatial domains and a spectrum of behavioral disorders constitute the associated features of PD-D [11]. Several tests have been recommended by the MDS task force (Table 5.3) The four-item Neuropsychiatric Inventory must be recommended to assess the behavioral symptoms of hallucinations, depression, delusions, and apathy. *Diagnosis of "probable" PD-D = Impairment in at least two of the four cognitive domains supported by the presence of at least one behavioral symptom.* If the clinical features are not considered "typical" (more consistent

Table 5.3 Tests proposed by the MDS task force to assess cognitive deficits in the clinical setting [24]

Cognitive domain	Proposed tests	Cutoff scores
Attention	Serial 7 s of the MMSE repeatedly subtract 7 starting at 100 months of the year backwards	Two or more incorrect responses Omission of two or more months
Executive function	Lexical fluency, e.g., list words beginning with S in 1 min Clock-drawing test: Draw clock with hands at "10 past 2"	Less than 9 words in a minute Inability to draw clock or show time
Visuo-constructive ability	MMSE pentagons: Copy two overlapping pentagons	Inability to draw pentagons
Memory	3-word recall of the MMSE: Free recall of three words	Missing at least one word

with AD), even in the presence of established PD, only "possible" PD-D should be diagnosed [11, 27].

Possible PDD

The diagnosis of "possible PD-D" (instead of a "probable PD-D") occurs when the time interval between the onset of motor and cognitive symptoms is not clearly defined, or it is difficult to distinguish between DLB and PD [27]. There may also be other medical or neurological comorbidities to rule out before making a PD diagnosis. Medical conditions such as systemic infections, dehydration, vitamin deficiencies, and toxic-metabolic etiologies associated with impairment in cognition and behavioral symptoms need to be excluded. In these situations, a reliable PD diagnosis is not possible. Cognitive impairment secondary to medications, especially those with anticholinergic action, dopamine replacement, and benzodiazepines, must also be considered. The diagnosis of dementia can be challenging, especially in the presence of major depressive disorder symptoms. However, in real-world scenarios, depression is frequently comorbid with Parkinson's disease and hence should not readily be considered as a criterion for exclusion [28].

Scales commonly used to screen for cognitive functions in PD include general-purpose scales and PD-specific scales [29]. The general-purpose scales include the Mini-Mental State Examination (MMSE), Montreal Cognitive Examination (MoCA), Addenbrooke's Cognitive Assessment (ACE), and Frontal Assessment Battery (FAB). PD-specific scales include Mini-Mental Parkinson and Parkinson Neuropsychometric Dementia Assessment (PANDA). More quantitative scales include the general ones like Alzheimer Disease Assessment Scale-Cognitive Section (ADAS-COG) and Mattis Dementia Rating Scale (DRS), and PD-specific ones include Scales for Outcomes in Parkinson's Disease-Cognition (SCOPA-COG) and Parkinson Disease-Cognitive Rating Scale (PD-CRS) [30]. Objective measures like these scales to assess cognitive function should be conducted on PD patients on initial evaluations and then semi-regularly to establish a known timeline for possible cognitive impairment.

Assessment of Neuropsychiatric Symptoms

To gather an accurate understanding of behavioral symptoms, it is important to conduct a thorough assessment by engaging in a semi-structured interview with the patient, their family, and any caregivers involved [31]. Psychotic symptoms are not always easy to identify, and specific questions about delusional thinking and visual hallucinations are needed. Visual hallucinations may include insects, animals, or people [21]. It is important to assess for depressive symptoms, including specifically lack of motivation, apathy, social withdrawal, sadness, and anhedonia.

Sleep disorders are common in PD-D [32, 33]. PD patients commonly experience various sleep disorders, such as insomnia, excessive sleepiness, restless legs syndrome, and REM sleep behavior disorder [34]. Sleep disruption in a patient with cognitive impairment or subtle signs of parkinsonism should increase the suspicion of an underlying neurodegenerative process [35]. RBD is a commonly encountered sleep disturbance that is characterized by acting out dreams, such as speaking, shouting, or moving during sleep. It can occur in patients without dementia and may precede the onset of the disease by many years, and it is significantly more frequent in PD-D patients [36]. Emergence of RBD symptoms in a patient with PD may signal the onset of cognitive dysfunction. RBD, especially when combined with hallucinations, has been found to predict cognitive decline in non-demented PD patients [37].

Neuropsychiatric Inventory (NPI) is the most commonly used assessment scale to evaluate behavioral and neuropsychiatric symptoms [38]. The recent version of the Unified Parkinson's Disease Rating Scale (UPDRS) can screen for specific neuropsychiatric symptoms that are common in PD-D, which include anxiety, depression, psychosis, apathy, and sleep disturbances [39].

Assessment of Functional Impairment

The functional impairment caused by motor symptoms is often aggravated by cognitive impairment [40]. Functional impairment is best assessed by directly asking the family members about the level of functioning before and after the onset of cognitive symptoms. The evaluation should include an assessment of functioning in both instrumental activities of daily living (I-ADLs) and basic ADLs. Impairment in the domains of social and occupational functioning should be assessed by lead questions. It is important to establish if the changes in functioning are due to motor or cognitive symptoms, which will in turn help with developing appropriate inter-

ventions. As most patients with Parkinson's are on medications, the ability to organize and remember his/her own medication schedule has been widely used to assess functional impairment [24]. The Pill Questionnaire is also useful as a basic screening tool for dementia, but the positive predictive value is noted to be low [41].

The prevalence of falls in PD is estimated to be 40–90% [42], and it increases with disease duration [43]. Gait disturbances can be continuous and episodic or paroxysmal [44]. Changes in the walking pattern that are present from one step to the next and present all the time are noted to be continuous disturbances. On the other hand, changes emerging in a random and inexplicable manner are noted to be paroxysmal. Festination, start hesitation, and freezing of gait (FOG) are episodic gait disturbances [45]. Both types of gait disturbances may be influenced by the cognitive changes associated with PD, and both are associated with an increased risk of falls. Gait abnormalities can predict the onset of dementia, and cognitive impairment can increase the risk of falls. Cognitive impairment and gait abnormalities are closely associated with each other, and recognition of this interrelationship will help in improving the management [46].

Patients who develop dementia are more vulnerable, especially regarding medical decision-making, research participation, and public safety issues [40]. Early discussion about future decisions should be initiated in a timely manner. Several ethically challenging situations might arise in the course of illness. They may fail to protect their own interests (failure to fully appreciate when providing informed consent in treatment and research), or there may be a need to protect others from patients' poor judgment and behaviors (e.g., continuing to drive despite clearly diminishing driving skills). As the disease progresses, with the development of cognitive impairment, patients can become increasingly vulnerable to manipulation and coercion and sometimes may act against their own best interests. The clinicians will have to exercise their best judgment balancing patient's autonomy and choices while ensuring that safety issues are addressed. Financial capacity concerns are a recurring issue in patients diagnosed with Parkinson's disease and related dementias. Additionally, clinicians must consider the need for referral to assess the patient's financial capacity and ascertain if they are vulnerable to financial exploitation or abuse by others. The accurate identification, assessment, and effective management of these financial capacity issues can significantly influence the financial and psychological well-being of both patients and their family members [47, 48]. Complex decision-making is often impaired, and a healthcare proxy or power of attorney for healthcare can be identified by the patient who can help with the decision-making, if they become unable to do so [40].

Visual, cognitive, and motor impairments can lead to unsafe driving in many patients [40]. History of recent crashes or near misses, being lost in familiar geographical places, and night-time difficulties in driving might indicate that driving capacity is impaired. Assessment of driving capacity should be done in a timely manner. Clinically, a simple battery using contrast sensitivity, Clinical Dementia Rating Scale, the UPDRS III, and disease duration, which has a sensitivity of 96%, can be used to decide which patients to refer for further multidisciplinary evaluation [49]. Periodic multidisciplinary evaluations in close cooperation with the patient, caregivers, and state authorities are needed to assess driving fitness and to offer alternative transportation methods in appropriate cases [50].

Laboratory Examinations and Neuroimaging

It is important to differentiate delirium from dementia and exclude other causes of dementia due to metabolic, vascular, endocrine, autoimmune, and toxic states [51]. Patients with PD are often elderly, and other causes of dementia can affect them. Hence, a workup including a basic metabolic profile, complete blood count with differential, folate level, vitamin B12 level, thyroid functions, and urinalysis should be performed in PD patients who develop changes in cognition or sensorium. Further array of investigations can be done based on the clinical presentation. Repeated structural imaging may not be necessary when the presentation is typical in a patient with long-standing PD. Conventional magnetic resonance imaging (MRI) holds limited utility in clinical practice of diagnostic purposes. Nonetheless, the progress made in structural and functional imaging has enhanced the capability of MRI to identify alterations in PD and distinguish it from other parkinsonian syndromes [52]. When an alternative diagnosis is suspected, imaging may be helpful to rule out other etiologies. The inclusion of CSF α-synuclein species as a component of a biomarker panel can offer utility in diagnosing dementia with Lewy bodies/PD-D. Furthermore, CSF levels of total α-synuclein were found to be lower in dementia with Lewy bodies and PD-D compared to Alzheimer's disease and control subjects [53]. This finding may help in differentiating AD from PD-D when combined with other established AD CSF markers such as β-amyloid 1–42 [54].

Differential Diagnosis

1. The onset, course, and pattern of neuropsychological and behavioral symptoms and the presence or absence of systemic and laboratory findings are important factors in deciding whether the patient is suffering from PD-D or from conditions that can mimic dementia. Other neurodegenerative disorders which may present with parkinsonism and dementia include dementia with Lewy bodies, progressive supranuclear palsy, corticobasal ganglionic degeneration, frontotemporal dementia–parkinsonism complex, and multiple system atrophy [55]. Other disorders that may present with features of parkinsonism and dementia include cerebrovascular disease [56], normal-pressure hydrocephalus [57], and drug intoxication with neuroleptics [57].

Although dementia with Lewy bodies (DLB) and PD-D share many clinical, neurochemical, and morphological features, both have been incorporated into DSM-5 as two separate entities

Table 5.4 Clinical overlap and dissimilarities between dementia with Lewy bodies (DLB) and Parkinson's disease with dementia (PDD) [58]

Overlap	Dissimilarities
Rigidity, akinesia Cognitive impairments: Frontal executive dysfunction Visual-constructive impairment Mild language impairment Mood disturbances (depression, anxiety) REM sleep behavior disorder (RBD), neuroleptic sensitivity	Some cognitive dysfunctions: Deficiencies of attention greater, episodic verbal memory tasks lower in DLB Tremor less frequent in DLB Motor performance: Slower walk and poorer balance in DLB Visual hallucinations more frequent in DLB; relative timing of dementia and parkinsonism (1-year rule); onset of dementia earlier in PDD Orthostatic hypotension more frequent in DLB, frontal/temporal associated cognitive subsets more severe in DLB, cognitive decline is faster in DLB/DLB + AD Delusions, visual hallucinations, and attentional fluctuation more frequent in DLB; visual hallucinations: Spontaneous in DLB; after L-dopa therapy in PDD, but also in drug-naive cases

of major neurocognitive disorders with Lewy bodies. The arbitrary distinction with regard to the time of onset of motor and cognitive symptoms determines the diagnosis of DLB vs. PD-D. DLB is characterized by early cognitive impairment, whereas PD-D has later onset of cognitive impairment that follows motor symptoms [58]. The umbrella term "Lewy body disorders" has been endorsed by some authors to include PD, PD-D, and DLB, which can help with continued practical use and direct efforts at developing drugs that target neurodegenerative mechanisms due to alpha-synuclein metabolism [59]. Table 5.4 enumerates the overlap and differences between DLB and PDD.

Treatments

In assessing patients with suspected cognitive impairment, clinicians should adopt a systematic approach. This involves conducting a compre-hensive mental status examination and engaging in interviews with informed individuals to iden-tify any functional deficits and ascertain the spe-cific cognitive domains affected [60]. It is important to differentiate and establish if the symptoms are the result of the natural course of the illness or due to other causes, which include medication side effects, comorbid mood distur-bances, and systemic and metabolic disturbances. The context in which the symptoms develop and the mode of onset should guide appropriate investigations. Any recent medication changes (introduction of new medications or recent changes in doses) should be carefully reviewed [61]. Modifying PD-D medication regimens requires careful balance, as improvements in psy-chotic symptoms may be accompanied by wors-ened motor symptoms. Medications that can adversely affect cognition, those with anticholin-ergic properties, benzodiazepines, and dopamine agonists, should be gradually discontinued. Once the obvious triggers for cognitive changes are excluded, appropriate non-pharmacological mea-sures need to be implemented. The severity, fre-quency, and burden of the symptom will help determine if pharmacological interventions are needed. It is important to emphasize that occa-sional transient hallucinations with fully pre-served insight or mild cognitive deficits may not need treatment. Unfortunately, polypharmacy is common and widely prevalent as multiple drugs to treat motor symptoms, neuropsychiatric symp-toms, and autonomic dysfunction. The risk and benefit ratio should be carefully reviewed prior to the initiation of any new medications [62]. As a rule, it is important to introduce one drug at a time at a low dose and titrate up as needed. Psychotropic medications often used to treat behavioral symptoms should be appropriately tapered and discontinued when sufficient symp-tom control is obtained [40]. The primary focus is on symptom management with the treatment of mood disorders, sleep disturbances, and behav-ioral disturbances that arise as the disease pro-gresses [63]. It is important to encourage general lifestyle modifications like a healthy diet, physi-cal activity, and social engagement that improve

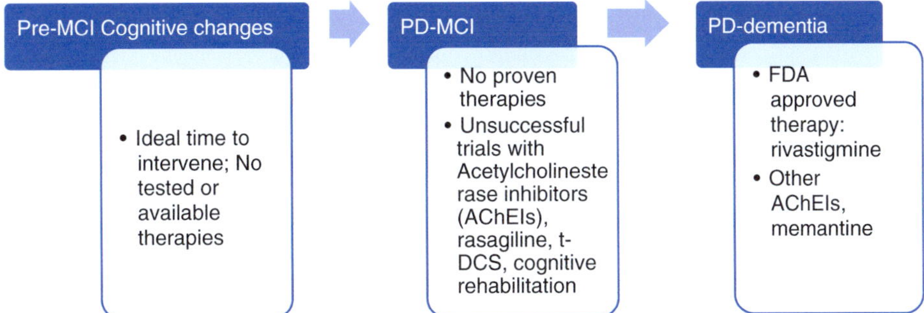

Fig. 5.2 Approach to treating cognitive impairment in Parkinson's disease [63]

quality of life. There are no current treatment approach differences between men and women, although PD is more common in men than women [9]. Figure 5.2 describes the approach to treating cognitive impairment in PD.

Non-pharmacological Management

There are very few studies that have investigated the effects of non-pharmacologic approaches on cognition in individuals with PD-D. Adequate information and education about the disease process should be provided to the patient and the family to alleviate concerns about visual hallucinations that may arise as the cognitive decline progresses [63]. Falls are very frequently associated with cognitive deficits in PD [64]. Hence, routine physiotherapy and exercise programs should be incorporated into the daily routine [40]. In addition to encouraging adequate mental and physical activity, triggers such as undue sensory stimuli and environmental factors should be identified and avoided. Cognitive training in the domains of attention, executive functions, memory, and visuospatial functions has shown significant benefits [65]. Improvement in executive functions is linked to passive cycling and physical exercise [66]. Repetitive magnetic stimulation (left dorsolateral prefrontal cortex

stimulation) has been shown to positively affect both depressive symptoms and cognitive symptoms [67]. Deep brain stimulation (DBS) of the nucleus basalis of Meynert (DBS-NBM) has not shown any promising results between treatment and control groups after 6 weeks [68]. The primary outcomes studied include primary cognitive outcomes such as Verbal Learning Test, verbal fluency, WAIS (Wechsler Adult Intelligence Scale)-III-digit span, Posner covert attention test, and simple and choice reaction times. Electroconvulsive therapy (ECT) is useful in alleviating the psychotic symptoms in PD. Significant improvements in psychotic symptoms after ECT have been reported in patients resistant to quetiapine [69]. ECT has also been shown to improve motor symptoms and could be promising in treating both psychosis and depression in PD [70]. A retrospective study revealed a significant improvement (nearly 50%) in the Brief Psychiatric Rating Scale (BPRS) as well as the Hamilton Depression Rating Scale (HDRS) after ECT in PD patients with psychosis and depression, respectively [71]. A systematic review concluded that ECT could be an effective treatment in addressing severe and treatment-refractory agitation and aggression in dementia, with few adverse consequences [72]. Figure 5.3 provides an overview of non-pharmacological interventions in PD-D.

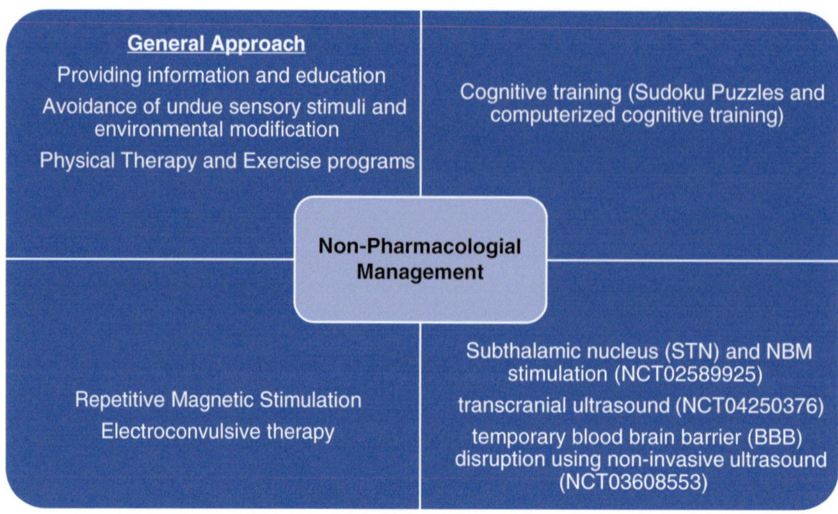

Fig. 5.3 Overview of non-pharmacological interventions in PD-D

Pharmacological Management

Cholinesterase Inhibitors

Cholinesterase inhibitors are the most frequently studied medications for PD-D. There is strong evidence that a profound cholinergic deficit is a consistent biochemical correlate of cognitive dysfunction in PD-D [73]. The enzyme, acetylcholinesterase, which breaks down acetylcholine in the synaptic cleft, is inhibited by cholinesterase inhibitors (ChE-Is). This leads to prolongation of the synaptic half-life of acetylcholine, and subsequently cholinergic activity is enhanced.

Rivastigmine is the only FDA-approved cholinesterase inhibitor for use in PD-D. The EXPRESS study looked at 541 patients with mild to moderate PD-D, and they were assigned to receive up to 12 mg/day of rivastigmine or placebo over 24 weeks [56]. Statistically significant improvements on rivastigmine treatment were noted on both primary endpoints (Alzheimer's Disease [AD] Assessment Scale-Cognitive Subscale [ADAS-cog] and Clinical Global Impression of Change scale) and secondary endpoints (Mini-Mental State Examination [MMSE], Neuropsychiatric Inventory [NPI], the clock drawing test, verbal fluency, and computer-based attention tests) when compared to placebo. Activities of daily living (ADL) scores showed a minimal worsening from baseline in patients on rivastigmine, whereas those on placebo had a statistically significantly worsening on ADL scores [74]. Rivastigmine was more frequently associated with the worsening of parkinsonian symptoms (27.3% versus 15.6% on placebo) primarily due to worsening of tremors (10.2% on rivastigmine versus 3.9% on placebo) [74].

Rivastigmine has also been reported to improve all aspects of attention. A 24-week, randomized, double-blind, placebo-controlled, multicenter study of rivastigmine assessed 487 patients with PD-D. The investigators completed an evaluation of attention on the Cognitive Drug Research computerized cognitive assessment system prior to dosing and 16 and 24 weeks following dosing of the medication [57]. Significant benefits of rivastigmine over placebo were seen in sustained attention, focused attention, consistency of responding, and central processing speed. The subgroup analysis suggested that patients with visual hallucinations seemed to obtain more benefit from rivastigmine when compared to placebo [75]. The presence of hallucinations also predicted better overall tolerability and titration to increasing doses of rivastigmine. When compared to the rivastigmine patch, rivastigmine capsules benefitted patients, especially when they had lower MMSE scores. However, there were no differences between the rivastigmine capsule and patch in terms of efficacy in persons with MMSE >21. When long-term safety of rivastigmine in PD-D was studied, the rate of progression of motor symptoms was in the range expected from natural progression, and no new or unexpected safety issues were seen to emerge [76].

In a large randomized, double-blind, placebo-controlled study of 550 patients with mild to moderate PD-D, donepezil was shown to demonstrate some benefits in cognition [77]. The three groups were randomized and received a placebo, donepezil 5 mg/day, or donepezil 10 mg/day for 24 weeks. The primary efficacy parameters were ADAS-Cog (Alzheimer's Disease Assessment Scale-Cognitive Subscale) and a global measure of change from baseline. Donepezil at a dose of 10 mg/day was shown to have statistically significant superiority on the global measures of change, but this was not so with the 5 mg/day dosing. The results also favored donepezil on some secondary measures, including the MMSE, Brief Test of Attention, and the Verbal Fluency Test. No differences from placebo were noted on the ADL scale Disability Assessment in Dementia and the NPI. Additionally, there was no worsening of motor symptoms on donepezil as seen by the Unified Parkinson's Disease Rating Scale (UPDRS) motor scores [77]. Treatment with cholinesterase inhibitors (ChEIs) may also have some benefits on several neuropsychiatric symptoms of PD-D, especially apathy, anxiety, sleep disturbance, and delusions [78]. Rivastigmine is started at an initial dose of 3 mg/day and titrated at 3 mg/month to a maximum of 12 mg/day; rivastigmine transdermal patch is started at 5 cm^2/day and titrated at 5 cm^2/month to a maximum of 10–15 cm^2/day, and donepezil is typically started at a dose of 5 mg/day and titrated upwards by 5 mg/month to a maximum of 10 mg/day [40].

NMDA Receptor Antagonist

Memantine, an uncompetitive antagonist of N-methyl-d-aspartate receptors, has been studied for use in PD-D. One study reported significant improvements in attentional performance involving information processing and verbal episodic recognition memory in both DLB and PD-D patients [79]. However, a meta-analytic study examining the effects of memantine on neuropsychological functioning revealed that it has minimal effects on cognition in PD-D and DLB and hence unlikely to have clinically significant improvements in cognition [80]. Memantine has also been shown to decrease RBD in patients with PD-D [81].

Antidopaminergic Drugs

Severe agitation and related behaviors are less likely to improve with ChEIs and may even get worse as the patient becomes more activated. The mainstay of treatment for psychotic and severe agitation in PD-D is antipsychotic medications [40]. There is a high prevalence of neuroleptic sensitivity to these medications in individuals with PD and PD-D, and it has important clinical implications. First-generation antipsychotics like haloperidol can provoke severe neuroleptic sensitivity and are hence contraindicated for use among people with PD and PD-D [82]. These reactions have also been observed with most of the atypical antipsychotics (risperidone, olanzapine, and aripiprazole). The risk vs. benefit ratio should be carefully assessed before starting treatment with a neuroleptic medication, given the increased sensitivity to these medications and the greater risk for cerebrovascular events, cardiovascular events, and also death.

Quetiapine is often used as a first-line treatment for psychosis in PD (PD-P) given the ease of use and its relative lack of worsening motor symptoms, even though the evidence for its efficacy is noted to be weak [83, 84]. There are no high-quality RCTs available for quetiapine for the treatment of psychosis in PD. Quetiapine had similar efficacy to clozapine in a clozapine-controlled trial that did not include a placebo arm [85]. Quetiapine can be started with a dose of 12.5 mg/d and can be titrated up to a maximum dose of 150 mg/d among individuals with PD-D. The commonly observed side effects for quetiapine include drowsiness and QT-prolongation [86].

Olanzapine was not found to be useful among individuals with PD-D in a low-quality study [87].

Clozapine is the only antipsychotic that has sufficient evidence from randomized, controlled trials to treat psychosis in PD. Clozapine is associated with various side effects, including anticholinergic effects, metabolic disturbances, and risk of agranulocytosis. During the initial 6 months of clozapine administration, weekly blood draws are necessary. This is followed by biweekly draws for the next 6 months, and then monthly draws throughout the remaining duration of treatment [88]. It may increase confusion due to the antimuscarinic properties in patients with dementia, and these may be dose dependent [89, 90]. In the PSYCLOPS (PSYchosis and CLOzapine in the treatment of Parkinsonism) trial on 60 patients with PD-P, clozapine (with a dose <50 mg/d) led to significant improvement in psychosis without aggravating the parkinsonian symptoms. The anti-tremor effect of clozapine was also reported in this study [89]. Clozapine is usually started at a dose of 6.25 mg/d and titrated up to 50 mg/d for the treatment of PD-P [91]. Clozapine is not associated with any extrapyramidal side effects, but its association with agranulocytosis and blood monitoring limits its use in real life.

Pimavanserin is a combined inverse agonist of the 5-HT$_{2A}$ and 5HT$_{2C}$ receptors [92]. It is the only FDA-approved drug for the treatment of PD-P, and it does not have dopamine-blocking property. Pimavanserin resulted in a significant improvement in psychosis in patients with PD in a large, randomized, placebo-controlled clinical trial over a 6-week period [93]. The study compared the scores on the Scale for Assessment of Positive Symptoms (SAPS) adapted for PD (SAPS-PD) between 90 patients who received a placebo vs. 95 patients who received pimavanserin. The groups that received pimavanserin had a significant decrease in the SAPS-PD score after 6 weeks when compared to the placebo. Additionally, there were no significant adverse events or treatment-associated worsening of motor symptoms. This study also found improvement in measures of nighttime sleep, daytime wakefulness, and caregiver burden with the use of pimavanserin. Pimavanserin was described as "clinically useful" for the treatment of PD-P in a recently published review commissioned by the International Movement Disorder Society [85]. The recommended dose for pimavanserin is 34 mg/day and can be taken with or without food. The current commercially available formulation does carry a boxed warning that patients with dementia taking antipsychotics have increased overall mortality even though, as compared to placebo, it was not associated with significant adverse events in the clinical trials [94]. Prolongation of QT interval is associated with pimavanserin and should be avoided in patients with known prolonged QT interval and a history of arrhythmias. Concomitant use with other QT-prolonging medications should also be avoided. Peripheral edema and confusion are the other rare side effects associated with pimavanserin [86].

Dopaminergic Drugs

Pramipexole was shown to be beneficial in PD patients without dementia who had depressive symptoms in a large, randomized, placebo-controlled trial [95]. However, psychosis and cognition can worsen when pramipexole is used in patients with PD-D.

Antidepressants

There are no randomized controlled studies of antidepressants in PD-D. A few studies have looked at antidepressant use in PD. A meta-analysis concluded that there was no statistical significance between active drug and placebo, although both had large effect sizes [76]. Increasing age and major depression appeared to predict better response. Amitriptyline was found to be efficacious in PD depression in one systematic review [31]. Tricyclics such as amitriptyline and nortriptyline may have larger effect sizes, but they should be avoided in PD-D patients because of their anticholinergic effects and hence the potential to worsen cognition. Selective serotonin reuptake inhibitors (SSRIs) or serotonin and noradrenaline reuptake inhibitors (SNRIs) should be preferred in these patients. Venlafaxine and paroxetine improved depression in patients with PD in a randomized trial [96]. There may be a worsening of PD tremor by up to 5% and parkinsonism in patients treated with SSRIs [85]. Worsening of RBD symptoms has been described in case reports of all classes of antidepressants [97].

Benzodiazepines and Melatonin

Clonazepam or melatonin, or a combination of these, has been found useful in the treatment of RBD in PD, although there is no evidence from RCTs [97]. Melatonin has shown benefits in the control of RBD symptoms in 10 out of 14 patients who did not respond to clonazepam or were able to tolerate it [98].

Disease-Modifying Agents

Repurposing of multiple pharmacologic agents is being tested for benefits in PD cognitive impairment. PD-D is characterized by aggregation of the protein α-synuclein in subcortical and cortical brain areas. β-Glucocerebrosidase (GCase; gene name GBA1) is one of the leading genetic risk factors. Studies in cell culture and animal models have shown that raising the levels of GCase can decrease the levels of α-synuclein. Ambroxol is a pharmacological chaperone for GCase and is able to raise the levels of GCase and could therefore be a disease-modifying treatment for PD-D [99]. Research is needed for both disease-modifying and symptomatic treatments in PD cognitive impairment. Ceftriaxone, an antibiotic with potential neuroprotective effect by reducing glutamatergic hyperactivity and excitotoxicity, is also being studied [63]. Other alternative agents tried include yokukansan, a herbal agent in Chinese medicine. There are reports that it improves behavioral symptoms without worsening cognitive function, ability to perform activities of daily living, or parkinsonism [100].

Evidence-Based Treatment

The 2019 Movement Disorder Society update on evidence-based treatments for non-motor symptoms of PD concluded that there is only sufficient evidence to support rivastigmine as efficacious for PD-D [70]. There is insufficient evidence for the efficacy of donepezil, galantamine, or memantine. The update identified rivastigmine as being clinically useful. The other cholinesterase inhibitors were classified as possibly useful, given their antidementia benefit outside PD. Memantine was labeled as being an investigational drug for PD-D. Table 5.5 summarizes the medications used to treat PD-D. Table 5.6 enumerates the treatment of behavioral symptoms in PD-D. Figure 5.4 provides a flowchart for clinical approach to individuals with suspected Parkinson's disease dementia.

Table 5.5 Summary of PD-D medications, indications, and adverse effects

Drug class	Indications	Adverse effects
Cholinesterase inhibitor	May improve cognition, balance, psychiatric symptoms, and gait in patients with PD-D	Nausea, vomiting, diarrhea, and anorexia. Use with caution in patients with severe bradycardia, peptic ulcer disease, or asthma
Antipsychotics	May be used for aggression, agitation, or psychotic conditions with varying effects Quetiapine may be considered as a first line due to lack of severe side effects Pimavanserin is a new atypical antipsychotic medication that is FDA approved for PD-P Clozapine has been shown to reduce psychotic symptoms in patients with PD-P, but it must be used with caution due to side effect profile	Worsening of metabolic abnormalities, extrapyramidal symptoms, or cognition Quetiapine: Drowsiness, increased appetite Pimavanserin: Possible QT prolongation, worsening of psychiatric symptoms Clozapine: Major side effect of agranulocytosis requiring frequent blood-level monitoring
Antidepressants	No direct studies for utility in PD-D, but may be used to treat comorbid major depressive disorder or anxiety disorders	Diarrhea, nausea vomiting, insomnia, dizziness. Possible weight gain or sexual dysfunction

(continued)

Table 5.5 (continued)

Drug class	Indications	Adverse effects
Benzodiazepines	No direct evidence for utility in PD-D but may be considered sparingly for treatment of RBD and disturbances in sleep–wake cycle	Excessive drowsiness, worsening dementia symptoms, increased risk of falls, confusion
NMDA receptor antagonist	Memantine is being investigated for use in people with PD-D with limited evidence	Dizziness, headache, confusion
Dopaminergic drugs	Limited evidence for efficacy in people with PD-D	Worsening of confusion, hallucinations, extrapyramidal side effects, or compulsive behaviors

Table 5.6 Summary of neuropsychiatric symptoms in Parkinson's disease dementia (PD-D) [101]

Symptom or disorder	Clinical description	Symptom management
Aggression/agitation	Mostly in the context of psychosis and can manifest as irritability, emotional lability, aberrant motor behaviors, and disinhibited behaviors. Occurs more often in severe cognitive decline—Lower MMSE scores, higher UPDRS and NPI scores. Associated with increased caregiver distress Occurs in 30–40% of PD-D patients	Ruling out other medical causes that can lead to exacerbation Consider decrease in PD medications and adjustments made to PD medications to minimize "off" periods Off-label use of antipsychotics, and benzodiazepines (should be used with caution in PD-D patients) Off-label use of cholinesterase inhibitors and antidepressants
Anxiety	More likely to occur in women and in patients with non-motor fluctuations (e.g., slowness of thinking, fatigue, and dysphoria) Common and comorbid with other mood disturbances	Antidepressants such as SSRIs Low-dose benzodiazepines (should be used with caution in PD-D patients) Subthalamic nucleus (STN) DBS may improve symptoms
Pseudobulbar affect	Episodes of involuntary expression of either crying or laughing that are repeated and brief that are typically incongruent with the patient's mood. May or may not be associated with a stimulus and happens in 5–10% of PD patients. Is easily misdiagnosed as depression	Only anecdotal evidence for SSRIs and mood stabilizers Educating patient and families about the difference between PBA and depression
Depression	Tends to increase with age and more severe illness process; is itself an independent risk factor for PDD; highly comorbid with anxiety. More likely to occur in women. Occurs in 30–60% of the PDD patients	SSRIs and SNRIs are helpful. Tricyclic antidepressants should be avoided due to a potentially significant adverse event Interaction of second-generation antidepressants and monoamine oxidase B inhibitors can lead to serotonin syndrome May benefit from stimulation of D2/D3 receptors. Use these medications with caution as studies excluded patients with dementia. The Subthalamic Nucleus (STN) Deep Brain stimulation (DBS) may improve symptoms
Psychosis	Tends to increase with age and more severe illness process and exposure to PD medications; associated with cognitive decline and development of dementia, and worsening of motor symptoms. Highly predictive of caregiver distress and institutionalization Often comorbid with mood, anxiety, sleep disturbances, and apathy Hallucinations can occur in up to 45–65% and delusions in 25–30%	Adjustment to PD medications followed using antipsychotic medications (quetiapine, clozapine, pimavanserin) Cholinesterase inhibitors have some evidence

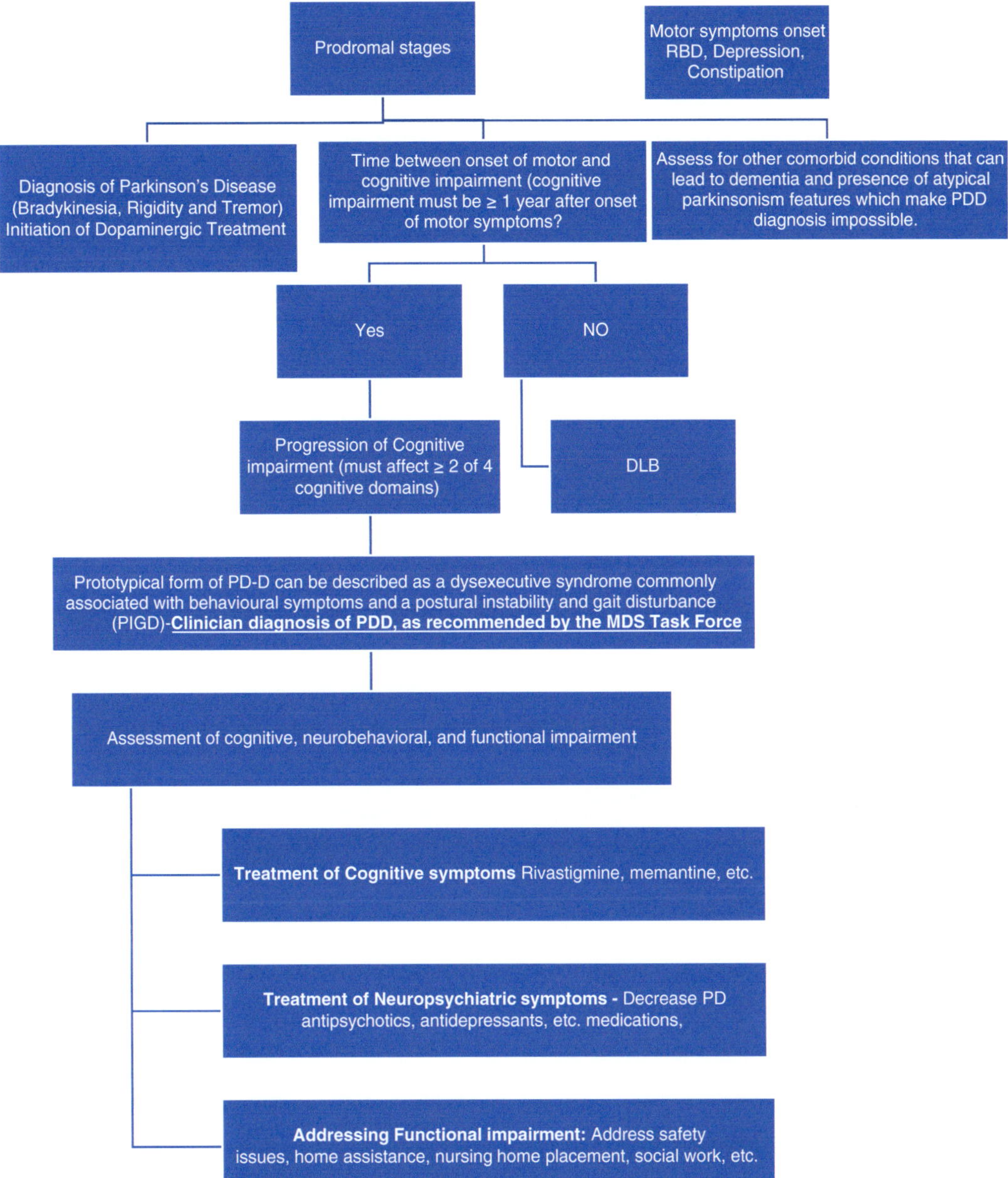

Fig. 5.4 Flowchart for clinical approach to suspected Parkinson's disease dementia

Conclusions

The management of patients with PD-D starts with early recognition and with excluding other causes of dementia or conditions that mimic dementia. The management plan should consider the whole symptom complex with careful assess-ment of the risks and benefits of medications. Patients who suffer from PD-D often have increased anxiety, depression, and possible epi-sodes of agitation and aggression. Families and caregivers should be made aware of possible comorbidities. It is essential to educate and involve patients and families in decision-making in a collaborative manner. Information on non-pharmacological methods, such as redirection, should be provided during aggressive episodes. Additionally, the importance of safety for caregivers and patients should be stressed to all involved in patient care. Early discussion with the patient and their family about decision-making and end-of-life care will help alleviate challenging ethical dilemmas that may arise. Given the progressive nature of the illness, periodic cognitive and neuropsychiatric assessments must be performed to initiate appropriate interventions and ensure that safety measures are in place. Early identification of neuropsychiatric symptoms that arise during the illness and initiating the appropriate pharmacological and non-pharmacological measures will lead to better outcomes.

References

1. Emre M. Introduction. In: Cognitive impairment and dementia in Parkinson's disease. 2nd ed; 2015. pp. 1–4.
2. Tysnes OB, Storstein A. Epidemiology of Parkinson's disease. J Neural Transm (Vienna) [Internet]. 2017;124(8):901–5. Available from: https://pubmed.ncbi.nlm.nih.gov/28150045/
3. Simon DK, Tanner CM, Brundin P. Parkinson disease epidemiology, pathology, genetics, and pathophysiology. Clin Geriatr Med [Internet]. 2020;36(1):1–12. https://pubmed.ncbi.nlm.nih.gov/31733690/.
4. Dorsey ER, Sherer T, Okun MS, Bloemd BR. The emerging evidence of the Parkinson pandemic. J Parkinsons Dis [Internet]. 2018;8(s1):S3–8. https://pubmed.ncbi.nlm.nih.gov/30584159/.
5. Kaltenboeck A, Johnson SJ, Davis MR, Birnbaum HG, Carroll CA, Tarrants ML, et al. Direct costs and survival of medicare beneficiaries with early and advanced Parkinson's disease. Parkinsonism Relat Disord [Internet]. 2012;18(4):321–6. Available from: https://pubmed.ncbi.nlm.nih.gov/22177623/
6. Wright Willis A, Evanoff BA, Lian M, Criswell SR, Racette BA. Geographic and ethnic variation in Parkinson disease: a population-based study of US Medicare beneficiaries. Neuroepidemiology [Internet]. 2010;34(3):143–51. https://pubmed.ncbi.nlm.nih.gov/20090375/.
7. Aarsland D, Kurz MW. The epidemiology of dementia associated with Parkinson disease. J Neurol Sci. 2010;289:289(1–2).
8. Williams-Gray CH, Mason SL, Evans JR, Foltynie T, Brayne C, Robbins TW, et al. The CamPaIGN study of Parkinson's disease: 10-year outlook in an incident population-based cohort. J Neurol Neurosurg Psychiatry. 2013;84(11):1258.
9. Chen S, Chen H, Wang K. The diagnostic criteria and treatment guideline for Parkinson's disease dementia (second version). Chin J Neurol. 2021;54(8)
10. Pedersen KF, Larsen JP, Tysnes OB, Alves G. Prognosis of mild cognitive impairment in early Parkinson disease: the Norwegian ParkWest study. JAMA Neurol. 2013;70(5):580.
11. Emre M, Aarsland D, Brown R, Burn DJ, Duyckaerts C, Mizuno Y, et al. Clinical diagnostic criteria for dementia associated with Parkinson's disease. Mov Disord. 2007;22:1689.
12. Dag Aarsland, Alexandra Bernadotte. Epidemiology of dementia associated with Parkinson's disease. In: Emre M, editor. Cognitive impairment and dementia in Parkinson's disease. 2nd ed; 2015. pp. 5–16.
13. Savica R, Grossardt BR, Bower JH, Boeve BF, Ahlskog JE, Rocca WA. Incidence of dementia with Lewy bodies and Parkinson disease dementia. JAMA Neurol. 2013;70(11):1396.
14. Riedel O, Schneider C, Klotsche J, Reichmann H, Storch A, Wittchen HU. The prevalence of Parkinson's disease, associated dementia, and depression in Dresden. Fortschritte der Neurologie. Psychiatrie. 2013;81(2):81.
15. Reid WGJ, Hely MA, Morris JGL, Broe GA, Adena M, Sullivan DJO, et al. A longitudinal study of Parkinson's disease: clinical and neuropsychological correlates of dementia. J Clin Neurosci. 1996;3(4):327.
16. Emre M. Dementia associated with Parkinson's disease. Lancet Neurol. 2003;2:229–37.
17. Kraybill ML, Larson EB, Tsuang DW, Teri L, McCormick WC, Bowen JD, et al. Cognitive differences in dementia patients with autopsy-verified AD, Lewy body pathology, or both. Neurology. 2005;64:2069.
18. Polymeropoulos MH, Lavedan C, Leroy E, Ide SE, Dehejia A, Dutra A, et al. Mutation in the alpha-synuclein gene identified in families with Parkinson's disease. Science [Internet]. 1997;276(5321):2045–7. https://pubmed.ncbi.nlm.nih.gov/9197268/.
19. Tanner CM, Goldman SM, Ross GW, Grate SJ. The disease intersection of susceptibility and exposure: chemical exposures and neurodegenerative disease risk. Alzheimers Dement [Internet]. 2014;10(3 Suppl). https://pubmed.ncbi.nlm.nih.gov/24924672/.
20. Ritz B, Ascherio A, Checkoway H, Marder KS, Nelson LM, Rocca WA, et al. Pooled analysis of tobacco use and risk of Parkinson disease. Arch Neurol [Internet]. 2007;64(7):990–7. https://pubmed.ncbi.nlm.nih.gov/17620489/.
21. Emre M. Diagnosis of dementia in Parkinson's disease. In: Emre M, editor. Cognitive impairment and dementia in Parkinson's disease. 2nd ed. Oxford: Oxford Academic; 2015; online ed. p. 275–88.

22. Emre M, editor. Cognitive impairment and dementia in Parkinson's disease, vol. 2015. 2nd ed. Oxford: Oxford Academic; 2015; online ed. p. 17–26.
23. Emre M. General features, mode of onset, and course of dementia in Parkinson's disease. In: Emre M, editor. Cognitive impairment and dementia in Parkinson's disease. 2nd ed. Oxford, online ed.: Oxford Academic; 2015. p. 17–26.
24. Dubois B, Burn D, Goetz C, Aarsland D, Brown RG, Broe GA, et al. Diagnostic procedures for Parkinson's disease dementia: recommendations from the Movement Disorder Society Task Force. Mov Disord. 2007;22:2314.
25. Hughes AJ, Daniel SE, Kilford L, Lees AJ. Accuracy of clinical diagnosis of idiopathic Parkinson's disease: a clinico-pathological study of 100 cases. J Neurol Neurosurg Psychiatry. 1992;55(3):181.
26. McKeith IG. Dementia with Lewy bodies. Br J Psychiatry. 2002;180:144.
27. Poewe W, Gauthier S, Aarsland D, Leverenz JB, Barone P, Weintraub D, et al. Diagnosis and management of Parkinson's disease dementia. Int J Clin Pract. 2008;62:1581.
28. Cummings JL. Depression and Parkinson's disease: a review. Am J Psychiatry. 1992;149(4):443.
29. Aarsland D, Batzu L, Halliday GM, Geurtsen GJ, Ballard C, Ray Chaudhuri K, et al. Parkinson disease-associated cognitive impairment. Nat Rev Dis Primers. 2021;7(1)
30. Emre M. Diagnosis of dementia in Parkinson's disease. In: Emre M, editor. Cognitive impairment and dementia in Parkinson's disease. 2nd ed. Oxford, 2015; online ed, Oxford Academic; 2015. p. 275–88.
31. Miyasaki JM, Shannon K, Voon V, Ravina B, Kleiner-Fisman G, Anderson K, et al. Practice parameter: evaluation and treatment of depression, psychosis, and dementia in Parkinson disease (an evidence-based review): report of the quality standards Subcommittee of the American Academy of Neurology. Neurology. 2006;66(7):996.
32. Rothman SM, Mattson MP. Sleep disturbances in Alzheimer's and Parkinson's diseases. NeuroMolecular Med. 2012;14:194.
33. Suzuki K, Miyamoto M, Miyamoto T, Iwanami M, Hirata K. Sleep disturbances associated with Parkinson's disease. Parkinson's Disease. 2011;2011:1.
34. Bollu PC, Sahota P. Sleep and Parkinson disease. Mo Med. 2017;114:5.
35. Chow M. Sleep in Parkinson's disease dementia. In: Dementia in Parkinson's disease—everything you need to know; 2022.
36. Marion MH, Qurashi M, Marshall G, Foster O. Is REM sleep behaviour disorder (RBD) a risk factor of dementia in idiopathic Parkinson's disease? J Neurol. 2008;255(2):192.
37. Vendette M, Gagnon JF, Décary A, Massicotte-Marquez J, Postuma RB, Doyon J, et al. REM sleep behavior disorder predicts cognitive impairment in Parkinson disease without dementia. Neurology. 2007;69(19):1843.
38. Cummings JL, Mega M, Gray K, Rosenberg-Thompson S, Carusi DA, Gornbein J. The neuropsychiatric inventory: comprehensive assessment of psychopathology in dementia. Neurology. 1994;44(12):2308.
39. Gallagher DA, Goetz CG, Stebbins G, Lees AJ, Schrag A. Validation of the MDS-UPDRS part I for nonmotor symptoms in Parkinson's disease. Mov Disord. 2012;27:27(1).
40. Emre M, Ford PJ, Bilgiç B, Uç EY. Cognitive impairment and dementia in Parkinson's disease: practical issues and management. Mov Disord. 2014;29:663.
41. Martinez-Martin P. Dementia in Parkinson's disease: usefulness of the pill questionnaire. Mov Disord. 2013;28(13):1832.
42. Pickering RM, Grimbergen YAM, Rigney U, Ashburn A, Mazibrada G, Wood B, et al. A meta-analysis of six prospective studies of falling in Parkinson's disease. Mov Disord. 2007;22(13):1892.
43. Kerr GK, Worringham CJ, Cole MH, Lacherez PF, Wood JM, Silburn PA. Predictors of future falls in Parkinson disease. Neurology. 2010;75(2):116.
44. Giladi N, Horak FB, Hausdorff JM. Classification of gait disturbances: distinguishing between continuous and episodic changes. Mov Disord. 2013;28:1469.
45. Bloem BR, Hausdorff JM, Visser JE, Giladi N. Falls and freezing of gait in Parkinson's disease: a review of two interconnected, episodic phenomena. Mov Disord. 2004;19:871.
46. Amboni M, Barone P, Hausdorff JM. Cognitive contributions to gait and falls: evidence and implications. Mov Disord. 2013;28:1520.
47. Marson DC. Clinical and ethical aspects of financial capacity in dementia: a commentary. Am J Geriatr Psychiatr. 2013;21(4):382.
48. Widera E, Steenpass V, Marson D, Sudore R. Finances in the older patient with cognitive impairment: 'He didn't want me to take over'. JAMA. 2011;305
49. Devos H, Vandenberghe W, Nieuwboer A, Tant M, de Weerdt W, Dawson JD, et al. Validation of a screening battery to predict driving fitness in people with Parkinson's disease. Mov Disord. 2013;28(5):671.
50. Uc EY. Driving in Parkinson's disease. In: Current clinical neurology; 2022.
51. Bevins EA, Peters J, Léger GC. The diagnosis and management of reversible dementia syndromes. Curr Treat Options Neurol. 2021;23
52. Pyatigorskaya N, Gallea C, Garcia-Lorenzo D, Vidailhet M, Lehericy S. A review of the use of magnetic resonance imaging in Parkinson's disease. Ther Adv Neurol Disord. 2014;7:206.
53. van Steenoven I, Majbour NK, Vaikath NN, Berendse HW, van der Flier WM, van de Berg WDJ, et al. α-Synuclein species as potential cerebrospinal fluid biomarkers for dementia with Lewy bodies. Mov Disord. 2018;33(11):1724.

54. Hall S, Öhrfelt A, Constantinescu R, Andreasson U, Surova Y, Bostrom F, et al. Accuracy of a panel of 5 cerebrospinal fluid biomarkers in the differential diagnosis of patients with dementia and/or parkinsonian disorders. Arch Neurol. 2012;69(11):1445.

55. Stamelou M, Quinn NP, Bhatia KP. 'Atypical' atypical parkinsonism: new genetic conditions presenting with features of progressive supranuclear palsy, corticobasal degeneration, or multiple system atrophy- A diagnostic guide. Mov Disord. 2013;28(9):1184.

56. Narasimhan M, Schwartz R, Halliday G. Parkinsonism and cerebrovascular disease. J Neurol Sci. 2022;433:120011.

57. Mostile G, Fasano A, Zappia M. Parkinsonism in idiopathic normal pressure hydrocephalus: is it time for defining a clinical tetrad? Neurol Sci. 2022;43:5201.

58. Jellinger KA, Korczyn AD. Are dementia with Lewy bodies and Parkinson's disease dementia the same disease? BMC Med. 2018;16(1):34.

59. Lippa CF, Duda JE, Grossman M, Hurtig HI, Aarsland D, Boeve BF, et al. DLB and PDD boundary issues: diagnosis, treatment, molecular pathology, and biomarkers. Neurology. 2007;68(11):812.

60. McCollum L, Karlawish J. Cognitive impairment evaluation and management. Med Clin North Am. 2020;104:807.

61. Goldman JG, Holden S. Treatment of psychosis and dementia in Parkinson's disease topical collection on movement disorders. Curr Treat Options Neurol. 2014;16(3):281.

62. Masopust J, Protopopová D, Vališ M, Pavelek Z, Klímová B. Treatment of behavioral and psychological symptoms of dementias with psychopharmaceuticals: a review. Neuropsychiatr Dis Treat. 2018;14:1211.

63. Sun C, Armstrong MJ. Treatment of Parkinson's disease with cognitive impairment: current approaches and future directions. Behav Sci. 2021;11

64. Morris R, Martini D, McBarron G, Mancini M, Horak F. The interplay between cholinergic activity, attention, and turning in Parkinson's disease. Movement Disorder. 2019;34.

65. París AP, Saleta HG, de la Cruz Crespo Maraver M, Silvestre E, Freixa MG, Torrellas CP, et al. Blind randomized controlled study of the efficacy of cognitive training in Parkinson's disease. Mov Disord. 2011;26(7):1251.

66. Ridgel AL, Kim CH, Fickes EJ, Muller MD, Alberts JL. Changes in executive function after acute bouts of passive cycling in Parkinson's disease. J Aging Phys Act. 2011;19(2):87.

67. Pal E, Nagy F, Aschermann Z, Balazs E, Kovacs N. The impact of left prefrontal repetitive transcranial magnetic stimulation on depression in Parkinson's disease: A randomized, double-blind, placebo-controlled study. Mov Disord. 2010;25(14):2311.

68. Gratwicke J, Zrinzo L, Kahan J, Peters A, Beigi M, Akram H, et al. Bilateral deep brain stimulation of the nucleus basalis of Meynert for Parkinson disease dementia a randomized clinical trial. JAMA Neurol. 2018;75(2):169.

69. Usui C, Hatta K, Doi N, Kubo S, Kamigaichi R, Nakanishi A, et al. Improvements in both psychosis and motor signs in Parkinson's disease, and changes in regional cerebral blood flow after electroconvulsive therapy. Prog Neuro-Psychopharmacol Biol Psychiatry. 2011;35(7):1704.

70. Grover S, Somani A, Sahni N, Mehta S, Choudhary S, Chakravarty RK, Rabha AM. Effectiveness of electroconvulsive therapy (ECT) in Parkinsonian symptoms: a case series. Innov Clin Neurosci. 2018;15(1–2):23–7.

71. Calderón-Fajardo H, Cervantes-Arriaga A, Llorens-Arenas R, Ramírez-Bermudez J, Ruiz-Chow Á, Rodríguez-Violante M. Electroconvulsive therapy in Parkinson's disease. Arq Neuropsiquiatr. 2015;73(10):856.

72. van den Berg JF, Kruithof HC, Kok RM, Verwijk E, Spaans HP. Electroconvulsive therapy for agitation and aggression in dementia: a systematic review. Am J Geriatr Psychiatr. 2018;26(4):419.

73. Tiraboschi P, Hansen LA, Alford M, Sabbagh MN, Schoos B, Masliah E, et al. Cholinergic dysfunction in diseases with LEWY bodies. Neurology. 2000;54(2):407.

74. Emre M, Aarsland D, Albanese A, Byrne EJ, Deuschl G, de Deyn PP, et al. Rivastigmine for dementia associated with Parkinson's disease. N Engl J Med. 2004;351(24):2509.

75. Burn D, Emre M, McKeith I, de Deyn PP, Aarsland D, Hsu C, et al. Effects of rivastigmine in patients with and without visual hallucinations in dementia associated with Parkinson's disease. Mov Disord. 2006;21(11):1899.

76. Emre M, Poewe W, de Deyn PP, Barone P, Kulisevsky J, Pourcher E, et al. Long-term safety of rivastigmine in Parkinson disease dementia: an open-label, randomized study. Clin Neuropharmacol. 2014;37(1):9.

77. Dubois B, Tolosa E, Katzenschlager R, Emre M, Lees AJ, Schumann G, et al. Donepezil in Parkinson's disease dementia: a randomized, double-blind efficacy and safety study. Mov Disord. 2012;27(10):1230–8.

78. Aarsland D, Mosimann UP, McKeith IG. Role of cholinesterase inhibitors in Parkinson's disease and dementia with Lewy bodies. J Geriatr Psychiatry Neurol. 2004;17:164.

79. Wesnes KA, Aarsland D, Ballard C, Londos E. Memantine improves attention and episodic memory in Parkinson's disease dementia and dementia with Lewy bodies. Int J Geriatr Psychiatry. 2015;30(1):46.

80. Brennan L, Pantelyat A, Duda JE, Morley JF, Weintraub D, Wilkinson JR, et al. Memantine and cognition in Parkinson's disease dementia/dementia with Lewy bodies: a meta-analysis. Mov Disord Clin Pract. 2016;3(2):161.

81. Larsson V, Aarsland D, Ballard C, Minthon L, Londos E. The effect of memantine on sleep behaviour in dementia with Lewy bodies and Parkinson's

disease dementia. Int J Geriatr Psychiatry. 2010;25(10):1030.

82. Aarsland D, Perry R, Larsen JP, McKeith IG, O'Brien JT, Perry EK, et al. Neuroleptic sensitivity in Parkinson's disease and Parkinsonian dementias. J Clin Psychiatry. 2005;66(5):504.

83. Morgante L, Epifanio A, Spina E, Zappia M, di Rosa AE, Marconi R, et al. Quetiapine and clozapine in parkinsonian patients with dopaminergic psychosis. Clin Neuropharmacol. 2004;27, 153(4):–6.

84. Fernandez HH, Okun MS, Rodriguez RL, Malaty IA, Romrell J, Sun A, et al. Quetiapine improves visual hallucinations in Parkinson disease but not through normalization of sleep architecture: results from a double-blind clinical-polysomnography study. Int J Neurosci. 2009;119(12):2196.

85. Seppi K, Weintraub D, Coelho M, Perez-Lloret S, Fox SH, Katzenschlager R, et al. The movement disorder society evidence-based medicine review update: treatments for the non-motor symptoms of Parkinson's disease. Mov Disord. 2011;26(Suppl. 3):S42.

86. Lenka A, Gomathinayagam V, Bahroo L. Approach to the management of psychosis in Parkinson's disease. Ann Movement Disorders. 2019;2:83.

87. Seppi K, Ray Chaudhuri K, Coelho M, Fox SH, Katzenschlager R, Perez Lloret S, et al. Update on treatments for nonmotor symptoms of Parkinson's disease—an evidence-based medicine review. Mov Disord. 2019;34:180.

88. Divac N, Stojanović R, Vujović KS, Medić B, Damjanović A, Prostran M. The efficacy and safety of antipsychotic medications in the treatment of psychosis in patients with Parkinson's disease. Behav Neurol. 2016;2016:4938154.

89. The Parkinson Study Group. Low-dose clozapine for the treatment of drug-induced psychosis in Parkinson's disease. The Parkinson Study Group. N Engl J Med. 1999;340(10):757.

90. Pollak P, Tison F, Rascol O, Destée A, Péré JJ, Senard JM, et al. Clozapine in drug induced psychosis in Parkinson's disease: a randomised, placebo controlled study with open follow up. J Neurol Neurosurg Psychiatry. 2004;75(5):689.

91. Hindle JV. The practical management of cognitive impairment and psychosis in the older Parkinson's disease patient. J Neural Transm. 2013;120:649.

92. Meltzer HY, Mills R, Revell S, Williams H, Johnson A, Bahr D, et al. Pimavanserin, a serotonin 2A receptor inverse agonist, for the treatment of Parkinson's disease psychosis. Neuropsychopharmacology. 2010;35(4):881.

93. Cummings J, Isaacson S, Mills R, Williams H, Chi-Burris K, Corbett A, et al. Pimavanserin for patients with Parkinson's disease psychosis: a randomised, placebo-controlled phase 3 trial. Lancet. 2014;383(9916):533.

94. Kales HC, Valenstein M, Kim HM, McCarthy JF, Ganoczy D, Cunningham F, et al. Mortality risk in patients with dementia treated with antipsychotics versus other psychiatric medications. Am J Psychiatry. 2007;164(10):1568.

95. Bxarone P, Poewe W, Albrecht S, Debieuvre C, Massey D, Rascol O, et al. Pramipexole for the treatment of depressive symptoms in patients with Parkinson's disease: a randomised, double-blind, placebo-controlled trial. Lancet Neurol. 2010;9(6):573.

96. Richard IH, McDermott MP, Kurlan R, Lyness JM, Como PG, Pearson N, et al. A randomized, double-blind, placebo-controlled trial of antidepressants in Parkinson disease. Neurology. 2012;78(16):1229.

97. St Louis EK, Boeve AR, Boeve BF. REM sleep behavior disorder in Parkinson's disease and other synucleinopathies. Mov Disord. 2017;32:645.

98. Boeve BF, Silber MH, Ferman TJ. Melatonin for treatment of REM sleep behavior disorder in neurologic disorders: results in 14 patients. Sleep Med. 2003;4(4):281.

99. Pasternak SH, Silveira C, Li Z, Bartha R, Borrie M, Wells J, et al. P1-067: Ambroxol as pharmacological chaperone targeting gba1 as a disease modifying treatment for parkinson's disease dementia: a phase 2 randomized, double-blind, placebo-controlled trial. Alzheimers Dement. 2018;14(7S_Part_5)

100. Kawanabe T, Yoritaka A, Shimura H, Oizumi H, Tanaka S, Hattori N. Successful treatment with Yokukansan for behavioral and psychological symptoms of parkinsonian dementia. Prog Neuro-Psychopharmacol Biol Psychiatry. 2010;34(2):284.

101. Mamikonyan E, Weintraub D. Neuropsychiatric symptoms in Parkinson's disease dementia. In: Emre M, editor. Cognitive impairment and dementia in Parkinson's disease. 2nd ed. Oxford: Oxford Academic; 2015. p. 47–68, online ed.

Rajesh R. Tampi and Deena J. Tampi

Epidemiology

Behavioral and psychological symptoms of dementia (BPSD) refer to a group of symptoms and behaviors commonly seen among individuals with dementia and that are unsafe and disruptive and impair their care in a given environment [1, 2]. BPSD occurs in over 90% of individuals with dementia at some point during the course of the illness and is noted across the various etiologies for dementia [3]. The various symptoms and behaviors that are seen among individuals with BPSD include agitation, aggression, depression, anxiety, apathy, psychosis (delusions and hallucinations), night-time behaviors, disinhibition (socially and sexually inappropriate behaviors), motor disturbances along with appetite, and eating problems [4]. The most common form of BPSD is apathy which is followed by depression, aggression, anxiety, and sleep disturbances [5].

Current evidence indicates that the individual symptoms of BPSD often vary over time and with the etiology of dementia, with many of these symptoms also occurring together [6, 7]. It has also been recognized that the relationship between a particular symptom of BPSD and factors like age, sex, premorbid personality, severity of illness, and severity of cognitive impairment may not continue over time [8]. Additionally, the progression of the symptoms of BPSD may not be linear.

The presence of BPSD is associated with faster progression of the illness [9]. BPSD is also associated with greater morbidity and mortality rates among individuals with dementia. Admissions to acute care facilities and skilled nursing facilities increase with the occurrence of BPSD. BPSD is also associated with longer lengths of acute care hospital stay. It also results in increased caregiver distress and depression. One-third of the cost for caring of individuals with dementia is associated with BPSD, and it occurs due to greater utilization of health services among these individuals [10].

Risk Factors Including Neurobiology

It has been noted among individuals with BPSD that the prevalence of irritability, anxiety, agitation, and aggression increases as the severity of dementia worsens [11]. The prevalence of depression on the other hand appears to remain stable across the various stages of dementia severity.

R. R. Tampi (✉)
Department of Psychiatry, Creighton University School of Medicine, Omaha, NE, USA

Department of Psychiatry, Yale School of Medicine, New Haven, CT, USA

D. J. Tampi
Behavioral Health Advisory Group, Princeton, NJ, USA

R. R. Tampi, D. J. Tampi (eds.), *Treatment of Psychiatric Disorders Among Older Adults*, https://doi.org/10.1007/978-3-031-55711-8_6

Apathy is the most common BPSD among individuals with Alzheimer's disease (AD). It is followed by depression, anxiety, irritability, agitation, and aggression. Depression is the most common BPSD in vascular dementia (VaD) followed by agitation and aggression, apathy, anxiety, and irritability. Anxiety is the most common BPSD in dementia with Lewy bodies (DLB) followed by depression, irritability, agitation, and aggression. Agitation and aggression are the most common BPSD among individuals with FTD followed by anxiety, irritability, and depression.

Progressive neurodegeneration among individuals with dementia is known to be associated with the development of apathy [8]. Better executive function, working memory, and visual memory are all associated with lower levels of depression. The association between global cognitive impairment, cardiovascular comorbidities, and depression has shown mixed results. Male sex, younger age of the individual, and younger age of onset of AD have shown associations with the occurrence of agitation. Male gender, caregiver burden, sadness, loss of functional abilities, and premorbid neuroticism all have shown an association with the development of aggression.

BPSD occurs due to the interaction between biological, psychological, social, and environmental factors [4, 9, 12–14]. Among the biological factors, Nowrangi et al. found reduced cholinergic receptor binding in the left frontal cortex and lower binding of dopamine transporter among individuals with AD who present with apathy [12]. The authors also found reduced metabolic activity in the anterior cingulate and orbitofrontal cortices of these individuals. Increased white matter hyperintensity in the frontal cortex has been noted among individuals with apathy [12]. A reduction in 5-HT1A receptors in the brain has been noted among individuals presenting with depression in AD [12]. Individuals with depression in AD have been noted to have reduced noradrenergic neurons in locus coeruleus and serotoninergic neurons in the raphe nucleus. In addition, reduced levels of gamma amino butyric acid (GABA) and greater numbers of GABA (A) receptors have been noted in the brains of these individuals who present with reduced cortical thickness in the entorhinal cortex and greater atrophy in the anterior cingulate cortex [12, 13]. Individuals with depression in AD present with reduced cerebral glucose metabolism in the frontal and parietal cortices [12].

Among individuals with AD, agitation and aggression have been associated with 5-HT2A receptor gene polymorphisms [12]. Grey matter atrophy in bilateral anterior cingulate and in the left insula has been associated with agitation in AD. The severity of agitation among these individuals is correlated with greater atrophy of frontal cortex, insula, amygdala, cingulate gyrus, and hippocampal regions [12]. Agitation in AD is also correlated with reduced metabolic activity in both cingulate cortices, right lateral temporal cortex, and right lateral frontal cortex [12]. Grey matter atrophy in bilateral anterior cingulate and right middle frontal gyri has been found to be associated with disinhibition [12].

Increased dopamine D3 receptor density in the nucleus accumbens, greater availability of striatal dopamine (D2/D3), and reduced density of serotonin receptors in the prosubiculum and the ventral temporal cortex have been noted among individuals who present with psychosis in AD [12]. These individuals also present with reduced perfusion in the right angular gyrus and in the right occipital lobe. Atrophy in neocortical, lateral frontal, lateral parietal, and anterior cingulate gyrus has been associated with psychosis in AD [12, 13].

Undiagnosed medical disorders like pain, constipation, hypothyroidism, urinary tract infection, pneumonia, and constipation have been noted among one-third of individuals who present with BPSD [9]. These conditions may precipitate or perpetuate symptoms of BPSD.

An association has been noted between premorbid neuroticism and development of BPSD [14]. Premorbid extraversion, openness, agreeableness, and conscientiousness are thought to be protective against the development of BPSD.

Negative communication styles including a harsh tone of voice, being angry, and yelling have been noted to exacerbate the symptoms of BPSD [9]. The lack of understanding of the illness may result in unrealistic caregiver expectations and that may lead to frustration and tension between the caregiver and the individual with dementia. BPSD can be precipitated and/or perpetuated by changes in routine, changes in environment, and an under- or overstimulating environment.

The possible biological, psychological, social and environmental factors associated with BPSD have been discussed in Table 6.1.

Table 6.1 Factors possibly associated with BPSD [4, 9, 12–14]

Biological factors	Psychological factors
Depression – Dysfunctions in monoaminergic, noradrenergic, and gamma-aminobutyric acid (GABA) neurotransmission – Reduction of entorhinal cortex thickness, atrophy in anterior cingulum, and decreased cerebral glucose in frontal and parietal cortex **Apathy** – Reduced dopamine transporter binding and lower cholinergic receptor binding – Reduced metabolic activity in anterior cingulate and orbitofrontal cortex plus functional deficits in medial and inferior frontal cortical regions **Agitation and aggression** – Deficits in cholinergic neurotransmission, increased D2/D3 receptor availability, and deficits in monoaminergic (5-HT2A) neurotransmission – Atrophy of cingulum and frontal gyrus; atrophy of insula, amygdala, and hippocampus; and reduced metabolic activity in temporal and frontal cortices and the cingulum **Psychotic symptoms** – Greater availability of striatal dopamine (D2/D3) and greater dopamine D3 receptor density within the nucleus accumbens – Lower density of serotonin receptors in the ventral temporal cortex and prosubiculum plus increased ratio of acetylcholinesterase when compared to serotonin – Lower cerebral blood flow to the angular gyrus and the occipital cortex plus greater atrophy of the neocortex, frontal and parietal cortices, and the cingulum **Additional factors** – Polymorphisms of apolipoprotein E4 allele – Acute medical illness – Untreated pain – Comorbid psychiatric disorders	• Premorbid neuroticism has a significant association with the development of BPSD • Premorbid conscientiousness, extraversion, openness, and agreeableness appear to be protective factors
Social factors	**Environmental factors**
• Caregiver factors – Distress – Fatigue – Depression – Non-empathetic caregiving style – Unrealistic expectations – Negative communication style • Limited financial and caregiver resources	• Inadequate living arrangements • Lack of daily routine or structure • Under- or overstimulation • Lack of exposure to sunlight

Assessment

When assessing individuals with BPSD, the evaluator should obtain a thorough psychiatric history [15]. In addition, comprehensive medical, family, personal, and social histories should be obtained. This should be followed by a complete mental status examination. A focused physical examination and appropriate laboratory evaluation will aid with identifying the underlying medical and/or neurological disorders that can precipitate or exacerbate BPSD including neurovascular disorders [16]. Collateral information that is obtained from family members, caregivers, and medical providers will assist with identifying the onset and course of BPSD [15]. In addition, this information will assist with identifying possible etiologies, risk factors, and prognostic factors for BPSD. There should also be a thorough assessment of environmental, caregiver, and other psychosocial factors as these can precipitate or exacerbate BPSD. The symptoms of BPSD can be quantified and qualified with the use of validated screening measures. Although there is no clear evidence for the superiority of any one screening instrument over the other, the Neuropsychiatric Interview-Clinician (NPI-C) stands out as the most efficient measure [17]. The DICE (describe, investigate, create, and evaluate) is an evidence-based and structured protocol for the assessment and management of individuals with BPSD [3, 18]. Figure 6.1 describes the assessment of BPSD.

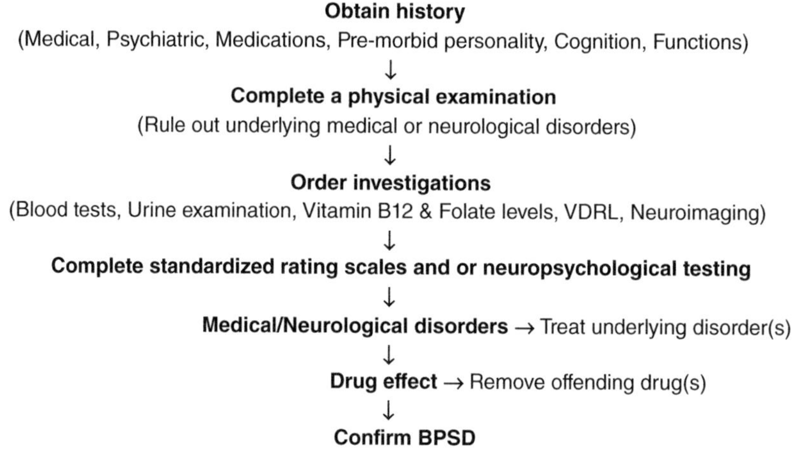

Fig. 6.1 Assessment of individuals with BPSD

Treatments

There are a number of studies that have evaluated the efficacy and tolerability of non-pharmacological and pharmacological strategies in the treatment of BPSD [9]. Non-pharmacological treatments are recommended as a first-line option for the treatment of BPSD in most situations [19].

Non-pharmacological

Brodaty and Arasartnam in their meta-analysis found that skill training for caregivers, education of caregivers, activity planning and environmental design, enhancing support for caregivers, self-care technique for caregivers, and collaborative care not only reduced the frequency and severity of BPSD (effect size = 0.34, $P < 0.01$), but also reduced the caregiver burden (effect size = 0.15, $P = 0.006$) [20]. These interventions lasted between 6 weeks and 24 months with a follow-up duration from 3 to 24 months.

In their network meta-analysis (NMA), Watt et al. found that among individuals with dementia who have agitation and aggression, multidisciplinary care [standardized mean difference (SMD) = −0.5], massage and touch therapy (SMD = −0.75), and music combined with massage and touch therapy (SMD = −0.91) were more efficacious clinically than usual care [21]. Recreation therapy was not found to be clinically more efficacious than usual care (SMD = −0.29). For combined aggression and agitation, and for physical aggression, the surface under the cumulative ranking curve (SUCRA) indicated that outdoor activities were the highest ranked treatment (SUCRA = 95%). Outdoor activities and massage and touch therapy were the highest ranked treatment for verbal aggression (SUCRA = 92%). The highest-ranking treatment for physical agitation (SUCRA = 90%) was exercise combined with activities of daily living (ADL) modification.

Leng et al. found that in a pairwise meta-analysis, when compared to control groups, benefits were noted for massage therapy [standardized mean difference *(SMD)* = −0.77], animal-assisted intervention (SMD = −0.47), personally tailored intervention (SMD = −0.39), and pet robot intervention (SMD = −0.38) [22]. For agitation in dementia, in a network meta-analysis, the investigators noted significant effects for massage therapy (SMD = −5.220), light therapy (SMD = −5.25), music therapy (SMD = −3.61), reminiscence therapy (SMD = −4.59), animal-assisted intervention (SMD = −3.14), and personally tailored intervention (SMD = −2.98). The probability of the efficacy for the management of agitation in dementia found massage therapy to be ranked 1 (43%) followed by animal-assisted intervention at rank 2 (16%), personally tailored intervention at rank 3 (18%), and pet robot intervention at rank 4 (11%). The duration of intervention period ranged from 10 days to 15 months, and the frequency of interventions ranged from 1 time a week to 21 times a week. The duration of each session ranged from 5 to 120 min.

In their meta-analysis, Meng et al. found that among individuals with BPSD, there was a small but significant benefit (SMD = −0.12, $P = 0.01$) noted for non-pharmacological interventions [23]. In addition, benefits of these interventions were also noted during the follow-up period of 10–96 weeks (SMD = −0.24, $P = 0.002$). Benefits were noted for caregiver reactions to BPSD (SMD = −0.27, $P = 0.001$). Tailored interventions that involved activities catering to the abilities and interests of individual with BPSD or the offer of education and support to the caregivers were more effective than standardized intervention (SMD = −0.24, $P = 0.04$) in reducing BPSD. The duration of these interventions ranged from 1 to 48 weeks, and the number of sessions ranged from 4 to 75.

The International Delphi consensus found the DICE (describe, investigate, create, and evaluate) approach and music therapy to be the most promising non-pharmacologic treatments for the management of BPSD [18]. The DICE approach evaluates BPSD using a structured method, which includes the assessment of underlying causes, planning of care, and follow-up monitoring along with the training and empowerment of caregivers [18].

Pharmacological

Atypical Antipsychotics

Efficacy

Kirkham et al. in their meta-analysis found that antipsychotics are commonly used among individuals with dementia with a pooled prevalence of 27.5% for any antipsychotic use [24]. Antipsychotic use is greater among individuals living at long-term care facilities when compared to persons living in the community (37.5% vs. 12.3%, $P < 0.001$) and among individuals with severe dementia when compared to individuals with mild or moderate dementia (45.1% vs. 6.7% vs. 12.2%, $P < 0.001$).

Although there are multiple studies evaluating the efficacy of atypical antipsychotics for the management of BPSD, only brexpiprazole is Food and Drug Administration (FDA) approved for the treatment of agitation among individuals with AD dementia in the United States [25]. In Australia, Canada, New Zealand, and the United Kingdom, risperidone is licensed for the treatment of severe BPSD [26].

The meta-analysis by Ballard and Waite found that risperidone had modest benefit in treating symptoms of BPSD including aggression and psychosis [27]. Olanzapine was found to be beneficial in treating aggression, anxiety, euphoria, and elation. Aripiprazole on the other hand was found to be beneficial in treating psychosis. Schneider et al. in their meta-analysis found efficacy for aripiprazole on the Brief Psychiatric Rating Scale (BPRS) and the Neuropsychiatric Inventory (NPI) change scores [28]. Benefits for aripiprazole were also noted on the Cohen-Mansfield Agitation Inventory (CMAI). Olanzapine did not show any benefit on the BPRS or NPI change scores. One trial of quetiapine showed benefit on the Clinical Global Impression of Change (CGIC), but no benefit on the Excited

Component of the Positive and Negative Syndrome Scale (PANSS-EC). Quetiapine did not show any benefit on the NPI psychosis subscale. Benefits on the Behavioral Pathology in Alzheimer's Disease Rating Scale (BEHAVE-AD), CMAI, and BEHAVE-AD psychosis subscale were noted for risperidone, but there were no benefits noted on the NPI psychosis subscale or the Clinical Global Impression Severity (CGIS) scale.

Yunusa et al. in their network meta-analysis (NMA) found that only aripiprazole was associated with improvements on the NPI when compared to placebo [29]. Improvements on the BPRS were noted for aripiprazole and quetiapine when compared to placebo. Improvements on the CMAI were identified for aripiprazole and risperidone when compared to placebo.

Pimavanserin, a selective 5-hydroxytryptamine (HT) 2A receptor inverse agonist/antagonist, is approved for the treatment of hallucinations and delusions associated with Parkinson's disease psychosis (PDP) in the United States [30, 31]. One RCT with two published papers evaluated the efficacy of pimavanserin (34 mg/day) for 12 weeks compared to placebo for the treatment of psychosis among individuals with AD [32, 33]. Benefit was noted for pimavanserin on the Neuropsychiatric Inventory-Nursing Home Version psychosis score (NPI-NH-PS) when compared to placebo at week 6, but not at week 12. Benefits were also noted for both hallucination and delusions among individuals with more severe symptoms at baseline (NPI-NH-PS ≥ 12). At 6 weeks or 12 weeks, the NPI-NH total scores did not differ between the two pimavanserin and placebo groups among individuals with mild psychotic symptoms (NPI-NH-PS < 12).

There are two randomized, double-blind, placebo-controlled, and parallel-arm studies that evaluated the use of brexpiprazole, an atypical antipsychotic that acts as a partial agonist at the serotonin 5-HT$_{1A}$ and dopamine D$_2$ receptors and as an antagonist at the serotonin 5-HT$_{2A}$ and noradrenaline α_{1B}/α_{2C} receptors among individuals with AD who present with agitation [34]. In the first study, participants were randomized to brexpiprazole 2 mg/day, brexpiprazole 1 mg/day, or placebo for 12 weeks. Benefit was noted for brexpiprazole 2 mg but not for 1 mg dosing on the CMAI total score when compared to placebo. There were no benefits noted for brexpiprazole 2 mg or 1 mg on the CGI-S. In the second study, participants were randomized to flexibly dosed brexpiprazole 0.5–2 mg/day or placebo for 12 weeks [34]. The investigators did not notice any benefits for brexpiprazole 0.5–2 mg dosing on the CMAI total score. However, on post hoc analyses, benefits on the CGI-S were noted among individuals who were titrated to brexpiprazole 2 mg/day dosing over the 4-week period. Brexpiprazole became the first drug to receive approval from the FDA for the treatment of agitation among individuals with AD dementia.

Adverse Effects

In this section, we review the data on major adverse effects (death, cerebrovascular adverse events (CVAEs), and decline in cognition) among individuals with dementia who were prescribed atypical antipsychotics.

The FDA in 2005 issued a public health advisory that there is an associated increase in mortality when individuals with BPSD are treated with atypical (second-generation) antipsychotics: aripiprazole, olanzapine, quetiapine, risperidone, clozapine, and ziprasidone [35]. The FDA identified 15 studies that indicated that there was a numerical increase in mortality among individuals treated with these drugs when compared to individuals receiving placebo. Most of the deaths were due to either heart-related events (e.g., heart failure and sudden death) or infections (mostly pneumonia). The manufacturers of these drugs were notified by the FDA to include a Boxed Warning in their labeling that described the risks and indicating that these drugs are not approved for the treatment of BPSD. The FDA subsequently extended the Boxed Warning to all antipsychotics [36].

Schneider et al. in their meta-analysis found that among individuals with BPSD, the odds of death were greater among individuals randomized to receive atypical antipsychotics when compared to those individuals receiving placebo [37]. There was no heterogeneity noted between trials of individuals with higher cognitive function (i.e., Mini-Mental State Examination score

>10) when compared to those with lower cognitive function, among individuals with psychosis of AD when compared with those trials that did not include individuals with psychosis, and among trials of inpatients when compared to outpatients.

Zhai et al. in their meta-analysis found that the risk of death was higher among individuals with AD who were prescribed antipsychotics when compared to those individuals who were not receiving antipsychotics [38]. The risk for mortality was similar among individuals with AD who were prescribed a typical versus atypical antipsychotics.

The NMA by Yunusa et al. found that none of the atypical antipsychotics are significantly different from placebo or from each other in the risk for death when they are used for the treatment of BPSD [29]. However, the SUCRA indicated that when compared to placebo, risperidone had the highest probability of safety on the mortality outcome followed by aripiprazole, quetiapine, and olanzapine.

Herrmann and Lanctot in their post hoc analyses found that the incidence rates for exposure-adjusted cerebrovascular adverse events (CVAEs) were significantly greater in the olanzapine group compared to the placebo group [39]. Among the risperidone-treated individuals, the rate of serious CVAEs, i.e., those causing death, life-threatening, requiring hospitalization, and leading to persistent disability, was greater when compared to the individuals receiving placebo. However, this difference was not statistically significant. The investigators found that the rates of nonserious CVAEs were significantly higher in the risperidone-treated group compared to the placebo group.

The meta-analysis Rao et al. found no significant difference in the relative risk (RR) for cerebrovascular accident (CVA) or stroke among individuals with dementia who were prescribed atypical vs. typical antipsychotics [40]. There were no differences noted for the risk for CVA among individuals with dementia who received atypical antipsychotics when compared to those not on any antipsychotics.

Yunusa et al. in their NMA found that olanzapine and risperidone were associated with a significantly greater risk of CVAEs when compared to placebo [29]. This risk was not found to be associated with aripiprazole or quetiapine. The investigators found that the risk of CVAEs was not significantly different between the antipsychotics. The highest probability of safety for CVAEs was for aripiprazole when compared to placebo. This was followed by quetiapine, risperidone, and olanzapine.

In the CATIE-AD trial, it was noted that there was a decline in cognition among individuals with AD who were treated with olanzapine, quetiapine, or risperidone when compared to individuals receiving placebo on multiple cognitive measures (Mini-Mental State Examination (MMSE), the BPRS cognitive subscale, and a cognitive summary score summarizing a change on 18 cognitive tests) [41].

In their meta-analysis, Wolf et al. found that the use of atypical antipsychotics resulted in cognitive worsening when compared to placebo [42]. The investigators found that the longer the duration of the trial, the greater was the cognitive impairment. They also noted that the higher the baseline cognition as measured by the MMSE, there was an associated greater decline in cognition with antipsychotic treatment.

Withdrawal

In a meta-analysis, Declercq et al. found that withdrawal of antipsychotics among individuals with dementia may not always result in a worsening of BPSD [43]. Individuals who presented with higher baseline BPSD symptoms benefited from the continuation of medications for 12 weeks. Two studies indicate that the withdrawal of antipsychotics among individuals with BPSD who had responded to treatment with antipsychotics for agitation or psychosis resulted in a higher risk for and shorter time to relapse of symptoms.

The meta-analysis by Pan et al. identified that among individuals with BPSD, the withdrawal of antipsychotics caused an increase in severity of BPSD [44]. However, this result was not statistically significant. There were a greater proportion of individuals who had a worsening of BPSD symptoms in the antipsychotic withdrawal group, and this result was statistically significant. The antipsychotic withdrawal group also had a greater proportion of participants with early study termination, but this result was not statistically significant. A lower proportion of participants died during the study period of 4 weeks to 1 year in the antipsychotic withdrawal group, but this result was not statistically significant.

Tariot et al. found that among individuals with psychosis related to AD, Parkinson's disease dementia (PDD), dementia with Lewy bodies (DLB), frontotemporal dementia (FTD), or vascular dementia (VaD) who had responded to pimavanserin, a switch to placebo caused an increase in likelihood of recurrence of psychosis when compared to individuals who were continued on pimavanserin [45]. The investigators found no significant differences in the rates of adverse effects between the two groups.

Acetylcholinesterase Inhibitors

Trinh et al. in their meta-analysis found that individuals with dementia who received acetylcholinesterase inhibitors did better by 1.72 points on the NPI scale when compared to individuals who received placebo [46]. Although small, this was a statistically significant benefit. In terms of improvements on the NPI, there was no difference noted between any of the three acetylcholinesterase inhibitors (donepezil, rivastigmine, and galantamine) when compared to placebo. This meta-analysis did not include tolerability data for the acetylcholinesterase inhibitors.

Memantine

Maidment et al. in their meta-analysis found that individuals who received memantine improved on the NPI scale by 1.99 points when compared to those individuals receiving placebo [47]. This was a small but statistically significant benefit ($P = 0.04$). This meta-analysis did not include tolerability data for memantine.

Antidepressants

In their meta-analysis, Seitz et al. found that individuals with dementia who received sertraline and fluoxetine did better than individuals receiving placebo on the CMAI (mean difference (MD) = −0.89, P < 0.001) [48]. There was no difference noted between the two groups on withdrawal due to adverse effects (RR = 1.07).

Anticonvulsants/Mood Stabilizers

Xiao et al. in their meta-analysis found that individuals with AD receiving mood stabilizers (valproate/divalproex, carbamazepine, and lithium) had a worsening on the NPI total score when compared to placebo (WMD = 3.71, P = 0.04) [49]. No effects were noted for the mood stabilizers on the BPRS total score (WMD = 0.83, P = 0.55), the CMAI total score (WMD = 5.09, P = 0.58), or the NPI/BPRS agitation subscale score (SMD = 0.30, P = 0.53) when compared to placebo. A decline on the MMSE scores with the use of mood stabilizers when compared to placebo (WMB = -0.89, P = 0.03) was also noted in this study.

Baillon et al. in their meta-analysis found that on the total BPRS scores, there was no difference noted between the valproate and placebo groups after 6 weeks of treatment (MD = 0.23) [50]. A meta-analysis of three studies of divalproex indicated that there were higher rates of adverse effects among individuals receiving divalproex sodium when compared to individuals receiving placebo (OR = 2.02).

Cannabinoids

A meta-analysis by Bhaji et al. found benefits for cannabinoids on the CMAI (SMD = −0.80), the NPI total score (SMD = −0.61), the NPI-Agitation/Aggression sub-score (SMD = −0.61), and the nocturnal motor activity scores (SMD = −1.05) [51]. The following associations were also noted: (1) larger effect size among individuals with higher baseline MMSE for the CMAI (P = 0.001), (2) larger greater effect sizes for older studies on the CMAI (P = 0.003), and (3) larger effect sizes for higher total daily doses of cannabinoids for the NPI total score (P < 0.001). On the NPI total and NPI-Agitation/Aggression sub-scores, larger effect sizes were noted for quasi-randomized studies when compared to randomized trial score (P = 0.001 and P = 0.047, respectively). Lethargy was the only adverse effect that was noted to be potentially related to cannabinoid use. As for changes in weight, systolic blood pressure, or diastolic blood pressure, there were relatively few reports. There were no reports of serious adverse events.

In their meta-analysis, Kuharic et al. did not find any benefit on the NPI/NPI-NH (MD = −1.97) for cannabinoids when compared to placebo [52]. Sedation/lethargy was more common among individuals on nabilone when compared to placebo (OR = 2.83). There were no other differences noted between the cannabinoids and placebo in other adverse effects.

Prazosin

Tampi et al. in their systematic review found that there was only one small published randomized controlled trial (RCT) of 22 individuals with AD that evaluated the use of prazosin among individuals with BPSD [53]. In this 8-week study, among individuals who completed the study, individuals receiving prazosin did better on the NPI and BPRS (P = 0.12 and P = 0.36, respectively) at the end of the study when compared to individuals receiving placebo. At the end of the study, the differences in CGIC between the prazosin and placebo groups were also statistically significant (P = 0.011). In the placebo group, 6 of the 11 participants showed some worsening of symptoms when compared to the prazosin group where all the participants were either doing the same or showing improvements. When compared to placebo, prazosin was well tolerated with no significant differences noted between the two groups on blood pressure changes, sedation, and hallucinations.

Propranolol

In a review of the literatures, Tampi et al. found a total of three case series; one randomized controlled trial and one case report were identified that evaluated the use of propranolol for the management of BPSD [54]. These studies indicated that propranolol improves BPSD, including agitation and aggression. Additionally, propranolol was found to be well tolerated with no significant bradycardia or hypotension noted among these studies.

Repetitive Transcranial Magnetic Stimulation (rTMS)

The meta-analysis by Vacas et al. found benefits for rTMS, among individuals with BPSD (overall effect = −0.58, P = 0.01) [55]. The only adverse effect noted from rTMS was minor tiredness.

Electroconvulsive Therapy (ECT)

van Den Berg in the systematic review noted clinical improvements in 88% of the individuals with BPSD who received ECT [56]. Symptoms that responded to ECT included agitation, aggression, yelling/screaming, and food intake. Maintenance ECT was recommended for 48% of the initial responders to ECT. The adverse effects were often mild and transient. Delirium (5%), severe postictal confusion (2%), and seizure (1%) were uncommon adverse effects.

A literature review by Tampi et al. identified 20 published reports on the use of ECT for BPSD [57]. Majority of these were case reports (40%), followed by retrospective chart reviews (25%) and case series (20%). The authors only identified one prospective cohort study, one case-control study, and one prospective observational study. The most common etiology for dementia in these reports was AD (40%) followed by unspecified dementia (15%) and vascular dementia (13%). The most common electrode placement was bitemporal, which was followed by right unilateral and bilateral electrode place-

ments. Over 90% of the individuals with BPSD had a positive response to ECT including those individuals with physical aggression and suicidal behaviors. The authors noted that adverse effects were uncommon. If adverse effects did occur, they were transient and mild. The most common adverse effects were postictal confusion/memory impairment seen in 15% of the individuals.

Evidence-Based Treatment Algorithm for Treating BPSD

There is growing evidence that indicates that non-pharmacological treatments including patient-centered care (PCC) should be considered first-line treatments for BPSD as there is significant evidence for their feasibility and benefits in this population. Available evidence indicates that the use of pharmacotherapy for the treatment of BPSD is constrained by the modest efficacy of these medications and the risk of serious adverse effects associated with their use.

Available evidence indicates that the use of pharmacotherapeutic agents has shown modest efficacy in the treatment of symptoms of BPSD including aggression, anxiety, euphoria, elation, agitation, and psychosis. However, there is no clear evidence for the superiority of any individual drug class over the others. Based on the available evidence, pharmacotherapy should only be used among individuals with BPSD when the symptoms are either severe or refractory and where non-pharmacological treatments either have failed to produce the desired benefit or are not safe or feasible to use given the urgency of the situation. Even in such situations, medications should be used at the minimum effective doses and for the shortest possible time period to manage the symptoms. The choice of medication is often determined by the urgency of the situation, the cluster of symptoms that are present, medical and psychiatric comorbidities, risk factors for adverse effects (e.g., CVAEs in VaD), evidence from previous medication trials in the individual, and the individual and/or caregiver choice.

The use of atypical antipsychotics in this population can be associated with serious adverse effects including greater risk for death, CVAEs, and possible cognitive decline. These adverse effects do not appear to be an individual drug effect, rather than a drug class effect and an age effect. Data, although limited, indicates that these adverse effects are more common at higher drug doses and when these drugs are used for longer periods of time.

There should always be regular benefit versus risk evaluations with close monitoring of risk factors and adverse effects with the use of these medications. Additionally, when using atypical antipsychotics among individuals with BPSD, it is prudent for clinicians to follow national guidelines like the American Psychiatric Association (APA) practice guideline or the European Academy of Neurology guidelines when prescribing these medications [58, 59].

Judicious combination of medications can be tried if symptoms of BPSD do not respond adequately to single-medication trials. Injudicious combinations of medications such as multiple medications of different classes should be avoided in order to minimize serious adverse effects. The medications that are ineffective in managing the symptoms must be tapered and discontinued, prior to starting any new medication trial. After about 3–4 months of clinical stability, the effective medication or medication combination can be tapered and discontinued if clinically feasible. In a significant number of individuals with BPSD, multiple different medication trials are often required either as monotherapy or in combination prior to achieving symptom control. In situations where the symptoms of BPSD are refractory to other medication classes, the use of cannabinoids, rTMS, or ECT should be seriously considered.

Figures 6.2 and 6.3 describe the proposed algorithms in the treatment of BPSD. Table 6.2 lists the medications and their doses that can used in the treatment of BPSD.

Fig. 6.2 Algorithm for treating emergent BPSD

Offer Risperidone: 0.25 mg-1.0 mg dose

Or Aripiprazole 2.0-5.0 mg dose

Or Quetiapine 25 mg-50 mg dose

or Olanzapine 2.5 mg-5 mg dose

Can repeat the dose in 30 min-60 min if needed

May need 1-2 repeat doses before the patient responds. **Avoid Benzos!**

❖ **If patient is refusing oral medications and is very agitated or aggressive**

Give IM Olanzapine: 2.5 mg-5.0 mg dose

Or IM Haloperidol: 0.5 mg-2.0 mg dose

Can repeat dose in 30 min-60 min if needed

May need 1-2 repeat doses before the patient responds. **Avoid Benzos!**

Fig. 6.3 Algorithm for treating non-emergent BPSD

- Start treatment with a cholinesterase inhibitor
- Add memantine if the patient has moderate to severe dementia
- If agitation persists, consider trial of SSRIs (sertraline or citalopram)
- If SSRI trials fail, consider trazodone
- If trazodone trial fails, consider brexpiprazole or risperidone or aripiprazole
- If risperidone and aripiprazole trials fail, consider quetiapine
- If quetiapine trial fails, use olanzapine
- If olanzapine trial fails, use carbamazepine
- If carbamazepine trial fails, consider propranolol or prazosin
- If propranolol and prazosin trials fail, consider cannabinoids
- If cannabinoid trial fails, try rTMS
- If rTMS trial fails, try ECT
- Consider combination therapy ONLY if monotherapy trials suboptimal*

Table 6.2 Medications for the management of BPSD

Class of medication	Name of medication and dosages
Antipsychotics	• Aripiprazole: 2 mg–10 mg/day • Olanzapine: 2.5 mg–10 mg/day • Quetiapine: 25 mg–200 mg/day • Risperidone: 0.25 mg–2 mg/day
Antidepressants	• Citalopram: 10 mg–20 mg/day • Escitalopram: 5 mg–20 mg/day • Mirtazapine: 7.5 mg–45 mg/day • Sertraline: 25 mg–200 mg/day
Mood stabilizers	• Carbamazepine: 200 mg–400 mg/day • Divalproex sodium: 250 mg–1000 mg/day • Oxcarbazepine: 300 mg–600 mg/day
Cognitive enhancers	• Donepezil: 5 mg–10 mg/day • Galantamine: 8 mg–24 mg/day • Rivastigmine: 3 mg–12 mg/day • Memantine: 10 mg–20 mg/day
Prazosin	• 1–6 mg/day
Propranolol	• 60–560 mg/day

Conclusions

BPSD is a group of noncognitive symptoms and behaviors that are commonly seen among individuals with dementia. Available evidence indicates that BPSD is associated with poorer outcomes among individuals with dementia and their caregivers. The neurobiology of BPSD indicates a complex interplay between the biological, psychological, social, and environmental factors. The assessment of individuals with BPSD should include a comprehensive history, focused physical examination, laboratory testing, and use of standardized rating scales to quantify and qualify the symptoms. Additionally, there should be a thorough evaluation of comorbid conditions, environmental stressors, and psychosocial factors that can precipitate and perpetuate the symptoms. The cornerstone for the treatment of individuals with BPSD is non-pharmacological interventions. Pharmacotherapy should only be used in situations where non-pharmacological interventions have been ineffective or are not feasible. There should also be close monitoring of risk factors and adverse effects to minimize negative outcomes when pharmacotherapy is being used to treat BPSD. Furthermore, the minimum effective doses of medications should be used for the shortest possible time period. For refractory BPSD, the use of cannabinoids, rTMS or ECT should be considered. Best results are often noted when pharmacotherapy is combined with non-pharmacological treatment strategies.

References

1. Cerejeira J, Lagarto L, Mukaetova-Ladinska EB. Behavioral and psychological symptoms of dementia. Front Neurol. 2012;3:73.
2. Bharucha AJ, Rosen J, Mulsant BH, Pollock BG. Assessment of behavioral and psychological symptoms of dementia. CNS Spectr. 2002;7(11):797–802.
3. Kales HC, Gitlin LN, Lyketsos CG, Detroit Expert Panel on Assessment and Management of Neuropsychiatric Symptoms of Dementia. Management of neuropsychiatric symptoms of dementia in clinical settings: recommendations from a multidisciplinary expert panel. J Am Geriatr Soc. 2014;62(4):762–9.
4. Kales HC, Gitlin LN, Lyketsos CG. Assessment and management of behavioral and psychological symptoms of dementia. BMJ. 2015;350:h369.
5. Zhao QF, Tan L, Wang HF, Jiang T, Tan MS, Tan L, Xu W, Li JQ, Wang J, Lai TJ, Yu JT. The prevalence of neuropsychiatric symptoms in Alzheimer's disease: systematic review and meta-analysis. J Affect Disord. 2016;190:264–71.
6. Vik-Mo AO, Giil LM, Ballard C, Aarsland D. Course of neuropsychiatric symptoms in dementia: 5-year longitudinal study. Int J Geriatr Psychiatry. 2018;33(10):1361–9.
7. Savva GM, Zaccai J, Matthews FE, Davidson JE, McKeith I, Brayne C, Medical Research Council Cognitive Function and Ageing Study. Prevalence, correlates and course of behavioural and psychological symptoms of dementia in the population. Br J Psychiatry. 2009;194(3):212–9.
8. Kolanowski A, Boltz M, Galik E, Gitlin LN, Kales HC, Resnick B, Van Haitsma KS, Knehans A, Sutterlin JE, Sefcik JS, Liu W, Petrovsky DV, Massimo L, Gilmore-Bykovskyi A, MacAndrew M, Brewster G, Nalls V, Jao YL, Duffort N, Scerpella D. Determinants of behavioral and psychological symptoms of dementia: a scoping review of the evidence. Nurs Outlook. 2017;65(5):515–29.
9. Gerlach LB, Kales HC. Managing behavioral and psychological symptoms of dementia. Clin Geriatr Med. 2020;36(2):315–27.
10. Beeri MS, Werner P, Davidson M, Noy S. The cost of behavioral and psychological symptoms of dementia (BPSD) in community dwelling Alzheimer's disease patients. Int J Geriatr Psychiatry. 2002;17(5):403–8.
11. Kwon CY, Lee B. Prevalence of behavioral and psychological symptoms of dementia in community-dwelling dementia patients: a systematic review. Front Psych. 2021;12:741059.
12. Nowrangi MA, Lyketsos CG, Rosenberg PB. Principles and management of neuropsychiatric symptoms in Alzheimer's dementia. Alzheimers Res Ther. 2015;7(1):12.
13. Ambrogio F, Martella LA, Odetti P, Monacelli F. Behavioral disturbances in dementia and beyond: time for a new conceptual frame? Int J Mol Sci. 2019;20(15):3647.
14. Young JJ, Balachandran S, Garg G, Balasubramaniam M, Gupta A, Tampi DJ, Tampi RR. Personality and the risk factors for developing behavioral and psychological symptoms of dementia: a narrative review. Neurodegener Dis Manag. 2019;9(2):107–18.
15. Bessey LJ, Walaszek A. Management of behavioral and psychological symptoms of dementia. Curr Psychiatry Rep. 2019;21(8):66.
16. Wolinsky D, Drake K, Bostwick J. Diagnosis and management of neuropsychiatric symptoms in Alzheimer's disease. Curr Psychiatry Rep. 2018;20(12):117.
17. Gitlin LN, Marx KA, Stanley IH, Hansen BR, Van Haitsma KS. Assessing neuropsychiatric symptoms in people with dementia: a systematic review of measures. Int Psychogeriatr. 2014;26(11):1805–48.
18. Kales HC, Lyketsos CG, Miller EM, Ballard C. Management of behavioral and psychological symptoms in people with Alzheimer's disease: an international Delphi consensus. Int Psychogeriatr. 2019;31(1):83–90.
19. Dyer SM, Harrison SL, Laver K, Whitehead C, Crotty M. An overview of systematic reviews of pharmacological and non-pharmacological interventions for the treatment of behavioral and psychological symptoms of dementia. Int Psychogeriatr. 2018;30(3):295–309.
20. Brodaty H, Arasaratnam C. Meta-analysis of non-pharmacological interventions for neuropsychiatric symptoms of dementia. Am J Psychiatry. 2012;169(9):946–53.
21. Watt JA, Goodarzi Z, Veroniki AA, Nincic V, Khan PA, Ghassemi M, Thompson Y, Tricco AC, Straus

SE. Comparative efficacy of interventions for aggressive and agitated behaviors in dementia: a systematic review and network meta-analysis. Ann Intern Med. 2019;171(9):633–42.

22. Leng M, Zhao Y, Wang Z. Comparative efficacy of non-pharmacological interventions on agitation in people with dementia: a systematic review and Bayesian network meta-analysis. Int J Nurs Stud. 2020;102:103489.

23. Meng X, Su J, Li H, Ma D, Zhao Y, Li Y, Zhang X, Li Z, Sun J. Effectiveness of caregiver non-pharmacological interventions for behavioural and psychological symptoms of dementia: an updated meta-analysis. Ageing Res Rev. 2021;71:101448.

24. Kirkham J, Sherman C, Velkers C, Maxwell C, Gill S, Rochon P, Seitz D. Antipsychotic use in dementia. Can J Psychiatr. 2017;62(3):170–81.

25. Tampi RR, Tampi DJ, Rogers K, Alagarsamy S. Antipsychotics in the management of behavioral and psychological symptoms of dementia: maximizing gain and minimizing harm. Neurodegener Dis Manag. 2020;10(1):5–8.

26. Yunusa I, El Helou ML. The use of risperidone in behavioral and psychological symptoms of dementia: a review of pharmacology, clinical evidence, regulatory approvals, and off-label use. Front Pharmacol. 2020;11:596.

27. Ballard C, Waite J. The effectiveness of atypical antipsychotics for the treatment of aggression and psychosis in Alzheimer's disease. Cochrane Database Syst Rev. 2006;(1):CD003476.

28. Schneider LS, Dagerman K, Insel PS. Efficacy and adverse effects of atypical antipsychotics for dementia: meta-analysis of randomized, placebo-controlled trials. Am J Geriatr Psychiatry. 2006;14(3):191–210.

29. Yunusa I, Alsumali A, Garba AE, Regestein QR, Eguale T. Assessment of reported comparative effectiveness and safety of atypical antipsychotics in the treatment of behavioral and psychological symptoms of dementia: a network meta-analysis. JAMA Netw Open. 2019;2(3):e190828.

30. Hacksell U, Burstein ES, McFarland K, Mills RG, Williams H. On the discovery and development of pimavanserin: a novel drug candidate for Parkinson's psychosis. Neurochem Res. 2014;39(10):2008–17.

31. Espay AJ, Guskey MT, Norton JC, Coate B, Vizcarra JA, Ballard C, Factor SA, Friedman JH, Lang AE, Larsen NJ, Andersson C, Fredericks D, Weintraub D. Pimavanserin for Parkinson's disease psychosis: effects stratified by baseline cognition and use of cognitive-enhancing medications. Mov Disord. 2018;33(11):1769–76.

32. Ballard C, Banister C, Khan Z, Cummings J, Demos G, Coate B, Youakim JM, Owen R, Stankovic S, Investigators ADP. Evaluation of the safety, tolerability, and efficacy of pimavanserin versus placebo in patients with Alzheimer's disease psychosis: a phase 2, randomised, placebo-controlled, double-blind study. Lancet Neurol. 2018;17(3):213–22.

33. Ballard C, Youakim JM, Coate B, Stankovic S. Pimavanserin in Alzheimer's disease psychosis: efficacy in patients with more pronounced psychotic symptoms. J Prev Alzheimers Dis. 2019;6(1):27–33.

34. Grossberg GT, Kohegyi E, Mergel V, Josiassen MK, Meulien D, Hobart M, Slomkowski M, Baker RA, McQuade RD, Cummings JL. Efficacy and safety of brexpiprazole for the treatment of agitation in Alzheimer's dementia: two 12-week, randomized, double-blind, placebo-controlled trials. Am J Geriatr Psychiatry. 2020;28(4):383–400.

35. Mittal V, Kurup L, Williamson D, Muralee S, Tampi RR. Risk of cerebrovascular adverse events and death in elderly patients with dementia when treated with antipsychotic medications: a literature review of evidence. Am J Alzheimers Dis Other Dement. 2011;26(1):10–28.

36. Rubino A, Sanon M, Ganz ML, Simpson A, Fenton MC, Verma S, Hartry A, Baker RA, Duffy RA, Gwin K, Fillit H. Association of the US Food and Drug Administration antipsychotic drug boxed warning with medication use and health outcomes in elderly patients with dementia. JAMA Netw Open. 2020;3(4):e203630.

37. Schneider LS, Dagerman KS, Insel P. Risk of death with atypical antipsychotic drug treatment for dementia: meta-analysis of randomized placebo-controlled trials. JAMA. 2005;294(15):1934–43.

38. Zhai Y, Yin S, Zhang D. Association between antipsychotic drugs and mortality in older persons with Alzheimer's disease: a systematic review and meta-analysis. J Alzheimers Dis. 2016;52(2):631–9.

39. Herrmann N, Lanctôt KL. Do atypical antipsychotics cause stroke? CNS Drugs. 2005;19(2):91–103. https://doi.org/10.2165/00023210-200519020-00001.

40. Rao A, Suliman A, Story G, Vuik S, Aylin P, Darzi A. Meta-analysis of population-based studies comparing risk of cerebrovascular accident associated with first- and second-generation antipsychotic prescribing in dementia. Int J Methods Psychiatr Res. 2016;25(4):289–98.

41. Vigen CL, Mack WJ, Keefe RS, Sano M, Sultzer DL, Stroup TS, Dagerman KS, Hsiao JK, Lebowitz BD, Lyketsos CG, Tariot PN, Zheng L, Schneider LS. Cognitive effects of atypical antipsychotic medications in patients with Alzheimer's disease: outcomes from CATIE-AD. Am J Psychiatry. 2011;168(8):831–9.

42. Wolf A, Leucht S, Pajonk FG. Do antipsychotics lead to cognitive impairment in dementia? A meta-analysis of randomised placebo-controlled trials. Eur Arch Psychiatry Clin Neurosci. 2017;267(3):187–98.

43. Declercq T, Petrovic M, Azermai M, Vander Stichele R, De Sutter AI, van Driel ML, Christiaens T. Withdrawal versus continuation of chronic antipsychotic drugs for behavioural and psychological symptoms in older people with dementia. Cochrane Database Syst Rev. 2013;(3):CD007726.

44. Pan YJ, Wu CS, Gau SS, Chan HY, Banerjee S. Antipsychotic discontinuation in patients with

dementia: a systematic review and meta-analysis of published randomized controlled studies. Dement Geriatr Cogn Disord. 2014;37(3–4):125–40.

45. Tariot PN, Cummings JL, Soto-Martin ME, Ballard C, Erten-Lyons D, Sultzer DL, Devanand DP, Weintraub D, McEvoy B, Youakim JM, Stankovic S, Foff EP. Trial of pimavanserin in dementia-related psychosis. N Engl J Med. 2021;385(4):309–19.

46. Trinh NH, Hoblyn J, Mohanty S, Yaffe K. Efficacy of cholinesterase inhibitors in the treatment of neuropsychiatric symptoms and functional impairment in Alzheimer disease: a meta-analysis. JAMA. 2003;289(2):210–6.

47. Maidment ID, Fox CG, Boustani M, Rodriguez J, Brown RC, Katona CL. Efficacy of memantine on behavioral and psychological symptoms related to dementia: a systematic meta-analysis. Ann Pharmacother. 2008;42(1):32–8.

48. Seitz DP, Adunuri N, Gill SS, Gruneir A, Herrmann N, Rochon P. Antidepressants for agitation and psychosis in dementia. Cochrane Database Syst Rev. 2011;(2):CD008191.

49. Xiao H, Su Y, Cao X, Sun S, Liang Z. A meta-analysis of mood stabilizers for Alzheimer's disease. J Huazhong Univ Sci Technolog Med Sci. 2010;30(5):652–8.

50. Baillon SF, Narayana U, Luxenberg JS, Clifton AV. Valproate preparations for agitation in dementia. Cochrane Database Syst Rev. 2018;10(10):CD003945.

51. Bahji A, Meyyappan AC, Hawken ER. Cannabinoids for the neuropsychiatric symptoms of dementia: a systematic review and meta-analysis. Can J Psychiatr. 2020;65(6):365–76.

52. Bosnjak Kuharic D, Markovic D, Brkovic T, Jeric Kegalj M, Rubic Z, Vuica Vukasovic A, Jeroncic A, Puljak L. Cannabinoids for the treatment of dementia. Cochrane Database Syst Rev. 2021;9(9):CD012820.

53. Tampi RR, Tampi DJ, Farheen SA, Adnan M, Dasarathy D. Prazosin for the management of behavioural and psychological symptoms of dementia. Drugs Context. 2022;11:2022-3-3.

54. Tampi RR, Tampi DJ, Farheen SA, Ochije SI, Joshi P. Propranolol for the management of behavioural and psychological symptoms of dementia. Drugs. Context. 2022;11:2022-8-3.

55. Vacas SM, Stella F, Loureiro JC, Simões do Couto F, Oliveira-Maia AJ, Forlenza OV. Noninvasive brain stimulation for behavioural and psychological symptoms of dementia: a systematic review and meta-analysis. Int J Geriatr Psychiatry. 2019;34(9):1336–45.

56. van den Berg JF, Kruithof HC, Kok RM, Verwijk E, Spaans HP. Electroconvulsive therapy for agitation and aggression in dementia: a systematic review. Am J Geriatr Psychiatry. 2018;26(4):419–34.

57. Tampi RR, Tampi DJ, Young J, Hoq R, Resnick K. The place for electroconvulsive therapy in the management of behavioral and psychological symptoms of dementia. Neurodegener Dis Manag. 2019;9:283–8.

58. Reus VI, Fochtmann LJ, Eyler AE, Hilty DM, Horvitz-Lennon M, Jibson MD, Lopez OL, Mahoney J, Pasic J, Tan ZS, Wills CD, Rhoads R, Yager J. The American Psychiatric Association practice guideline on the use of antipsychotics to treat agitation or psychosis in patients with dementia. Am J Psychiatry. 2016;173(5):543–6.

59. Frederiksen KS, Cooper C, Frisoni GB, Frölich L, Georges J, Kramberger MG, Nilsson C, Passmore P, Mantoan Ritter L, Religa D, Schmidt R, Stefanova E, Verdelho A, Vandenbulcke M, Winblad B, Waldemar G. A European Academy of Neurology guideline on medical management issues in dementia. Eur J Neurol. 2020;27(10):1805–20.

Badr Ratnakaran, Darlon Jan,
Laureen Raelly-Muze, Ty Owens,
and Sophia Wang

Introduction

Mild neurocognitive disorder (MiND) is defined as a transitional stage between healthy aging and dementia (also called major neurocognitive disorder, MND). Several other terms have been used to describe the cognitive impairments associated with this preclinical stage, including mild cognitive impairment (MCI), cognitive impairment no dementia (CIND), age-associated/consistent memory impairment, age-associated cognitive decline, benign senescent forgetfulness, questionable dementia, malignant senescent forgetfulness, and late-life forgetfulness [1]. Much of the literature on MiND has described the syndrome as MCI, and these terms will be used as approximate synonyms in this chapter. The criteria to determine the diagnosis of MiND have expanded over time from specifically diagnosing early memory impairments that precede the development of Alzheimer's dementia to diagnosing early signs of any mild cognitive symptoms that may progress to a wide range of neurodegenerative processes [2, 3]. The International Consensus Criteria for MCI correspond closely to the expanded Mayo Criteria [2], NIA-AA criteria, and "mild neurocognitive disorder" from the DSM-5 [4]. The key diagnostic criteria for the diagnosis of MCI include:

1. Cognitive decline, as determined by self and/or informant report and impairment on objective cognitive measures and/or decline in function over time on objective cognitive tasks
2. Preserved functioning in basic activities of daily living [activities of daily living (ADLs), e.g., eating, dressing, washing] and minimal interference with instrumental ADLs (IADLs) (e.g., managing finances, functioning outside familiar environments)

B. Ratnakaran (✉) · D. Jan
Department of Psychiatry, Carilion Clinic-Virginia Tech Carilion School of Medicine,
Roanoke, VA, USA

L. Raelly-Muze
Long School of Medicine, University of Texas Health Science Center at San Antonio,
San Antonia, TX, USA
e-mail: raellymuze@livemail.uthscsa.edu

T. Owens
Department of Neurology, Indiana University School of Medicine, Indianapolis, IN, USA
e-mail: owensty@iu.edu

S. Wang
Department of Psychiatry, Indiana University School of Medicine, Indianapolis, IN, USA

Department of Psychiatry, Indiana Alzheimer's Disease Research Center, Indiana University School of Medicine, Indianapolis, IN, USA
e-mail: sophwang@iupui.edu

© The Author(s), under exclusive license to Springer Nature Switzerland AG 2024
R. R. Tampi, D. J. Tampi (eds.), *Treatment of Psychiatric Disorders Among Older Adults*,
https://doi.org/10.1007/978-3-031-55711-8_7

Further diagnostic specification discriminates between the presence and absence of objective memory impairment (amnestic versus non-amnestic) and whether impairments are observed in single versus multiple cognitive domains (single domain versus multiple domains) [2]. The classification of MCI is labeled using both categorizations, resulting in four primary descriptions for MCI: amnestic MCI (aMCI) single domain, aMCI multiple domain, non-amnestic MCI (naMCI) single domain, and naMCI multiple domain.

The Diagnostic and Statistical Manual of Mental Disorders, Fifth Edition, Text Revision (DSM-5-TR), defines MiND as modest cognitive decline from baseline in one or more cognitive domains: complex attention, executive function, learning and memory, language, perceptual-motor, or social cognition [4]. This decline should be based on information from the patient, a knowledgeable informant, or a clinician, and with impairment in cognitive performance on standardized neuropsychological or other quantified clinical assessment. The decline should not interfere with the capacity to perform daily activities independently (e.g., paying bills, managing medications) and does not occur in the context of delirium or other psychiatric disorders. MiND includes MCI as well as diagnoses that used terms to define cognitive impairments associated with preclinical stage of MND as described above including age-associated cognitive decline and questionable dementia. MCI primarily applies to older adults, while MiND includes all age groups [1].

Epidemiology

Research into the prevalence of MiND varies as studies use retrospective, prospective, or cross-sectional study designs, various diagnostic criteria, or a variety of their adaptations [5]. In a recent meta-analysis of 66 articles, the overall prevalence of MiND was found to be 15.56% in community-dwelling adults aged 50 years and older [6]. The prevalence rates of aMCI and naMCI were found to be 10.3% and 8.72%, respectively. Gillis et al. in their systematic review found the incidence of MiND per 1000 years to be 22.5 for older adults aged 75–79 years, 40.9 for ages 80–84 years, and 60.1 for 85 years and above [7]. McGrattan et al., in their systematic review, found the prevalence of MiND in low- and middle-income countries ranging from 6.1% to 30.4%, with the prevalence of aMCI ranging from 0.6% to 22.3% [8]. The Mayo Clinic study of aging evaluated a random sample of nearly 3000 older adults aged 70–89 in Olmsted County, Minnesota, who were non-demented or had MiND at the time of study [9]. The prevalence of MiND in this study was 16% in the non-demented study participants with the ratio of aMCI to naMCI found to be 2:1. The LIFE-ADULT-Study assessed 1080 dementia-free older adults aged 60–79 years in Leipzig, Germany, and found the total prevalence of MiND to be 20.3% [10].

Etiology and Risk Factors

MiND was originally conceptualized as a precursor to Alzheimer's dementia [11]. However, not all cases of MiND progress to MND, and multiple other etiologies have been recognized as sources of mild cognitive decline, including vascular disease, Lewy body disease, frontotemporal degeneration, substance/medication use, traumatic brain injury, HIV infection, Parkinson's disease, and Huntington's disease [4]. While most sources of MCI are neurodegenerative and typically convert to MND, there are cases of MiND where treatable conditions (see Table 7.1) underly the cognitive impairment which, when addressed, can lead to the reversal of MiND back to normal cognition for age [12–14].

Following age as the largest risk for the conversion of MiND to MND, other important risk factors for developing MCI/MND are male sex, presence of apolipoprotein E4 allele genotype, family history of cognitive impairment, and vascular risk factors including hypertension and stroke [14]. These and other risk factors for developing MiND are provided in Table 7.2 [14–

Table 7.1 Reversible causes of MiND

Polypharmacy
Medications like benzodiazepines, anticholinergics, antihypertensives, steroid, and anticonvulsants
Hypotension
Depression
Late-onset schizophrenia
Endocrine disorders like hypo/hyperthyroidism and hypo/hyperparathyroidism
Collagen vascular diseases like systemic lupus erythematosus and sarcoidosis
Nutritional deficiencies including iron, vitamin B1, B12, and B6, and folate deficiency
Hypo/hyperglycemia
Dehydration
Visual/hearing loss
Obstructive sleep apnea
Chronic obstructive pulmonary disease
Normal pressure hydrocephalus
Central nervous system tumors and space-occupying lesions
Subdural hematoma
Infections like neurosyphilis, meningitis, HIV
Atrial fibrillation

Table 7.2 Risk factors for developing MiND

Older age
Male sex
Lower education status
Apoprotein E ε4 allele genotype
Family history of cognitive impairment
Hypertension
Hyperlipidemia
Coronary artery disease
Stroke
Obesity
Chronic obstructive pulmonary disease
Depression
Diabetes mellitus
Sedentary lifestyle

Table 7.3 Risk factors for conversion of MiND to MND

Older age
Amnestic type of mild cognitive impairment
Apolipoprotein E4 allele genotype
Cerebrovascular disease
Depression
Use of anticholinergic drugs
Insomnia
Social isolation
Global and medial temporal atrophy and increased rate of atrophy on neuroimaging
White matter hyperintensity volume on neuroimaging
Glucose hypometabolism in temporal and parietal lobes on PET scan
Lower levels of β-amyloid (1–42) (Aβ42) protein in cerebrospinal fluid
Elevated levels of total tau and phosphorylated tau protein in cerebrospinal fluid
Lower cognitive test scores
Higher Alzheimer's Disease Assessment Scale (ADAS) cognitive subscale scores

tion, it is 21.9% [19]. Based on the subtype MCI, aMCI subtype has been found to have 8.5 times higher risk of converting to MND when compared to naMCI group [20]. Other risk factors for conversion of MiND to MND are provided in Table 7.3 [17, 21–25]. A meta-analysis of community-based studies estimated the conversion rate of MiND to normal to be 25% [26]. However, conversion rates have been found to range from 8 to 59% due to differences in study methodology, sample size, definition of MiND, and follow-up period [27]. Important factors related to reversion to normal include impairment of cognition in a single domain, high cognitive test scores, absence of apolipoprotein E4 allele genotype, and greater hippocampus volume on neuroimaging [14].

Assessment

The diagnosis of MiND is mainly a clinical diagnosis, and laboratory testing or neuroimaging alone should not become the basis of the diagnosis. Essential components of history gathering include interview with the patient, interview with collateral sources (e.g., family, close friends who will have observed the patient's behavior), review

17]. Higher educational status has been found to be protective in developing MiND [18].

The annual rate of progression of patients with MiND to MND is 5–10% when compared to 1–2% of the incidence of MND per year in the general population [19]. Conversion rates from MiND to MND can vary based on definitions of MiND and the setting. The conversion rates in specialty settings like a memory disorder clinic are estimated to be 39.2%, and in general popula-

of relevant medical records, and review of neuropsychological testing. When characterizing the cognitive complaint, information is gathered about the initial presentation of symptoms, domain or domains of cognitive change experienced (e.g., memory loss, language, executive function), onset of symptoms (e.g., acute versus insidious/gradual, presence of co-occurring conditions that may correlate with onset), duration of symptoms, and progression of symptom course and severity. Informant interview is also essential as patients may lack awareness of their own cognitive and functional declines (i.e., anosognosia) or lack the ability to fully recall their history [28].

Care should also be taken to assess for reversible causes of MiND as listed in Table 7.1. A medication review, mental status examination, and a physical and neurological examination should be done during the encounter. Structural neuroimaging of the brain, such as MRI and CT scan, can help in assessing structural abnormalities related to MiND. MRI is preferable over CT scan due to its higher structural resolution, which can be useful for assessing abnormalities like white matter hyperintensities. Neuroimaging of the brain in patients with MiND due to Alzheimer's disease (AD) has shown findings of hippocampal, medial temporal atrophy, and entorhinal atrophy [29–31]. Patients with MiND and a hippocampal volume at or below 25th percentile have a high risk of progression to MND [32]. Volumetric changes on neuroimaging have been noted in the prefrontal cortex, anterior temporal regions, insula, anterior cingulate, and striatum in patients with MiND related to frontotemporal dementia (FTD) [33]. White matter hyperintensities in the brain or ischemic small-vessel changes are suggestive of vascular dementia (VaD), and presence of underlying medical conditions like normal-pressure hydrocephalus and central nervous system tumors can be assessed on neuroimaging. *Single-photon emission computed tomography* (SPECT) and fluorodeoxyglucose-positron emission tomography (FDG-PET) scans can identify areas of hypoperfusion and glucose hypometabolism in the brain, which can be early predictors of neurodegenerative pathologies, which underly MCI and dementia. Abnormalities particularly in the temporoparietal cortices are

known risk factors for conversion of MiND to MND [31]. FDG-PET scan is considered more sensitive than magnetic resonance imaging (MRI) and SPECT in detecting MiND [34, 35].

Biomarkers such as elevated cerebrospinal fluid (CSF) total tau and phosphorylated tau proteins, reduced CSF Aβ42 levels, and Aβ42 deposition in the brain on amyloid PET imaging have been helpful in the early detection of MiND related to AD [14]. However, there is a lack of standardization in techniques used to identify these biomarkers along with inconsistencies in cutoff points of these biomarkers for diagnosis [14]. The diagnostic cutoffs for many of these biomarkers have been mostly examined in research cohorts who are predominantly highly educated non-Hispanic White older adults with few medical or psychiatric comorbidities; therefore, it is not what the clinical implications are for more racially and ethnically diverse individuals with multiple comorbidities and living in communities with a higher area deprivation index. The European Union Joint Program—Neurodegenerative Disease Research—recommended that CSF biomarkers related to the diagnosis of MiND can be used to predict conversion to Alzheimer's disease 3 years later, but the group did not provide recommendations on the use of specific CSF biomarker as the evidence was limited to recommend a CSF biomarker over the other [36]. The Alzheimer's Association has recommended using PET scan in patients with progressive unexplained MiND, atypical presentation of possible AD, or early onset of progressive MND. They also recommended that the amyloid PET scan should not be used in asymptomatic individuals, typical presentation, and progression of MND, in patients identified with known apolipoprotein E allele, or to assess the severity of cognitive impairment [37].

In addition to neuroimaging and biomarker studies, several standardized clinical tools are available to help with diagnostic accuracy and consistency. The Clinical Dementia Rating (CDR) was developed to help standardize clinical staging of MND and summarizes in a single score changes in memory, orientation, judgment/problem-solving, engagement in community affairs (e.g., shopping, socializing), function at home/participation in hobbies, and personal care, with a global CDR score of 0.5 corresponding to MiND [38]. Other instruments elicit information about neuropsychiatric symptoms (e.g., agitation, hallucinations) via self-report questionnaire (NPI-Q) or brief structured interview (MINI) [39, 40]. Depression symptoms may cause mild cognitive symptoms, although mood changes may also reflect prodromal symptoms of neurodegenerative disease [41, 42]. Additionally, depression or anxiety may result from adjustment to loss of cognitive and adaptive function and other related life stressors [43, 44]. These psychiatric comorbidities are common in MiND and need to be carefully assessed to help determine their relationship to the presenting cognitive symptoms.

Brief cognitive screeners, such as the Montreal Cognitive Assessment (MOCA), Mini-Mental State Examination (MMSE), and Mini-Cog, are frequently used in primary care and neurology settings to help determine if additional follow-up is required to better characterize cognitive function for individuals with concern of MiND [45]. There are also an increasing number of digital cognitive screening tools and apps (e.g., digital clock, computerized National Institute of Health Toolbox Cognition Battery), though research is ongoing to determine whether these screening tools are equivalent to those done by paper and pencil [46].

These cognitive screening instruments commonly use predetermined cutoff scores to help guide the need for further evaluation. However, scores below cutoff require additional assessment (e.g., neuropsychological assessment) to confirm a diagnosis of MiND or MND; conversely, patients with scores in the normal range (particularly those with high educational levels) may have cognitive impairments that may be identified using more sensitive measures [47]. Demographic factors, such as educational attainment, may also affect score interpretation. For example, individuals with high education may score in the normal range despite cognitive decline when compared to their baseline, while individuals with less educational attainment may score below cutoff, but do not necessarily have cognitive deficits. Clinical judgment is essential when interpreting cutoff scores, and scores should always be interpreted in the context of the patient's clinical history. In cases where there is a question of true cognitive impairment or presence of psychiatric comorbidities, referral for comprehensive neuropsychological evaluation is indicated.

Comprehensive neuropsychological evaluations help characterize cognitive function across multiple domains of functioning, clarify diagnosis, and guide further treatment recommendations. Crucially, neuropsychological evaluations provide objective evidence of cognitive impairment and are an essential tool for distinguishing between a person who has subjective cognitive complaints but normal cognitive functioning and a person who is experiencing early signs of cognitive decline.

Treatments

Non-pharmacological

The strongest evidence for treatments for MiND is non-pharmacological interventions like physical activity and cognitive intervention. Hu et al. reviewed non-pharmacological interventions in people with MiND to determine their effectiveness [48]. Three types of physical activity (aerobic, muscle-strengthening, and mind-body) were compared, and all improved cognitive function in those with MiND. They found no difference in effectiveness between the types of activity, although other studies have shown that muscle training might be more effective than aerobic and mind-body exercises [49]. Overall, studies have also shown that patients undergoing cognitive training, a guided practice incorporating standardized tasks intended to improve cognitive domains, show improvements in memory [50, 51]. However, Liang suggested that cognitive stimulation, which focuses on the general improvement of individual cognitive behavior through engaging in a group-oriented social setting, was more effective than cognitive training and rehabilitation, which relies on the patient's personally relevant goals [52, 53]. Psychotherapeutic interventions that have been studied for the treatment of MiND include interpersonal therapy, coping strategies, and mindfulness training [54], but these interventions alone did not show any significant changes in cognitive function. Burgener et al. studied the combined benefits of cognitive behavioral therapy and tai chi exercises and reported small improvements in the global measure of cognitive function [55].

Due to increasing evidence connecting environmental factors to MiND and overall health, lifestyle interventions are often recommended to MiND patients. In 2020, The Lancet published a report identifying 12 modifiable risk factors that account for 40% of worldwide dementias [56]. Among those factors were cardiovascular risk, diabetes, weight control, diet, and social interaction. Increased social contact and participation in social activities throughout life have shown protective effects against MiND, but the specifics regarding the type and amount of participation are still unclear [57]. Studies have also shown that participating in cognitively stimulating activities such as reading magazines, playing music, and craft making was also linked with lower odds of having MiND [58]. Cardiovascular risk can be decreased through smoking cessation and blood pressure regulation. The Systolic Blood Pressure Intervention Trial-Memory and Cognition in Decreased Hypertension (SPRINT-MIND) trial was a randomized clinical trial that included 9361 adults with hypertension, aged 50 years and older, who underwent either intensive treatment (systolic blood pressure goal of <120 mmHg) or standard treatment (systolic blood pressure goal of <140 mmHg) followed by cognitive assessment. Although the study was terminated early, analysis showed that intensive treatment was associated with a reduced risk of MiND and the combined risk of MiND and probable MND [59].

The Mediterranean-DASH Diet Intervention for Neurodegenerative Delay (MIND) diet was associated with the reduced incidence of AD by 53% and may contribute to improved cognitive performance [60]. The MIND diet focuses on plant-based foods with protective effects against MND while limiting red meat, sugar, cheese, butter, and fried foods. It includes ten healthy food groups: leafy green vegetables, other vegetables, berries, whole grains, fish, poultry, beans, nuts,

wine, and olive oil. However, the Finnish Geriatric Intervention Study to Prevent Cognitive Impairment and Disability (FINGER) trial assessed a multidomain lifestyle intervention to prevent cognitive decline [61]. The 2-year study tested the efficacy of an intervention consisting of nutritional guidance, exercise, cognitive training, social activity, and intensive monitoring and management of metabolic and vascular risk factors. In comparison to the control who received general health advice, the intervention group showed improved cognition and a decreased risk for cognitive decline demonstrating the benefits of a multidomain approach [61].

Jiang et al., in their meta-analysis of nine studies of repetitive transcranial magnetic stimulation (rTMS) for MiND, showed significant improvement in global cognitive function [standardized mean difference (SMD) 2.09, 95% CI: 0.94–3.24] and memory (SMD 0.44, 95% CI: 0.16–0.7) [62]. The meta-analysis also found that rTMS targeting the left hemisphere improved global cognitive function, and rTMS targeting the bilateral hemispheres, high-frequency rTMS, and ≥20 times rTMS treatments could improve global cognitive function and memory. However, the number of studies included in the meta-analysis was low, and they were assessed by the authors to be of low- to moderate-quality evidence. Despite the limitations, rTMS can be a promising non-pharmacological intervention for the management of MiND, when more positive results become available from more studies. This would also open possibilities for other noninvasive brain stimulation therapies such as transcranial direct current stimulation (tDCS).

Pharmacological

Historically, several medications have been utilized to alleviate the symptoms of MCI as pharmacological agents available for the treatment of MCI are limited [63–65]. Acetylcholinesterase inhibitors and NMDA antagonists are often utilized for dementia treatment for preservation of memory functioning. Donepezil, rivastigmine, and galantamine are intended to enhance cognitive function through enhancement of cholinergic function. Dementia, such as AD, causes cortical cholinergic dysfunction. Other cognitive enhancers, such as memantine, attempt to improve cognitive function through glutamate modulation. This is thought to decrease excitatory NDMA activation, which increases neuronal damage in dementias, resulting in a neuroprotective effect. These benefits noted in MND treatment have not been shown in MiND patients. Older adults were not found to have improvement on cognitive testing, nor were delays in the progression of MCI to dementia noted [63, 66]. These findings have been consistent over numerous meta-analyses and systematic reviews of cognitive enhancer trials ranging from several months to years [63, 66–69].

Usage of antihypertensives and diabetic medications in MND trials is sparse, and, overall, no benefit was noted in cognitive testing or delaying of disease progression [63]. No reduction in risks for MiND or MND was noted in adults with normal cognition with either intensive or standard glucose control [60]. No differences were also noted with fenofibrates [63]. Some benefit in the reduction of all-cause dementia was noted with statins in a meta-analysis, with a possible decreased risk in the progression to AD [70]. Interestingly, this meta-analysis noted no benefit in the reduction of vascular dementia (VaD).

NSAIDs were also not noted to improve cognitive test performance in AD, although no trials were performed for MiND. The Alzheimer's Disease Anti-Inflammatory Prevention Trial (ADAPT) compared naproxen, celecoxib, and placebo treatment over 15 months and noted no difference in dementia incident and testing results over 8 and 4 years [71]. Aspirin use was similarly without noted benefit during follow-up after 4 years [72].

Estrogen has been proposed as a possible treatment for MCI, though research has not shown that estrogen replacement/supplementation has improved cognitive test performance. The Women's Health Initiative Memory Study (WHIMS) noted an overall increased incidence of MCI or dementia in the estrogen group, though this was noted to be present on an aggregate whole as opposed to individual outcomes [73]. Use of estrogen with progestin similarly increased

the risks for dementia without change in cognitive test performance. It should be noted that for both estrogen and estrogen with progestin use, increase in cardiovascular risks was noted. The use of selective estrogen receptor modulator, raloxifene, at 60 mg or 120 mg daily, resulted in a decrease in MiND, although the strength of the evidence was noted to be low [74, 75]. No difference in memory, attention, processing, or executive function when compared to placebo groups was noted for dementia testing. Testosterone use was not noted to have differences compared to controls with regard to cognitive test performance [76]. The overall strength of evidence for hormonal therapy use for dementia and MCI is generally low [63].

Use of ginkgo biloba was also not shown to prevent cognitive decline in MiND, though some studies noted improvement in the management of neuropsychiatric symptoms and activities of daily living [68, 77, 78]. EGb761, an extract of ginkgo biloba, was noted to have some statistical significance in the improvement of cognitive function and quality-of-life measures for mild to moderate MND as well as MiND compared to placebo trials [78]. Meta-analysis of EGb761 noted beneficial results for the management of behavioral and psychiatric symptoms associated with MND, although no benefit was noted in the progression of MND [78]. These benefits were noted at 240 mg/day in a dose-dependent fashion [78]. Safety concerns from increased inhibition of platelet aggregation from ginkgolide B, a platelet-activating factor (PAF) antagonist, were not noted at recommended therapeutic doses and in doses up to 480 mg/day [78]. PAF inhibition was noted at 600 mg/day, though no changes in bleeding time were observed. Similarly, coadministration of EGb761 with warfarin or aspirin did not inhibit platelet aggregation or increase bleeding time.

Overall, Chinese herbal medicines were not beneficial for MCI. A meta-analysis review of Chinese herbal medicines noted potential neuroprotective benefit with Chinese herbal medicines (e.g., *Acorus tatarinowii*, *Polygala tenuifolia*), though there was no significant difference in MMSE score results compared to donepezil or other options such as SSRIs or hypertensive medications. Additionally, the study sample sizes were small, and studies were not methodically rigorous [64].

Nootropics are medications in a broad sense that positively affect cognition [79]. These medications include piracetam, oxiracetam, lecithin, citicoline, acetyl-carnitine, cerebrolysin, docosahexaenoic acid, and phospholipase A2. Many of these medications have been used to treat cognitive impairment related to cerebrovascular accidents and traumatic brain injury, but the evidence for their use in the treatment of MiND is low [79]. Souvenaid, a dietary supplement that has been marketed as a medical food product for individuals with MiND consisting of a special patented composition of omega-3 fatty acids, vitamins, minerals, trace elements, and choline [80]. However, a recent Cochrane review found that after 2 years of treatment, Souvenaid did not reduce the risk of progression of MiND to MND [80].

Prior to 2021, five medications were approved by the Food and Drug Administration (FDA) for the treatment of AD: donepezil, galantamine, rivastigmine, memantine, and a combination of donepezil and memantine. The next drug to be FDA approved since 2003 for MND was the anti-amyloid therapy, aducanumab, on June seventh, 2021. Notably, this drug was approved through an accelerated approval pathway and was later approved for use in MiND [14]. PET imaging studies have suggested that a critical mass of amyloid burden must be reached before tau spread; consequently, it is thought that the specific targeting of amyloid should reduce downstream cognitive decline. Aducanumab is a recombinant IgG1 anti-Aβ monoclonal antibody [65, 81]. It was noted to bind with greater affinity to soluble and insoluble Aβ amyloid aggregates compared to monomers ($>$10,000-fold selectivity). It is suggested that it prevents Aβ aggregation with studies showing reduced Aβ plaque size [82]. Two major trials, studies 301 and 302, were performed on ~1650 participants each to assess the efficacy of aducanumab in reducing cognitive decline [65]. Apolipoprotein E epsilon 4 (ApoEe4) carriers made up 66–70% of the participants in these two studies. Participants were assessed to be positive for brain amyloid pathology and have a diagnosis of early symptomatic AD. Studies 301 and 302 tested aducanumab at dosages of 3 mg/kg for a low-dose titration over 8 weeks and a 6 mg/kg and a 10 mg/kg titration for high dose over 24 weeks for study 301, whereas study 302 looked at 6 mg/kg over 24 weeks titration for a low dose and 10 mg/kg over 24 weeks titration for a high dose [65]. These studies identified a target titration dose of 10 mg/kg for efficacy, with lower dosages possibly without benefit with ongoing risk of amyloid-related imaging abnormalities (ARIAs) [83] Aducanumab is infused once a month, with the first two infusions at 1 mg/kg. Third and fourth infusions are at 3 mg/kg, fifth and sixth infusions at 6 mg/kg, and seventh infusion and beyond at 10 mg/kg. MRI imaging is recommended within 1 year of initiation with a subsequent MRI prior to the fifth infusion, seventh infusion, and 12th infusion. MRIs are recommended throughout the process if signs or symptoms suggestive of ARIA occur. In the advent of ARIA, treatment is recommended to be halted and may be resumed after repeat MRI in 1 month's time that shows resolution of ARIA-E (ARIA with edema) or stabilization of ARIA-H (ARIA with intracerebral hemorrhage). Trails 301 and 302 noted that ARIA was more frequent in ApoEe4 carriers and was noted to occur earlier during treatment. ARIA events were rare in the placebo group, suggesting this to be associated with aducanumab [65]. MRI studies with concerns for ARIA are recommended to include T1, T2, or fluid-attenuated inversion recovery (FLAIR), T2 gradient recalled echo (GRE), or susceptibility-weighted imaging (SWI) and diffusion-weighted imaging (DWI) [83]. Though there are no explicit studies into management with missed doses, recommendations are to restart at the previous lower dose for three or more missed infusions [83].

Overall findings noted no clear delay in clinical progression of cognitive or functional decline in the studies. Several concerns ranging from early termination of the studies for "futility" to sporadic unblinding to variable distribution of the enrollment were identified [65]. Furthermore, an increased risk for cerebral edema and intracerebral hemorrhage was noted to be greater in ApoEe4 carriers early during treatment. Additionally, the results from study 302 conflicted with the results for study 301 [65]. A major outcome goal, reduction in Clinical Dementia Rating-Sum of Boxes (CDR-SB) global score, was not noted when compared to placebo in study 301 but was noted for high-dose aducanumab in study 302, a group that also noted severe symptoms possibly due to high dosages of the medication. Currently, the post-approval trial is not planned to be complete until 2030 [65]. Some of the other anti-amyloid agents being studied at this time include BAN2401 (lecanemab), solanezumab, and donanemab [81, 82]. Lecanemab is a humanized IgG1 version of a mouse monoclonal antibody that selectively binds to soluble $A\beta$ protofibrils, reducing protofibrils in the brain and CSF. A phase III randomized, double-blind trial of lecanemab known as Clarity AD (NCT03887455) recently published its results in late 2022 [79]. This study found less decline on measures of cognition and function based on the CDR-SB scores at 18 months. In this study, 1.2% of participants receiving lecanemab reported infusion-related reactions, and 0.8% of participants receiving the medication reported ARIA-E [79]. As the phase III trial results have just recently been released for lecanemab, recommended dosages are not established at this time. The trials were performed with a dosage of 10 mg/kg, suggesting that this may be the future recommended targeted dosage [84]. Although initial studies suggested that incidences of ARIA on MRI were like those of placebo, later trials suggest a nearly 10% incidence at 10 mg/kg [85]. Like aducanumab, lecanemab is administered intravenously. Although no deaths were reported in the phase III trial results, a subsequent case report showed that a patient with mild cognitive impairment who was treated in the extension phase of a trial of lecanemab developed multiple cerebral hemorrhages during infusion of t-PA for acute stroke and died [86]. This points to the need for additional guidance about relative and absolute contraindications for lecanemab and other anti-amyloid agents.

Solanezumab is a humanized monoclonal antibody that improves $A\beta$ clearance from the central nervous systems via sequestration of $A\beta$ from the central nervous system to the plasma. It is currently in a phase II/III trial, although some previous trials were terminated due to failure to reduce cognitive decline [82]. It was also shown to be ineffective in preclinical AD [87]. Donanemab is also a humanized antibody that facilitates $A\beta$ clearance. Some studies have noted a reduction in amyloid on PET scans by the 24th week. Some studies have noted no difference in global tau levels when compared to placebo, whereas other studies note a slowing of tau level accumulation. Although ARIA-H and -E were noted with donanemab, all-cause mortality was lower than placebo, and no difference in serious adverse events compared to placebo groups was noted [88]. ARIA was identified in 27% of the treatment group, with ~6% of the individuals developing ARIA-E. Similar to lecanemab, ARIA risk was higher among individuals who were homozygous for ApoE4, and the ARIA usually resolved spontaneously [85].

Many trials are ongoing for new medications for MiND and MND, and the list of FDA-approved medications for these disorders will change in the future. A list of disease-modifying anti-amyloid medications that have been studied for MiND is mentioned in Table 7.4 [82, 88, 89]. As new developments occur, it will be important for clinicians to discuss individual risks and benefits with patients. Risk factors such as increased risk of ARIA-A are present with those with APOE4 genotypes [85]. ARIA was generally not observed in doses below 3 mg/kg for aducanumab [85]. Additionally, certain subgroups were noted to have greater efficacy with anti-amyloid agents. Given the current evidence, providers should inform the patients and their families that these medications slow cognitive and functional decline but do not cure dementia or MCI. Furthermore, race and ethnic response differences to these medications are currently not well known. There are also logistical issues with the use of aducanumab and lecanemab as both these medications are administered via intravenous infusion. Consequently, patients will require reliable transportation as well as supportive family/friends who can accompany the patient for these infusions. In addition, these infusions occur over

Table 7.4 Anti-amyloid medications that have been studied for MiND

Anti-amyloid agents	Current status	Method of delivery	Mechanism
Aducanumab	FDA approved in 2021	Infusion	IgG1 to aggregated soluble and insoluble Aβ
Lecanemab	FDA approved in January 2023 for priority review	Infusion	IgG1 to Aβ protofibrils
Gantenerumab	Phase 3—unsuccessful with AD	Subcutaneous	IgG1 antibody to Aβ aggregates
Solanezumab	Phase III	Infusion	IgG1 antibody to soluble monomeric Aβ
Crenezumab	Discontinued for AD	Infusion	IgG4 antibody to both monomeric and aggregated forms of Aβ
Donanemab	Accelerated approval rejected	Infusion	Selective to existing amyloid deposits through N-terminal pyroglutamate

the course of many months with extensive monitoring/imaging possibly required, especially if there is occurrence of ARIA.

The management of the symptoms of MiND will depend on both the causes of the MiND and the management of any comorbidities that have a substantial impact on the individual's ability to live independently or cause increased caregiver burden [90, 91]. In situations such as MiND related to vascular risk factors, modification of various vascular risks through cardiovascular health potentially reduces the risks of further MiND progression from these causes. Hypertension management is generally advised in reducing the risk of MiND related to vascular risk factors. Similarly, treatment of Parkinson's disease (PD) is likely to benefit management of PD-related MiND. Use of dopaminergic medication such as levodopa or dopamine agonists was noted to improve both cognition and overall functioning. Atomoxetine along with clozapine, and second-generation tricyclic antidepressants, was found to enhance attention and help manage/control some psychosis and depressed mood with MiND associated with PD. Medication side effects should always be considered when dealing with the older adults who have MiND [91]. The supplementation of vitamin D has not shown much benefit in MCI management [92].

Two common major comorbidities associated with MiND are depression and anxiety. The estimates of depression and anxiety within the MiND population range from 60 to 70% [93]. In addition to the decreased quality of life associated with depression and anxiety, these comorbidities were also associated with negative effects on cognition and increased progression of MiND to MND [93]. In addition to psychotherapy for the management of MiND, the use of antidepressants like selective serotonin reuptake inhibitors (SSRIs) and selective serotonin-norepinephrine reuptake inhibitors (SNRIs) is a preferred medication choice if pharmacological management is desired for the management of depression and anxiety. SSRIs were also noted to have some benefit in improving cognition in AD although no reduction in the amyloid burden was noted among these individuals [94, 95].

Some key considerations when selecting pharmacological agents for the management of MiND include minimizing adverse drug-drug interactions as well as anticholinergic effects of various medications contributing to cognitive impairment. Anticholinergic agents should also be avoided in combination with the cholinesterase inhibitors that were described earlier in the chapter. A list of the medications to be avoided can be found on the Beers criteria for potentially inappropriate medication use in older adults [96].

Evidence-Based Treatment Algorithm

Once the diagnosis of MiND is made, healthcare providers should plan to discuss this diagnosis with the patient and their family members/caregivers. They should also discuss the management plans and available supports and community resources. Patients' cognition and functioning should be monitored via routine follow-up appointments every 6–12 months [97]. Although patients with MiND are at high risk for developing MND, they should also be educated that in some cases of MiND, symptoms can remain stable or improve. Patients should have a medical evaluation for reversible causes of MiND, and an attempt to wean patients from medications that can contribute to cognitive impairment should be initiated. Structural neuroimaging like a computerized tomography (CT) scan or an MRI scan of the brain can assess for abnormalities in the brain including atrophy, tumors, or strokes. For atypical cases, FDG-PET scan can assess regional metabolic patterns in the brain and assist with distinguishing MiND due to AD and FTD. Availability and cost considerations should be made when deciding between structural neuroimaging and functional neuroimaging like an FDG-PET scan. Providers should also counsel patients that currently there are no accepted biomarkers available for the identification of MiND. They can also provide the option of referring patients to organizations that conduct biomarker research related to MiND.

There are multiple guidelines that are available for the treatment of MiND from various medical societies and expert workgroups from different countries [98]. A summary of guidelines from important national medical societies and work groups available in English is mentioned in Table 7.5. The guidelines are not updated in terms of pharmacological treatment of MiND, as all of them do not address the newly approved medications. Non-pharmacologic interventions for MiND, including physical exercise, cognitive training, and control of cardiovascular risk factors, are highly recommended in many of these treatment guidelines. Non-pharmacologic interventions are relatively safe and inexpensive and have well-established evidence in reducing the risk of progression of MiND to MND. Healthcare providers can choose to provide acetylcholinesterase inhibitors for patients with MiND, but they should first discuss with patients and their families that it will be an off-label prescription and it has low strength of evidence for treatment efficacy. Safety and costs should be considered in the decision-making process for using the newer FDA-approved medications for MiND, along with the evidence of its limited clinical benefit. An algorithm for the treatment of MiND has been provided in Fig. 7.1.

Table 7.5 Summary of important treatment guidelines of MiND available in English from medical societies and work groups

Name of society/workgroup	Pharmacological treatment	Control of cardiovascular risk factors	Physical activity and cognitive activation	Treatment of psychiatric/ behavioral symptoms
Asian Clinical Expert Group on Neurocognitive Disorders [78]	Recommend use of EGb761	Not mentioned	Not mentioned	Not mentioned
Dementia Australia [99]	Not recommended	Recommended	Recommended	Recommended
British Association for Psychopharmacology [100]	Not recommended	Not mentioned	Not mentioned	Not mentioned
Canadian Consensus Conferences on the Diagnosis and Treatment of Dementia [101]	Not mentioned	Recommended	Recommended	Recommended
American Academy of Neurology [102]	May choose to offer acetylcholinesterase inhibitors as off-label use	Recommended	Recommended	Recommended
World Health Organization [103]	Not mentioned	Recommended	Recommended	Not recommended

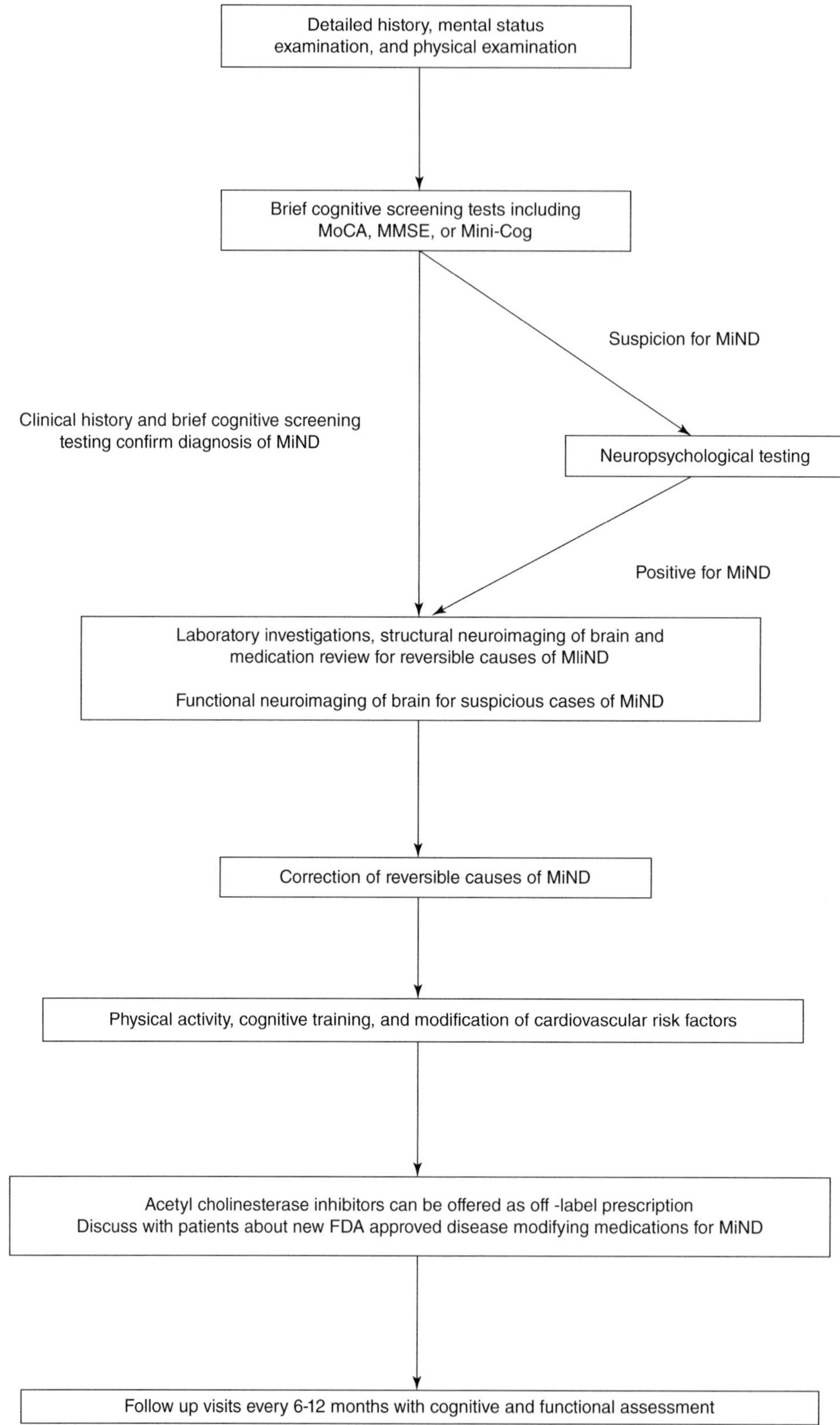

Fig. 7.1 Algorithm for the management of MiND

Conclusion

As the population ages, there is a need for early identification and monitoring of the cognitive and functional impairment of MiND. Although many patients with MiND do progress to MND, workup and treatment of reversible causes of MiND are crucial as it can significantly improve cognitive and functional impairment. Even those patients who have MiND which remains relatively stable can require additional support, especially as they experience functional decline due to medical comorbidities. Physical exercise, cognitive training, and control of cardiovascular risk factors are essential interventions in the management of patients with MiND. The other major development in the field of MiND therapeutics is the recent approval of new disease-modifying medications, including anti-amyloid antibodies. Major challenges include the notable risk of ARIA-E and the intensive nature of treatment and monitoring for ARIA-E, which requires subspecialty access and follow-up. Key questions about the risks and benefits and their use in diverse populations require further investigation and will need to be answered before these classes of disease-modifying therapeutics for MiND can be scaled up.

References

1. Stokin GB, Krell-Roesch J, Petersen RC, Geda YE. Mild neurocognitive disorder: an old wine in a new bottle. Harv Rev Psychiatry. 2015;23(5):368–76.
2. Petersen RC. Mild cognitive impairment as a diagnostic entity. J Intern Med. 2004;256(3):183–94.
3. Petersen RC, Smith GE, Waring SC, Ivnik RJ, Tangalos EG, Kokmen E. Mild cognitive impairment: clinical characterization and outcome. Arch Neurol. 1999;56(3):303–8.
4. American Psychiatric Association. Neurocognitive disorders. Diagnostic and statistical manual of mental disorders, fifth edition, text revision. Washington, DC: American Psychiatric Association; 2022. p. 867–732.
5. Petersen RC. Mild cognitive impairment. Continuum (Minneap Minn). 2016;22(2 Dementia):404–18.
6. Bai W, Chen P, Cai H, Zhang Q, Su Z, Cheung T, Jackson T, Sha S, Xiang YT. Worldwide prevalence of mild cognitive impairment among community dwellers aged 50 years and older: a meta-analysis and systematic review of epidemiology studies. Age Ageing. 2022;51(8):afac173.
7. Gillis C, Mirzaei F, Potashman M, Ikram MA, Maserejian N. The incidence of mild cognitive impairment: a systematic review and data synthesis. Alzheimers Dement (Amst). 2019;11:248–56.
8. McGrattan AM, Zhu Y, Richardson CD, Mohan D, Soh YC, Sajjad A, van Aller C, Chen S, Paddick SM, Prina M, Siervo M, Robinson LA, Stephan BCM. Prevalence and risk of mild cognitive impairment in low and middle-income countries: a systematic review. J Alzheimers Dis. 2021;79(2):743–62.
9. Roberts RO, Geda YE, Knopman DS, Cha RH, Pankratz VS, Boeve BF, Ivnik RJ, Tangalos EG, Petersen RC, Rocca WA. The Mayo Clinic study of aging: design and sampling, participation, baseline measures and sample characteristics. Neuroepidemiology. 2008;30(1):58–69.
10. Luck T, Then FS, Schroeter ML, Witte V, Engel C, Loeffler M, Thiery J, Villringer A, Riedel-Heller SG. Prevalence of DSM-5 mild neurocognitive disorder in dementia-free older adults: results of the population-based LIFE-adult-study. Am J Geriatr Psychiatry. 2017;25(4):328–39.
11. Morris JC. Mild cognitive impairment is early-stage Alzheimer disease: time to revise diagnostic criteria. Arch Neurol. 2006;63(1):15–6.
12. Burke D, Sengoz A, Schwartz R. Potentially reversible cognitive impairment in patients presenting to a memory disorders clinic. J Clin Neurosci. 2000;7(2):120–3.
13. Muangpaisan W, Petcharat C, Srinonprasert V. Prevalence of potentially reversible conditions in dementia and mild cognitive impairment in a geriatric clinic. Geriatr Gerontol Int. 2012;12(1):59–64.
14. Sanford AM. Mild cognitive impairment. Clin Geriatr Med. 2017;33(3):325–37.
15. Luck T, Luppa M, Briel S, Riedel-Heller SG. Incidence of mild cognitive impairment: a systematic review. Dement Geriatr Cogn Disord. 2010;29(2):164–75.
16. Ganguli M, Fu B, Snitz BE, Hughes TF, Chang CC. Mild cognitive impairment: incidence and vascular risk factors in a population-based cohort. Neurology. 2013;80(23):2112–20.
17. Lara E, Martín-María N, De la Torre-Luque A, Koyanagi A, Vancampfort D, Izquierdo A, Miret M. Does loneliness contribute to mild cognitive impairment and dementia? A systematic review and meta-analysis of longitudinal studies. Ageing Res Rev. 2019;52:7–16.
18. Tervo S, Kivipelto M, Hänninen T, Vanhanen M, Hallikainen M, Mannermaa A, Soininen H. Incidence and risk factors for mild cognitive impairment: a population-based three-year follow-up study of cognitively healthy elderly subjects. Dement Geriatr Cogn Disord. 2004;17(3):196–203.
19. Mitchell AJ, Shiri-Feshki M. Rate of progression of mild cognitive impairment to dementia—meta-

analysis of 41 robust inception cohort studies. Acta Psychiatr Scand. 2009;119(4):252–65.

20. Espinosa A, Alegret M, Valero S, Vinyes-Junqué G, Hernández I, Mauleón A, Rosende-Roca M, Ruiz A, López O, Tárraga L, Boada M. A longitudinal follow-up of 550 mild cognitive impairment patients: evidence for large conversion to dementia rates and detection of major risk factors involved. J Alzheimers Dis. 2013;34(3):769–80.

21. Artero S, Ancelin ML, Portet F, Dupuy A, Berr C, Dartigues JF, Tzourio C, Rouaud O, Poncet M, Pasquier F, Auriacombe S, Touchon J, Ritchie K. Risk profiles for mild cognitive impairment and progression to dementia are gender specific. J Neurol Neurosurg Psychiatry. 2008;79(9):979–84.

22. Li JQ, Tan L, Wang HF, Tan MS, Tan L, Xu W, Zhao QF, Wang J, Jiang T, Yu JT. Risk factors for predicting progression from mild cognitive impairment to Alzheimer's disease: a systematic review and meta-analysis of cohort studies. J Neurol Neurosurg Psychiatry. 2016;87(5):476–84.

23. Sluimer JD, van der Flier WM, Karas GB, van Schijndel R, Barnes J, Boyes RG, Cover KS, Olabarriaga SD, Fox NC, Scheltens P, Vrenken H, Barkhof F. Accelerating regional atrophy rates in the progression from normal aging to Alzheimer's disease. Eur Radiol. 2009;19(12):2826–33.

24. Hansson O, Zetterberg H, Buchhave P, Londos E, Blennow K, Minthon L. Association between CSF biomarkers and incipient Alzheimer's disease in patients with mild cognitive impairment: a follow-up study. Lancet Neurol. 2006;5(3):228–34.

25. Mattsson N, Zetterberg H, Hansson O, Andreasen N, Parnetti L, Jonsson M, Herukka SK, van der Flier WM, Blankenstein MA, Ewers M, Rich K, Kaiser E, Verbeek M, Tsolaki M, Mulugeta E, Rosén E, Aarsland D, Visser PJ, Schröder J, Marcusson J, de Leon M, Hampel H, Scheltens P, Pirttilä T, Wallin A, Jönhagen ME, Minthon L, Winblad B, Blennow K. CSF biomarkers and incipient Alzheimer disease in patients with mild cognitive impairment. JAMA. 2009;302(4):385–93.

26. Canevelli M, Grande G, Lacorte E, Quarchioni E, Cesari M, Mariani C, Bruno G, Vanacore N. Spontaneous reversion of mild cognitive impairment to normal cognition: a systematic review of literature and meta-analysis. J Am Med Dir Assoc. 2016;17(10):943–8.

27. Chung JY, Yoon HJ, Kim H, Choi KY, Lee JJ, Lee KH, Seo EH. Reversion from mild cognitive impairment to normal cognition: false-positive error or true restoration thanks to cognitive control ability? Neuropsychiatr Dis Treat. 2019;15:3021–32.

28. Mondragón JD, Maurits NM, De Deyn PP. Functional neural correlates of Anosognosia in mild cognitive impairment and Alzheimer's disease: a systematic review. Neuropsychol Rev. 2019;29(2):139–65.

29. Risacher SL, Saykin AJ, West JD, Shen L, Firpi HA, McDonald BC. Alzheimer's disease neuroimaging initiative (ADNI). Baseline MRI predictors of conversion from MCI to probable AD in the ADNI cohort. Curr Alzheimer Res. 2009;6(4):347–61.

30. Heister D, Brewer JB, Magda S, Blennow K, McEvoy LK. Alzheimer's disease neuroimaging initiative. Predicting MCI outcome with clinically available MRI and CSF biomarkers. Neurology. 2011;77(17):1619–28.

31. Yuan Y, Gu ZX, Wei WS. Fluorodeoxyglucose-positron-emission tomography, single-photon emission tomography, and structural MR imaging for prediction of rapid conversion to Alzheimer disease in patients with mild cognitive impairment: a meta-analysis. AJNR Am J Neuroradiol. 2009;30(2):404–10.

32. Jack CR Jr, Wiste HJ, Vemuri P, Weigand SD, Senjem ML, Zeng G, Bernstein MA, Gunter JL, Pankratz VS, Aisen PS, Weiner MW, Petersen RC, Shaw LM, Trojanowski JQ, Knopman DS. Alzheimer's disease neuroimaging initiative. Brain beta-amyloid measures and magnetic resonance imaging atrophy both predict time-to-progression from mild cognitive impairment to Alzheimer's disease. Brain. 2010;133(11):3336–48.

33. Jiskoot LC, Panman JL, Meeter LH, Dopper EGP, Donker Kaat L, Franzen S, van der Ende EL, van Minkelen R, Rombouts SARB, Papma JM, van Swieten JC. Longitudinal multimodal MRI as prognostic and diagnostic biomarker in presymptomatic familial frontotemporal dementia. Brain. 2019;142(1):193–208.

34. Karow DS, McEvoy LK, Fennema-Notestine C, Hagler DJ Jr, Jennings RG, Brewer JB, Hoh CK, Dale AM. Alzheimer's disease neuroimaging initiative. Relative capability of MR imaging and FDG PET to depict changes associated with prodromal and early Alzheimer disease. Radiology. 2010;256(3):932–42.

35. Wicklund M, Petersen RC. Emerging biomarkers in cognition. Clin Geriatr Med. 2013;29(4):809–28.

36. Herukka SK, Simonsen AH, Andreasen N, Baldeiras I, Bjerke M, Blennow K, Engelborghs S, Frisoni GB, Gabryelewicz T, Galluzzi S, Handels R, Kramberger MG, Kulczyńska A, Molinuevo JL, Mroczko B, Nordberg A, Oliveira CR, Otto M, Rinne JO, Rot U, Saka E, Soininen H, Struyfs H, Suardi S, Visser PJ, Winblad B, Zetterberg H, Waldemar G. Recommendations for cerebrospinal fluid Alzheimer's disease biomarkers in the diagnostic evaluation of mild cognitive impairment. Alzheimers Dement. 2017;13(3):285–95.

37. Johnson KA, Minoshima S, Bohnen NI, Donohoe KJ, Foster NL, Herscovitch P, Karlawish JH, Rowe CC, Carrillo MC, Hartley DM, Hedrick S, Pappas V, Thies WH, Alzheimer's Association, Society of Nuclear Medicine and Molecular Imaging, Amyloid Imaging Taskforce. Appropriate use criteria for amyloid PET: a report of the Amyloid Imaging Task Force, the Society of Nuclear Medicine and Molecular Imaging, and the Alzheimer's Association. Alzheimers Dement. 2013;9(1):e-1–16.

38. Morris JC. Clinical dementia rating: a reliable and valid diagnostic and staging measure for dementia of the Alzheimer type. Int Psychogeriatr. 1997;9(S1):173–6.

39. Kaufer DI, Cummings JL, Ketchel P, Smith V, MacMillan A, Shelley T, et al. Validation of the NPI-Q, a brief clinical form of the Neuropsychiatric Inventory. J Neuropsychiatry Clin Neurosci. 2000;12(2):233–9.

40. Sheehan DV, Lecrubier Y, Sheehan KH, Amorim P, Janavs J, Weiller E, et al. The Mini-International Neuropsychiatric Interview (M.I.N.I.): the development and validation of a structured diagnostic psychiatric interview for DSM-IV and ICD-10. J Clin Psychiatry. 1998;59(Suppl 20):22–33;quiz 4–57.

41. Brommelhoff JA, Gatz M, Johansson B, McArdle JJ, Fratiglioni L, Pedersen NL. Depression as a risk factor or prodromal feature for dementia? Findings in a population-based sample of Swedish twins. Psychol Aging. 2009;24(2):373–84.

42. Byers AL, Yaffe K. Depression and risk of developing dementia. Nat Rev Neurol. 2011;7(6):323–31.

43. Tonga JB, Eilertsen D-E, Solem IKL, Arnevik EA, Korsnes MS, Ulstein ID. Effect of self-efficacy on quality of life in people with mild cognitive impairment and mild dementia: the mediating roles of depression and anxiety. Am J Alzheimers Dis Other Dement. 2020;35:1533317519885264.

44. Regan B, Varanelli L. Adjustment, depression, and anxiety in mild cognitive impairment and early dementia: a systematic review of psychological intervention studies. Int Psychogeriatr. 2013;25(12):1963–84.

45. Ismail Z, Rajji TK, Shulman KI. Brief cognitive screening instruments: an update. Int J Geriatr Psychiatry. 2010;25(2):111–20.

46. Chan JYC, Yau STY, Kwok TCY, Tsoi KKF. Diagnostic performance of digital cognitive tests for the identification of MCI and dementia: a systematic review. Ageing Res Rev. 2021;72:101506.

47. Ciesielska N, Sokołowski R, Mazur E, Podhorecka M, Polak-Szabela A, Kędziora-Kornatowska K. Is the Montreal Cognitive Assessment (MoCA) test better suited than the Mini-Mental State Examination (MMSE) in mild cognitive impairment (MCI) detection among people aged over 60? Meta-analysis. Psychiatr Pol. 2016;50(5):1039–52.

48. Hu M, Hu H, Shao Z, et al. Effectiveness and acceptability of non-pharmacological interventions in people with mild cognitive impairment: overview of systematic reviews and network meta-analysis. J Affect Disord. 2022;311:383–90.

49. Wang S, Yin H, Wang X, et al. Efficacy of different types of exercises on global cognition in adults with mild cognitive impairment: a network meta-analysis. Aging Clin Exp Res. 2019;31(10):1391–400.

50. Liang JH, Shen WT, Li JY, et al. The optimal treatment for improving cognitive function in elder people with mild cognitive impairment incorporating Bayesian network meta-analysis and systematic review. Ageing Res Rev. 2019;51:85–96.

51. Wang YQ, Jia RX, Liang JH, et al. Effects of non-pharmacological therapies for people with mild cognitive impairment. A Bayesian network meta-analysis. Int J Geriatr Psychiatry. 2020;35(6):591–600.

52. Woods B, Aguirre E, Spector AE, Orrell M. Cognitive stimulation to improve cognitive functioning in people with dementia. Cochrane Database Syst Rev. 2012;(2):CD005562.

53. Clare L, Woods RT, Moniz Cook ED, Orrell M, Spector A. Cognitive rehabilitation and cognitive training for early-stage Alzheimer's disease and vascular dementia. Cochrane Database Syst Rev. 2003;(4):CD003260.

54. Rodakowski J, Saghafi E, Butters MA, Skidmore ER. Non-pharmacological interventions for adults with mild cognitive impairment and early stage dementia: an updated scoping review. Mol Asp Med. 2015;43-44:38–53.

55. Burgener SC, Yang Y, Gilbert R, Marsh-Yant S. The effects of a multimodal intervention on outcomes of persons with early-stage dementia. Am J Alzheimers Dis Other Dement. 2008;23(4):382–94.

56. Livingston G, Huntley J, Sommerlad A, et al. Dementia prevention, intervention, and care: 2020 report of the Lancet Commission. Lancet. 2020;396(10248):413–46.

57. Marioni RE, Proust-Lima C, Amieva H, et al. Social activity, cognitive decline and dementia risk: a 20-year prospective cohort study. BMC Public Health. 2015;15:1089.

58. Geda YE, Topazian HM, Roberts LA, Roberts RO, Knopman DS, Pankratz VS, Christianson TJ, Boeve BF, Tangalos EG, Ivnik RJ, Petersen RC. Engaging in cognitive activities, aging, and mild cognitive impairment: a population-based study. J Neuropsychiatry Clin Neurosci. 2011;23(2):149–54.

59. SPRINT MIND Investigators for the SPRINT Research Group, Williamson JD, Pajewski NM, et al. Effect of intensive vs standard blood pressure control on probable dementia: a randomized clinical trial. JAMA. 2019;321(6):553–61.

60. Morris MC, Tangney CC, Wang Y, Sacks FM, Bennett DA, Aggarwal NT. MIND diet associated with reduced incidence of Alzheimer's disease. Alzheimers Dement. 2015;11(9):1007–14.

61. Ngandu T, Lehtisalo J, Solomon A, et al. A 2 year multidomain intervention of diet, exercise, cognitive training, and vascular risk monitoring versus control to prevent cognitive decline in at-risk elderly people (FINGER): a randomised controlled trial. Lancet. 2015;385(9984):2255–63.

62. Jiang L, Cui H, Zhang C, Cao X, Gu N, Zhu Y, Wang J, Yang Z, Li C. Repetitive transcranial magnetic stimulation for improving cognitive function in patients with mild cognitive impairment: a systematic review. Front Aging Neurosci. 2021;12:593000.

63. Fink HA, Jutkowitz E, McCarten JR, Hemmy LS, Butler M, Davila H, Ratner E, Calvert C, Barclay TR, Brasure M, Nelson VA, Kane RL. Pharmacologic interventions to prevent cognitive decline, mild cognitive impairment, and clinical Alzheimer-type dementia: a systematic review. Ann Intern Med. 2018;168(1):39–51.

64. Dong L, May BH, Feng M, et al. Chinese herbal medicine for mild cognitive impairment: a systematic review and meta-analysis of cognitive outcomes. Phytother Res. 2016;30(10):1592–604.

65. Tampi RR, Forester BP, Agronin M. Aducanumab: evidence from clinical trial data and controversies. Drugs Context. 2021;10:2021-7-3.

66. Tricco AC, Soobiah C, Berliner S, et al. Efficacy and safety of cognitive enhancers for patients with mild cognitive impairment: a systematic review and meta-analysis. CMAJ. 2013;185(16):1393–401.

67. Assaf G, Tanielian M. Mild cognitive impairment in primary care: a clinical review. Postgrad Med J. 2018;94(1117):647–52. https://doi.org/10.1136/postgradmedj-2018-136035.

68. Bensadon BA, Odenheimer GL. Current management decisions in mild cognitive impairment. Clin Geriatr Med. 2013;29(4):847–71.

69. Eshkoor SA, Hamid TA, Mun CY, Ng CK. Mild cognitive impairment and its management in older people. Clin Interv Aging. 2015;10:687–93.

70. Chu CS, Tseng PT, Stubbs B, et al. Use of statins and the risk of dementia and mild cognitive impairment: a systematic review and meta-analysis. Sci Rep. 2018;8(1):5804.

71. ADAPT-FS Research Group. Follow-up evaluation of cognitive function in the randomized Alzheimer's disease anti-inflammatory prevention trial and its follow-up study. Alzheimers Dement. 2015;11(2):216–25.e1.

72. Kang JH, Cook N, Manson J, Buring JE, Grodstein F. Low dose aspirin and cognitive function in the women's health study cognitive cohort. BMJ. 2007;334(7601):987.

73. Espeland MA, Rapp SR, Shumaker SA, Brunner R, Manson JE, Sherwin BB, Hsia J, Margolis KL, Hogan PE, Wallace R, Dailey M, Freeman R, Hays J, Women's Health Initiative Memory Study. Conjugated equine estrogens and global cognitive function in postmenopausal women: Women's Health Initiative Memory Study. JAMA. 2004;291(24):2959–68.

74. Nickelsen T, Lufkin EG, Riggs BL, Cox DA, Crook TH. Raloxifene hydrochloride, a selective estrogen receptor modulator: safety assessment of effects on cognitive function and mood in postmenopausal women. Psychoneuroendocrinology. 1999;24(1):115–28.

75. Yaffe K, Krueger K, Cummings SR, Blackwell T, Henderson VW, Sarkar S, Ensrud K, Grady D. Effect of raloxifene on prevention of dementia and cognitive impairment in older women: the Multiple Outcomes of Raloxifene Evaluation (MORE) randomized trial. Am J Psychiatry. 2005;162(4):683–90.

76. Resnick SM, Matsumoto AM, Stephens-Shields AJ, Ellenberg SS, Gill TM, Shumaker SA, Pleasants DD, Barrett-Connor E, Bhasin S, Cauley JA, Cella D, Crandall JP, Cunningham GR, Ensrud KE, Farrar JT, Lewis CE, Molitch ME, Pahor M, Swerdloff RS, Cifelli D, Anton S, Basaria S, Diem SJ, Wang C, Hou X, Snyder PJ. Testosterone treatment and cognitive function in older men with low testosterone and age-associated memory impairment. JAMA. 2017;317(7):717–27.

77. Langa KM, Levine DA. The diagnosis and management of mild cognitive impairment: a clinical review. JAMA. 2014;312(23):2551–61.

78. Kandiah N, Ong PA, Yuda T, Ng LL, Mamun K, Merchant RA, Chen C, Dominguez J, Marasigan S, Ampil E, Nguyen VT, Yusoff S, Chan YF, Yong FM, Krairit O, Suthisisang C, Senanarong V, Ji Y, Thukral R, Ihl R. Treatment of dementia and mild cognitive impairment with or without cerebrovascular disease: expert consensus on the use of Ginkgo biloba extract, EGb 761®. CNS Neurosci Ther. 2019;25(2):288–98.

79. Colucci L, Bosco M, Rosario Ziello A, Rea R, Amenta F, Fasanaro AM. Effectiveness of nootropic drugs with cholinergic activity in treatment of cognitive deficit: a review. J Exp Pharmacol. 2012;4:163–72.

80. Burckhardt M, Watzke S, Wienke A, Langer G, Fink A. Souvenaid for Alzheimer's disease. Cochrane Database Syst Rev. 2020;12(12):CD011679.

81. Tolar M, Abushakra S, Hey JA, Porsteinsson A, Sabbagh M. Aducanumab, gantenerumab, BAN2401, and ALZ-801-the first wave of amyloid-targeting drugs for Alzheimer's disease with potential for near term approval. Alzheimers Res Ther. 2020;12(1):95.

82. Decourt B, Boumelhem F, Pope ED 3rd, Shi J, Mari Z, Sabbagh MN. Critical appraisal of amyloid lowering agents in AD. Curr Neurol Neurosci Rep. 2021;21(8):39.

83. Cummings J, Aisen P, Apostolova LG, Atri A, Salloway S, Weiner M. Aducanumab: appropriate use recommendations. J Prev Alzheimers Dis. 2021;8(4):398–410.

84. van Dyck CH, Swanson CJ, Aisen P, Bateman RJ, Chen C, Gee M, Kanekiyo M, Li D, Reyderman L, Cohen S, Froelich L, Katayama S, Sabbagh M, Vellas B, Watson D, Dhadda S, Irizarry M, Kramer LD, Iwatsubo T. Lecanemab in early Alzheimer's disease. N Engl J Med. 2023;388(1):9–21.

85. Withington CG, Turner RS. Amyloid-related imaging abnormalities with anti-amyloid antibodies for the treatment of dementia due to Alzheimer's disease. Front Neurol. 2022;13:862369.

86. Reish NJ, Jamshidi P, Stamm B, Flanagan ME, Sugg E, Tang M, Donohue KL, McCord M, Krumpelman C, Mesulam MM, Castellani R, Chou SH. Multiple

cerebral hemorrhages in a patient receiving lecanemab and treated with t-PA for stroke. N Engl J Med. 2023;388(5):478–9.

87. National Institute of Aging. NIA statement on study results suggesting solanezumab does not reduce cognitive decline in people at risk for developing Alzheimer's; 2023. https://www.nia.nih.gov/news/nia-statement-study-results-suggesting-solanezumab-does-not-reduce-cognitive-decline-people. Accessed 19 Mar 2023.

88. Rashad A, Rasool A, Shaheryar M, Sarfraz A, Sarfraz Z, Robles-Velasco K, Cherrez-Ojeda I. Donanemab for Alzheimer's disease: a systematic review of clinical trials. Healthcare (Basel). 2022;11(1):32.

89. Ostrowitzki S, Bittner T, Sink KM, Mackey H, Rabe C, Honig LS, Cassetta E, Woodward M, Boada M, van Dyck CH, Grimmer T, Selkoe DJ, Schneider A, Blondeau K, Hu N, Quartino A, Clayton D, Dolton M, Dang Y, Ostaszewski B, Sanabria-Bohórquez SM, Rabbia M, Toth B, Eichenlaub U, Smith J, Honigberg LA, Doody RS. Evaluating the safety and efficacy of crenezumab vs placebo in adults with early Alzheimer disease: two phase 3 randomized placebo-controlled trials. JAMA Neurol. 2022;79(11):1113–21.

90. Anderson ND. State of the science on mild cognitive impairment (MCI). CNS Spectr. 2019;24(1):78–87.

91. Jongsiriyanyong S, Limpawattana P. Mild cognitive impairment in clinical practice: a review article. Am J Alzheimers Dis Other Dement. 2018;33(8):500–7.

92. Gil Martínez V, Avedillo Salas A, Santander BS. Vitamin supplementation and dementia: a systematic review. Nutrients. 2022;14(5):1033.

93. Orgeta V, Qazi A, Spector A, Orrell M. Psychological treatments for depression and anxiety in dementia and mild cognitive impairment: systematic review and meta-analysis. Br J Psychiatry. 2015;207(4):293–8.

94. Han F, Bonnett T, Brenowitz WD, Teylan MA, Besser LM, Chen YC, Chan G, Cao KG, Gao Y, Zhou XH. Estimating associations between antidepressant use and incident mild cognitive impairment in older adults with depression. PLoS One. 2020;15(1):e0227924.

95. Bouter Y, Bouter C. Selective serotonin reuptake inhibitor-treatment does not show beneficial effects on cognition or amyloid burden in cognitively impaired and cognitively normal subjects. Front Aging Neurosci. 2022;14:883256.

96. Bhattacharjee S, Lee JK, Patanwala AE, Vadiei N, Malone DC, Knapp SM, Lo-Ciganic WH, Burke WJ. Extent and predictors of potentially inappropriate antidepressant use among older adults with dementia and major depressive disorder. Am J Geriatr Psychiatry. 2019;27(8):794–805.

97. Porsteinsson AP, Isaacson RS, Knox S, Sabbagh MN, Rubino I. Diagnosis of early Alzheimer's disease: clinical practice in 2021. J Prev Alzheimers Dis. 2021;8(3):371–86.

98. Kasper S, Bancher C, Eckert A, Förstl H, Frölich L, Hort J, Korczyn AD, Kressig RW, Levin O, Palomo MSM. Management of mild cognitive impairment (MCI): the need for national and international guidelines. World J Biol Psychiatry. 2020;21(8):579–94.

99. Woodward M, Brodaty H, McCabe M, Masters CL, Naismith SL, Morris P, Rowe CC, Walker P, Yates M. Nationally informed recommendations on approaching the detection, assessment, and management of mild cognitive impairment. J Alzheimers Dis. 2022;89(3):803–9.

100. O'Brien JT, Holmes C, Jones M, Jones R, Livingston G, McKeith I, Mittler P, Passmore P, Ritchie C, Robinson L, Sampson EL, Taylor JP, Thomas A, Burns A. Clinical practice with anti-dementia drugs: a revised (third) consensus statement from the British Association for Psychopharmacology. J Psychopharmacol. 2017;31(2):147–68.

101. Ismail Z, Black SE, Camicioli R, Chertkow H, Herrmann N, Laforce R Jr, Montero-Odasso M, Rockwood K, Rosa-Neto P, Seitz D, Sivananthan S, Smith EE, Soucy JP, Vedel I, Gauthier S, CCCDTD5 Participants. Recommendations of the 5th Canadian consensus conference on the diagnosis and treatment of dementia. Alzheimers Dement. 2020;16(8):1182–95.

102. Petersen RC, Lopez O, Armstrong MJ, Getchius TSD, Ganguli M, Gloss D, Gronseth GS, Marson D, Pringsheim T, Day GS, Sager M, Stevens J, Rae-Grant A. Practice guideline update summary: mild cognitive impairment: report of the guideline development, dissemination, and implementation Subcommittee of the American Academy of Neurology. Neurology. 2018;90(3):126–35.

103. World Health Organization. Risk Reduction of cognitive decline and dementia: WHO Guidelines; 2019. https://apps.who.int/iris/bitstream/handle/10665/312180/9789241550543-eng.pdf. Accessed 20 Feb 2023.

Delirium

8

Rosalyn Chi, Sophia Wang, and Babar Khan

Epidemiology

Delirium is defined by the *Diagnostic and Statistical Manual of Mental Disorders, fifth edition (DSM-5)*, as "a disturbance in attention … accompanied by reduced awareness of the environment" [1]. The onset of delirium is an acute change from baseline, usually occurring over hours to days, and tends to have a fluctuating course.

Delirium transiently affects cognitive functioning across multiple domains, resulting in difficulties with memory and recall, language expression and comprehension, and visuospatial perception. Delirium will often include emotional disturbances, such as symptoms of anxiety or depression, and behavioral changes, including agitation and impulsivity. Changes in the sleep-wake cycle are also noted in the form of sleep loss, reduced arousal, or reversal of the usual circadian rhythm sleep pattern. Delirium may also be hypoactive, hyperactive, or mixed with regard to psychomotor activity [2].

According to the *International Statistical Classification of Diseases and Related Health Problems (ICD-11)*, delirium can be differentiated from dementia in that delirium is acute in onset and transient and tends to wax and wane compared with the gradual onset and progressive nature of dementia [3]. The ICD-11 also considers delirium to be diagnostically distinct from altered mental states due to brain injury from trauma or other precipitating neurologic events, such as a stroke or intracranial bleed.

The prevalence of delirium in the community is lower than in hospital or acute care settings. One systematic review estimated an overall point prevalence of delirium of 0.7% for people aged $\geq$60 years, though this estimate was based on only a few studies, and there was variation between studies on the assessments used for diagnosing delirium [4]. A cohort study by Davis et al. created and validated a study-specific algorithm for diagnosing delirium in older adults $\geq$65 years in the general population; using this algorithm, they reported a period prevalence of 5.6% [5].

Delirium is much more common in the hospital setting. One study found that delirium was present on hospital admission in 12% of older patients [6], while others have reported occurrence rates of 14–58% in older hospitalized medical patients [7]. One systematic review found that 10–31% of older patients were noted to have delirium on admission, with incidence rates of

R. Chi (✉) · B. Khan
Department of Internal Medicine, Division of Pulmonary, Critical Care, Sleep, and Occupational Medicine, Indiana University School of Medicine, Indianapolis, IN, USA
e-mail: rchi@iu.edu; bakhan@iu.edu

S. Wang
Department of Psychiatry, Indiana University School of Medicine, Indianapolis, IN, USA
e-mail: sophwang@iupui.edu

new-onset delirium per admission ranging from 3% to 29% [8]. Delirium is especially prevalent in the intensive care unit (ICU) setting, where estimates range from 31% to over 80% of older ICU patients eventually developing delirium [9–13]. Delirium is also prevalent in older hospitalized patients undergoing surgery of any kind, with over 40% developing postoperative delirium [14, 15].

Numerous studies have found that the development of delirium during hospitalization is associated with worse functional outcomes and long-term disability [6, 16–19]. Delirium has also been associated with higher morbidity and mortality rates both during hospitalization and after discharge [10, 20–23]. Delirium has also been associated with persistent cognitive dysfunction in up to 70% of patients after discharge [24–28]. Delirium is recognized as a significant in-hospital risk factor for the development of post-ICU syndrome, or PICS, defined as new or worsening long-term impairments in physical, cognitive, or mental health functioning among ICU survivors [29, 30].

Although delirium is usually defined as an acute transient process, there is evidence to suggest that delirium may persist to discharge and beyond. A systematic review by Cole et al. noted that across 18 studies, 44.7% were noted to have persistent delirium at the time of discharge, though this number had declined to 32.8%, 25.6%, and 21% at 1, 3, and 6 months, respectively [31]. Furthermore, patients with persistent delirium had worse clinical outcomes in terms of cognitive and physical functioning, nursing home placement, and mortality compared to patients who had recovered from delirium. According to a systematic review by Dasgupta et al., risk factors for persistent delirium included dementia, higher delirium severity, hypoactive symptoms, hypoxia, and a higher number of medical diagnoses [32].

It is estimated that the healthcare costs associated with delirium range from $16,303 to $64,421 per patient, cumulatively reaching as high as $152 billion annually [33, 34]. One study found that the 30-day cumulative cost of delirium in the ICU was $17,838 per patient and would have been closer to approximately $22,500, except for the cost savings due to delirium-associated early mortality [35]. Despite its profound clinical and economic consequences, delirium in the hospital is often underrecognized, with one study revealing that the diagnosis of delirium was missed by the primary team in more than 60% of inpatients who were referred for palliative care [36].

Risk Factors

Delirium can have various etiologies and is often multifactorial. According to the *DSM-5*, delirium can be triggered by medical illness, use of or withdrawal from certain medications or recreational substances, or other unknown factors [1]. Maldonado has proposed a "system integration failure" hypothesis that posits that delirium is the result of neurotransmitter imbalances and an integration failure of neural networks that occurs after an acute insult in the presence of certain patient-specific physiologic characteristics (referred to as "substrates") that confer a cognitive vulnerability and predisposition to delirium [37].

Certain predisposing risk factors are known to be associated with delirium. Older age and a prior history of dementia are two of the most commonly cited risk factors [38–42]. Other medical comorbidities and illness-specific risk factors that have been found to be associated with delirium include alcoholism, hypertension, smoking history, illness severity, and metabolic and lab abnormalities such as low arterial pH, elevated creatinine, and elevated bilirubin [11, 13, 42–45].

Treatment-related risk factors for delirium have also been identified, particularly related to the use of certain medications. The most consistently identified medications associated with delirium in research studies are benzodiazepines [11–13, 39, 42] and corticosteroids [46–49]. Anticholinergic medications have also been found to be deliriogenic [50–52], though a couple of studies have failed to find a clear association [53, 54]. Benzodiazepines, corticosteroids, and anticholinergics are all listed on the American Geriatric Society 2019 Beers Criteria as medications that are typically best avoided in older adults due to the potential for inducing or worsening delirium [55].

Studies examining the use of opiates have yielded inconsistent results. One study by Dubois et al. found that morphine and epidural use were associated with delirium. However, Ouimet et al. found that sedatives and analgesia increased the risk of delirium only when used to induce coma but not with any other use [11], while Pandharipande et al. found that fentanyl increased the risk of delirium in the surgical ICU, but morphine reduced the risk of delirium [12]. A systematic review of postoperative analgesia and its effects on delirium found that with the exception of meperidine, more frequently used opioids such as morphine, fentanyl, and hydromorphone were not associated with higher rates of postoperative delirium [56]. Other studies have found that untreated pain and lower doses of analgesia after elective surgery in older adults were associated with a higher risk of delirium [57–59].

Environmental risk factors may also play an important role. In the hospital setting, sleep disturbances triggered by machine noise, patient care activities, certain medications, and critical illnesses can lead to circadian rhythm disruptions that may contribute to the development of delirium. Studies show that ICU patients have profound disruptions in sleep, from sleep fragmentation to decreased rapid eye movement (REM) sleep to reduced sleep quantity [60–62]. One study found a significant association between severe REM sleep reduction and delirium in the critically ill patient population [63]. Outside of the hospital setting, sleep disturbances have been associated with hallucinations in patients with neurodegenerative disorders [64, 65]. It is unclear whether delirium is a result or a cause of sleep disturbances [66], although interventions targeted at improving sleep hygiene in the ICU setting have been shown to reduce the incidence of delirium [67, 68], suggesting a causal relationship.

The risk factors associated with postoperative delirium in older surgical patients differ from delirium in nonsurgical patients in important ways. Older surgical patients are exposed to the additional stressors of anesthesia and surgery, which may contribute to the risk of delirium via different mechanisms as compared to nonsurgical illness. Research involving older patients undergoing elective surgery has provided valuable insights into the delirium risk factors specific to anesthesia and surgery by allowing for preoperative baseline assessments of cognitive function and serial bloodwork prior to the onset of delirium.

A growing body of evidence suggests that intraoperative and post-procedural blood transfusions may be associated with postoperative delirium. Whitlock et al. found that in cardiothoracic surgery patients, intraoperative blood transfusion was an independent risk factor for postoperative delirium [69]. Behrends et al. found that in older adults undergoing major noncardiac surgery, intraoperative blood transfusion of more than 1 L was the most strongly associated predictor of delirium on the first postoperative day [70]. An electronic health record study of postoperative ICU patients found that blood transfusions were one of the factors associated with postoperative delirium [71]. The 2018 Clinical Practice Guidelines for the Prevention and Management of Pain, Agitation/Sedation, Delirium, Immobility, and Sleep Disruption in Adult Patients in the ICU, also known as the PADIS guidelines, found strong evidence for only two modifiable risk factors for delirium: blood transfusion and benzodiazepine use [72].

Risk factors related to the depth and method of anesthesia administration may contribute to delirium. Numerous studies suggest that elderly patients require substantially lower doses of sedative and anesthetic medications than younger patients to achieve the same effect [73–75]. When administered anesthetics in the OR, compared to younger patients, elderly patients spent a higher proportion of time in burst suppression on EEG and have higher suppression ratios on bispectral index (BIS) monitoring [76, 77], indicative of oversedation. There is evidence to suggest that oversedation of elderly patients under anesthesia contributes to postoperative delirium. A number of research studies have found that using BIS or EEG monitoring to guide anesthesia and target lighter sedation goals was associated with a lower incidence of delirium and subsequent cognitive impairment [78–81], although the recent ENGAGES trial failed to find a difference in postoperative delirium rates when using EEG-guided anesthesia [82].

There is conflicting evidence regarding the type of anesthetic used and its impact on delirium. A Cochrane review found modest evidence to suggest that peripheral nerve blocks could reduce the risk of delirium in patients with hip fractures [83], while a recent systematic review and meta-analysis of randomized controlled trials found that regional nerve blocks were effective in preventing delirium only in patients without preexisting cognitive impairment [84]. One major randomized controlled clinical trial failed to find a difference between regional and general anesthesia in reducing postoperative delirium rates [85]. Finally, the question of whether intravenous anesthesia with propofol may be superior to inhalational anesthesia in reducing postoperative delirium is still uncertain. A Cochrane systematic review aimed at answering this question was unable to reach definitive conclusions based on the included studies [86].

Assessment

Several diagnostic screening tools have been developed to allow for easy and reliable detection of delirium in the hospital setting. The Confusion Assessment Method (CAM) is a 10-item screening instrument developed by Inouye et al. to detect delirium in the general medicine ward setting, with a sensitivity of 94–100%, specificity of 90–95%, and high inter-observer reliability [87]. The CAM can be abbreviated into its short form by focusing on only the first four features which, if present, is sufficient to meet the criteria for delirium.

Despite the strengths of the CAM as a delirium screening tool, its interview-based nature made it challenging to use in the ICU setting, especially in mechanically ventilated nonverbal patients. Therefore, there was a need for delirium

screening tools that could be used specifically in the ICU population. The CAM was adapted for the ICU setting by Ely et al., which became known as the CAM-ICU [88]. The CAM-ICU was demonstrated to have good interrater reliability and validity among ICU patient populations, even in mechanically ventilated nonverbal patients [89]. Another commonly used tool is the Intensive Care Delirium Screening Checklist (ICDSC), a tool developed by Bergeron et al. and validated in medical and surgical ICU patients [90]. The ICDSC asks about specific DSM-based symptoms such as sleep disruptions, inappropriate moods, and psychotic symptoms, which are not explicitly addressed in the CAM-ICU. Both assessment tools have been discussed for use in delirium screening in the 2018 PADIS guidelines [91]. A systematic review and meta-analysis by Gusmao-Flores et al. found that CAM-ICU had higher sensitivity and specificity than the ICDSC [92], though another systematic review by Neto et al. found that the ICDSC had better sensitivity, though lower specificity, than the CAM-ICU [92, 93].

Other assessment tools have been developed to ascertain not just the presence of delirium but its severity as well. The CAM-S is based on the CAM but ascribes a score of 0–2 on each of the items to yield a total score and can be administered in either short- or long-form versions [94]. The Delirium Rating Scale-Revised-98 (DRS-R-98) is a 16-item scale, which yields a total score ranging from 0 to 39 points and has been shown to have high sensitivity and specificity as well as good reliability and validity [95]. However, the use of either the CAM-S or the DRS-R-98 in mechanically ventilated patients is limited by the inability to ascertain the patient's language and thought processes in detail. The CAM-ICU-7, developed by Khan et al., is a 7-point rating scale derived from the CAM-ICU and Richmond Agitation Sedation Scale (RASS) assessments, and it has been shown to have high internal reliability, strong correlation with the DRS-R-98, and good predictive validity for outcomes such as mortality and discharge to home [96]. However, at this time, assessment of delirium severity is not routinely done in the clinical setting, and its use is mostly limited to research studies.

Research studies have examined the role of serum and cerebrospinal fluid biomarkers in delirium, including pro-inflammatory cytokines and chemokines (such as IL-1, IL-6, IL-8, IL-10, TNFα, IFN-γ, CCL-2), biomarkers specific to neurodegeneration (such as amyloid-β and tau proteins), biomarkers indicative of neural injury (such as S100β and neurofilament light chain), and biomarkers associated with endothelial injury (such as PAI-1, E-selectin, and VEGF). Numerous studies have found correlations between various biomarkers and the presence and severity of delirium [97–100]. However, although these studies have provided important clues as to the pathophysiologic mechanisms underlying delirium, no single biomarker has been noted to have a consistent diagnostic or predictive utility for delirium.

Delirium has been associated with certain anatomical changes on neuroimaging. A study by Gunther et al. found more global brain atrophy, more volume loss in the superior frontal lobes, and smaller hippocampal volumes on brain MRI in ICU survivors with a longer duration of delirium, and these findings correlated with worse cognitive and executive functioning at 3- and 12-month follow-up visits [101]. A recent study by Sprung et al. found decreased hippocampal volumes and increased cortical thinning on brain MRI in ICU patients compared to hospitalized non-ICU patients and that these changes were more pronounced in ICU patients with delirium compared to those without delirium [102]. However, despite these intriguing findings, neuroimaging is not considered a mainstay of delirium workup or treatment and is of little clinical benefit, except in ruling out a primary neurologic etiology of altered mental status.

Research studies have also found certain electroencephalogram (EEG) findings that are correlated with delirium. A recent systematic review of 31 studies found that delirium was associated with generalized slowing of the EEG, along with reduced measures of functional connectivity between brain regions [103]. Across many of the included studies, delirium was consistently associated with a decrease in alpha power (normally associated with attention and consciousness) and increase in delta power (a pathologic EEG finding associated with reduced cognitive function), and several studies found increased burst suppression duration prior to the onset of delirium [103, 104]. However, while research to characterize pathognomonic EEG markers for delirium is still actively ongoing, EEG is currently not used to diagnose or manage delirium and is only clinically useful in ruling out seizure activity as a cause of altered mentation.

One important diagnostic consideration is the clinical overlap between depression and delirium, particularly hypoactive delirium. Both conditions can manifest similarly, with reduced psychomotor activity, cognitive impairment, sleep disturbances, and impaired concentration or inattention. Further complicating the picture is the frequent co-occurrence of both conditions, with numerous studies showing an association between delirium and increased depressive symptomatology on subsequent follow-up [105–107]. Studies suggest that a considerable proportion of hospitalized patients with delirium are initially misdiagnosed with and referred to psychiatry consult services for depression, with estimates ranging from 6% to 52% [108–110]. However, certain clinical features can help distinguish between the two. Delirium typically has a more acute onset with a fluctuating course in the setting of medical illness, more profound changes in awareness, and psychotic symptoms related to their immediate environment, whereas the features of depression are more sustained, with more complex psychosis related to guilt or nihilism, and are usually associated with psychological stress [111]. Some patients who exhibit both delirium and depression may need to be treated for both, in which case, avoidance of pharmacologic agents with anticholinergic properties or other mechanisms that can exacerbate delirium is of utmost importance.

Treatment

Non-pharmacologic

The approach to managing delirium is largely non-pharmacological and usually involves an integrated multimodal approach. One highly effective program for managing delirium in older adults in the inpatient setting is the Hospital Elder Life Program (HELP), a model of care developed by Inouye et al. that focuses on a series of targeted interventions designed to reduce delirium and prevent cognitive and functional decline during hospitalization [112]. The program is overseen by an interdisciplinary team comprised of a geriatrician, a nurse specialist, an operations specialist/volunteer coordinator, and trained volunteers. Core interventions include daily orientation of the patient, overcoming vision or auditory barriers, encouraging cognitive stimulation and early mobilization, assisting with feeds, and optimizing sleep. Interdisciplinary rounds, geriatric nursing assessments, provider education, and quality assurance procedures are also important components of the model that promote coordination of care.

Since its inception, HELP has become a very successful reference model for delirium prevention in the hospital setting. It has been modified for older adults in the surgical setting [113] and adapted in hospitals and healthcare systems internationally [114–119]. It has also been expanded to allow for the participation of family members and caregivers in HELP interventions [120]. Numerous studies have supported the clinical and economic benefits of HELP and other similar multicomponent non-pharmacological delirium interventions [121, 122]. A clinical trial found that implementation of HELP led to a significant reduction in new delirium cases, delirium episodes, and total days with delirium, although there was no effect on delirium severity once delirium had occurred [123]. Adaptation of the HELP model in a 40-bed inpatient unit in a community hospital resulted in a 35.3% reduction in delirium rates and significant cost savings of approximately $600,000 over 6 months [124]. When the same hospital later expanded the program to six inpatient units, cost savings were estimated to be more than $7.3 million per year, with lower rates of delirium, shorter lengths of stay, and greater satisfaction among patients, their families, and nursing staff [125]. Another community hospital found that the HELP program reduced delirium episode rates by 40% and shortened length of stay by 2 days, resulting in cost savings of $841,000 over 9 months [126].

Many of the same principles underlying the HELP program have been adapted to the ICU setting in what is now termed the "ABCDEF" bundle [127, 128]. The "ABCDEF" bundle is a non-pharmacologic multicomponent protocol that promotes evidence-based interdisciplinary strategies to prevent or mitigate delirium in the ICU setting. The "ABCDEF" acronym stands for **A**ssess and treat pain, **B**oth spontaneous awakening and breathing trials, **C**hoice of Sedation, **D**elirium monitoring and treatment, **E**arly mobility and exercise, and **F**amily engagement. The **D**elirium monitoring and treatment portion involves an array of tactics that include addressing pain, frequently reorienting the patient to date and place, providing visual or hearing aids as needed, reducing sleep interruptions, and promoting daytime wakefulness to preserve circadian rhythms. As with the HELP model, the ABCDEF bundle has been shown to reduce delirium and substantially improve patient outcomes. A prospective cohort study of over 15,000 adult ICU patients in 68 hospitals found that complete adherence to the ABCDEF bundle performance significantly reduced the likelihood of numerous clinical outcomes, including hospital death within 7 days, next-day mechanical ventilation, coma, delirium, use of physical restraints, ICU readmission, and discharge to a facility other than home [129].

Pharmacologic

Although the mainstay of delirium treatment is largely non-pharmacologic, medications are sometimes used to address the side effects of delirium, such as agitation or insomnia. As neurotransmitter imbalances have been posited to play a key role in the pathophysiology of delirium [37], research studies have examined whether the use of certain medications that affect neurotransmitter signaling, particularly with regard to dopamine and acetylcholine, can effectively treat or even prevent delirium. First-generation and atypical antipsychotics, such as haloperidol, risperidone, olanzapine, and quetiapine, work by blocking dopamine receptors and are commonly used to treat agitation in delirious patients. However, studies generally have not shown a substantial benefit of antipsychotics in preventing delirium or reducing its severity [130–133], and evidence suggests that they may even worsen delirium symptoms in terminally ill adult patients [134]. Furthermore, the FDA issued a black box warning in 2003 for the use of antipsychotics in elderly patients with dementia-related psychosis or agitation, due to the increased risks of cerebrovascular events and death noted in clinical trials [135]. Given that dementia is a strong risk factor for delirium, this poses a dilemma for the inpatient clinician having to manage agitation in delirious patients with a history of dementia. In general, the use of antipsychotics should be reserved for severe agitation posing an immediate risk of harm to self or others, after carefully considering and discussing the risks versus benefits with family members, using the lowest effective dose, and closely monitoring the patient for prolonged QT or potential arrhythmias with regular ECGs or telemetry [136].

Similarly, the use of cholinesterase inhibitors such as rivastigmine and donepezil to prevent or treat delirium has also been well studied, based on the hypothesis that impaired cholinergic neurotransmission might play a key role in the development of delirium [137]. There is evidence to support this hypothesis, with a recent study by Hughes et al. finding that higher plasma acetylcholinesterase levels were associated with increased odds of same-day delirium in critically ill patients with respiratory failure or shock [138]. However, a Cochrane systematic review found insufficient evidence to support or refute its use in treating delirium in non-ICU settings, although only one study of 15 patients comparing rivastigmine to placebo met the criteria for inclusion

[139]. A more inclusive systematic review by Tampi et al. evaluated 7 randomized controlled trials involving acetylcholinesterase inhibitors for delirium in older adults and similarly concluded a lack of efficacy of acetylcholinesterase inhibitors in preventing or treating delirium [140]. One randomized controlled trial examining rivastigmine or placebo as an adjunct to haloperidol in adult ICU patients with delirium found that the duration of delirium was actually 2 days longer in the rivastigmine group, and in a more worrisome development, mortality was noted to be nearly three times higher in the rivastigmine group compared to placebo, prompting the trial to be halted early [141]. However, a recent retrospective cohort study found that prehospital use of donepezil in patients with dementia reduced delirium prevalence and led to improved clinical outcomes in terms of in-hospital and 90-day mortality, ICU length of stay, and duration of mechanical ventilation [142]. It is possible that the preventative benefit of cholinesterase inhibitors may be limited to patients with preexisting dementia already on medication prior to admission, with limited or no benefit to its acute use in treating delirium in the hospital.

Research studies have found evidence that dexmedetomidine may offer some benefit in preventing or mitigating delirium compared to other sedative medications. In the MENDS trial, Pandharipande et al. found that dexmedetomidine infusion for sedation in mechanically ventilated patients was associated with more days alive without delirium or coma and more time at sedation-level targets when compared to lorazepam infusion [143]. Another systematic review by Pereira et al. found that dexmedetomidine use for sedation was associated with a lower incidence of delirium when compared to propofol use [144]. A systematic review and meta-analysis by Flükiger et al. found that dexmedetomidine was associated with a reduced incidence and duration of delirium compared with placebo, standard sedatives, and haloperidol [145]. Finally, a meta-analysis performed in a Cochrane systematic review by Burry et al. concluded that there was evidence to suggest that dexmedetomidine may shorten delirium duration compared to placebo, though the effect was small and only seen in pairwise analyses

[146]. However, routine use of dexmedetomidine is limited by side effects such as bradycardia and hypotension, its availability in intravenous form only, and the fact that dexmedetomidine does not offer the same depth of sedation as propofol or other sedative medications.

As poor sleep hygiene and disruptions in circadian rhythms are known triggers for delirium, it had been hypothesized that melatonin or melatonin receptor agonists might have a protective effect on delirium. However, results have been mixed. A 2016 Cochrane systematic review did not find clear evidence that melatonin use had any effect on delirium in hospitalized non-ICU patients, but two more recent meta-analyses found that melatonin was associated with a reduced incidence of delirium in surgical and ICU patients [147, 148].

The question of whether de-prescribing efforts reduce the incidence or severity of delirium has also been investigated. A randomized clinical trial by Khan et al. examined a pharmacist-driven multicomponent bundle in the ICU designed to reduce exposure to anticholinergic medications and benzodiazepines and to offer low-dose haloperidol as an alternative, but the use of this bundle did not result in fewer delirium/coma-free days or reduction in delirium severity at 1 week [133]. However, the intervention also did not achieve a significant reduction in benzodiazepine or anticholinergic medication use in the intervention group compared with the usual care group, which may have affected the results [149]. It is possible that de-prescribing efforts to reduce delirium risk may be more beneficial after discharge or in the outpatient setting. One systematic review of medication withdrawal trials in older adults, many of which were done in nursing homes, concluded that withdrawal of benzodiazepines improved cognitive functioning, though these studies did not specifically examine delirium [150]. The same systematic review also noted that antipsychotic withdrawal trials generally did not demonstrate any differences in behavioral, psychiatric, cognitive, or functional measures after cessation of antipsychotics.

Evidence-Based Treatment Algorithm

Figure 8.1 provides a general evidence-based approach to the management of delirium in the hospital setting. This approach involves

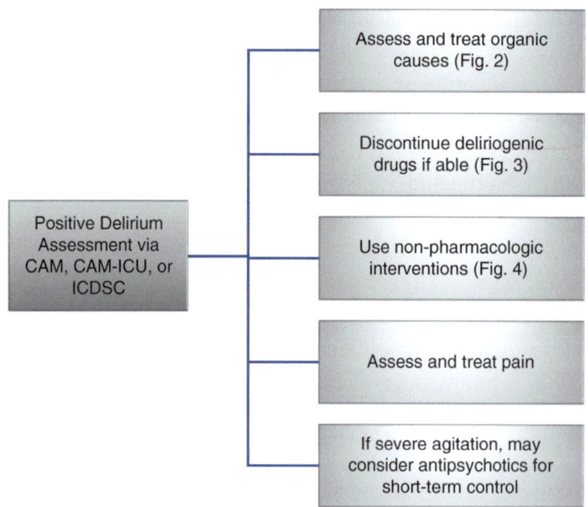

Fig. 8.1 Approach to the hospitalized patient with delirium

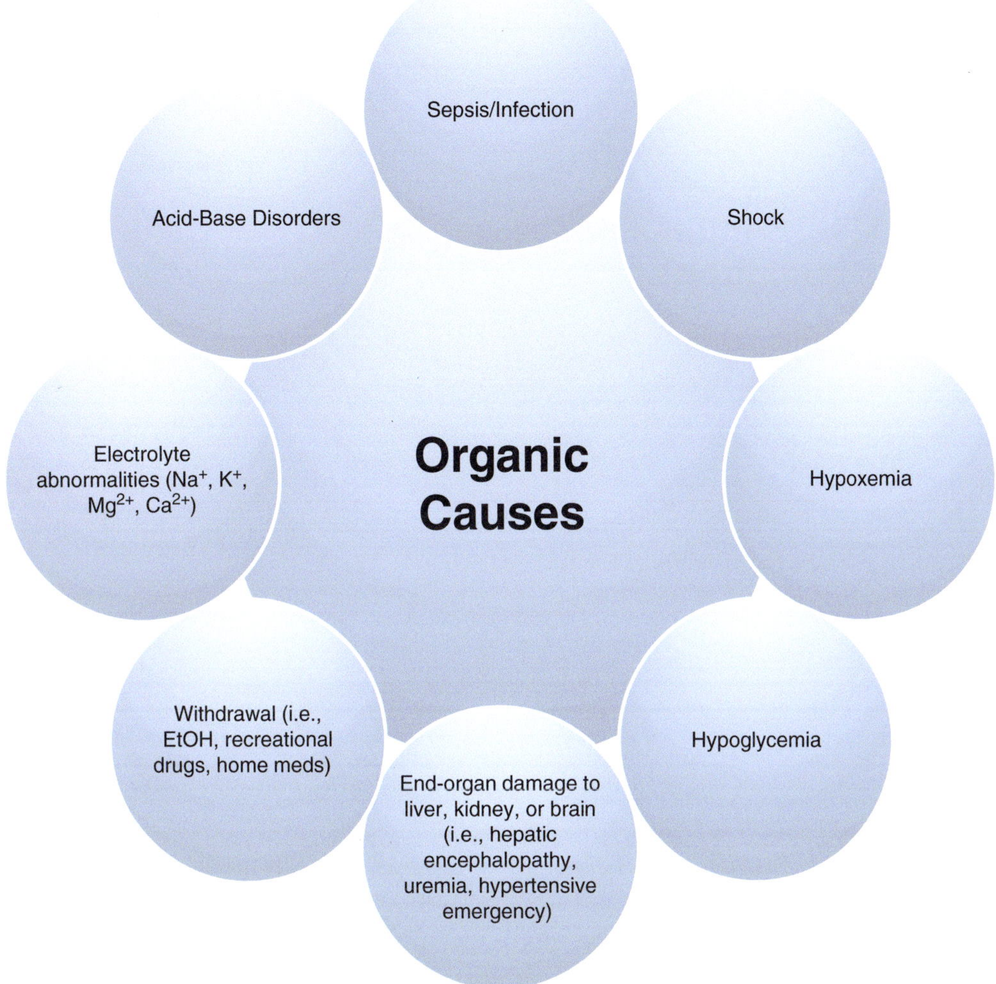

Fig. 8.2 Organic causes of delirium

addressing medical conditions or organic etiologies of delirium (Fig. 8.2), minimizing or eliminating deliriogenic medications (Fig. 8.3), and non-pharmacologic interventions targeted towards orienting the patient and optimizing the environment (Fig. 8.4). Other specific treatment algorithms are also available to clinicians, such as the ICU Delirium Protocol available on ICUdelirium.org, a helpful Web resource developed by the Critical Illness, Brain Dysfunction, and Survivorship (CIBS) Center at Vanderbilt University [151]. The American Geriatrics Society CoCare website also provides a wealth of resources that can assist with institutional implementation of the HELP model [152].

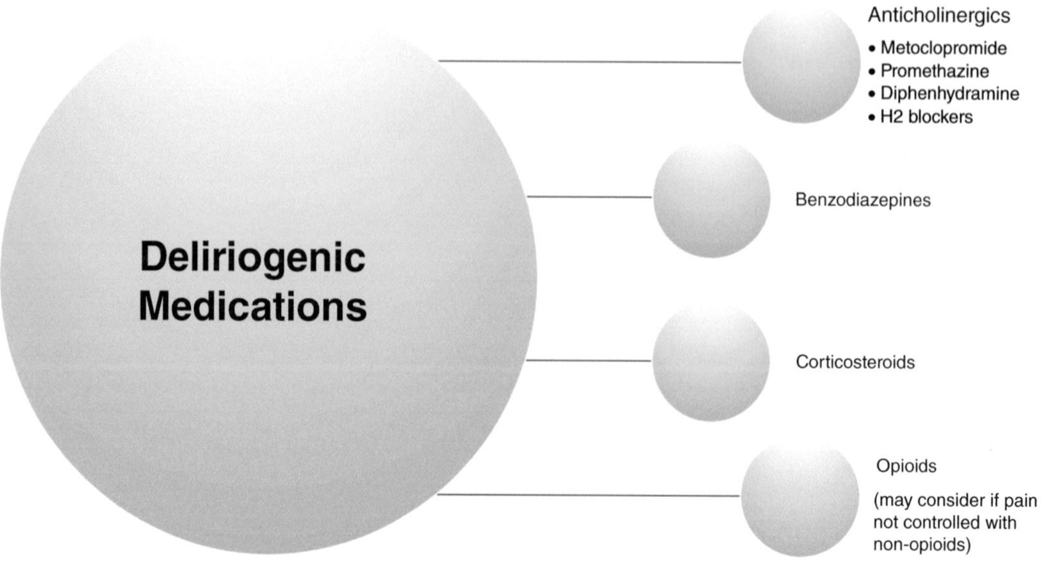

Fig. 8.3 Medications that may contribute to delirium

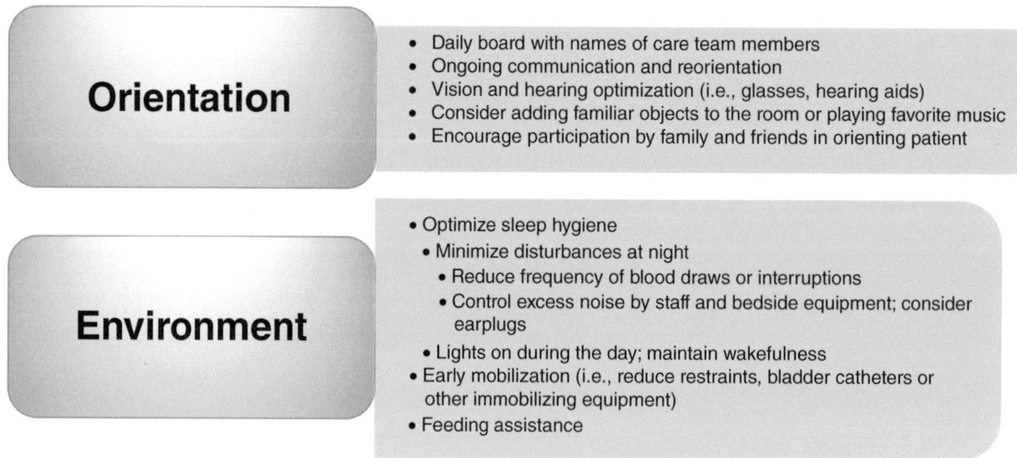

Consider the use of a well-established, validated multicomponent bundle:
- HELP model (general inpatient setting)
- ABCDEF bundle (ICU setting)

Fig. 8.4 Non-pharmacologic interventions for delirium

Conclusion

Delirium is highly prevalent among older hospitalized and postoperative patients but remains underrecognized and undertreated despite deleterious long-term consequences. Because of its multifactorial etiology and lack of effective pharmacologic treatment, a multimodal non-pharmacologic approach such as the HELP model or ABCDEF bundle is the accepted standard of care for delirium management, but the implementation of these approaches varies widely across hospitals. Clinicians and hospitals must prioritize delirium recognition and management by incorporating validated delirium screening tools and treatment protocols into routine inpatient care to improve outcomes and minimize the harmful effects of delirium.

References

1. APA. Neurocognitive disorders. Diagnostic and statistical manual of mental disorders. DSM Library. 5th ed. Washington, DC: American Psychiatric Association Publishing; 2022.
2. Peterson JF, Pun BT, Dittus RS, Thomason JW, Jackson JC, Shintani AK, et al. Delirium and its motoric subtypes: a study of 614 critically ill patients. J Am Geriatr Soc. 2006;54(3):479–84.
3. WHO. 6D70 delirium. International statistical classification of diseases and related health problems. 11th ed. World Health Organization; 2019.
4. Davis DH, Kreisel SH, Muniz Terrera G, Hall AJ, Morandi A, Boustani M, et al. The epidemiology of delirium: challenges and opportunities for population studies. Am J Geriatr Psychiatry. 2013;21(12):1173–89.
5. Davis DH, Barnes LE, Stephan BC, MacLullich AM, Meagher D, Copeland J, et al. The descriptive epidemiology of delirium symptoms in a large population-based cohort study: results from the Medical Research Council Cognitive Function and Ageing Study (MRC CFAS). BMC Geriatr. 2014;14:87.
6. Inouye SK, Rushing JT, Foreman MD, Palmer RM, Pompei P. Does delirium contribute to poor hospital outcomes? A three-site epidemiologic study. J Gen Intern Med. 1998;13(4):234–42.
7. Inouye SK. The dilemma of delirium: clinical and research controversies regarding diagnosis and evaluation of delirium in hospitalized elderly medical patients. Am J Med. 1994;97(3):278–88.
8. Siddiqi N, House AO, Holmes JD. Occurrence and outcome of delirium in medical in-patients: a systematic literature review. Age Ageing. 2006;35(4):350–64.
9. Brummel NE, Jackson JC, Pandharipande PP, Thompson JL, Shintani AK, Dittus RS, et al. Delirium in the ICU and subsequent long-term disability among survivors of mechanical ventilation. Crit Care Med. 2014;42(2):369–77.
10. Ely EW, Shintani A, Truman B, Speroff T, Gordon SM, Harrell FE Jr, et al. Delirium as a predictor of mortality in mechanically ventilated patients in the intensive care unit. JAMA. 2004;291(14):1753–62.
11. Ouimet S, Kavanagh BP, Gottfried SB, Skrobik Y. Incidence, risk factors and consequences of ICU delirium. Intensive Care Med. 2007;33(1):66–73.
12. Pandharipande P, Cotton BA, Shintani A, Thompson J, Pun BT, Morris JA Jr, et al. Prevalence and risk factors for development of delirium in surgical and trauma intensive care unit patients. J Trauma. 2008;65(1):34–41.
13. Pisani MA, Murphy TE, Van Ness PH, Araujo KL, Inouye SK. Characteristics associated with delirium in older patients in a medical intensive care unit. Arch Intern Med. 2007;167(15):1629–34.
14. Jin Z, Hu J, Ma D. Postoperative delirium: perioperative assessment, risk reduction, and management. Br J Anaesth. 2020;125(4):492–504.
15. Robinson TN, Raeburn CD, Tran ZV, Angles EM, Brenner LA, Moss M. Postoperative delirium in the elderly: risk factors and outcomes. Ann Surg. 2009;249(1):173–8.
16. Marcantonio ER, Flacker JM, Michaels M, Resnick NM. Delirium is independently associated with poor functional recovery after hip fracture. J Am Geriatr Soc. 2000;48(6):618–24.
17. McCusker J, Cole M, Dendukuri N, Belzile E, Primeau F. Delirium in older medical inpatients and subsequent cognitive and functional status: a prospective study. CMAJ. 2001;165(5):575–83.
18. Quinlan N, Rudolph JL. Postoperative delirium and functional decline after noncardiac surgery. J Am Geriatr Soc. 2011;59(Suppl 2):S301–4.
19. Rudolph JL, Inouye SK, Jones RN, Yang FM, Fong TG, Levkoff SE, et al. Delirium: an independent predictor of functional decline after cardiac surgery. J Am Geriatr Soc. 2010;58(4):643–9.
20. Pisani MA, Kong SY, Kasl SV, Murphy TE, Araujo KL, Van Ness PH. Days of delirium are associated with 1-year mortality in an older intensive care unit population. Am J Respir Crit Care Med. 2009;180(11):1092–7.
21. Pandharipande P, Jackson J, Ely EW. Delirium: acute cognitive dysfunction in the critically ill. Curr Opin Crit Care. 2005;11(4):360–8.
22. Inouye SK, Schlesinger MJ, Lydon TJ. Delirium: a symptom of how hospital care is failing older persons and a window to improve quality of hospital care. Am J Med. 1999;106(5):565–73.
23. Leslie DL, Zhang Y, Holford TR, Bogardus ST, Leo-Summers LS, Inouye SK. Premature death associated with delirium at 1-year follow-up. Arch Intern Med. 2005;165(14):1657–62.
24. Fong TG, Davis D, Growdon ME, Albuquerque A, Inouye SK. The interface between delirium and dementia in elderly adults. Lancet Neurol. 2015;14(8):823–32.
25. Davis DH, Muniz Terrera G, Keage H, Rahkonen T, Oinas M, Matthews FE, et al. Delirium is a strong risk factor for dementia in the oldest-old: a population-based cohort study. Brain. 2012;135(Pt 9):2809–16.
26. Pandharipande PP, Girard TD, Jackson JC, Morandi A, Thompson JL, Pun BT, et al. Long-term cognitive impairment after critical illness. N Engl J Med. 2013;369(14):1306–16.

27. Fong TG, Tulebaev SR, Inouye SK. Delirium in elderly adults: diagnosis, prevention and treatment. Nat Rev Neurol. 2009;5(4):210–20.

28. Girard TD, Jackson JC, Pandharipande PP, Pun BT, Thompson JL, Shintani AK, et al. Delirium as a predictor of long-term cognitive impairment in survivors of critical illness. Crit Care Med. 2010;38(7):1513–20.

29. Lee M, Kang J, Jeong YJ. Risk factors for post-intensive care syndrome: a systematic review and meta-analysis. Aust Crit Care. 2020;33(3):287–94.

30. Mikkelsen ME, Still M, Anderson BJ, Bienvenu OJ, Brodsky MB, Brummel N, et al. Society of Critical Care Medicine's international consensus conference on prediction and identification of long-term impairments after critical illness. Crit Care Med. 2020;48(11):1670–9.

31. Cole MG, Ciampi A, Belzile E, Zhong L. Persistent delirium in older hospital patients: a systematic review of frequency and prognosis. Age Ageing. 2009;38(1):19–26.

32. Dasgupta M, Hillier LM. Factors associated with prolonged delirium: a systematic review. Int Psychogeriatr. 2010;22(3):373–94.

33. Leslie DL, Inouye SK. The importance of delirium: economic and societal costs. J Am Geriatr Soc. 2011;59(Suppl 2):S241–3.

34. Leslie DL, Marcantonio ER, Zhang Y, Leo-Summers L, Inouye SK. One-year health care costs associated with delirium in the elderly population. Arch Intern Med. 2008;168(1):27–32.

35. Vasilevskis EE, Chandrasekhar R, Holtze CH, Graves J, Speroff T, Girard TD, et al. The cost of ICU delirium and coma in the intensive care unit patient. Med Care. 2018;56(10):890–7.

36. de la Cruz M, Fan J, Yennu S, Tanco K, Shin S, Wu J, et al. The frequency of missed delirium in patients referred to palliative care in a comprehensive cancer center. Support Care Cancer. 2015;23(8):2427–33.

37. Maldonado JR. Delirium pathophysiology: an updated hypothesis of the etiology of acute brain failure. Int J Geriatr Psychiatry. 2018;33(11):1428–57.

38. Canet E, Amjad S, Robbins R, Lewis J, Matalanis M, Jones D, et al. Differential clinical characteristics, management and outcome of delirium among ward compared with intensive care unit patients. Intern Med J. 2019;49(12):1496–504.

39. Tachibana M, Inada T, Ichida M, Kojima S, Shioya M, Wakayama K, et al. Factors associated with the severity of delirium. Hum Psychopharmacol. 2021;36(5):e2787.

40. Ryan DJ, O'Regan NA, Caoimh RO, Clare J, O'Connor M, Leonard M, et al. Delirium in an adult acute hospital population: predictors, prevalence and detection. BMJ Open. 2013;3(1):e001772.

41. McNicoll L, Pisani MA, Zhang Y, Ely EW, Siegel MD, Inouye SK. Delirium in the intensive care unit: occurrence and clinical course in older patients. J Am Geriatr Soc. 2003;51(5):591–8.

42. Pandharipande P, Shintani A, Peterson J, Pun BT, Wilkinson GR, Dittus RS, et al. Lorazepam is an independent risk factor for transitioning to delirium in intensive care unit patients. Anesthesiology. 2006;104(1):21–6.

43. Dubois MJ, Bergeron N, Dumont M, Dial S, Skrobik Y. Delirium in an intensive care unit: a study of risk factors. Intensive Care Med. 2001;27(8):1297–304.

44. Aldemir M, Ozen S, Kara IH, Sir A, Bac B. Predisposing factors for delirium in the surgical intensive care unit. Crit Care. 2001;5(5):265–70.

45. Gravante F, Giannarelli D, Pucci A, Gagliardi AM, Mitello L, Montagna A, et al. Prevalence and risk factors of delirium in the intensive care unit: an observational study. Nurs Crit Care. 2021;26(3):156–65.

46. Warrington TP, Bostwick JM. Psychiatric adverse effects of corticosteroids. Mayo Clin Proc. 2006;81(10):1361–7.

47. Schreiber MP, Colantuoni E, Bienvenu OJ, Neufeld KJ, Chen KF, Shanholtz C, et al. Corticosteroids and transition to delirium in patients with acute lung injury. Crit Care Med. 2014;42(6):1480–6.

48. Cole JL. Steroid-induced sleep disturbance and delirium: a focused review for critically ill patients. Fed Pract. 2020;37(6):260–7.

49. Wu Z, Li H, Liao K, Wang Y. Association between dexamethasone and delirium in critically ill patients: a retrospective cohort study of a large clinical database. J Surg Res. 2021;263:89–101.

50. Egberts A, Moreno-Gonzalez R, Alan H, Ziere G, Mattace-Raso FUS. Anticholinergic drug burden and delirium: a systematic review. J Am Med Dir Assoc. 2021;22(1):65–73 e4.

51. Oudewortel L, van der Roest HG, Onder G, Wijnen VJM, Liperoti R, Denkinger M, et al. The Association of Anticholinergic Drugs and Delirium in nursing home patients with dementia: results from the SHELTER study. J Am Med Dir Assoc. 2021;22(10):2087–92.

52. Pasina L, Rizzi B, Nobili A, Recchia A. Anticholinergic load and delirium in end-of-life patients. Eur J Clin Pharmacol. 2021;77(9):1419–24.

53. Pasina L, Colzani L, Cortesi L, Tettamanti M, Zambon A, Nobili A, et al. Relation between delirium and anticholinergic drug burden in a cohort of hospitalized older patients: an observational study. Drugs Aging. 2019;36(1):85–91.

54. Wolters AE, Zaal IJ, Veldhuijzen DS, Cremer OL, Devlin JW, van Dijk D, et al. Anticholinergic medication use and transition to delirium in critically ill patients: a prospective cohort study. Crit Care Med. 2015;43(9):1846–52.

55. By the American Geriatrics Society Beers Criteria Update Expert P. American Geriatrics Society 2019 updated AGS beers criteria(R) for potentially inappropriate medication use in older adults. J Am Geriatr Soc. 2019;67(4):674–94.

56. Fong HK, Sands LP, Leung JM. The role of postoperative analgesia in delirium and cognitive decline in

elderly patients: a systematic review. Anesth Analg. 2006;102(4):1255–66.

57. Lynch EP, Lazor MA, Gellis JE, Orav J, Goldman L, Marcantonio ER. The impact of postoperative pain on the development of postoperative delirium. Anesth Analg. 1998;86(4):781–5.

58. Duggleby W, Lander J. Cognitive status and postoperative pain: older adults. J Pain Symptom Manag. 1994;9(1):19–27.

59. Morrison RS, Magaziner J, Gilbert M, Koval KJ, McLaughlin MA, Orosz G, et al. Relationship between pain and opioid analgesics on the development of delirium following hip fracture. J Gerontol A Biol Sci Med Sci. 2003;58(1):76–81.

60. Elliott R, McKinley S, Cistulli P, Fien M. Characterisation of sleep in intensive care using 24-hour polysomnography: an observational study. Crit Care. 2013;17(2):R46.

61. Friese RS, Diaz-Arrastia R, McBride D, Frankel H, Gentilello LM. Quantity and quality of sleep in the surgical intensive care unit: are our patients sleeping? J Trauma. 2007;63(6):1210–4.

62. Watson PL, Pandharipande P, Gehlbach BK, Thompson JL, Shintani AK, Dittus BS, et al. Atypical sleep in ventilated patients: empirical electroencephalography findings and the path toward revised ICU sleep scoring criteria. Crit Care Med. 2013;41(8):1958–67.

63. Trompeo AC, Vidi Y, Locane MD, Braghiroli A, Mascia L, Bosma K, et al. Sleep disturbances in the critically ill patients: role of delirium and sedative agents. Minerva Anestesiol. 2011;77(6):604–12.

64. Sinforiani E, Terzaghi M, Pasotti C, Zucchella C, Zambrelli E, Manni R. Hallucinations and sleep-wake cycle in Alzheimer's disease: a questionnaire-based study in 218 patients. Neurol Sci. 2007;28(2):96–9.

65. Sinforiani E, Zangaglia R, Manni R, Cristina S, Marchioni E, Nappi G, et al. REM sleep behavior disorder, hallucinations, and cognitive impairment in Parkinson's disease. Mov Disord. 2006;21(4):462–6.

66. McGuire BE, Basten CJ, Ryan CJ, Gallagher J. Intensive care unit syndrome: a dangerous misnomer. Arch Intern Med. 2000;160(7):906–9.

67. Litton E, Carnegie V, Elliott R, Webb SA. The efficacy of earplugs as a sleep hygiene strategy for reducing delirium in the ICU: a systematic review and meta-analysis. Crit Care Med. 2016;44(5):992–9.

68. Tonna JE, Dalton A, Presson AP, Zhang C, Colantuoni E, Lander K, et al. The effect of a quality improvement intervention on sleep and delirium in critically ill patients in a surgical ICU. Chest. 2021;160(3):899–908.

69. Whitlock EL, Torres BA, Lin N, Helsten DL, Nadelson MR, Mashour GA, et al. Postoperative delirium in a substudy of cardiothoracic surgical patients in the BAG-RECALL clinical trial. Anesth Analg. 2014;118(4):809–17.

70. Behrends M, DePalma G, Sands L, Leung J. Association between intraoperative blood transfusions and early postoperative delirium in older adults. J Am Geriatr Soc. 2013;61(3):365–70.

71. Romanauski TR, Martin EE, Sprung J, Martin DP, Schroeder DR, Weingarten TN. Delirium in postoperative patients admitted to the intensive care unit. Am Surg. 2018;84(6):875–80.

72. Devlin JW, Zaal IJ, Slooter AJ. Clarifying the confusion surrounding drug-associated delirium in the ICU. Crit Care Med. 2014;42(6):1565–6.

73. Cardin F, Andreotti A, Martella B, Terranova C, Militello C. Current practice in colonoscopy in the elderly. Aging Clin Exp Res. 2012;24(3 Suppl):9–13.

74. Patanwala AE, Christich AC, Jasiak KD, Edwards CJ, Phan H, Snyder EM. Age-related differences in propofol dosing for procedural sedation in the Emergency Department. J Emerg Med. 2013;44(4):823–8.

75. Hernandez-Perez AL, Gallardo-Hernandez AG, Ordonez-Espinosa G, Martinez-Carrillo B, Bermudez-Ochoa MG, Revilla-Monsalve C, et al. Significant and safe reduction of propofol sedation dose for geriatric population undergoing pacemaker implantation: randomized clinical trial. Aging Clin Exp Res. 2018;30(10):1233–9.

76. Besch G, Liu N, Samain E, Pericard C, Boichut N, Mercier M, et al. Occurrence of and risk factors for electroencephalogram burst suppression during propofol-remifentanil anaesthesia. Br J Anaesth. 2011;107(5):749–56.

77. Schwartz AE, Tuttle RH, Poppers PJ. Electroencephalographic burst suppression in elderly and young patients anesthetized with isoflurane. Anesth Analg. 1989;68(1):9–12.

78. Chan MT, Cheng BC, Lee TM, Gin T, Group CT. BIS-guided anesthesia decreases postoperative delirium and cognitive decline. J Neurosurg Anesthesiol. 2013;25(1):33–42.

79. Evered LA, Chan MTV, Han R, Chu MHM, Cheng BP, Scott DA, et al. Anaesthetic depth and delirium after major surgery: a randomised clinical trial. Br J Anaesth. 2021;127(5):704–12.

80. Oliveira CR, Bernardo WM, Nunes VM. Benefit of general anesthesia monitored by bispectral index compared with monitoring guided only by clinical parameters. Systematic review and meta-analysis. Braz J Anesthesiol. 2017;67(1):72–84.

81. Punjasawadwong Y, Chau-In W, Laopaiboon M, Punjasawadwong S, Pin-On P. Processed electroencephalogram and evoked potential techniques for amelioration of postoperative delirium and cognitive dysfunction following non-cardiac and non-neurosurgical procedures in adults. Cochrane Database Syst Rev. 2018;5(5):CD011283.

82. Wildes TS, Mickle AM, Ben Abdallah A, Maybrier HR, Oberhaus J, Budelier TP, et al. Effect of electroencephalography-guided anesthetic administration on postoperative delirium among older adults undergoing major surgery: the ENGAGES randomized clinical trial. JAMA. 2019;321(5):473–83.

83. Guay J, Kopp S. Peripheral nerve blocks for hip fractures in adults. Cochrane Database Syst Rev. 2020;11(11):CD001159.

84. Kim CH, Yang JY, Min CH, Shon HC, Kim JW, Lim EJ. The effect of regional nerve block on perioperative delirium in hip fracture surgery for the elderly: a systematic review and meta-analysis of randomized controlled trials. Orthop Traumatol Surg Res. 2022;108(1):103151.

85. Li T, Li J, Yuan L, Wu J, Jiang C, Daniels J, et al. Effect of regional vs general anesthesia on incidence of postoperative delirium in older patients undergoing hip fracture surgery: the RAGA randomized trial. JAMA. 2022;327(1):50–8.

86. Miller D, Lewis SR, Pritchard MW, Schofield-Robinson OJ, Shelton CL, Alderson P, et al. Intravenous versus inhalational maintenance of anaesthesia for postoperative cognitive outcomes in elderly people undergoing non-cardiac surgery. Cochrane Database Syst Rev. 2018;8(8):CD012317.

87. Inouye SK, van Dyck CH, Alessi CA, Balkin S, Siegal AP, Horwitz RI. Clarifying confusion: the confusion assessment method. A new method for detection of delirium. Ann Intern Med. 1990;113(12):941–8.

88. Ely EW, Margolin R, Francis J, May L, Truman B, Dittus R, et al. Evaluation of delirium in critically ill patients: validation of the Confusion Assessment Method for the Intensive Care Unit (CAM-ICU). Crit Care Med. 2001;29(7):1370–9.

89. Ely EW, Inouye SK, Bernard GR, Gordon S, Francis J, May L, et al. Delirium in mechanically ventilated patients: validity and reliability of the confusion assessment method for the intensive care unit (CAM-ICU). JAMA. 2001;286(21):2703–10.

90. Bergeron N, Dubois MJ, Dumont M, Dial S, Skrobik Y. Intensive Care Delirium Screening Checklist: evaluation of a new screening tool. Intensive Care Med. 2001;27(5):859–64.

91. Devlin JW, Skrobik Y, Gelinas C, Needham DM, Slooter AJC, Pandharipande PP, et al. Clinical practice guidelines for the prevention and management of pain, agitation/sedation, delirium, immobility, and sleep disruption in adult patients in the ICU. Crit Care Med. 2018;46(9):e825–e73.

92. Gusmao-Flores D, Salluh JI, Chalhub RA, Quarantini LC. The confusion assessment method for the intensive care unit (CAM-ICU) and intensive care delirium screening checklist (ICDSC) for the diagnosis of delirium: a systematic review and meta-analysis of clinical studies. Crit Care. 2012;16(4):R115.

93. Neto AS, Nassar AP Jr, Cardoso SO, Manetta JA, Pereira VG, Esposito DC, et al. Delirium screening in critically ill patients: a systematic review and meta-analysis. Crit Care Med. 2012;40(6):1946–51.

94. Inouye SK, Kosar CM, Tommet D, Schmitt EM, Puelle MR, Saczynski JS, et al. The CAM-S: development and validation of a new scoring system for delirium severity in 2 cohorts. Ann Intern Med. 2014;160(8):526–33.

95. Trzepacz PT, Mittal D, Torres R, Kanary K, Norton J, Jimerson N. Validation of the Delirium Rating Scale-revised-98: comparison with the delirium rating scale and the cognitive test for delirium. J Neuropsychiatry Clin Neurosci. 2001;13(2):229–42.

96. Khan BA, Perkins AJ, Gao S, Hui SL, Campbell NL, Farber MO, et al. The confusion assessment method for the ICU-7 delirium severity scale: a novel delirium severity instrument for use in the ICU. Crit Care Med. 2017;45(5):851–7.

97. Toft K, Tontsch J, Abdelhamid S, Steiner L, Siegemund M, Hollinger A. Serum biomarkers of delirium in the elderly: a narrative review. Ann Intensive Care. 2019;9(1):76.

98. Khan BA, Zawahiri M, Campbell NL, Boustani MA. Biomarkers for delirium—a review. J Am Geriatr Soc. 2011;59(Suppl 2):S256–61.

99. Dunne SS, Coffey JC, Konje S, Gasior S, Clancy CC, Gulati G, et al. Biomarkers in delirium: a systematic review. J Psychosom Res. 2021;147:110530.

100. Khan BA, Perkins AJ, Prasad NK, Shekhar A, Campbell NL, Gao S, et al. Biomarkers of delirium duration and delirium severity in the ICU. Crit Care Med. 2020;48(3):353–61.

101. Gunther ML, Morandi A, Krauskopf E, Pandharipande P, Girard TD, Jackson JC, et al. The association between brain volumes, delirium duration, and cognitive outcomes in intensive care unit survivors: the VISIONS cohort magnetic resonance imaging study*. Crit Care Med. 2012;40(7):2022–32.

102. Sprung J, Warner DO, Knopman DS, Petersen RC, Mielke MM, Jack CR Jr, et al. Brain MRI after critical care admission: a longitudinal imaging study. J Crit Care. 2021;62:117–23.

103. Boord MS, Moezzi B, Davis D, Ross TJ, Coussens S, Psaltis PJ, et al. Investigating how electroencephalogram measures associate with delirium: a systematic review. Clin Neurophysiol. 2021;132(1):246–57.

104. Palanca BJA, Guay CS. Associations between delirium and electroencephalographic markers: notes from the field. Clin Neurophysiol. 2021;132(1):210–1.

105. Fann JR, Alfano CM, Roth-Roemer S, Katon WJ, Syrjala KL. Impact of delirium on cognition, distress, and health-related quality of life after hematopoietic stem-cell transplantation. J Clin Oncol. 2007;25(10):1223–31.

106. Slor CJ, Witlox J, Jansen RW, Adamis D, Meagher DJ, Tieken E, et al. Affective functioning after delirium in elderly hip fracture patients. Int Psychogeriatr. 2013;25(3):445–55.

107. Witlox J, Slor CJ, Jansen RW, Kalisvaart KJ, van Stijn MF, Houdijk AP, et al. The neuropsychological sequelae of delirium in elderly patients with hip fracture three months after hospital discharge. Int Psychogeriatr. 2013;25(9):1521–31.

108. Farrell KR, Ganzini L. Misdiagnosing delirium as depression in medically ill elderly patients. Arch Intern Med. 1995;155(22):2459–64.

109. Nicholas LM, Lindsey BA. Delirium presenting with symptoms of depression. Psychosomatics. 1995;36(5):471–9.
110. Yamada K, Hosoda M, Nakashima S, Furuta K, Awata S. Psychiatric diagnosis in the elderly referred to a consultation-liaison psychiatry service in a general geriatric hospital in Japan. Geriatr Gerontol Int. 2012;12(2):304–9.
111. O'Sullivan R, Inouye SK, Meagher D. Delirium and depression: inter-relationship and clinical overlap in elderly people. Lancet Psychiatry. 2014;1(4):303–11.
112. Inouye SK, Bogardus ST Jr, Baker DI, Leo-Summers L, Cooney LM Jr. The hospital elder life program: a model of care to prevent cognitive and functional decline in older hospitalized patients. Hospital elder life program. J Am Geriatr Soc. 2000;48(12):1697–706.
113. Chen CC, Saczynski J, Inouye SK. The modified Hospital Elder Life Program: adapting a complex intervention for feasibility and scalability in a surgical setting. J Gerontol Nurs. 2014;40(5):16–22.
114. Deeken F, Sanchez A, Rapp MA, Denkinger M, Brefka S, Spank J, et al. Outcomes of a delirium prevention program in older persons after elective surgery: a stepped-wedge cluster randomized clinical trial. JAMA Surg. 2022;157(2):e216370.
115. Kojaie-Bidgoli A, Sharifi F, Maghsoud F, Alizadeh-Khoei M, Jafari F, Sadeghi F. The Modified Hospital Elder Life Program (HELP) in geriatric hospitalized patients in internal wards: a double-blind randomized control trial. BMC Geriatr. 2021;21(1):599.
116. Yue J, Tabloski P, Dowal SL, Puelle MR, Nandan R, Inouye SK. NICE to HELP: operationalizing National Institute for Health and Clinical Excellence guidelines to improve clinical practice. J Am Geriatr Soc. 2014;62(4):754–61.
117. Strijbos MJ, Steunenberg B, van der Mast RC, Inouye SK, Schuurmans MJ. Design and methods of the Hospital Elder Life Program (HELP), a multicomponent targeted intervention to prevent delirium in hospitalized older patients: efficacy and cost-effectiveness in Dutch health care. BMC Geriatr. 2013;13:78.
118. Honda M. The key factors for implementation of Hospital Elder Life Program into Japanese hospitals. Nihon Ronen Igakkai Zasshi. 2013;50(5):641–3.
119. Bakker FC, Persoon A, Schoon Y, Olde Rikkert MG. Hospital elder life program integrated in dutch hospital care: a pilot. J Am Geriatr Soc. 2013;61(4):641–2.
120. Rosenbloom-Brunton DA, Henneman EA, Inouye SK. Feasibility of family participation in a delirium prevention program for hospitalized older adults. J Gerontol Nurs. 2010;36(9):22–33; quiz 4–5.
121. Hshieh TT, Yue J, Oh E, Puelle M, Dowal S, Travison T, et al. Effectiveness of multicomponent nonpharmacological delirium interventions: a meta-analysis. JAMA Intern Med. 2015;175(4):512–20.
122. Burton JK, Craig LE, Yong SQ, Siddiqi N, Teale EA, Woodhouse R, et al. Non-pharmacological interventions for preventing delirium in hospitalised non-ICU patients. Cochrane Database Syst Rev. 2021;7(7):CD013307.
123. Inouye SK, Bogardus ST Jr, Charpentier PA, Leo-Summers L, Acampora D, Holford TR, et al. A multicomponent intervention to prevent delirium in hospitalized older patients. N Engl J Med. 1999;340(9):669–76.
124. Rubin FH, Williams JT, Lescisin DA, Mook WJ, Hassan S, Inouye SK. Replicating the hospital elder life program in a community hospital and demonstrating effectiveness using quality improvement methodology. J Am Geriatr Soc. 2006;54(6):969–74.
125. Rubin FH, Neal K, Fenlon K, Hassan S, Inouye SK. Sustainability and scalability of the hospital elder life program at a community hospital. J Am Geriatr Soc. 2011;59(2):359–65.
126. Zaubler TS, Murphy K, Rizzuto L, Santos R, Skotzko C, Giordano J, et al. Quality improvement and cost savings with multicomponent delirium interventions: replication of the Hospital Elder Life Program in a community hospital. Psychosomatics. 2013;54(3):219–26.
127. Marra A, Ely EW, Pandharipande PP, Patel MB. The ABCDEF bundle in critical care. Crit Care Clin. 2017;33(2):225–43.
128. Morandi A, Brummel NE, Ely EW. Sedation, delirium and mechanical ventilation: the 'ABCDE' approach. Curr Opin Crit Care. 2011;17(1):43–9.
129. Pun BT, Balas MC, Barnes-Daly MA, Thompson JL, Aldrich JM, Barr J, et al. Caring for critically ill patients with the ABCDEF bundle: results of the ICU liberation collaborative in over 15,000 adults. Crit Care Med. 2019;47(1):3–14.
130. Burry L, Mehta S, Perreault MM, Luxenberg JS, Siddiqi N, Hutton B, et al. Antipsychotics for treatment of delirium in hospitalised non-ICU patients. Cochrane Database Syst Rev. 2018;6(6):CD005594.
131. Girard TD, Exline MC, Carson SS, Hough CL, Rock P, Gong MN, et al. Haloperidol and ziprasidone for treatment of delirium in critical illness. N Engl J Med. 2018;379(26):2506–16.
132. Nikooie R, Neufeld KJ, Oh ES, Wilson LM, Zhang A, Robinson KA, et al. Antipsychotics for treating delirium in hospitalized adults: a systematic review. Ann Intern Med. 2019;171(7):485–95.
133. Khan BA, Perkins AJ, Campbell NL, Gao S, Farber MO, Wang S, et al. Pharmacological management of delirium in the intensive care unit: a randomized pragmatic clinical trial. J Am Geriatr Soc. 2019;67(5):1057–65.
134. Finucane AM, Jones L, Leurent B, Sampson EL, Stone P, Tookman A, et al. Drug therapy for delirium in terminally ill adults. Cochrane Database Syst Rev. 2020;1(1):CD004770.
135. Jeste DV, Blazer D, Casey D, Meeks T, Salzman C, Schneider L, et al. ACNP white paper: update on use of antipsychotic drugs in elderly persons with dementia. Neuropsychopharmacology. 2008;33(5):957–70.

136. Glass OM, Hermida AP, Hershenberg R, Schwartz AC. Considerations and current trends in the management of the geriatric patient on a consultation-liaison service. Curr Psychiatry Rep. 2020;22(5):21.

137. van Gool WA, van de Beek D, Eikelenboom P. Systemic infection and delirium: when cytokines and acetylcholine collide. Lancet. 2010;375(9716):773–5.

138. Hughes CG, Boncyk CS, Fedeles B, Pandharipande PP, Chen W, Patel MB, et al. Association between cholinesterase activity and critical illness brain dysfunction. Crit Care. 2022;26(1):377.

139. Yu A, Wu S, Zhang Z, Dening T, Zhao S, Pinner G, et al. Cholinesterase inhibitors for the treatment of delirium in non-ICU settings. Cochrane Database Syst Rev. 2018;6(6):CD012494.

140. Tampi RR, Tampi DJ, Ghori AK. Acetylcholinesterase inhibitors for delirium in older adults. Am J Alzheimers Dis Other Dement. 2016;31(4):305–10.

141. van Eijk MM, Roes KC, Honing ML, Kuiper MA, Karakus A, van der Jagt M, et al. Effect of rivastigmine as an adjunct to usual care with haloperidol on duration of delirium and mortality in critically ill patients: a multicentre, double-blind, placebo-controlled randomised trial. Lancet. 2010;376(9755):1829–37.

142. Lieberman OJ, Lee S, Zabinski J. Donepezil treatment is associated with improved outcomes in critically ill dementia patients via a reduction in delirium. Alzheimers Dement. 2022:1742.

143. Pandharipande PP, Pun BT, Herr DL, Maze M, Girard TD, Miller RR, et al. Effect of sedation with dexmedetomidine vs lorazepam on acute brain dysfunction in mechanically ventilated patients: the MENDS randomized controlled trial. JAMA. 2007;298(22):2644–53.

144. Pereira JV, Sanjanwala RM, Mohammed MK, Le ML, Arora RC. Dexmedetomidine versus propofol sedation in reducing delirium among older adults in the ICU: a systematic review and meta-analysis. Eur J Anaesthesiol. 2020;37(2):121–31.

145. Flukiger J, Hollinger A, Speich B, Meier V, Tontsch J, Zehnder T, et al. Dexmedetomidine in prevention and treatment of postoperative and intensive care unit delirium: a systematic review and meta-analysis. Ann Intensive Care. 2018;8(1):92.

146. Burry L, Hutton B, Williamson DR, Mehta S, Adhikari NK, Cheng W, et al. Pharmacological interventions for the treatment of delirium in critically ill adults. Cochrane Database Syst Rev. 2019;9(9):CD011749.

147. Campbell AM, Axon DR, Martin JR, Slack MK, Mollon L, Lee JK. Melatonin for the prevention of postoperative delirium in older adults: a systematic review and meta-analysis. BMC Geriatr. 2019;19(1):272.

148. Khaing K, Nair BR. Melatonin for delirium prevention in hospitalized patients: a systematic review and meta-analysis. J Psychiatr Res. 2021;133:181–90.

149. Campbell NL, Perkins AJ, Khan BA, Gao S, Farber MO, Khan S, et al. Deprescribing in the pharmacologic management of delirium: a randomized trial in the intensive care unit. J Am Geriatr Soc. 2019;67(4):695–702.

150. Iyer S, Naganathan V, McLachlan AJ, Le Couteur DG. Medication withdrawal trials in people aged 65 years and older: a systematic review. Drugs Aging. 2008;25(12):1021–31.

151. ICU Delirium: Resource downloads [Internet]. Nashville (TN): Critical Illness Brain Dysfunction and Survivorship (CIBS) Center; c2023 [cited 2023 Feb 24]. https://www.icudelirium.org/medical-professionals/downloads/resources-by-category.

152. AGS CoCare—HELP: American Geriatrics Society; c2023 [cited 2023 Feb 26]. https://help.agscocare.org/.

Part II

Depressive Disorders and Bipolar and Related Disorders

Depressive Disorders

Rajesh R. Tampi and Deena J. Tampi

Introduction

Major depressive disorder (MDD) is described in the Diagnostic and Statistical Manual of Mental Disorders, Fifth Edition (DSM-5), as a condition that is characterized by the presence of depressed mood or marked loss of interest or pleasure in activities [1]. Changes in sleep, energy, concentration, appetite, weight (changes in 5% of total body weight), and psychomotor activity are additional symptoms that can be associated with MDD. Feelings of inappropriate guilt or worthlessness and recurrent thoughts of death or suicide can also occur among individuals with MDD. An individual should have depressed mood or marked loss of interest or pleasure in activities in addition to four associated symptoms to meet the criteria for an MDD. Additionally, these symptoms should have occurred during the same 2-week period. Furthermore, these symptoms should cause clinically significant distress or impairments in social, occupational, or other areas of functioning. Also, these symptoms should not be attributable to the psychological effects of substances or medical conditions. Depression that occurs among individuals ≥65 years of age who have not had a previous history of depression is often referred to as "late-life depression" (LLD) [2].

Depressive symptoms are seen in approximately 30% and 45% of older adults [3, 4]. However, MDD is only seen in approximately 2% of community-dwelling older adults [3, 5]. Approximately 6–9% of older individuals who attend primary care clinics present with MDD [6]. MDD is seen in 10–12% of older adults who are admitted to acute care hospitals [6]. Among older adults who live at nursing homes, MDD is seen among 12–14% of individuals [2].

When compared to young adults, older adults with MDD are less likely to have a family history of depression [3, 7]. However, these individuals present with more agitation, hypochondriasis, and somatic symptoms and psychotic symptoms than younger individuals [8, 9]. Older individuals with MDD have less guilt and loss of sexual interest when compared to younger individuals [8].

Approximately 25–50% of admissions to inpatient geriatric psychiatry units are due to MDD with psychotic features [10]. Delusions that are commonly seen among older adults with MDD include nihilistic, somatic, or poverty-based delusions. Older individuals who have MDD with psychotics features present with higher rates of insomnia, somatic symptoms,

R. R. Tampi (✉)
Department of Psychiatry, Creighton University
School of Medicine, Omaha, NE, USA

Department of Psychiatry, Yale School of Medicine,
New Haven, CT, USA

D. J. Tampi
Behavioral Health Advisory Group,
Princeton, NJ, USA

diurnal variation of mood, and poor insight into their illness [3, 10]. Hallucinations tend to appear less frequently than delusions among these individuals. Older adults with MDD and psychotic features have frequent recurrences of symptoms and hospitalizations [3]. Being single, widowed, or living alone is a risk factor for the development of MDD with psychotic features among older individuals [10]. Possible reasons for why psychotic symptoms are common among older adults with MDD include age-related deterioration of the cortical areas of the brain, neurochemical changes that are associated with aging, comorbid medical conditions, social isolation, sensory deficits, cognitive decline, and polypharmacy [9].

Among older adults, depression and dementia are two conditions that share an important relationship and have similar presentations [11, 12]. Approximately, 20–50% of older adults with depression develop cognitive deficits including executive dysfunction and deficits in information processing and visuospatial functioning [13–15]. Among older individuals, cognitive deficits that are often seen during an episode of depression and tend to improve with the treatment of the depressive episode are called "depressive pseudodementia" or "depression-associated dementia" [2, 4]. Depressive symptoms can also be the presenting symptom of dementia among older adults. Available evidence indicates that depression may be a prodrome for the onset of dementia and an independent risk factor for dementia [16]. Individuals who present with depression-associated dementia when compared to primary dementia have an acute onset of symptoms, presence of significant guilt or self-reproach, diurnal variations in mood, poor effort on cognitive testing, significant impairment in both registration and recall, absence of deficits in multiple cognitive domains, and improvement of symptoms with sleep deprivation [17].

Risk Factors and Neurobiology

Depression among older adults occurs due to the interplay between the different biological, psychological, and sociological factors [18].

Approximately 25% of older individuals who are post-cerebrovascular accident develop MDD [19]. These individuals often present with the co-localization of atrophy and ischemic lesions in the frontostriatal, limbic, and subcortical regions of the brain [2, 3]. Psychomotor retardation, reduced interest in activities, and poor insight into their illness are often seen among these individuals [2]. MDD is also seen among approximately 40% of older adults with Parkinson's disease [19]. Furthermore, MDD is seen in approximately 25% older individuals who are post-myocardial ischemia (MI) [20, 21]. Medications that can cause depression among older adults include the following: antihypertensive medications—methyldopa, reserpine, clonidine, and hydralazine; antiparkinson drugs—levodopa; anticancer drugs—tamoxifen, vinblastine, and vincristine; hormonal agents—estrogen and progesterone; benzodiazepines; corticosteroids; and cimetidine [2].

Psychological factors that can result in depression and suicidal ideation among older adults include neuroticism, pessimistic thinking, and less open attitudes to new experiences [22–24]. Isolation, bereavement, functional decline, and disability are associated with the development of depression among older adults [3, 25]. Social factors that result in depression among older individuals include prolonged caregiving, behavioral issues in the person receiving care, and when the caregiver has limited social supports [26]. Personal and environmental factors can alter the impact of psychosocial risk factors on depression among older adults [26].

Additional risk factors for the development of depression among community-dwelling older individuals include a prior history of depression, female gender, sleep disturbance, bereavement, and presence of disability [27].

Consequences

Among older adults, the occurrence of depression can result in numerous poor outcomes. The occurrence of morbidity among older adults with depression is approximately 1.5–3 times greater than among older individuals without depression [1]. Comorbid anxiety disorders and substance use disorders are also more common among older adults with depression [28]. Chronic diseases such as arthritis and heart diseases are more common among older people with depression when compared to older adults without depression. These individuals also have greater risk for developing inflammatory disorders, bone resorption, cancer, heart disease, and death from heart disease [29–31]. The risk for Alzheimer's disease (AD) and vascular dementia (VaD) is also greater among older adults with depression when compared to older adults who are not depressed [32]. There is a bidirectional relationship between depression and medical comorbidities with depression worsening the outcomes for comorbid medical conditions, and these disorders worsening the outcomes for depression [33]. Older adults with depression have an approximately 15% greater lifetime risk for suicide when compared to age-matched controls [1]. Approximately 1 in 10 of these individuals die annually from completed suicides.

Suicides are five times higher among older people with depression when compared to the general population [21]. Approximately 75% of the individuals who complete suicide have symptoms of depression and visit their primary care physician within the preceding month [7]. Approximately $5.4 billion is lost each year from the economy due to suicides resulting from depression [34]. The presence of medical and psychiatric comorbidities, substance use disorders, certain personality traits, and severe social stressors are all risk factors for suicide among older adults who are depressed [2, 3, 19, 35].

Significant reduction in workplace productivity and greater healthcare utilization are seen among older individuals with depression [28, 36, 37]. Each year, the direct medical cost for depression is approximately $26.1 billion, and the yearly financial loss to the workplace is approximately $51.5 billion [34].

Assessment

Almost 50% of older people with MDD go undiagnosed [38, 39]. A common reason for this underdiagnosis is because their primary physi-

cian is the person who completes the initial assessment for depression in a majority of cases. In addition, many older adults do not report the classic depressive symptoms, but they present with numerous somatic complaints [33]. Additionally, a significant number of individuals also report cognitive problems and/or functional impairments.

Among older adults, the evaluation of depression starts with a comprehensive history, which should be obtained from the individuals and also from a reliable collateral source/informant [3]. In addition, these individuals should have a thorough mental status examination, a focused physical examination, appropriate laboratory testing, and a psychosocial assessment. As these older individuals with depression have higher rates of medical comorbidities when compared to age-matched controls, a focused physical examination becomes an important part of the assessment of depression among older adults to identify the medical comorbidities [37].

Appropriate laboratory examination for older adults with depression includes a complete blood count (CBC); a complete metabolic panel (CMP); liver function test (LFT); thyroid function tests including TSH, T4, T3, and thyroid-binding globulin (TBG); vitamin B12 and folate levels; syphilis screening tests including RPR or VDRL and HIV testing; and a urine drug screen (UDS). These tests can identify common medical comorbidities and substance use disorders that can cause and/or exacerbate depressive symptoms among older adults [33].

Standardized screening instruments can assist with evaluating the severity of depression, identifying suicidal ideation and psychotic symptoms [40]. They can also help with assessing the response of the depressive symptoms to the prescribed treatments. The Geriatric Depression Scale [GDS], the Cornell Scale for Depression in Dementia [CSDD], the Hamilton Rating Scale for Depression [HAM-D], Montgomery-Asberg Depression Rating Scale [MADRS], and the Zung Self-Rating Depression Scale [SDS] are the common screening tools for depression among older adults. Although not specific to older adults, the Brief Psychiatric Rating Scale [BPRS] is often used to detect and rate the severity of psy-

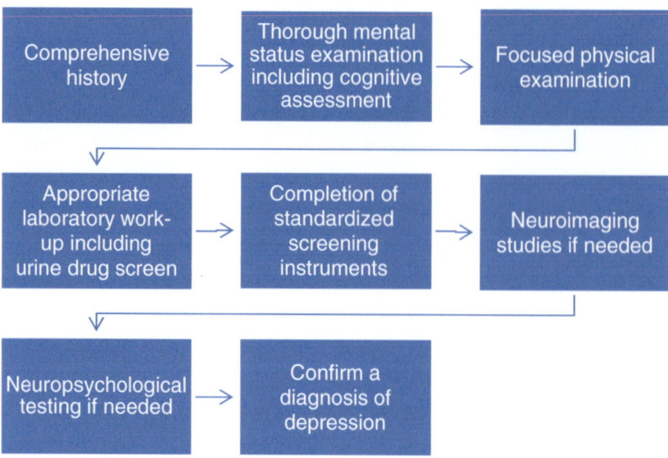

Fig. 9.1 Workup for depression among older adults

chopathology among older adults with depression and psychotic symptoms. When compared to GDS, HAM-D is thought to be a less sensitive instrument in identifying depressive symptoms among older adults [41, 42].

Neuroimaging studies can assist with identifying cerebral pathology that results in cognitive impairment, increases the burden of illness, and worsens prognosis among older individuals with depression [43, 44]. Neuropsychological testing can assist with identifying the extent, severity, and etiologies for depressive symptoms in addition to evaluating the extent and severity of cognitive impairment [45]. Figure 9.1 describes the workup for depression among older adults.

Prognosis

Depression is known to have a chronic and relapsing course [46]. Approximately 25% of older adults with depression will attain full remission of symptoms with or without any treatment, whereas about 25% will never achieve any treatment response [3]. The rest of the older individuals with depression will have a waxing-and-waning course. Poor prognostic factors include the presence of psychotic symptoms, comorbid medical disorders, physical disability, and limited or absent social supports [3, 10]. Among older people with depression, an important risk factor for limited treatment response and poor antidepressant tolerability is the presence of comorbid medical conditions [46].

Treatments

Psychotherapy, pharmacotherapy, electroconvulsive therapy (ECT), and transcranial magnetic stimulation (TMS) have shown good benefit for the treatment of depression among older individuals [47–49]. Aerobic and supervised group exercise regimens may also improve depressive symptoms among older people [50].

Psychotherapy

Among older adults with depression, benefits have been noted for cognitive behavioral therapy (CBT), reminiscence therapy (RT), brief dynamic therapy (BDT), problem-solving therapy (PST), and the combination of medication and interpersonal psychotherapy (IPT) [51–55]. Large effect sizes have been noted for CBT and RT, with moderate effect sizes being identified for psychodynamic therapy, psychoeducation, physical exercise, and supportive interventions [53]. CBT has been noted to be more effective than wait list controls, but no significant treatment differences have been noted between CBT and psychodynamic therapy [54]. In one meta-analysis, the treatment difference between psychotherapy and control groups was noted to be 0.64, and the number needed to treat (NNT) was 3 [65]. There are no significant differences noted whether the therapy is being delivered in the individual format, in groups, or via a bibliotherapy format [52]. Older individuals with depression who have greater baseline levels of anxiety, increased levels of stress, underlying personality disorders, and reduced self-rated health scores often have a poorer response to therapy [55].

Pharmacotherapy

In the treatment of older adults with depression, there are no significant differences noted in efficacy between the various antidepressant classes [6]. These include selective serotonin reuptake inhibitors [SSRIs], mirtazapine, bupropion, and tricyclic antidepressants [TCAs]. One study found that the NNT was 8 for all the antidepressants combined [6]. When compared to placebo, bupropion, mirtazapine, serotonin norepinephrine reuptake inhibitors (SNRIs), and SSRIs have been found to have greater but modest efficacy in the treatment of symptoms of depression among older adults [56]. In the treatment of depression among older adults, no significant difference in efficacy or adverse effects has been noted for dual-action antidepressants like SNRIs or TCAs, when compared to single-action antidepressants like the SSRIs [57].

For the treatment of depression among older adults, SSRIs are often considered first-line drugs given their efficacy and fairly benign adverse effect profile [19]. Nausea, diarrhea, anxiety, and sleep disturbance are the most common side effects of SSRIs among older individuals [58]. Among older adults with depression, both venlafaxine and duloxetine (SNRIs) have shown good efficacy and tolerable adverse effect profile [59, 60]. When used in the treatment of older adults with depression, mirtazapine has been found to have a similar efficacy to paroxetine, but with a better adverse effect profile [61]. The most common adverse effects for mirtazapine are increased appetite and sedation when used to treat older adults with depression [61].

For the treatment for depression among older adults, TCAs are not identified as first-line drugs due to their significant adverse effect profile despite overall good efficacy [7, 14]. Among the TCAs, secondary amine TCAs like nortriptyline and desipramine are considered as being safer than tertiary amine TCAs including imipramine and amitriptyline [7, 14]. Among older adults with depression who have risk factors for suicide, TCAs should be prescribed with caution as these drugs are lethal in overdoses [14]. Sedation, orthostatic-hypotension, tachycardia, dry mouth, visual problems, dizziness, and weight gain are the commonly reported adverse effects from the TCAs.

Data from one RCT indicated that older adults with depression who were treated with vortioxetine had greater rates of remission when compared to individuals who received placebo [62]. Nausea was the more common adverse effect in the drug group when compared to the placebo group. Individuals who received vortioxetine did better than individuals who received placebo on two cognitive tests. Quetiapine XR monotherapy was noted in one RCT to be effective in improving symptoms of depression among older adults as early as week 1 when compared to placebo [63]. Somnolence, headache, dry mouth, and dizziness were the common adverse events (>10% of participants) noted in the quetiapine XR group.

One RCT found that the addition of aripiprazole resulted in a greater proportion of participants in the aripiprazole group attaining and maintaining remission when compared to individuals receiving the addition of placebo among individuals ≥60 years in age who did not achieve remission from symptoms of depression with the use of venlafaxine [64]. For remission with the addition of aripiprazole, the odds ratio [OR] was 2.0 ($P = 0.03$), and the number needed to treat [NNT] was 6.6. The most common adverse effects with the addition of aripiprazole when compared to the addition of placebo were akathisia (26% versus 12%) and parkinsonism (17% versus 2%), respectively.

Lavretsky et al. compared treatment responses among three groups of individuals who received either methylphenidate + placebo, citalopram + placebo, or citalopram + methylphenidate in an RCT of older individuals who had been diagnosed with MDD [65]. In all three groups, significant improvements were noted for depression severity and cognitive performance. However, individuals in the citalopram + methylphenidate group showed greater improvements in depression severity and global improvements when compared to individuals in the other groups. Additionally, the rate of improvement in the citalopram + methylphenidate group was higher than the citalopram + placebo group in the first 4 weeks of the trial. No significant differences in cognitive improvement or the number of side effects were noted between the three groups.

At the present time, there is a lack of published evidence regarding the efficacy of vilazodone, levomilnacipran, and brexpiprazole among older adults with depression [66].

Ketamine and esketamine have been found to be beneficial in the treatment of depression among older individuals [67]. Ketamine is an N-methyl-D-aspartate receptor (NMDAR) antagonist, and esketamine is an enantiomer of ketamine with a higher affinity for NMDAR [68]. Evidence suggests both NMDAR inhibition-dependent and NMDAR inhibition-independent mechanisms having a role to play in the mechanism of action of ketamine as an antidepressant. Two controlled studies have evaluated the use of ketamine for depression among older people [69, 70]. Significant reduction in depressive symptoms with repeated subcutaneous ketamine use was noted among older adults with depression in the first study [69]. However, in the second study, participants did not achieve significant improvements in the primary outcome measure, but a decrease in depression scores with a higher response and remission rates was noted in the esketamine group when compared to the placebo group [70]. Adverse effects usually lasted only a few hours and resolved spontaneously with the use of ketamine. Perceptual disturbance, derealization, altered body perception, and altered time perception were the common adverse effects noted with the use of ketamine. It was noted that

the dissociative symptoms were dose related. Systolic and diastolic blood pressures and heart rate showed a transient increase with ketamine use but resolved spontaneously in a few hours. Among individuals receiving ketamine palpitations, flushing, dizziness, fatigue/sleepiness/poor concentration/spacing out, and paresthesia were also noted, but they resolved spontaneously. Neither trial indicated any cognitive decline with the use of ketamine.

Evidence indicates that the rate and speed of response among older adults with depression are similar either when there is augmentation of the standard antidepressant treatment with lithium or with another agent (an additional antidepressant, buspirone, or aripiprazole) or with the switch from one antidepressant class to a different class [71–77].

Among older adults with psychotic depression, evidence from controlled studies indicates efficacy for the use of nortriptyline, imipramine, mifepristone, a combination of fluoxetine and olanzapine, and electroconvulsive therapy [78]. The vast majority of individuals with psychotic depression often do not require treatment with antipsychotics for >4 months [79].

Electroconvulsive Therapy

Electroconvulsive therapy [ECT] has been found to be an effective treatment for the treatment of depression among older adults [80, 81]. It is particularly effective especially in situations where the symptoms of depression have not adequately responded to psychotherapy and/or pharmacotherapy [80]. A faster resolution of symptoms is also noted with the use of ECT in these situations [82]. Both unilateral and bilateral ECTs have shown efficacy in the treatment of depression among older adults [80]. Unilateral ECT is often the preferred modality for short-term treatments [≤5], whereas bilateral ECT is preferred for longer term treatments [≥3 weeks] [80]. The adverse effects of ECT among older adults with depression have been noted to be mild and transient

[83]. Unilateral ECT has been noted to provide better cognitive outcomes when compared to bilateral ECT. A reduction in cognitive adverse effects from the use of ECT among older adults with depression has been noted with the use of right unilateral and bitemporal lead placements, the use of brief pulse stimulus, and the use of dose titration of stimulus [84]. Among older adults, the use of ECT can result in transient and mild hypertension plus tachycardia [80].

Repetitive Transcranial Magnetic Stimulation

Repetitive transcranial magnetic stimulation (rTMS) is FDA approved for the treatment of depression among adults who have failed at least one medication trial [85]. Advantages to rTMS include the lack of need for anesthesia, lack of induction of seizures, and absence of any significant cognitive adverse effects [84]. The most common adverse effects of rTMS include discomfort caused by scalp or facial muscle twitching and headaches, with seizures being the rare adverse effect [85]. Age ($\leq$55 years versus $\geq$55 years) has not been identified as a predictor of response to rTMS when used among individuals with depression [86]. Possible predictors of response to rTMS include a failure to respond to one adequate trial of an antidepressant medication in the current episode, the absence of a comorbid anxiety disorder, a higher baseline depression severity, female gender, and a shorter duration of illness (<2 years) [86]. Among individuals with LLD, one study found that the remission rates were significantly higher with the use of active rTMS when compared to sham rTMS (40.0% vs. 14.8%) and with a number needed to treat of 4 [49]. The investigators did not find any changes in the measures of executive functioning, and no serious adverse events were noted with the use of active rTMS. Only pain was significantly more common in the active rTMS group (16.0% vs. 0%) with the rest of the adverse effect profiles being similar between the two treatment groups.

Vagal Nerve Stimulation

Vagal nerve stimulation (VNS) is FDA approved for the adjunctive and long-term treatment for recurrent or chronic major depressive episode among individuals $\geq$18 years in age who have had an inadequate response to $\geq$4 adequate antidepressant trials [84]. The response rates for the treatment of depression among individuals who received adjunctive VNS treatment were 31% after 3 months, 44% after 1 year, and 42% after 2 years, and the remission rates were 15% at 3 months, 27% at 1 year, and 22% at 2 years in one study [87]. In this study >80% of the individuals were continuing to receive VNS at 2 years. Available evidence does not indicate any controlled trials of VNS among older adults with depression.

Expert Consensus Guideline for Treatment of Depression

Appropriate first-line treatments for minor depressive episodes among older adults per an expert consensus guideline include antidepressant alone, psychotherapy alone, or the combination of an antidepressant medication with psychotherapy [19]. The most widely recommended first-line treatment for more severe depressive episodes includes the combination of an antidepressant medication with psychotherapy. An appropriate alternative first-line treatment for these more severe episodes is treatment with an antidepressant alone. As per this guideline, first-line agents are SSRIs especially citalopram and sertraline and extended-release venlafaxine for the treatment of depression among older adults. TCAs, bupropion, and mirtazapine are considered as second-line agents. An adequate trial of an antidepressant is the use of maximally tolerated dose of one antidepressant for 4–7 weeks, prior to switching to another medication.

ECT is considered an alternate treatment for more severe depressive episodes among older adults, especially when the individual has failed adequate trials of ≥2 antidepressants [19]. The presence of any acute suicide/homicide risk and any contraindication for the use of antidepressants or other psychotropic medications are additional reasons for using ECT among depressed older adults.

The combination of an antidepressant and an antipsychotic medication is recommended as first-line treatment for the treatment of psychotic depression among older individuals [19]. If the response to pharmacotherapy is inadequate, a trial of ECT should be considered. First-line agents include SSRIs and venlafaxine with TCAs being considered as alternative drugs. Atypical antipsychotics including risperidone, olanzapine, and quetiapine are first-line agents, with ziprasidone being a second-line agent for use among older people [19].

First-line psychotherapies among older individuals with depression include CBT, supportive psychotherapy (ST), IPT, and PST. Among older adults with a first major depressive episode, treatment for an additional 1 year after the remission of symptoms is considered to be the adequate duration of treatment. Among those individuals who have had recurrent episodes (≥3) of depression, longer term treatment (≥3 years) is recommended [19].

Pharmacogenetics in the Treatment of Depression Among Depression Among Older Adults

Even among older individuals, pharmacogenetic testing may provide invaluable information on how medications should be prescribed to treat psychiatric disorders [88]. But data from two controlled trials that evaluated the effects of pharmacogenetic screening on antidepressant treatment response among older adults did not support the clinical use of currently available pharmacogenetic testing to guide the treatment with antidepressants [89, 90]. According to a recent systematic review, pharmacogenetic testing should be considered among older adults with depression who have failed one antidepressant

treatment trial or among individuals who have experienced intolerable adverse effects [91].

Collaborative Treatments

Older adults are more likely to accept treatment for depression when it is offered in the primary care setting [92]. The involvement of a skilled and empathic care manager appears to improve the treatment success among older individuals [93]. Collaborative care also appears to improve symptoms of depression among older adults [92, 94]. The Improving Mood-Promoting Access to Collaborative Treatment [IMPACT] program appeared to improve symptoms of depression, physical functioning, and quality of life among older adults [95]. The Prevention of Suicide in Primary Care Elderly: Collaborative Trial [PROSPECT] found that the collaboration between trained clinicians and primary care physicians along with the implementation of a comprehensive depression management program improved outcomes among older adults with depression [96]. When compared to individuals receiving usual care, individuals in the intervention group had an earlier, greater, and faster resolution of symptoms of depression along and a faster rate of reduction in suicidal ideation [97, 98].

Algorithm

Tampi and Tampi have proposed an algorithm for the treatment of depression among older adults based on current evidence [99]. The authors indicate that for mild symptoms of depression, either psychotherapy (CBT, ST, IPT, PST, RT, or BDT) or pharmacotherapy (first line: SSRIs especially citalopram and sertraline and extended-release venlafaxine; second line: TCAs, bupropion, and mirtazapine) can be used to treat symptoms. For moderate symptoms of depression, psychotherapy (CBT, ST, IPT, PST, RT, or BDT) in combination with pharmacotherapy (first line: SSRIs especially citalopram and sertraline and extended-release venlafaxine; second line: TCAs, bupropion, and mirtazapine) is recommended for the treatment of symptoms. For severe depression, it is recommended that psychotherapy (CBT, ST, IPT, PST, RT, or BDT) in combination with pharmacotherapy (first line: SSRIs especially citalopram and sertraline and extended-release venlafaxine; second line: TCAs, bupropion, and mirtazapine) be used for the treatment of symptoms. Additionally, ECT (unilateral or bilateral) can be used when there is inadequate response to pharmacotherapy, when there is need for a faster resolution of symptoms, when the individual is suicidal, or when there are contraindications for pharmacotherapy. Among individuals who present with a severe depressive episode with psychotic features, antidepressants (first line: SSRIs and venlafaxine; second line: TCAs) in combination with antipsychotics (first line: risperidone, olanzapine, and quetiapine; second line: ziprasidone) or ECT (unilateral or bilateral) should be used when there is inadequate response to pharmacotherapy, when there is need for a faster resolution of symptoms, when the individual is suicidal, or when there are contraindications for pharmacotherapy. Among individuals who present with treatment-resistant depression, augmentation of an antidepressant with lithium or another agent (a second antidepressant, buspirone, or aripiprazole), switching from one antidepressant medication class to another, switching to ketamine or esketamine, augmenting with rTMS, or augmenting with ECT should be considered [99].

Conclusions

Depression is not an uncommon condition among older people. This condition is often underdiagnosed among older adults. Depression is associated with worse outcomes including greater rates of morbidity and mortality among older adults. A comprehensive history, a focused physical examination, and appropriate laboratory workup are crucial in identifying depression among older adults. Psychotherapy, pharmacotherapy, ketamine/esketamine, ECT, and rTMS have been found to be efficacious in the treatment of depression among older individuals. The early identification of depression and prompt treatment will help improve outcomes in this population.

References

1. Depressive Disorders. American Psychiatric Association. Desk reference to the diagnostic criteria from DSM-5. Washington, DC: American Psychiatric Publishing; 2013. p. 93–114.
2. Alexopoulos GS. Depression in the elderly. Lancet. 2005;365(9475):1961–70.
3. Fountoulakis KN, O'Hara R, Iacovides A, et al. Unipolar late-onset depression: a comprehensive review. Ann Gen Hosp Psychiatry. 2003;2(1):11.
4. Alexopoulos GS. New concepts for prevention and treatment of late-life depression. Am J Psychiatry. 2001;158(6):835–8.
5. Harman JS, Schulberg HC, Mulsant BH, et al. The effect of patient and visit characteristics on diagnosis of depression in primary care. J Fam Pract. 2001;50(12):1068.
6. Taylor WD, Doraiswamy PM. A systematic review of antidepressant placebo-controlled trials for geriatric depression: limitations of current data and directions for the future. Neuropsychopharmacology. 2004;29(12):2285–99.
7. Dunner DL. Treatment considerations for depression in the elderly. CNS Spectr. 2003;8(12 Suppl 3):14–9.
8. Hegeman JM, Kok RM, van der Mast RC, Giltay EJ. Phenomenology of depression in older compared with younger adults: meta-analysis. Br J Psychiatry. 2012 Apr;200(4):275–81.
9. Thorpe L. The treatment of psychotic disorders in late life. Can J Psychiatry. 1997;42(Suppl 1):19S–27S.
10. Gournellis R, Lykouras L, Fortos A, et al. Psychotic (delusional) major depression in late life. Int J Geriatr Psychiatry. 2001;16(11):1085–91.
11. Raskind MA. The clinical interface of depression and dementia. J Clin Psychiatry. 1998;59(Suppl 10):9–12.
12. Wang S, Blazer DG. Depression and cognition in the elderly. Annu Rev Clin Psychol. 2015;11:331–60.
13. Yaffe K, Blackwell T, Gore R, et al. Depressive symptoms and cognitive decline in nondemented elderly women: a prospective study. Arch Gen Psychiatry. 1999;56(5):425–30.
14. Comijs HC, Jonker C, Beckman AT, Deeg DJ. The association between depressive symptoms and cognitive decline in community-dwelling elderly persons. Int J Geriatr Psychiatry. 2001;16(4):361–7.
15. Wilson RS, Barnes LL, Mendes de Leon CF, et al. Depressive symptoms, cognitive decline, and risk of AD in older persons. Neurology. 2002;59(3):364–70.
16. Bennett S, Thomas AJ. Depression and dementia: cause, consequence or coincidence? Maturitas. 2014 Oct;79(2):184–90.

17. Reynolds CF 3rd, Smith GS, Dew MA, et al. Accelerating symptom-reduction in late-life depression: a double-blind, randomized, placebo-controlled trial of sleep deprivation. Am J Geriatr Psychiatry. 2005;13(5):353–8.

18. Weisenbach SL, Kumar A. Current understanding of the neurobiology and longitudinal course of geriatric depression. Curr Psychiatry Rep. 2014 Sep;16(9):463.

19. Alexopoulos GS, Katz IR, Reynolds CF, et al. Pharmacotherapy of depression in older patients: a summary of the expert consensus guidelines. J Psychiatr Pract. 2001;7(6):361–76.

20. Frasure-Smith N, Lesperance F, Talajic M. Depression following myocardial infarction. Impact on 6-month survival. JAMA. 1993;270(15):1819–25.

21. Carney RM, Freedland KE. Depression, mortality, and medical morbidity in patients with coronary heart disease. Biol Psychiatry. 2003;54(3):241–7.

22. Katon W, Lin E, von Korff M, et al. The predictors of persistence of depression in primary care. J Affect Disord. 1994;31(2):81–90.

23. Lynch TR, Johnson CS, Mendelson T, et al. New onset and remission of suicidal ideation among a depressed adult sample. J Affect Disord. 1999;56(1):49–54.

24. Duberstein PR. Openness to experience and completed suicide across the second half of life. Int Psychogeriatr. 1995;7(2):183–98.

25. Bruce ML. Psychosocial risk factors for depressive disorders in late life. Biol Psychiatry. 2002;52(3):175–84.

26. Clyburn LD, Stones MJ, Hadjistavropoulos T, Tuokko H, et al. Predicting caregiver burden and depression in Alzheimer's disease. J Gerontol B Psychol Sci Soc Sci. 2000;55(1):S2–S13.

27. Cole MG, Dendukuri N. Risk factors for depression among elderly community subjects: a systematic review and meta-analysis. Am J Psychiatry. 2003 Jun;160(6):1147–56.

28. Goff VV. Depression: a decade of progress, more to do. NHPF Issue Brief. 2002;786:1–14.

29. Hall CA, Reynolds-III CF. Late-life depression in the primary care setting: challenges, collaborative care, and prevention. Maturitas. 2014 Oct;79(2):147–52.

30. Michelson D, Stratakis C, Hill L, et al. Bone mineral density in women with depression. N Engl J Med. 1996;335(16):1176–81.

31. Ferketich AK, Schwartzbaum JA, Frid DJ, et al. Depression as an antecedent to heart disease among women and men in the NHANES I study. National Health and Nutrition Examination Survey. Arch Intern Med. 2000;160(9):1261–8.

32. Diniz BS, Butters MA, Albert SM, et al. Late-life depression and risk of vascular dementia and Alzheimer's disease: systematic review and meta-analysis of community-based cohort studies. Br J Psychiatry. 2013 May;202(5):329–35.

33. Glover J, Srinivasan S. Assessment of the person with late-life depression. Psychiatr Clin North Am. 2013 Dec;36(4):545–60.

34. Greenberg PE, Kessler RC, Birnbaum HG, et al. The economic burden of depression in the United States: how did it change between 1990 and 2000? J Clin Psychiatry. 2003 Dec;64(12):1465–75.

35. Turvey CL, Conwell Y, Jones MP, et al. Risk factors for late-life suicide: a prospective, community-based study. Am J Geriatr Psychiatry. 2002;10(4):398–406.

36. Johnson J, Weissman MM, Klerman GL. Service utilization and social morbidity associated with depressive symptoms in the community. JAMA. 1992;267(11):1478–83.

37. Croghan TW, Obenchain RL, Crown WE. What does treatment of depression really cost? Health Aff (Millwood). 1998;17(4):198–208.

38. Mulsant BH, Ganguli M. Epidemiology and diagnosis of depression in late life. J Clin Psychiatry. 1999;60(Suppl 20):9–15.

39. Unutzer J, Katon W, Russo J, et al. Patterns of care for depressed older adults in a large-staff model HMO. Am J Geriatr Psychiatry. 1999;7(3):235–43.

40. Mulkeen A, Zdanys K, Muralee S, et al. Screening tools for late-life depression: a review. Depression Mind Body. 2008;3(4):150–7.

41. Lichtenberg PA, Marcopulos BA, Steiner DA, et al. Comparison of the Hamilton Depression Rating Scale and the Geriatric Depression Scale: detection of depression in dementia patients. Psychol Rep (United States). 1992;70:515–21.

42. Clayton AH, Holroyd S, Sheldon-Keller A. Geriatric Depression Scale vs Hamilton Rating Scale for Depression in a sample of anxiety patients. Clin Gerontol. 1997;17:3–13.

43. Benjamin S, Steffens DC. Structural neuroimaging of geriatric depression. Psychiatr Clin North Am. 2011 Jun;34(2):423–35.

44. Gunning FM, Smith GS. Functional neuroimaging in geriatric depression. Psychiatr Clin North Am. 2011 Jun;34(2):403–22.

45. McClintock SM, Minto L, Denney DA, Bailey KC, Cullum CM, Dotson VM. Clinical neuropsychological evaluation in older adults with major depressive disorder. Curr Psychiatry Rep. 2021;23(9):55.

46. Mitchell AJ, Subramaniam H. Prognosis of depression in old age compared to middle age: a systematic review of comparative studies. Am J Psychiatry. 2005;162(9):1588–601.

47. Mulsant BH, Blumberger DM, Ismail Z, et al. A systematic approach to pharmacotherapy for geriatric major depression. Clin Geriatr Med. 2014 Aug;30(3):517–34.

48. Knöchel C, Alves G, Friedrichs B, et al. Treatment-resistant late-life depression: challenges and perspectives. Curr Neuropharmacol. 2015;13(5):577–91.

49. Kaster TS, Daskalakis ZJ, Noda Y, Knyahnytska Y, Downar J, Rajji TK, Levkovitz Y, Zangen A, Butters MA, Mulsant BH, Blumberger DM. Efficacy, tolerability, and cognitive effects of deep transcranial magnetic stimulation for late-life depression: a prospective randomized controlled trial. Neuropsychopharmacology. 2018 Oct;43(11):2231–8.

50. Sjosten N, Kivela SL. The effects of physical exercise on depressive symptoms among the aged: a systematic review. Int J Geriatr Psychiatry. 2006;21(5):410–8.
51. Mackin RS, Areán PA. Evidence-based psychotherapeutic interventions for geriatric depression. Psychiatr Clin North Am. 2005;28(4):805–20, vii–viii.
52. Cuijpers P, van Straten A, Smit F. Psychological treatment of late-life depression: a meta-analysis of randomized controlled trials. Int J Geriatr Psychiatry. 2006 Dec;21(12):1139–49.
53. Pinquart M, Duberstein PR, Lyness JM. Effects of psychotherapy and other behavioral interventions on clinically depressed older adults: a meta-analysis. Aging Ment Health. 2007 Nov;11(6):645–57.
54. Wilson KC, Mottram PG, Vassilas CA. Psychotherapeutic treatments for older depressed people. Cochrane Database Syst Rev. 2008;(1):CD004853.
55. Kiosses DN, Leon AC, Areán PA. Psychosocial interventions for late-life major depression: evidence-based treatments, predictors of treatment outcomes, and moderators of treatment effects. Psychiatr Clin North Am. 2011;34(2):377–401, viii.
56. Nelson JC, Delucchi K, Schneider LS. Efficacy of second generation antidepressants in late-life depression: a meta-analysis of the evidence. Am J Geriatr Psychiatry. 2008;16(7):558–67.
57. Mukai Y, Tampi RR. Treatment of depression in the elderly: a review of the recent literature on the efficacy of single- versus dual-action antidepressants. Clin Ther. 2009 May;31(5):945–61.
58. Tollefson GD, Bosomworth JC, Heiligenstein JH, et al. A double-blind, placebo-controlled clinical trial of fluoxetine in geriatric patients with major depression. The Fluoxetine Collaborative Study Group. Int Psychogeriatr. 1995;7(1):89–104.
59. Allard P, Gram L, Timdahl K, et al. Efficacy and tolerability of venlafaxine in geriatric outpatients with major depression: a double-blind, randomised 6-month comparative trial with citalopram. Int J Geriatr Psychiatry. 2004;19(12):1123–30.
60. Nelson JC, Wohlreich MM, Mallinckrodt CH, et al. Duloxetine for the treatment of major depressive disorder in older patients. Am J Geriatr Psychiatry. 2005;13(3):227–35.
61. Schatzberg AF, Kremer C, Rodrigues HE, et al. Double-blind, randomized comparison of mirtazapine and paroxetine in elderly depressed patients. Am J Geriatr Psychiatry. 2002;10(5):541–50.
62. Katona C, Hansen T, Olsen CK. A randomized, double-blind, placebo-controlled, duloxetine-referenced, fixed-dose study comparing the efficacy and safety of Lu AA21004 in elderly patients with major depressive disorder. Int Clin Psychopharmacol. 2012 Jul;27(4):215–23.
63. Katila H, Mezhebovsky I, Mulroy A, Berggren L, Eriksson H, Earley W, Datto C. Randomized, double-blind study of the efficacy and tolerability of extended release quetiapine fumarate (quetiapine XR) monotherapy in elderly patients with major depressive disorder. Am J Geriatr Psychiatry. 2013 Aug;21(8):769–84.
64. Lenze EJ, Mulsant BH, Blumberger DM, Karp JF, Newcomer JW, Anderson SJ, Dew MA, Butters MA, Stack JA, Begley AE, Reynolds CF 3rd. Efficacy, safety, and tolerability of augmentation pharmacotherapy with aripiprazole for treatment-resistant depression in late life: a randomised, double-blind, placebo-controlled trial. Lancet. 2015;386(10011):2404–12.
65. Lavretsky H, Reinlieb M, St Cyr N, Siddarth P, Ercoli LM, Senturk D. Citalopram, methylphenidate, or their combination in geriatric depression: a randomized, double-blind, placebo-controlled trial. Am J Psychiatry. 2015 Jun;172(6):561–9.
66. Patel K, Abdool PS, Rajji TK, Mulsant BH. Pharmacotherapy of major depression in late life: what is the role of new agents? Expert Opin Pharmacother. 2017 Apr;18(6):599–609.
67. Subramanian S, Lenze EJ. Ketamine for depression in older adults. Am J Geriatr Psychiatry. 2021 Sep;29(9):914–6.
68. Gupta A, Dhar R, Patadia P, Funaro M, Bhattacharya G, Farheen SA, Tampi RR. A systematic review of ketamine for the treatment of depression among older adults. Int Psychogeriatr. 2021 Feb;33(2):179–91.
69. George D, Gálvez V, Martin D, Kumar D, Leyden J, Hadzi-Pavlovic D, Harper S, Brodaty H, Glue P, Taylor R, Mitchell PB, Loo CK. Pilot randomized controlled trial of titrated subcutaneous ketamine in older patients with treatment-resistant depression. Am J Geriatr Psychiatry. 2017 Nov;25(11):1199–209.
70. Ochs-Ross R, Daly EJ, Zhang Y, Lane R, Lim P, Morrison RL, Hough D, Manji H, Drevets WC, Sanacora G, Steffens DC, Adler C, McShane R, Gaillard R, Wilkinson ST, Singh JB. Efficacy and safety of esketamine nasal spray plus an oral antidepressant in elderly patients with treatment-resistant depression-TRANSFORM-3. Am J Geriatr Psychiatry. 2020 Feb;28(2):121–41.
71. Kamholz BA, Mellow AM. Management of treatment resistance in the depressed geriatric patient. Psychiatr Clin North Am. 1996;19(2):269–86.
72. Whyte EM, Basinski J, Farhi P, et al. Geriatric depression treatment in nonresponders to selective serotonin reuptake inhibitors. J Clin Psychiatry. 2004;65(12):1634–41.
73. Flint AJ, Rifat SL. The effect of sequential antidepressant treatment on geriatric depression. J Affect Disord. 1996;36(3–4):95–105.
74. Dew MA, Whyte EM, Lenze EJ, et al. Recovery from major depression in older adults receiving augmentation of antidepressant pharmacotherapy. Am J Psychiatry. 2007 Jun;164(6):892–9.
75. Karp JF, Whyte EM, Lenze EJ, et al. Rescue pharmacotherapy with duloxetine for selective serotonin reuptake inhibitor nonresponders in late-life depression: outcome and tolerability. J Clin Psychiatry. 2008 Mar;69(3):457–63.

76. Rutherford B, Sneed J, Miyazaki M, et al. An open trial of aripiprazole augmentation for SSRI non-remitters with late-life depression. Int J Geriatr Psychiatry. 2007 Oct;22(10):986–91.

77. Sheffrin M, Driscoll HC, Lenze EJ, et al. Pilot study of augmentation with aripiprazole for incomplete response in late-life depression: getting to remission. J Clin Psychiatry. 2009 Feb;70(2):208–13.

78. Shamsi A, Cichon D, Obey J, et al. Pharmacotherapy for late-life depression with psychotic features: a review of literature of randomized control trials. Curr Psychiatry Rev. 2010 Aug;6(3):219–22.

79. Rothschild AJ, Duval SE. How long should patients with psychotic depression stay on the antipsychotic medication? J Clin Psychiatry. 2003 Apr;64(4):390–6.

80. van der Wurff FB, Stek ML, et al. The efficacy and safety of ECT in depressed older adults: a literature review. Int J Geriatr Psychiatry. 2003;18(10):894–904.

81. Kellner CH, Husain MM, Knapp RG, et al. A novel strategy for continuation ECT in geriatric depression: phase 2 of the PRIDE study. Am J Psychiatry. 2016;173(11):1110–8.

82. Spaans HP, Sienaert P, Bouckaert F, et al. Speed of remission in elderly patients with depression: electroconvulsive therapy v. medication. Br J Psychiatry. 2015 Jan;206(1):67–71.

83. Kumar S, Mulsant BH, Liu AY, et al. Systematic review of cognitive effects of electroconvulsive therapy in late-life depression. Am J Geriatr Psychiatry. 2016 Jul;24(7):547–65.

84. McDonald WM. Neuromodulation treatments for geriatric mood and cognitive disorders. Am J Geriatr Psychiatry. 2016 Dec;24(12):1130–41.

85. Riva-Posse P, Hermida AP, McDonald WM. The role of electroconvulsive and neuromodulation therapies in the treatment of geriatric depression. Psychiatr Clin North Am. 2013 Dec;36(4):607–30.

86. Lisanby SH, Husain MM, Rosenquist PB, et al. Daily left prefrontal repetitive transcranial magnetic stimulation in the acute treatment of major depression: clinical predictors of outcome in a multisite, randomized controlled clinical trial. Neuropsychopharmacology. 2009 Jan;34(2):522–34.

87. Nahas Z, Marangell LB, Husain MM, et al. Two-year outcome of vagus nerve stimulation (VNS) for treatment of major depressive episodes. J Clin Psychiatry. 2005 Sep;66(9):1097–104.

88. Bigos KL. Invited perspective on pharmacogenetics in late-life depression. Am J Geriatr Psychiatry. 2020 Jun;28(6):630–2.

89. Greden JF, Parikh SV, Rothschild AJ, et al. Impact of pharmacogenomics on clinical outcomes in major depressive disorder in the GUIDED trial: a large, patient- and rater-blinded, randomized, controlled study. J Psychiatr Res. 2019 Apr;111:59–67.

90. van der Schans J, Hak E, Postma M, et al. Effects of pharmacogenetic screening for CYP2D6 among elderly starting therapy with nortriptyline or venlafaxine: a pragmatic randomized controlled trial (CYSCE trial). J Clin Psychopharmacol. 2019;39(6):583–90.

91. Marshe VS, Islam F, Maciukiewicz M, et al. Pharmacogenetic implications for antidepressant pharmacotherapy in late-life depression: a systematic review of the literature for response, pharmacokinetics and adverse drug reactions. Am J Geriatr Psychiatry. 2020 Jun;28(6):609–29.

92. Bartels SJ, Coakley EH, Zubritsky C, et al. Improving access to geriatric mental health services: a randomized trial comparing treatment engagement with integrated versus enhanced referral care for depression, anxiety, and at-risk alcohol use. Am J Psychiatry. 2004;161(8):1455–62.

93. Hunkeler EM, Meresman JF, Hargreaves WA, et al. Efficacy of nurse telehealth care and peer support in augmenting treatment of depression in primary care. Arch Fam Med. 2000;9(8):700–8.

94. Sherbourne CD, Wells KB, Duan N, et al. Long-term effectiveness of disseminating quality improvement for depression in primary care. Arch Gen Psychiatry. 2001;58(7):696–703.

95. Hunkeler EM, Katon W, Tang L, et al. Long term outcomes from the IMPACT randomised trial for depressed elderly patients in primary care. BMJ. 2006;332(7536):259–63.

96. Mulsant BH, Alexopoulos GS, Reynolds CF, et al. Pharmacological treatment of depression in older primary care patients: the PROSPECT algorithm. Int J Geriatr Psychiatry. 2001;16(6):585–92.

97. Bruce ML, Ten Have TR, Reynolds CF, et al. Reducing suicidal ideation and depressive symptoms in depressed older primary care patients: a randomized controlled trial. JAMA. 2004;291(9):1081–91.

98. Alexopoulos GS, Katz IR, Bruce ML, et al. Remission in depressed geriatric primary care patients: a report from the PROSPECT study. Am J Psychiatry. 2005;162(4):718–2.

99. Tampi RR, Tampi DJ. The Management of Depression Among Older Adults. Psychiatr Times. 2022;38(4):22–5.

Bipolar Disorders 10

Rajesh R. Tampi and Deena J. Tampi

Introduction

Bipolar disorder (BD) is described in the Diagnostic and Statistical Manual of Mental Disorders, Fifth Edition (DSM-5), as a condition that presents with recurrent and/or cyclical episodes of mania or hypomania and depression [1]. The DSM-5 describes two subtypes of BD: the bipolar I disorder (BD-I) which is characterized by manic episodes in addition to major depressive and/or hypomanic episodes and bipolar II disorder (BD-II) which is characterized by at least one hypomanic episode and at least one major depressive episode without any manic episodes. BD can also occur among older adults, although its prevalence is not as common as among younger people [2]. With the increase in the population of older adults, it is projected that the number of cases of OABD will also increase significantly over the next few decades [3]. One Australian study found that between 1980 and 1998, the relative frequency of late-onset bipolar disorder increased from 1% to 11% [4].

Epidemiology

Older age bipolar disorder (OABD) is defined by the International Society for Bipolar Disorders (ISBD) Task Force as BD occurring among people ≥ 50 years in age [5]. Approximately one-quarter of all cases of BD occurs among people ≥ 60 years and about 1 in 10 cases occurs among individuals ≥ 70 years of age [6].

Available evidence indicates that the point prevalence of OABD is between 0.1% and 0.5%, and its lifetime prevalence is between 0.5% and 1.0% [7]. Among older adults who are diagnosed with a mood disorder, approximately 1 in 10 to 1 in 4 individuals have BD [8, 9]. Approximately 70% of individuals with OABD are women [10]. About 8–10% of all geriatric inpatient admissions and 6% of all geriatric psychiatry outpatient visits are by individuals with OABD [10]. In the emergency department, among all older individuals who are seen for a psychiatric assessment, approximately 17% have a diagnosis of BD. The prevalence of BD among older adults living in different settings are as follows: residential care psychiatric programs (approximately 17.4%), nursing homes (approximately 3%), and chronic institutional setting (approximately 9.7%).

R. R. Tampi (✉)
Department of Psychiatry, Creighton University School of Medicine, Omaha, NE, USA

Department of Psychiatry, Yale School of Medicine, New Haven, CT, USA

D. J. Tampi
Behavioral Health Advisory Group, Princeton, NJ, USA

R. R. Tampi, D. J. Tampi (eds.), *Treatment of Psychiatric Disorders Among Older Adults*, https://doi.org/10.1007/978-3-031-55711-8_10

Comparison Between OABD and Early-Onset Bipolar Disorder (EOBD)

Among individuals with OABD, depression is often the most common presenting symptom instead of either hypomania or mania [11–13]. Among these individuals, the episodes of depression are often recurrent and severe [14]. The period of latency between the initial and subsequent mood episodes is often longer among individuals with OABD, when compared to people with EOBD [12]. When compared to people with EOBD, individuals with OABD are less likely to have a family history of mood disorders [11, 15]. When compared to age-matched controls, individuals with OABD also have more stressful life events (SLE) [16].

Cerebrovascular diseases and other neurological conditions are more common among people with OABD, when compared to individuals with EOBD [7]. Vascular changes in the right cerebral hemisphere are associated with manic symptoms, and depressive symptoms are associated with vascular changes in the left cerebral hemisphere, among individuals with OABD [17, 18]. Greater number of cardiovascular and metabolic disorders are seen among individuals with OABD, and these comorbid conditions result in poor clinical outcomes, including a worsening of the risk for suicides [19–22]. Individuals with OABD on an average have about 3–4 medical comorbidities [23].

Greater white matter hyperintensities particularly in the frontal, parietal, and putaminal areas of the brain are noted among people with OABD [24–26]. Some studies also indicate that individuals with OABD have greater cortical sulcal widening and lateral ventricle-brain ratio when compared to people with EOBD [27, 28]. People with OABD also have more morphological abnormalities as seen in neuroimaging studies of the brain, when compared to individuals with EOBD [18].

When compared to age-matched controls, people with OABD have more psychiatric comorbidities [29]. But the rates of psychiatric comorbidities are lower than what is commonly seen among individuals with EOBD. The most common comorbid psychiatric disorder among individuals with OABD is alcohol use disorder with a 12-month and lifetime prevalence rates of 38.1% and 38.1%, respectively. This is followed by panic disorder (12-month and lifetime prevalence rates of 11.9% and 19%), generalized anxiety disorder (12-month and lifetime prevalence rates of 9.5% and 20.5%), and dysthymia (12-month and lifetime prevalence rates of 7.1% and 15.5%). Older women with OABD have a greater rate of panic disorder when compared to age-matched controls, and older men have greater rates of alcohol use disorder. When compared to individuals with EOBD, the risk for suicides among individuals with OABD is lower [3].

A significant number of individuals with OABD also present with some form of cognitive impairment [30]. When compared to age-matched controls, impairments have been noted on the Mini-Mental State Examination (MMSE) scores and the Mattis Dementia Rating Scale (DRS) scores among these individuals. But no correlation has been noted between the Young Mania Rating Scale (YMRS) scores and the cognitive impairments noted among individuals with OABD [30]. When compared to individuals with EOBD, people with OABD also show poorer functioning on psychomotor activity and cognitive flexibility [31]. The scores on MMSE and DRS are ≥ 1 standard deviation (SD) below the mean among approximately half of the individuals with OABD when compared to people with EOBD [32]. Increased number of vascular risk factors and a greater number of hospital admissions are associated with greater cognitive impairment among individuals with OABD [33].

A recent meta-analysis found that individuals with OABD who were euthymic did worse than healthy controls on verbal learning and verbal and visual delayed memory (Hedge's g, −0.77 to −0.89; $P < 0.001$) [34]. These individuals also displayed statistically significant deficits in processing speed, working memory, immediate memory, cognitive flexibility, verbal fluency, psychomotor function, executive functions, attention, inhibition, and recognition (Hedge's g, −0.52 to −0.76; $P < 0.001$). There were no deficits noted in language and visuo-construction domains among individuals with OABD.

Individuals with OABD also utilize approximately four times the total amount of mental health services and are four times as likely to have psychiatric hospitalizations when compared to age-matched controls [35].

Differences Between OABD, BD-I, and BD-II

A cross-sectional analysis of the Global Aging and Geriatric Experiments in Bipolar Disorder (GAGE-BD) database found that after adjustment for study cohort, BD-I individuals were more likely to have a history of psychiatric hospitalization ($P < 0.001$) and current use of antipsychotics ($P = 0.003$), whereas BD-II individuals often had a late onset ≥50 years ($P = 0.008$) and more current severe depression ($P = 0.041$) [36]. However, BD-I and BD-II individuals did not differ in terms of general functioning, cognitive impairment, or somatic burden. The investigators opined that the distinction between BD-I and BD-II is not the best way to subtype individuals with OABD.

Diagnosis

The diagnosis of OABD can be made via a psychiatric diagnostic assessment [7]. A psychiatric diagnostic assessment includes a comprehensive history, a thorough mental status examination, a focused physical examination, and appropriate laboratory testing. Mood symptoms that occur due to comorbid medical and/or neurological disorders or as a sequelae to prescribed or illicit drug use must be promptly identified and treated before making the

diagnosis of OABD [7]. Common laboratory tests that are conducted as a part of the workup for OABD include a complete blood count, a complete metabolic panel, a thyroid panel, vitamin B12 and folate levels, rapid plasma reagin (RPR)/Venereal Disease Research Laboratory (VDRL) test, human immunodeficiency virus (HIV) testing, urine analysis, culture, and urine drug screen. Neuroimaging studies like computerized tomography (CT) scans or magnetic resonance imaging (MRI) are obtained in situations where there are questions regarding cerebrovascular disease resulting in mood symptoms and/or cognitive deficits.

Although not specific for use among individuals with OABD, the Mood Disorder Questionnaire (MDQ) is a common screening tool used for bipolar disorder [37]. This screening instrument has good sensitivity and specificity for detecting a lifetime history of mania or hypomania, but there is the potential for overdiagnosis of BD with its use [37, 38]. Although not specific for use among older adults, screening tools like the Bipolar Spectrum Diagnostic Scale (BSDS), the Hypomanic Personality Scale (HPS), the Bipolar Depression Rating Scale (BDRS), and the Young Mania Rating Scale (YMRS) can quantify and qualify the symptoms of BD and also assist with monitoring their progress during treatment [39–42]. The most widely used clinical assessment tool for the diagnosis of BD among adults is the Structured Clinical Interview from the DSM-IV, and it can also assist with the diagnosis of OABD [39]. Finally, the diagnosis of BD can be confirmed by using the DSM-5 criteria [1]. Figure 10.1 describes the workup among individuals with OABD.

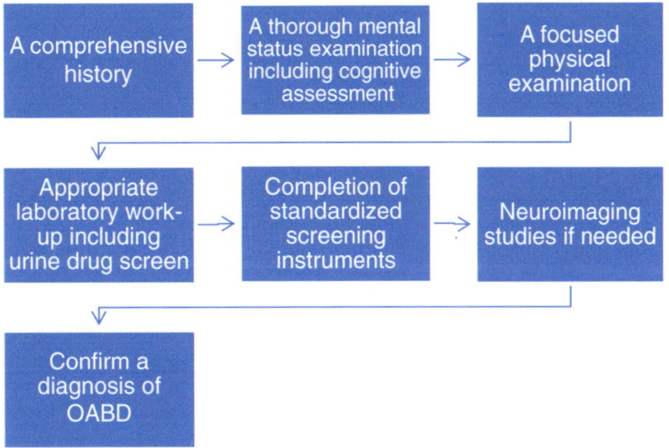

Fig. 10.1 Workup among individuals with OABD [7, 37–42]

Treatments

Nonpharmacological Treatments

Among individuals with OABD, the evidence for using specific psychotherapies is limited [3]. However, medication adherence skill training (MAST-BD) has been shown to improve adherence to medications, ability to manage medications, symptom of depression, energy, and social functioning among these individuals [43]. Improvements in patient satisfaction, follow-through rates, and good tolerability to treatment have been noted among individuals with OABD with the use of a manual-based medical care model (BCM) that included self-management sessions focusing on the control of BD symptoms, healthy habits, provider engagement, telephone-based care coordination, reinforcement of self-management goals, and guideline education that focused on medical issues in BD [44].

Pharmacological Treatments

Available evidence indicates efficacy for lithium, anticonvulsants, antipsychotics, antidepressants, and ECT for the treatment of individuals with OABD [45, 46]. Among people with OABD, the general principles for the pharmacotherapy are similar to those among individuals with EOBD. However, individuals with OABD require closer monitoring for adverse effects from the drugs that are used to treat their symptoms and for drug-drug interactions. Individuals with OABD often have multiple comorbid medical conditions and are generally being treated with multiple medication classes. In the next section of the chapter, we describe some of the common medications and medication classes that have been used among individuals with OABD.

Lithium

For the treatment of people with OABD, lithium remains the prototypical drug [45, 47–49]. It is most useful among those individuals who present with euphoric manic symptoms and among those people who have limited comorbid conditions. Lithium is also the drug of choice for monotherapy maintenance treatment among individuals with OABD [50]. The use of lithium may reduce the risk for suicide and cognitive decline among individuals with OABD [51, 52]. Prior to starting treatment with lithium among people with OABD, thyroid, renal, and cardiac functions should be evaluated [45, 49, 53]. These individuals are more prone to experiencing adverse effects with its use, have multiple comorbidities, and take multiple different medications. When lithium is co-prescribed with thiazide and loop diuretics, angiotensin-converting enzyme (ACE) inhibitors, and nonsteroidal anti-inflammatory drugs (NSAIDs), there should be close monitoring for lithium toxicity [45, 53, 54]. Sedation, weight gain, edema, hypothyroidism, renal dysfunction, gait abnormalities, and cognitive dysfunction are the most common adverse effects with the use of lithium [45, 49, 54]. The daily lithium dose that is recommended among individuals with OABD is approximately 1/4th to ½ of the adult daily dose [45]. Among individuals with OABD, the targeted lithium levels are between 0.4 mEq/L and 0.7 mEq/L.

Anticonvulsants

Data regarding the efficacy of anticonvulsants for the treatment of OABD from controlled studies is significantly limited [45]. Although there is no clear evidence that it is more efficacious or has better tolerability than lithium, valproic acid (VPA) preparations are being increasingly used among individuals with OABD [45, 47, 55]. As VPA preparations may cause serious adverse effects by interacting with drugs like warfarin, phenytoin, and phenobarbital and acetylsalicylic acid, caution must be exercised with the co-prescription of these drugs [45]. When compared to individuals with EOBD, therapeutic levels of VPA can be achieved among individuals with OABD by using lower daily dose of VPA [45, 55]. A combination of lithium and VPA may be particularly beneficial among people with OABD who have had partial response to lithium or VPA monotherapy or have a rapid cycling type of illness [56, 57].

In a 9-week randomized controlled trial (RCT) that evaluated the efficacy of lithium carbonate and divalproex among individuals ≥60 years in age with bipolar I disorder presenting with manic, hypomanic, or mixed episodes, the investigators noted that the cumulative response rates in the lithium and divalproex groups at weeks 3 and 9 were 62.5% and 57.1% ($P = 0.37$) and 78.6% and 73.2% ($P = 0.31$), respectively [58]. The cumulative remission rates in the lithium and divalproex groups at weeks 3 and 9 were 45.5% and 43.8% ($P = 0.74$) and 69.6% and 63.4% ($P = 0.29$), respectively. The targeted lithium and VPA serum concentrations were 0.80–0.99 mEq/L and 80–99 µg/mL, respectively. The attrition rates in the lithium and divalproex groups at weeks 3 and 9 were 14% and 51% and 18% and 44%, respectively. The rates of tremors were greater in the group receiving lithium when compared to divalproex, but the rates of sedation were similar between the two groups.

When compared to placebo, the use of lamotrigine was found to delay the time to intervention for any mood episode and for a depressive episode among people ≥55 years in age with bipolar I disorder [59]. Additionally, there was delayed time to intervention for any manic/hypomanic/mixed episodes with the use of lithium when compared to placebo in the same study. Among the lamotrigine group, back pain and headaches were the common adverse effects, whereas in the lithium group, the most adverse effects were dyspraxia, tremor, xerostomia, headache, infection, amnesia, dizziness, diarrhea, nausea, and fatigue. Lamotrigine has also shown a better cognitive profile when compared to other anticonvulsant mood stabilizers, among individuals with OABD [45].

Although there are no controlled trials for carbamazepine among individuals with OABD, data from mixed aged population studies indicate that for the treatment of acute mania and for the maintenance treatment among individuals with BD, carbamazepine appears to be inferior to both lithium and VPA [45, 60–62]. Carbamazepine should be reserved for the treatment of individuals who present with nonclassical or atypical features of BD [45]. Carbamazepine has also been found to be less well tolerated than other anticonvulsant mood stabilizers and causes significant drug-drug interactions among people with OABD [45].

As there are no controlled studies evaluating the efficacy and tolerability of gabapentin, oxcarbazepine, topiramate, and zonisamide among individuals with OABD, their routine use cannot be recommended among these people [45].

Antipsychotics

The United States Food and Drug Administration (FDA) has approved aripiprazole, asenapine, olanzapine, quetiapine, quetiapine extended release (XR), risperidone, and ziprasidone for the treatment of BD [63]. Olanzapine-fluoxetine combination (OFC), quetiapine, and lurasidone are approved for the acute treatment of bipolar depression [64]. Lurasidone is approved as a monotherapy and as an adjunct to lithium or divalproex therapy, and the OFC and quetiapine are approved as a monotherapy for acute treatment of bipolar depression. Lumateperone is the latest antipsychotic medication to be FDA approved for the treatment of depressive episodes associated with bipolar I or II disorder among adults, both as monotherapy and as adjunctive therapy with lithium or valproate [65].

Among people ≥55 years in age who had manic episodes as part of BD, quetiapine 400–800 mg a day was found to beneficial when compared to placebo, with symptomatic improvements noted from baseline to day 21 in a post hoc analysis of pooled data from two quetiapine monotherapy trials [66]. From day 4 of treatment, the investigators noted sustained reductions in mania scores. Dry mouth, somnolence, postural hypotension, insomnia, weight gain, and dizziness were the most common adverse effects in the quetiapine group in this analysis.

Investigators evaluated the efficacy of lurasidone for BD among older adults using data from a post hoc analysis of two 6-week placebo-controlled, randomized, double-blind trials of lurasidone [67]. One was a monotherapy trial, and the other was an adjunctive agent to lithium or valproate. Both trials included people who were ≥55 years in age and met the DSM-IV-TR criteria for bipolar I depression. In the first trial (monotherapy), the investigators evaluated the use of fixed flexible doses of lurasidone 20–60 mg a day or 80–120 mg a day when compared to placebo. In the second study, flexible doses of lurasidone 20–120 mg a day were used as an adjunct to either lithium or valproate and were compared to placebo. In both trials, a mean change at week 6 on the Montgomery-Åsberg Depression Rating Scale (MADRS) total score was the primary endpoint. The mean change in the MADRS total score was significantly more in the lurasidone group when compared to the placebo group (effect size = 0.83, P = 0.003) at week 6 in the first study. The mean change in the MADRS total score was not significantly different between the lurasidone and placebo groups (effect size = 0.26, P = 0.398) at week 6 in the second study. The investigators did not find any difference in the rates of discontinuation due to adverse events between the lurasidone and placebo groups in both studies: monotherapy study (6.8% vs. 6.9%) and the adjunctive therapy study (3.8% vs. 7.1%), respectively.

In an open-label study of 11 individuals who had acute manic episode and a mean age of 67.7 years who were consecutively admitted to a geriatric psychiatry unit, oral asenapine 10 mg twice was prescribed as monotherapy for 4 weeks [68]. At week 4, the investigators found improvements in manic symptoms in all the participants in the study, with remission of symptoms being noted in 7 of the 11 individuals. The adverse effects noted in the study were as follows: mild sedation (n = 3), rash (n = 1), and edema (n = 1). Following the discontinuation of the drug, all the adverse effects resolved quickly.

Investigators found that in a prospective open-label trial of asenapine among individuals aged ≥60 years and who had inadequate responses to other BD treatments, the use of asenapine resulted in significant improvements in the Brief Psychiatric Rating Scale (BPRS, P < 0.05), the Clinical Global Impression Scale, bipolar version (CGI-BP, P < 0.01), the CGI-BP mania subscale (P < 0.05), and depression subscale (P < 0.01) from baseline to week 12 [69]. In this study, the mean dose of asenapine was 11.2 mg a day. The most common adverse effect in this study was gastrointestinal discomfort that was seen in 33% of the participants. The other adverse effects that were noted included restlessness (13%), tremors (13%), cognitive difficulties (13%), and sluggishness (13%).

Clozapine has been found to be effective for the treatment of manic episodes with psychosis among three older men with BD who were institutionalized [70]. These individuals had not responded adequately to treatment with lithium, valproate, benzodiazepines, or antipsychotics either as monotherapy or as combination treatments. Among these people, sustained improvement in symptoms was noted over a period of 11 months, and there were no significant adverse effects noted among these individuals.

In a retrospective cohort study of individuals 65–89 years in age with a diagnosis of bipolar I or II disorder and receiving either lithium or an atypical antipsychotic medication, the most common antipsychotics that were prescribed were aripiprazole and quetiapine (33% each), followed by risperidone (17%), olanzapine (13%), and lurasidone (4%) [71]. All of the individuals on lithium had discontinued treatment when compared to 83.33% of individuals on atypical antipsychotics (P = 0.03) by the end of the data collection period. The days to discontinuation did not differ between the two groups (P = 0.998). Additionally, the discontinuation of treatment due to adverse effects was similar between the two groups (P = 0.523). Discontinuation due to perceived lack of efficacy (P = 0.80) and loss to follow up (P = 0.448) were similar between the two groups. In the lithium group, tremor was the most commonly reported adverse effect (40%). This was followed by renal failure (30%), toxicity (20%), and bloating/swelling (10%). In the atypical antipsychotic group, extrapyramidal symptoms (EPSs, 50%) and sedation (33%) were the most common adverse effects. This was followed by restlessness and hallucinations (17%). There were no significant QTc interval changes noted in either group. In the lithium group, hospitalizations due to BD occurred in 14% of the individuals, whereas 11% of the individuals in the atypical antipsychotic group were hospitalized.

Analysis of cross-sectional data from 16 studies among individuals $\geq$50 years in age with BD [the Global Aging & Geriatric Experiments in Bipolar Disorder Database (GAGE-BD)] found that 46.6% of these individuals were using antipsychotics [72]. Antipsychotics appeared to be prescribed to individuals who were younger ($P = 0.01$), who were less likely to be employed ($P < 0.001$), who had more psychiatric hospitalizations ($P = 0.009$), and those who were less likely to be prescribed lithium ($P < 0.001$). Majority (93%) of these individuals were prescribed atypical antipsychotics (93%).

There should be a risk-benefit analysis done prior to the prescription of antipsychotics to older adults [73]. These medications can increase the risk for cerebrovascular adverse events and deaths in this population, especially among those individuals who have dementia.

Antidepressants

A population-based retrospective cohort study by Schaffer et al. found that the prescription of antidepressants reduced the likelihood of admissions for manic/mixed episodes (adjusted rate ratio [aRR] = 0.5) among individuals $\geq$66 years in age with BD when compared to individuals who did not receive an antidepressant during the same time period [74]. However, these medications did not reduce the likelihood of depressive episodes (aRR = 0.7) in this population.

Electroconvulsive Therapy

Among individuals with OABD, there are no controlled studies of electroconvulsive therapy (ECT) [45, 75]. However, reports indicate that ECT is a safe and effective treatment among older individuals with severe or refractory mania [76]. Among older adults with BD, ECT is often used when quick treatment response is required and/or when the symptoms are refractory to pharmacotherapy. It is also an effective treatment where the individual with BD is at imminent suicide or homicide risk [45]. Additionally, ECT can be highly effective in situations where the older individual with BD presents with severe agitation, catatonia, or psychosis. ECT can also be used in situations where the individual's medical condition is unstable [45]. For the treatment of depressive episodes, both right unilateral and bilateral ECT have been noted to have equal efficacy [45, 77]. However, bilateral ECT is associated with longer postictal recovery period and greater memory impairments.

Treatment Algorithm

For the treatment of individuals with OABD, Tampi et al. have proposed a treatment algorithm [78]. A minimum of 3–4 weeks' trial for the medication that is chosen initially to treat the symptoms of OABD is recommended [45]. An appropriate combination of medications can be used when monotherapy has not been deemed beneficial. Among individuals who have responded adequately to a medication or medication combinations, these should be continued for at least the next 6–12 months. Among individuals whose symptoms are in remission, an initial gradual taper and discontinuation of adjunctive medications could be attempted after a period of 12 months [79]. Decreased response to treatment among individuals with OABD is thought to be due to limited treatment compliance and comorbid substance use disorder and/or medical disorders [5]. Table 10.1 enumerates the possible treatment options for OABD [78].

Table 10.1 Possible treatment options for OABD [3, 43–77]

Manic episodes	**Lithium** **Useful for:** Manic episode Maintenance treatment **Dose:** 1/4th to ½ the adult dose of drug Level: 0.4–0.7 mEq/L **Tolerability:** Less well tolerated than among younger individuals	**Anticonvulsant mood stabilizers** **Useful for:** Mixed episodes Rapid cycling episodes Individuals with comorbid medical and psychiatric disorders Maintenance treatment **Dose:** 1/4th to ½ the adult dose of drug **Tolerability:** Less well tolerated than among younger individuals	**Atypical antipsychotics** **Useful for:** Manic episode Maintenance treatment **Dose:** 1/4th to ½ the adult dose of drug **Tolerability:** Less well tolerated than among younger individuals Risk for metabolic syndrome with prolonged use Risk for cerebrovascular events and death among older individuals with dementia
Depressive episodes	**Lithium** **Useful for:** Maintenance treatment **Dose:** 1/4th to ½ the adult dose of drug **Levels:** 0.4–0.7 mEq/L **Tolerability:** Less well tolerated than among younger individuals	**Anticonvulsant mood stabilizers** **Useful for:** Lamotrigine is better for depressive episodes than mania **Dose:** 1/4th to ½ the adult dose of drug **Levels:** ½–¾ the adult levels **Tolerability:** Less well tolerated than among younger individuals	**Atypical antipsychotics** **Useful for:** Acute treatment of bipolar depression Lurasidone as a monotherapy and as an adjunct to lithium or divalproex treatment Olanzapine-fluoxetine combination and quetiapine as monotherapy **Dose:** 1/4th to ½ the adult dose of drug **Tolerability:** Less well tolerated than among younger individuals Risk for metabolic syndrome with prolonged use Risk for cerebrovascular events and death among older individuals with dementia
Partial response	**Electroconvulsive therapy** **Useful for:** Refractory symptoms Psychotic symptoms Catatonic symptoms Severe agitation Individuals who are actively suicidal and/or homicidal **Efficacy:** Bilateral = right unilateral **Tolerability:** Bilateral < right unilateral	**Psychosocial therapies** **Useful for:** Adjunctive treatment with medications **Tolerability:** Well tolerated among older adults	

Conclusion

Among the older adult population, BD is not an uncommon disorder. Older individuals with BD have greater burden of medical comorbidities, but less family history of BD. These individuals present with greater morbidity, worse outcomes, and higher rates of utilization of services when compared to age-matched controls. It is crucial to rule out underlying medical conditions and effects of prescribed medication or substances of abuse when assessing individuals with OABD, as they may precipitate or perpetuate symptoms of BD. Available evidence indicates that medication classes that are used to treat younger individuals with BD are also effective among individuals with OABD. Psychosocial treatments are beneficial as adjunctive treatment among these individuals. ECT is often highly effective among refractory cases of OABD.

References

1. Bipolar and related disorders. In: Diagnostic and statistical manual of mental disorders. DSM Library. American Psychiatric Association; 2013. Accessed 23 Dec 2022. doi: https://doi.org/10.1176/appi.books.9780890425596.dsm03.
2. Montes JM, Alegria A, Garcia-Lopez A, et al. Understanding bipolar disorder in late life: clinical and treatment correlates of a sample of elderly outpatients. J Nerv Ment Dis. 2013;201(8):674–9.
3. Dols A, Beekman A. Older Age Bipolar Disorder. Clin Geriatr Med. 2020;36(2):281–96.
4. Almeida OP, Fenner S. Bipolar disorder: similarities and differences between patients with illness onset before and after 65 years of age. Int Psychogeriatr. 2002;14(3):311–22.
5. Sajatovic M, Strejilevich SA, Gildengers AG, et al. A report on older-age bipolar disorder from the International Society for Bipolar Disorders Task Force. Bipolar Disord. 2015;17(7):689–704.
6. Sajatovic M, Blow FC, Ignacio RV, Kales HC. Age-related modifiers of clinical presentation and health service use among veterans with bipolar disorder. Psychiatr Serv. 2004;55(9):1014–21.
7. Sajatovic M, Chen P. Geriatric bipolar disorder. Psychiatr Clin North Am. 2011;34(2):319–33. vii
8. Depp CA, Jin H, Mohamed S, Kaskow J, Moore DJ, Jeste DV. Bipolar disorder in middle-aged and elderly adults: is age of onset important? J Nerv Ment Dis. 2004;192(11):796–9.
9. Yassa R, Nair V, Nastase C, Camille Y, Belzile L. Prevalence of bipolar disorder in a psychogeriatric population. J Affect Disord. 1988;14(3):197–201.
10. Depp CA, Jeste DV. Bipolar disorder in older adults: a critical review. Bipolar Disord. 2004;6(5):343–67.
11. Stone K. Mania in the elderly. Br J Psychiatry. 1989;155:220–4.
12. Shulman KI, Tohen M, Satlin A, Mallya G, Kalunian D. Mania compared with unipolar depression in old age. Am J Psychiatry. 1992;149(3):341–5.
13. Tohen M, Shulman KI, Satlin A. First-episode mania in late life. Am J Psychiatry. 1994;151(1):130–2. https://doi.org/10.1176/ajp.151.1.130.
14. García-López A, Ezquiaga E, De Dios C, Agud JL. Depressive symptoms in early- and late-onset older bipolar patients compared with younger ones. Int J Geriatr Psychiatry. 2017;32(2):201–7.
15. Hays JC, Krishnan KR, George LK, Blazer DG. Age of first onset of bipolar disorder: demographic, family history, and psychosocial correlates. Depress Anxiety. 1998;7(2):76–82.
16. Beyer JL, Kuchibhatla M, Cassidy F, Krishnan KRR. Stressful life events in older bipolar patients. Int J Geriatr Psychiatry. 2008;23(12):1271–5.
17. Robinson RG, Starkstein SE. Current research in affective disorders following stroke. J Neuropsychiatry Clin Neurosci. 1990;2(1):1–14.
18. Steffens DC, Krishnan KR. Structural neuroimaging and mood disorders: recent findings, implications for classification, and future directions. Biol Psychiatry. 1998;43(10):705–12.
19. Gildengers AG, Whyte EM, Drayer RA, et al. Medical burden in late-life bipolar and major depressive disorders. Am J Geriatr Psychiatry. 2008;16(3):194–200.
20. Kilbourne AM, Post EP, Nossek A, Drill L, Cooley S, Bauer MS. Improving medical and psychiatric outcomes among individuals with bipolar disorder: a randomized controlled trial. Psychiatr Serv. 2008;59(7):760–8.
21. McIntyre RS, Konarski JZ, Soczynska JK, et al. Medical comorbidity in bipolar disorder: implications for functional outcomes and health service utilization. Psychiatr Serv. 2006;57(8):1140–4.
22. Juurlink DN, Herrmann N, Szalai JP, Kopp A, Redelmeier DA. Medical illness and the risk of suicide in the elderly. Arch Intern Med. 2004;164(11):1179–84.
23. Lala SV, Sajatovic M. Medical and psychiatric comorbidities among elderly individuals with bipolar disorder: a literature review. J Geriatr Psychiatry Neurol. 2012;25(1):20–5.
24. Subramaniam H, Dennis MS, Byrne EJ. The role of vascular risk factors in late onset bipolar disorder. Int J Geriatr Psychiatry. 2007;22(8):733–7.
25. Lloyd AJ, Moore PB, Cousins DA, et al. White matter lesions in euthymic patients with bipolar disorder. Acta Psychiatr Scand. 2009;120(6):481–91.
26. Tamashiro JH, Zung S, Zanetti MV, et al. Increased rates of white matter hyperintensities in late-onset bipolar disorder. Bipolar Disord. 2008;10(7):765–75.

27. Sarnicola A, Kempton M, Germanà C, et al. No differential effect of age on brain matter volume and cognition in bipolar patients and healthy individuals. Bipolar Disord. 2009;11(3):316–22.

28. Young RC, Nambudiri DE, Jain H, de Asis JM, Alexopoulos GS. Brain computed tomography in geriatric manic disorder. Biol Psychiatry. 1999;45(8):1063–5.

29. Goldstein BI, Herrmann N, Shulman KI. Comorbidity in bipolar disorder among the elderly: results from an epidemiological community sample. Am J Psychiatry. 2006;163(2):319–21.

30. Young RC, Murphy CF, Heo M, Schulberg HC, Alexopoulos GS. Cognitive impairment in bipolar disorder in old age: literature review and findings in manic patients. J Affect Disord. 2006;92(1):125–31.

31. Schouws SNTM, Comijs HC, Stek ML, et al. Cognitive impairment in early and late bipolar disorder. Am J Geriatr Psychiatry. 2009;17(6):508–15.

32. Gildengers AG, Butters MA, Seligman K, et al. Cognitive functioning in late-life bipolar disorder. Am J Psychiatry. 2004;161(4):736–8.

33. Schouws SNTM, Stek ML, Comijs HC, Beekman ATF. Risk factors for cognitive impairment in elderly bipolar patients. J Affect Disord. 2010;125(1–3):330–5.

34. Montejo L, Torrent C, Jiménez E, et al. Cognition in older adults with bipolar disorder: an ISBD task force systematic review and meta-analysis based on a comprehensive neuropsychological assessment. Bipolar Disord. 2022;24(2):115–36.

35. Bartels SJ, Forester B, Miles KM, Joyce T. Mental health service use by elderly patients with bipolar disorder and unipolar major depression. Am J Geriatr Psychiatry. 2000;8(2):160–6.

36. Beunders AJM, Klaus F, Kok AAL, et al. Bipolar I and bipolar II subtypes in older age: results from the Global Aging and Geriatric Experiments in Bipolar Disorder (GAGE-BD) project. Bipolar Disord. 2022;25:43.

37. Hirschfeld RM, Williams JB, Spitzer RL, et al. Development and validation of a screening instrument for bipolar spectrum disorder: the Mood Disorder Questionnaire. Am J Psychiatry. 2000;157(11):1873–5.

38. Zimmerman M, Ruggero CJ, Galione JN, et al. Detecting differences in diagnostic assessment of bipolar disorder. J Nerv Ment Dis. 2010;198(5):339–42.

39. Baldassano CF. Assessment tools for screening and monitoring bipolar disorder. Bipolar Disord. 2005;7(Suppl 1):8–15.

40. Picardi A. Rating scales in bipolar disorder. Curr Opin Psychiatry. 2009;22(1):42–9.

41. Berk M, Malhi GS, Cahill C, et al. The Bipolar Depression Rating Scale (BDRS): its development, validation and utility. Bipolar Disord. 2007;9(6):571–9.

42. Young RC, Biggs JT, Ziegler VE, Meyer DA. A rating scale for mania: reliability, validity and sensitivity. Br J Psychiatry. 1978;133:429–35.

43. Depp CA, Lebowitz BD, Patterson TL, et al. Medication adherence skills training for middle-aged and elderly adults with bipolar disorder: development and pilot study. Bipolar Disord. 2007;9(6):636–45.

44. Kilbourne AM, Post EP, Nossek A, et al. Service delivery in older patients with bipolar disorder: a review and development of a medical care model. Bipolar Disord. 2008;10(6):672–83.

45. Aziz R, Lorberg B, Tampi RR. Treatment for late-life bipolar disorder. Am J Geriatr Pharmacother. 2006;4(4):347–64.

46. Dols A, Kessing LV, Strejilevich SA, et al. Do current national and international guidelines have specific recommendations for older adults with bipolar disorder? A brief report. Int J Geriatr Psychiatry. 2016;31(12):1295–300.

47. Fotso Soh J, Klil-Drori S, Rej S. Using lithium in older age bipolar disorder: special considerations. Drugs Aging. 2019;36(2):147–54.

48. Sajatovic M. Treatment of bipolar disorder in older adults. Int J Geriatr Psychiatry. 2002;17(9):865–73.

49. Sajatovic M, Madhusoodanan S, Coconcea N. Managing bipolar disorder in the elderly: defining the role of the newer agents. Drugs Aging. 2005;22(1):39–54.

50. Shulman KI, Almeida OP, Herrmann N, et al. Delphi survey of maintenance lithium treatment in older adults with bipolar disorder: an ISBD task force report. Bipolar Disord. 2019;21(2):117–23.

51. Kessing LV, Søndergård L, Kvist K, et al. Suicide risk in patients treated with lithium. Arch Gen Psychiatry. 2005;62(8):860–6.

52. Kessing LV, Forman JL, Andersen PK. Does lithium protect against dementia? Bipolar Disord. 2010;12(1):87–94.

53. American Psychiatric Association. Practice guideline for the treatment of patients with bipolar disorder (revision). Am J Psychiatry. 2002;159(Suppl 4):1–50.

54. Shulman KI, Rochon P, Sykora K, et al. Changing prescription patterns for lithium and valproic acid in old age: shifting practice without evidence. BMJ. 2003;326(7396):960–1.

55. Chen ST, Altshuler LL, Melnyk KA, et al. Efficacy of lithium vs. valproate in the treatment of mania in the elderly: a retrospective study. J Clin Psychiatry. 1999;60(3):181–6.

56. Schneider AL, Wilcox CS. Divalproate augmentation in lithium-resistant rapid cycling mania in four geriatric patients. J Affect Disord. 1998;47(1–3):201–5.

57. Goldberg JF, Sacks MH, Kocsis JH. Low-dose lithium augmentation of divalproex in geriatric mania. J Clin Psychiatry. 2000;61(4):304.

58. Young RC, Mulsant BH, Sajatovic M, et al. GERI-BD: a randomized double-blind controlled trial of lithium and divalproex in the treatment of mania in older patients with bipolar disorder. Am J Psychiatry. 2017;174(11):1086–93.

59. Sajatovic M, Gyulai L, Calabrese JR, et al. Maintenance treatment outcomes in older patients

with bipolar I disorder. Am J Geriatr Psychiatry. 2005;13(4):305–11.

60. Sajatovic M, Chen P. Geriatric bipolar disorder. Psychiatr Clin North Am. 2011;34(2):319–33.

61. Greil W, Kleindienst N, Erazo N, et al. Differential response to lithium and carbamazepine in the prophylaxis of bipolar disorder. J Clin Psychopharmacol. 1998;18(6):455–60.

62. Vasudev K, Goswami U, Kohli K. Carbamazepine and valproate monotherapy: feasibility, relative safety and efficacy, and therapeutic drug monitoring in manic disorder. Psychopharmacology. 2000;150(1):15–23.

63. Atypical Antipsychotic Medications: Use in adults. https://www.cms.gov/Medicare-Medicaid-Coordination/Fraud-Prevention/Medicaid-Integrity-Education/Pharmacy-Education-Materials/Downloads/atyp-antipsych-adult-factsheet11-14.pdf. Accessed 14 Aug 2022.

64. McIntyre RS, Cha DS, Kim RD, Mansur RB. A review of FDA-approved treatment options in bipolar depression. CNS Spectr. 2013;18(Suppl 1):4–20. quiz 21

65. Caplyta. https://www.accessdata.fda.gov/drugsatfda_docs/label/2021/209500s005s006lbl.pdf. Accessed 2 Jan 2023.

66. Sajatovic M, Calabrese JR, Mullen J. Quetiapine for the treatment of bipolar mania in older adults. Bipolar Disord. 2008;10(6):662–71.

67. Sajatovic M, Forester BP, Tsai J, et al. Efficacy of Lurasidone in adults aged 55 years and older with bipolar depression: post hoc analysis of 2 double-blind, placebo-controlled studies. J Clin Psychiatry. 2016;77(10):e1324–31.

68. Baruch Y, Tadger S, Plopski I, Barak Y. Asenapine for elderly bipolar manic patients. J Affect Disord. 2013;145(1):130–2.

69. Sajatovic M, Dines P, Fuentes-Casiano E, et al. Asenapine in the treatment of older adults with bipolar disorder. Int J Geriatr Psychiatry. 2015;30(7):710–9.

70. Shulman RW, Singh A, Shulman KI. Treatment of elderly institutionalized bipolar patients with clozapine. Psychopharmacol Bull. 1997;33(1):113–8.

71. Burton C, Mathys M, Gutierrez E. Comparison of lithium to second generation antipsychotics for the treatment of bipolar disorder in older veterans. Psychiatry Res. 2021;303:114063.

72. Chen P, Eyler LT, Gildengers A, et al. Demographic and clinical characteristics of antipsychotic drug-treated older adults with bipolar disorder from the Global Aging & Geriatric Experiments in Bipolar Disorder Database (GAGE-BD). Psychopharmacol Bull. 2022;52(2):8–33.

73. Mittal V, Kurup L, Williamson D, et al. Risk of cerebrovascular adverse events and death in elderly patients with dementia when treated with antipsychotic medications: a literature review of evidence. Am J Alzheimers Dis Other Dement. 2011;26(1):10–28.

74. Schaffer A, Mamdani M, Levitt A, et al. Effect of antidepressant use on admissions to hospital among elderly bipolar patients. Int J Geriatr Psychiatry. 2006;21(3):275–80.

75. McDonald WM. Neuromodulation treatments for geriatric mood and cognitive disorders. Am J Geriatr Psychiatry. 2016;24(12):1130–41.

76. Wilkins KM, Ostroff R, Tampi RR. Efficacy of electroconvulsive therapy in the treatment of non-depressed psychiatric illness in elderly patients: a review of the literature. J Geriatr Psychiatry Neurol. 2008;21(1):3–11.

77. Fraser RM, Glass IB. Unilateral and bilateral ECT in elderly patients. A comparative study. Acta Psychiatr Scand. 1980;62:13–31.

78. Tampi RR, Joshi P, Bhattacharya G, Gupta S. Evaluation and treatment of older-age bipolar disorder: a narrative review. Drugs. Context. 2021;10:2021-1-8.

79. Young RC, Gyulai L, Mulsant BH, et al. Pharmacotherapy of bipolar disorder in old age: review and recommendations. Am J Geriatr Psychiatry. 2004;12(4):342–57.

Part III

Sleep-Wake Disorders

Insomnia

Manju Pillai and Seetha Chandrasekhara

Introduction

Insomnia is defined as difficulty falling asleep, staying asleep, or returning to sleep after an early-morning awakening at least three nights per week over a minimum of 3 months and occurs despite adequate opportunity to sleep. In addition, sleep disturbance results in significant distress as well as impairments in mood, behavior, social/interpersonal relationships, and/or academic/occupational performance [1, 2]. The Diagnostic and Statistical Manual of Mental Disorders, 5th Edition (DSM5), criteria for insomnia are outlined in Table 11.1. Consequences of poor sleep are not just limited to the previously noted impairments to daily living though. Cognitive impairments (e.g., memory deficits and limited attention); impairments to balance, ambulation, and vision; increased risk of developing depression, heart disease, hypertension, myocardial infarction, stroke, and diabetes; and also a general higher incidence of mortality are all seen in older adults with inadequate sleep [3–18].

M. Pillai
Temple University Hospital, Philadelphia, PA, USA
e-mail: manju.pillai@tuhs.temple.edu

S. Chandrasekhara (✉)
Department of Psychiatry, Lewis Katz School of Medicine at Temple University,
Philadelphia, PA, USA
e-mail: tuc32963@temple.edu

Table 11.1 DSM-5 criteria for insomnia disorder

Complaint with sleep quality or quantity with at least one of the following: – Difficulty initiating sleep – Difficulty maintaining sleep – Awakening in early morning and unable to return to sleep
Causes significant distress or functional impairment
At least three nights per week
Present for at least 3 months
Difficulty with sleep occurs even with sufficient sleep opportunity
Not due to another sleep-wake disorder
Not due to effects of a substance or medication
Coexisting medical/mental disorders do not explain insomnia

*Specifiers: with non-sleep disorder mental comorbidity, with other medical comorbidity, with other sleep disorder
**Episodic (at least 1 month but less than 3 months), persistent (longer than 3 months), recurrent (at least two episodes within 1 year)

Epidemiology

According to a survey by the American Academy of Sleep Medicine (AASM), 28% of adults in the United States reported having insomnia that negatively impacted their daily lives [19]. When looking at just adults aged 60 years or older, as many as 50% report symptoms consistent with insomnia [20]. Insomnia is often a persistent condition, even in those who had been in remission. In a cohort study by Morin et al., 37.5% of adults with baseline insomnia continued to report

R. R. Tampi, D. J. Tampi (eds.), *Treatment of Psychiatric Disorders Among Older Adults*,
https://doi.org/10.1007/978-3-031-55711-8_11

insomnia at each of the annual follow-ups for the 5-year period. Those who had achieved remission had greater chance of relapse (OR 2.04, 95% CI 1.23–3.37) than to improve over the next year [1].

Normal Sleep Cycle

With the help of electroencephalographic (EEG) recordings, sleep has been divided into several distinct stages that are cycled through during the night. Broadly, sleep is divided into rapid eye movement (REM) sleep and non-rapid eye-movement (NREM) sleep. NREM is then further divided into three stages—N1, N2, and N3. Stage N1 accounts for 4–16% of total time asleep and is the first stage entered at sleep onset as well as when following an episode of arousal from another stage of sleep; on EEG, this stage is characterized by the presence of theta brain waves [21]. Stage N2 accounts for 45–55% of total time asleep and, on EEG, is characterized by the presence of sleep spindles and k-complexes. Stage N3 is also referred to as slow-wave sleep (SWS). Previously, N3 was further divided into N3 and N4, but these stages were combined when the AASM released their standard guidelines in 2007 [22]. On EEG, delta brain waves characterize this stage. Finally, REM accounts for 20–25% of total time asleep and is the stage of sleep where brain metabolism is the highest and in which there is spontaneous rapid eye moves (similar to the awake state) but with paralysis of skeletal muscles. EEG for REM will look similar to when awake—mixed-frequency, low-amplitude brain waves—though with low muscle tone [21]. Characteristics of the stages in the normal sleep cycle are listed in Table 11.2.

Throughout the night, one will cycle through the various stages of NREM and REM sleep in discrete periods referred to as sleep cycles. One sleep cycle accounts for 70–100 min of NREM sleep and 10–20 min of REM sleep for a total cycle length of 90–110 min. This cycle will start with N1 and end with REM sleep, and each cycle will be separated by either a brief arousal (which will then be followed by return to N1) or transition into light NREM sleep (stage N2). Over the

Table 11.2 Normal sleep cycle

Sleep stage	Characteristics
N1	– 4–16% total sleep time (TST) – Electroencephalogram (EEG)—theta waves present
N2	– 45–55% TST – EEG—theta waves, sleep spindles, K-complexes
N3	– 4–31% TST – Slow-wave sleep – EEG—delta waves present
REM	– 20–25% TST – EEG—beta waves present, low amplitude (may be mixed similar to wakefulness) – Eye movement with low skeletal muscle tone – Highest brain metabolism
Total sleep cycle	– 90–110 min per cycle (70–100-min NREM, 10–20-min REM) – Cycles separated by brief arousals or transition to N2 – 3–6 cycles per night (more NREM in first half, more REM in second half)

"*N*" Non-rapid eye movement (NREM) sleep, "*REM*" Rapid eye movement sleep

course of total sleep time, one will go through 3–6 sleep cycles, and with each successive cycle, the time spent in NREM sleep will decrease while time in REM sleep will increase. Overall, one will spend the most time in NREM sleep in the first half of the night, and in REM sleep in the second half of the night [21, 23].

Neurobiology of Sleep

The circadian rhythm is determined by the circadian clock located in the suprachiasmatic nucleus (SCN). This determines whether an individual will run on a 24-h clock or a less common variation. Within the SCN, the positive and negative feedback regulating the transcription of several genes (*Per, Cry, Clock,* and *Bmal1*) maintains this circadian rhythm; the timing is based on how long it takes for the transcription and translation of proteins from the *Per* and *Cry* genes to exert negative feedback on transcription until the level of protein production falls low enough again to encourage the process to start over—this process takes approximately 24 h [24–29]. Light is sensed by special receptors in the retina which sends the information to the SCN and then to the pineal gland which suppresses secretion of melatonin. When the light stimulus is no longer sensed, the suppression of melatonin is removed and melatonin is secreted once again. Melatonin synthesis increases as environmental light decreases with maximum secretion occurring at 2–4 AM [25, 26].

Sleep also requires communication and balance between two systems, an ascending arousal system and a sleep-promoting one [26]. The ascending arousal system comprises two groups of neurons that send projections to the hypothalamus and subsequently the cortex. The first group is cholinergic neurons in the pons-midbrain junction (active during wakefulness and REM sleep). The second group (also active during wakefulness) includes noradrenergic neurons of the locus coeruleus, serotonergic neurons of the raphe nucleus, dopaminergic neurons of the periaqueductal gray, and histaminergic neurons in the tuberomammillary nucleus. The sleep-promoting system involves the ventrolateral preoptic nucleus (VLPO) (active during REM sleep), which uses gamma-aminobutyric acid (GABA) and galanin to send inhibitory signals to the areas of the ascending arousal system [26]. This communication is reciprocal though, as the ascending arousal system also sends inhibitory projections to the VLPO [26–29]. There is also another system, the orexin system, that uses orexin-A and orexin-B to maintain wakefulness. These neuropeptides are produced in cells of the lateral hypothalamus, which then project to the regions of the ascending arousal system. During sleep, the VLPO turns off the orexin neurons [25–29].

Risk Factors for Insomnia Among Older Adults

As a normal part of aging, there are several sleep-related changes that are to be expected: N1 increases, SWS decreases (more common in men than women), REM latency as well as percentage of time spent in REM sleep decreases, and total

Table 11.3 Sleep changes in older adults

↑ Stage N1 increases
↓ Slow-wave sleep decreases (men > women)
↓ REM latency
↓ Total percentage in REM
↓ Total sleep time (decreases 30–60 min)
↑ Fragmented sleep (more brief arousals)
↑ Phase advancing (sleeping earlier, waking up earlier)

"*N*" Non-rapid eye movement (NREM) sleep, "*REM*" Rapid eye movement sleep

sleep time (TST) decreases by 30 min to 1 h by age 60 and then plateaus. Sleep also becomes more fragmentated with brief arousals [30–32]. Another expected change is referred to as a phase advance, resulting in sleep time occurring earlier in the evening and wake time occurring earlier in the morning [23]. Expected sleep changes in older adults are listed in Table 11.3.

Older adults with no health complaints may still find themselves dealing with poor sleep. Factors contributing to the issue, specific to this population, include the lack of a fixed schedule which affects consistent sleep and wake times and decreased regular exercise or exposure to natural light impacting the maintenance of the circadian rhythm. Another factor to consider is the resistance to the natural phase advance expected at this age. Older adults may try to stay up later due to the belief that it is too early to go to sleep, despite the earlier bedtime coinciding with their peak sleepiness [23, 33].

Other factors contributing to poor sleep and development of insomnia can be understood using the three-factor model by Spielman et al.—predisposing conditions, precipitating circumstances, and perpetuating factors. Predisposing conditions are present before the development of insomnia and lower the threshold for triggering a sleep disturbance [34]. Predisposing conditions include traits associated with perfectionism and neuroticism; female sex and age over 45; lower levels of educational attainment or lower income; being divorced, separated, or widowed; reduced physical activity; tobacco and alcohol use; and genetic variants in clock genes. A precipitating circumstance is the stressor that pushes someone from normal sleep into acute insomnia. This includes acute life stressors, presence of medical or psychiatric conditions, and medications [31–36].

The presence or number of acute life stressors alone does not predict the likelihood of an individual developing an acute sleep disorder. The major factor was how stressful the event was perceived by the individual [36]. A non-exhaustive list of medications that affect sleep includes glucocorticoids, decongestants, beta-blockers, cholinesterase inhibitors, selective serotonin reuptake inhibitors (SSRIs), and anti-androgen agents [33, 37]. Medical and psychiatric conditions that affect sleep include congestive heart failure, chronic obstructive pulmonary disease, asthma, chronic renal failure, anemia, arthritis, prostatic hypertrophy, gastroesophageal reflux disease, hyperthyroidism, diabetes, dementia, stroke, Parkinson's disease, depression, anxiety, schizophrenia, and mania along with substance use and/or withdrawal [23, 33, 37, 38].

The presence of predisposing and precipitating factors accounts for the development of acute insomnia, but the persistence of insomnia beyond this also requires perpetuating factors. These are behavioral or cognitive changes that can occur in response to acute insomnia and sustain the sleep disturbance resulting in the conversion to chronic insomnia [32, 34]. Examples of perpetuating factors include spending extended time in bed trying to force sleep, napping during the day, an irregular sleep-wake schedule, worrying about sleep leading to increased arousal around bedtime, and unhelpful beliefs about sleep and insomnia [32, 39, 40].

Assessment

Insomnia is a clinical diagnosis made by assessing a person's sleep history and their medical, psychiatric, and substance use history. For the sleep history, individuals should be asked about the onset, development, and current pattern of their specific sleep complaint. This includes time of sleep onset, total sleep time, number of awakenings throughout the night, wake time after each awakening, and waking time. Sleep during weekdays compared to weekends (or workdays compared to days off) along with pre-sleep conditions (sleep hygiene) and daytime consequences (effect on mood, behavior, work, interpersonal relationships) needs to be included. Other important questions to be asked include clarifying other sleep-related symptoms, past and present medication use, and past and present treatments for sleep complaint [32–34, 38, 41].

Standardized scales are utilized in the assessment process. In the AASM guidelines for evaluation and management of chronic insomnia, the Epworth Sleepiness Scale, a 2-week sleep log, as well as a sleep diary should be completed [41]. The sleep diary would encompass sleep prior to starting treatment, during active treatment to assess treatment response, and after a relapse [34, 41]. Two other scales that can be utilized to screen and monitor treatment response include the Insomnia Severity Index (ISI) and the Pittsburgh Sleep Quality Index (PSQI). The ISI is a seven-item scale that measures subjective symptoms and negative outcomes of insomnia over a 2-week period with questions incorporating both the International Classification of Diseases-10th Revision (ICD-10) and DSM-5 criteria. The PSQI is a 24-item questionnaire that assesses seven domains of sleep over a 1-month period. Questions include responses from self-report along with a room or bed partner. Both scales are commonly used and have shown good reliability [33, 42, 43].

A physical examination and mental status examination are also recommended to rule out associated medical or psychiatric conditions that could contribute to sleep difficulties. Polysomnography or multiple sleep latency testing are not indicated unless there is suspicion for sleep apnea or a movement disorder [38, 41]. The assessment process including history and exam is listed in Fig. 11.1.

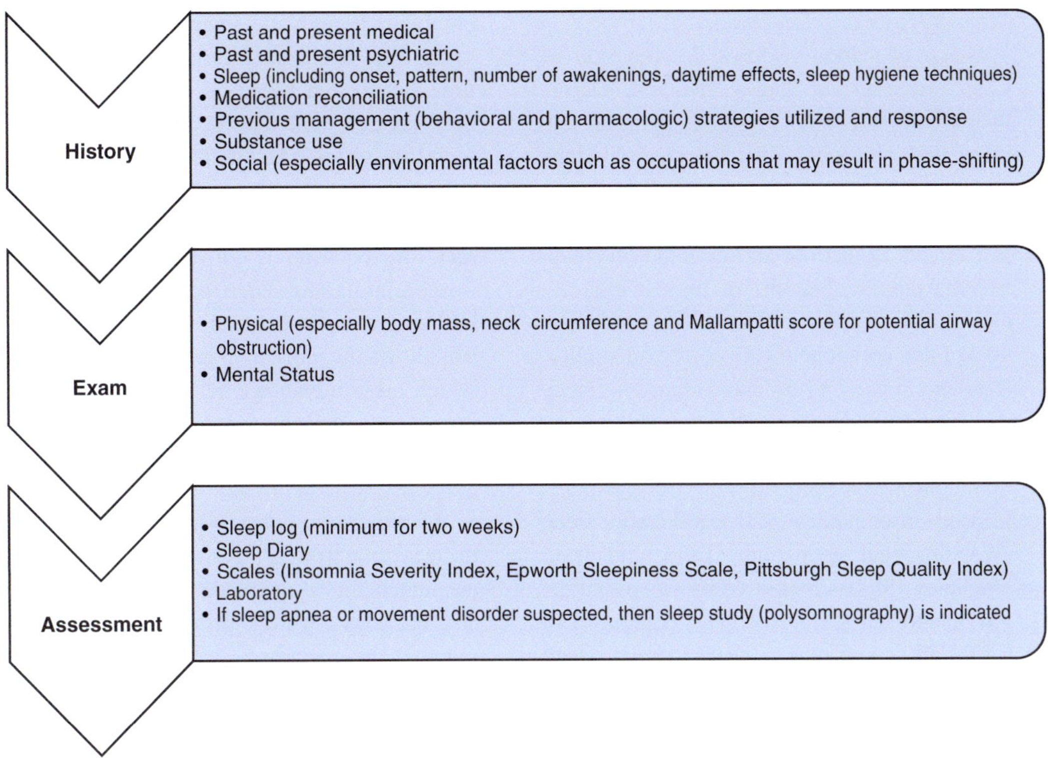

Fig. 11.1 Assessment of insomnia in older adults

Treatment

Non-pharmacological treatments are recommended as first line for adults with chronic insomnia [44, 45]. Pharmacological treatments may be considered on a short-term basis as an alternative or adjunctive treatment [45]. That said, some medication may be associated with harmful side effects in older adults and therefore require close monitoring.

Non-pharmacological

The first-line treatment for insomnia is cognitive behavioral therapy for insomnia (CBT-I). Both the AASM and the American College of Physicians (ACP) based this recommendation on its safety and efficacy profile. Studies have found that CBT-I administered alone or in conjunction with pharmacological treatment improves quality and quantity of sleep. Additionally, unlike pharmacotherapy, the results from CBT-I persist for up to at least 2 years after treatment has been completed [44–46]. A long-term study by Castronovo et al. found that the effects of CBT-I persisted for up to 10 years after treatment completion [47]. They also noted that participants who had utilized CBT techniques alone in response to a relapse reported lower scores on the ISI than those who had utilized hypnotic medications alone. CBT-I is provided by a therapist over 4–8 weekly sessions and encompasses sleep education, sleep hygiene, stimulus control, sleep restriction, cognitive therapy, and relaxation techniques to target the perpetuating factors of chronic insomnia [48].

1. *Sleep Hygiene and Education*

   Sleep education reviews the function of sleep, process and stages involved, factors that affect sleep, and natural changes that occur with aging [42, 49]. The sleep hygiene component reviews the optimal bedroom environment (dark, cool, and quiet), the negative effects of alcohol and caffeine on sleep, and the positive benefits of regular exercise and an appropriate diet on sleep [38]. The goal of this component is to correct misunderstandings a person may have regarding sleep and how to promote it. A meta-analysis by Chung et al. found that sleep hygiene education alone was associated with improvements in sleep-onset latency (SOL), wake after sleep (WASO), total sleep time (TST), and sleep efficiency (SE) as measured by sleep diaries, PSQI, and ISI [50]. However, compared to CBT-I and mindfulness-based therapy, sleep hygiene education alone was found to be less effective. Sleep hygiene and education are not recommended to treat chronic insomnia alone but are part of the introduction to the other components of CBT-I [42].

2. *Stimulus Control*

   The purpose of this component is to increase the ability of the bed and bedroom to serve as a cue for sleep. To strengthen this association, the bed and bedroom are reserved solely for sleep and sexual intercourse with all other activities being restricted to outside of the bedroom [39, 41]. Sleeping outside of the bedroom is also discouraged, as are daytime naps. The final instruction is for the individual to leave the bed if they cannot fall asleep within 15–20 min. They then should engage in a non-stimulating activity outside of the bedroom until they feel sleepy, at which time they may again try to go to sleep [39, 51].

3. *Sleep Restriction*

   The core goal of sleep restriction is to increase SE (the time spent sleeping compared to the time spent in bed). Using the data obtained through the sleep log, a consistent wake time is selected and the person's bedtime is adjusted based on the time at which they actually fall asleep. In the beginning, their time spent in bed will be reduced to coincide with the times in which they are likely to sleep. As the SE goal (usually set at ≥85%) is met, the bedtime is moved up by 15-min increments and the sleep window is increased. Utilizing sleep restriction with stimulus control allows the individual to build a sleep debt, which takes advantage of the body's natural homeostatic drive towards the sleep state [39, 51].

4. *Cognitive Restructuring*

   As previously noted, a large component of the transition from acute to chronic insomnia is accounted for by perpetuating factors, which also includes cognitive distortions (or inaccurate beliefs) regarding sleep. With cognitive restructuring, the therapist challenges these beliefs by testing their validity against evidence and the person's real-life experience. Once they can identify their cognitive distortions, they are taught alternative responses to replace their previous maladaptive ones [39, 51].

5. *Relaxation*

   This component of CBT-I utilizes techniques like guided imagery, progressive muscle relaxation, and deep breathing techniques to calm anxiety and help reach a more sleep-promoting state [38, 39].

Pharmacological

There are many medications utilized for sleep, with few that are Food and Drug Administration (FDA) approved for an indication of insomnia. In the community, many medications are used off-label, usually taking advantage of side effects that increase sedation. A list of medications including starting doses, maximum doses, and associated adverse effects is located at the end of the section in Table 11.4.

Table 11.4 Medications for insomnia in older adults

Medication class	Indication	Starting dose	Maximum dose	Adverse effects
Dual orexin receptor antagonists	FDA approved: Sleep onset Sleep maintenance	Suvorexant 10 mg Lemborexant 5 mg	Suvorexant 20 mg Lemborexant 10 mg	Fatigue, somnolence, dry mouth, complex sleep-related behavior, falls
Benzodiazepines	FDA approved: Short term (<1 week) Sleep onset Sleep maintenance	Temazepam 7.5 mg Triazolam 0.125 mg	Temazepam 30 mg Triazolam 0.25 mg	Opioid-related overdose, withdrawal, dizziness, falls, hallucinations, memory impairment, confusion
GABA receptor agonists	FDA approved: Short term (<1 week) Sleep onset Sleep maintenance	Zolpidem 5 mg Zaleplon 5 mg Eszopiclone 1 mg	Zolpidem 10 mg Zaleplon 10 mg Eszopiclone 3 mg	Dizziness, falls, hallucinations, memory impairment, confusion, gastrointestinal, headaches, parasomnias
Melatonin and melatonin receptor agonists	FDA approved: Sleep onset	Melatonin 1 mg Ramelteon 8 mg	Melatonin 3 mg Ramelteon 8 mg	Dizziness, nausea, headache
Tricyclic antidepressant	FDA approved: Sleep maintenance	Doxepin 3 mg	Doxepin 6 mg	Somnolence, dizziness (6 mg) Rebound insomnia (25–50 mg)
Atypical antidepressant	Off-label	Trazodone 25 mg	Trazodone 200 mg	Sedation, nausea, dizziness, weight gain, dry mouth, orthostasis, priapism (rare)
Anticonvulsant	Off-label	Tiagabine 4 mg	Tiagabine 8 mg	Dizziness, lethargy, nausea, gait dysfunction, confusion (8 mg)
Second-generation antipsychotics	Off-label	Olanzapine (O) 5 mg Quetiapine (Q) 25 mg	Olanzapine 10 mg Quetiapine 100 mg	Weight gain, metabolic syndrome, orthostasis, prolonged QTc, lowered seizure threshold, increased cerebrovascular accidents, periodic limb movements (Q), withdrawal (Q)
Tetracyclic antidepressant	Off-label	Mirtazapine 7.5 mg	Mirtazapine 30 mg	Sedation, dry mouth, dizziness, constipation, restless leg syndrome, periodic limb movements, neutropenia (rare)

FDA Food and Drug Administration, *GABA* Gamma-aminobutyric acid

Medications with the Food and Drug Administration (FDA) Approval for Insomnia

Dual Orexin Receptor Antagonists

Efficacy

Suvorexant is an orexin receptor antagonist with FDA approval for the treatment of sleep-onset and/or sleep-maintenance insomnia at doses of 10–20 milligrams (mg) [52]. In two 3-month randomized controlled clinical trials (RCTs), Herring et al. found that when compared to placebo, suvorexant was superior in improving sleep onset and increasing total sleep time. In older adults taking suvorexant 15 mg, subjective time to sleep onset was reduced by 5–7 min and subjective total sleep time was increased by

10–16 min [53]. At a dose of 30 mg, subjective time to sleep onset (sTSO) decreases by 8 min and subjective total sleep time (sTST) increases by 20 min, though this dosage does not have FDA approval.

Lemborexant is the second orexin receptor antagonist to be FDA approved for the treatment of sleep-onset and/or sleep-maintenance insomnia [54]. In an RCT by Murphy et al. investigating efficacy in adults 19–80 years of age, lemborexant improved SE by 0.3% (2.5 mg) to 8.9% (25 mg), decreased sSOL by 3.2 (1 mg) to 18.5 (10 mg) minutes, and decreased WASO by 21.5 min (25 mg) when compared to placebo [55]. In a phase 3 RCT in adults aged 55 and older, lemborexant was found to improve latency to the onset of persistent sleep (LPS) as well as SE and WASO when compared to placebo. Lemborexant 5 mg decreased LPS by 19.5 min, increased SE by 12.9%, and decreased WASO by 43.9 min in the first half of the night and by 27.2 in the second half of the night. Lemborexant 10 mg decreased LPS by 21.5 min, increased SE by 14.1%, and decreased WASO by 46.4 min in the first half of the night and by 28.8 min in the second half of the night. These results were collected on the last two nights of a 30-day period [56].

Adverse Effects

In a 1-year study assessing safety and efficacy, Michelson et al. found that 69% of participants experienced adverse events when taking suvorexant 30 mg when compared to 64% in the placebo control group [57]. The most commonly reported side effects were somnolence, fatigue, and dry mouth. Reports of somnolence were most common in the first 3 months of the study and decreased by month 6. Out of the 521 study participants in the suvorexant group, one reported a complex sleep-related behavior (specifically somnambulism), three reported hypnagogic hallucinations, and one reported hypnopompic hallucinations. In this study, 2.3% of the treatment group reported a fall when compared to 3.1% in the placebo group. In the 3-month study following individuals taking suvorexant 15/20 mg, there were no reports of complex sleep-related behav-

iors or hypnopompic hallucinations, and the rate of reports of somnolence and dry mouth was comparable to the placebo control group [53]. The most common adverse effect of lemborexant is somnolence, which is dose dependent increasing to a reported rate of 22% at 25 mg [55]. In subjects taking 15 mg, there were reports of potential cataplexy. There are also reports of sleep paralysis with lemborexant 5 and 10 mg.

Withdrawal

When compared to placebo, those taking suvorexant did not demonstrate any symptoms concerning withdrawal as assessed by the Tyrer Withdrawal Symptom Questionnaire [57]. When compared to placebo, those taking lemborexant 5–10 mg reported less withdrawal symptoms as assessed by the Tyrer Benzodiazepine Withdrawal Symptom Questionnaire [56].

Benzodiazepines and Gamma-Aminobutyric Acid (GABA) Receptor Agonists

Efficacy

Benzodiazepines and GABA receptor agonists that are FDA approved for insomnia include triazolam, estazolam, temazepam, flurazepam, quazepam, eszopiclone, zaleplon, and zolpidem [58]. A network meta-analysis by Wang et al. found that with short-term treatment (i.e., <1 week), benzodiazepines had a significant effect on improving sleep latency, total sleep time, sleep efficiency, and wake time after sleep onset [59]. Benzodiazepine receptor agonists had a similar effect on all sleep parameters, though in contrast to benzodiazepines, they showed improvement in both the short-term and long-term treatment groups. A meta-analysis by Rosner et al. found that eszopiclone (doses 1–3 mg) decreased SOL by 12 min, reduced WASO by 17 min, and increased TST by 28 min compared to placebo. In adults aged 64 and older, eszopiclone was found to reduce SOL by 11.41 min, decrease WASO by 22.16 min, and increase TST by 27.01 min when compared to placebo [60].

Adverse Effects

In a systematic review analyzing the efficacy and safety of eszopiclone, zaleplon, and zolpidem, Scharner et al. noted multiple adverse events reported including dizziness, falls, memory impairment, hallucinations, and confusion [61]. Particularly, studies on zolpidem use demonstrated a significant relationship between its use and an increased risk of hip fracture.

A study by Hernandez et al. found that benzodiazepine use increased the risk of opioid-related overdose five times in the first 90 days of concurrent use [62]. Boon et al. noted that the combined use of opioids and benzodiazepines increases the risk of death or serious harm in a dose-dependent manner [63]. Participants receiving methadone as an opioid replacement therapy were at a higher risk for severe adverse respiratory events with concomitant benzodiazepine use compared to individuals with concurrent buprenorphine and benzodiazepine use. In a meta-analysis by Lucchetta et al., an association between the use of benzodiazepines and development of dementia was suggested [64]. There was insufficient data to determine any differences in the effect of short-acting and long-acting benzodiazepines or the role of dose and/or duration of treatment.

Withdrawal

In participants taking benzodiazepines for longer than a 1-month period, approximately 50% will develop a physical dependence, with a greater risk in those taking benzodiazepines with a shorter half-life [65]. Timing of withdrawal symptoms is also dependent on the half-life of the particular agent, occurring 2–3 days after cessation in short-acting formulations and within 5–10 days in longer acting formulations. Withdrawal symptoms vary from symptom rebound (i.e., anxiety and/or insomnia), weakness, flu-like symptoms, hypertension, and tachycardia to hallucinations, delirium, and seizures. To prevent seizures and avoid severe withdrawal symptoms, individuals should be slowly tapered off benzodiazepines over the course of 4–8 weeks [65].

Melatonin Receptor Agonists

Ramelteon is a melatonin receptor agonist working on the MT1 and MT2 receptors. It is FDA approved for the treatment of sleep-onset insomnia at a dose of 8 mg [66]. A meta-analysis by Kuriyama et al. noted that ramelteon demonstrated statistically significant improvement in sSL (−4.6 min), sleep quality, LPS (−9.36 min), TST (+7.26 min), and SE (+4.3%) although the clinical effect is minimal. Compared to placebo, individuals taking ramelteon reported increased somnolence [relative risk (RR) = 1.97, CI 1.21–3.20] [67]. There are no reports of rebound insomnia or withdrawal symptoms following treatment discontinuation [66, 68].

Tasimelteon is a melatonin MT1/MT2 receptor agonist that currently only has FDA approval for the treatment of non-24-h sleep-wake disorder [69]. There is currently a lack of evidence for its role in managing primary insomnia [70].

Doxepin

Efficacy

Doxepin is a tricyclic antidepressant with FDA approval for sleep-maintenance insomnia at doses of 3–6 mg [71]. In a systematic review by Yeung et al., older adults assigned to take doxepin 3 mg showed statistically significant improvement in TST, SE, and ISI score on nights 1, 29, and 85 [72]. Compared to placebo, there were no significant differences in the incidence of adverse effects at 1 mg/3 mg. At 6 mg, there was an increase in reports of somnolence and dizziness. There were no reports of withdrawal effects at doses of 1–6 mg of doxepin. Incidence of rebound insomnia was greater than placebo in participants taking doxepin 25–50 mg.

Medications Used Off-Label for Insomnia

Trazodone

Trazodone is a serotonin antagonist and reuptake inhibitor with FDA approval for the treatment of major depression. However, it is widely prescribed off-label as a sleep aid [73]. In a meta-analysis of seven RCTs, Yi et al. found that trazodone was not more effective than placebo for improvement in SE, SL, TST, or WASO. It was found to significantly reduce the number of awakenings compared to placebo though [74]. Additionally, individuals evaluated with the PSQI reported improvements in perceived sleep quality when compared to placebo. Still, the two studies utilizing the PSQI were investigating insomnia secondary to unipolar/bipolar depression and opioid dependence. One RCT by Camargos et al. found that trazodone 50 mg administered to participants aged 60 or older with probable Alzheimer's disease (AD) (baseline MMSE score 11) increased TST by 42.5 min and SE by 8.5% when compared to placebo [75].

Tiagabine

Tiagabine is a selective GABA reuptake inhibitor that was approved for the treatment of focal (partial) seizures [76]. A study by Mathias et al. found that tiagabine 5 mg administered to ten older adults resulted in increased sleep efficiency by 2.6–5.6% and SWS by 16.6–43.6 min. There were no significant changes in SOL, TST, or number of awakenings (NA) [77].

In an RCT of 24 healthy adults aged 62 and older, tiagabine 4 mg was noted to increase TST by 11.7 min and SWS by 15.2 min and decrease WASO by 12.3 min compared to placebo. There was no significant effect on SOL. Tiagabine 8 mg was also noted to increase SWS by 42.5 min and decrease SWS latency by 17.9 min, but this dose was also associated with significantly increased reports of adverse events (lethargy, dizziness, and unsteady gait).

An RCT by Walsh et al. investigating the effect of tiagabine in 232 adults (mean age 44.3) found that tiagabine between 4 and 10 mg had no significant effects on SE, NA, TST, LPS, or WASO [78]. Tiagabine 6 mg was associated with a 7.1-min decrease in N1 and a 31.7-min increase in SWS; tiagabine 8 mg was associated with a 7.3-min decrease in N1, a 39.6-min increase in SWS, and a 2.1-min decrease in REM sleep; tiagabine 10 mg was associated with a 15.5-min reduction in N1, a 52.9-min increase in SWS, and a 9.9-min decrease in REM sleep. Tiagabine 4 mg and 6 mg were tolerated similar to placebo, while doses of 8 mg and 10 mg were associated with increased adverse events—dizziness and nausea.

An RCT by Roth et al. found that in older adults with primary insomnia, tiagabine 2 mg was equivalent to placebo with no significant improvements in any sleep parameter [76]. Tiagabine 4 mg did not affect TST, WASO, SE, NA, or LPS; this dose was associated with an 11-min decrease in N1 sleep and a 20-min increase in SWS. Tiagabine 6 mg and 8 mg were found to be associated with a decrease in the number of 30-s awakenings by 2 and 1, respectively; they were also associated with decreased time in N1 (10.6 min and 17.5 min, respectively), increased time in SWS (38 min, 46.9 min), and decreased time in REM sleep (6.1 min, 13.9 min). These doses did not affect WASO, LPS, TST, or SE. Tolerability of tiagabine 2–6 mg was equal to placebo. Tiagabine 8 mg was associated with increased adverse events (confusion, nausea, and dizziness).

Second-Generation Antipsychotics

Efficacy

Olanzapine is an atypical antipsychotic with FDA approval for the treatment of schizophrenia, bipolar disorder, and agitation associated with schizophrenia/bipolar disorder [79]. In 2000, Sharpley et al. found that a dose of olanzapine 5 mg or 10 mg at bedtime in healthy adults increased TST (by 25 min) and SE (by 5%) and decreased wake time (by 13 min/3%) in comparison to placebo [80]. In 2002, Staner et al. investigated the effects of olanzapine 10 mg on sleep in healthy adults over 8 days and found that it decreased SOL and increased SE [81]. More recent studies have only investigated the effects of olanzapine on sleep in individuals with schizophrenia and/or bipolar disorder.

Quetiapine is another atypical antipsychotic with FDA approval for the treatment of schizophrenia, bipolar disorder with manic features, and depressive features and also as maintenance adjunctive treatment of bipolar disorder [82]. In 2004, Cohrs et al. investigated the effects of quetiapine 25 mg and 100 mg on sleep compared to placebo in healthy subjects [83]. Administration of quetiapine 25 mg/100 mg increased SE by 6/6.2% and increased TST by 28 min/30 min compared with placebo. In participants taking quetiapine 100 mg, a significant increase in periodic limb movements was observed. In 2016, Rock et al. studied the effect of quetiapine XL 150 mg on healthy volunteers over a period of 7 days [84]. Subjects taking quetiapine XL 150 mg had increased TST by 60 min compared to placebo. In 2017, Karsten et al. investigated the efficacy of quetiapine 50 mg for transient insomnia over a period of 3 days and found an increase in TST (average of 21 min) and decrease in SL, WASO, and NA [85].

Adverse Effects

Adverse effects for second-generation antipsychotics commonly include weight gain and development of metabolic syndrome, orthostatic hypotension, lowering of seizure threshold, QTc prolongation, and increased cerebrovascular events [86]. In a meta-analysis by Rognoni et al. evaluating metabolic and cardiovascular side effects of second-generation antipsychotics, olanzapine was associated with the greatest weight gain (excluding clozapine) and greatest increase in cholesterol and fasting glucose [86]. Quetiapine was noted to be associated with the greatest increase in both systolic and diastolic blood pressure. Cates et al. investigated the metabolic effects of low-dose quetiapine (<200 mg at bedtime) and found an increase in weight by an average of 4.9 pounds and an increase in BMI by 0.8 points. Two-thirds of participants gained weight with 60% gaining 1–10 lbs, 17% gaining 11–20 lbs, and 25% gaining greater than 20 pounds [87].

Withdrawal

A systematic review by Monahan et al. found reports of fatigue, headache, nausea/vomiting, palpitations, tachycardia, dizziness, lightheadedness, hypertension, orthostatic hypertension, involuntary movements, dysphoria, anxiety, and irritability following abrupt cessation of quetiapine use [88]. They found no correlation between the dosage (ranging from 25 mg to 1800 mg) and the severity of symptoms reported. If upon cessation or dose reduction, withdrawal is suspected, it is recommended to reinstate the previous dose and gradually taper the medication.

Mirtazapine

In an RCT by Karsten et al., the authors found that mirtazapine 7.5 mg was associated with increased TST and decreased number of awakenings compared to placebo when used for transient insomnia over a period of 3 days [85]. In a study comparing mirtazapine 30 mg with placebo in a group of healthy volunteers, Aslan et al. found an increase in SE and decreased number of awakenings and their durations [89]. Mirtazapine has been associated with dizziness, somnolence, dry mouth, constipation, and rarely neutropenia (which resolved on treatment discontinuation) [90]. In a few individuals, there is an increased risk for restless leg syndrome and/or periodic limb movements [91].

Diphenhydramine

In a 14-day RCT, Glass et al. found that diphenhydramine 50 mg administered to study participants aged 70–89 years reduced the number of awakenings compared to placebo [92]. There were no significant differences in SOL, TST, or sleep quality when compared to placebo. Due to lack of safety and efficacy data, the AASM Guidelines for treatment of insomnia do not recommend the use of diphenhydramine [45]. With first-generation antihistamines, in which diphenhydramine is included, tolerance to sedation begins to develop by days 3–4 of continuous use. Antagonism of the muscarinic receptors can cause constipation, urinary retention, confusion, and dry eyes/mouth [93]. The AGS Beers Criteria recommend avoiding the use of first-generation antihistamines in older adults because of these potential side effects [94].

Melatonin

A meta-analysis by Ferracioli-Oda et al. found that exogenous melatonin reduced SL by 7 min and increased TST by 8 min when compared to placebo with higher doses being associated with greater effect [95]. Melatonin is generally regarded as safe and well tolerated with most side effects spontaneously resolving within a few days or upon termination of treatment [96]. The most commonly reported side effects are headache, dizziness, and daytime sleepiness (associated with the prolonged-release formulations). Less common side effects include nightmares, agitation, and palpitations. The more severe side effects were noted to be associated with doses much higher than what is commonly prescribed and may have been confounded in individuals taking other medications.

Evidence-Based Treatment Algorithm for Treating Insomnia

The ACP and the AASM have released guidelines addressing evaluation and treatment of chronic insomnia in adults [44, 45]. There is currently no expert guideline for the treatment of insomnia in older adults specifically. So, one would need to utilize the recommendations of the ACP and AASM in the context of the guidelines from the American Geriatrics Society (AGS) Beers Criteria for potentially inappropriate medication use. Please refer to Fig. 11.2 for the management of insomnia.

In a network meta-analysis (NMA) by Chiu et al., the safety and efficacy of eszopiclone, doxepin, zaleplon, temazepam, suvorexant, ramelteon, and zolpidem were compared against each other and against placebo [97]. The authors found that zaleplon, ramelteon, doxepin, and suvorexant were significantly superior to placebo in improving objective sleep-onset latency (as determined by PSG). Of this, ramelteon was superior to suvorexant and eszopiclone, while zaleplon was superior to doxepin, suvorexant, and eszopiclone. For WASO, only zolpidem ER and suvorexant were significantly superior to placebo. For SE, doxepin, eszopiclone, suvorexant, zolpidem ER, and temazepam were superior to placebo, with doxepin and eszopiclone being superior to ramelteon. For TST, eszopiclone, suvorexant, and doxepin were significantly superior to placebo. Regarding safety, triazolam was associated with significantly increased adverse events compared to zaleplon. The authors concluded that in light of both safety and efficacy, low-dose doxepin was optimal for increasing sleep duration and efficiency in older adults with insomnia.

According to an NMA from Samara et al., the authors found that food supplement (containing melatonin 5 mg, magnesium, and zinc), diazepam, promethazine, propiomazine, temazepam, doxepin, and eszopiclone were superior to placebo in improving TST [98]. For SOL, diazepam, propiomazine, promethazine, doxepin, eszopiclone, temazepam, chlormethiazole, ramelteon, and suvorexant were better than placebo. For sleep quality, food supplement, propiomazine, melatonin, temazepam, eszopiclone, and doxepin were better than placebo. Zolpidem, temazepam, propiomazine, and diphenhydramine were better than placebo in reducing the number of awakenings. Suvorexant, melatonin, esmirtazapine (not FDA approved in the USA), doxepin, zolpidem, and eszopiclone reduced WASO.

Crescenzo et al. also analyzed data as an NMA, and the authors found that for acute treatment of insomnia, benzodiazepines, doxylamine,

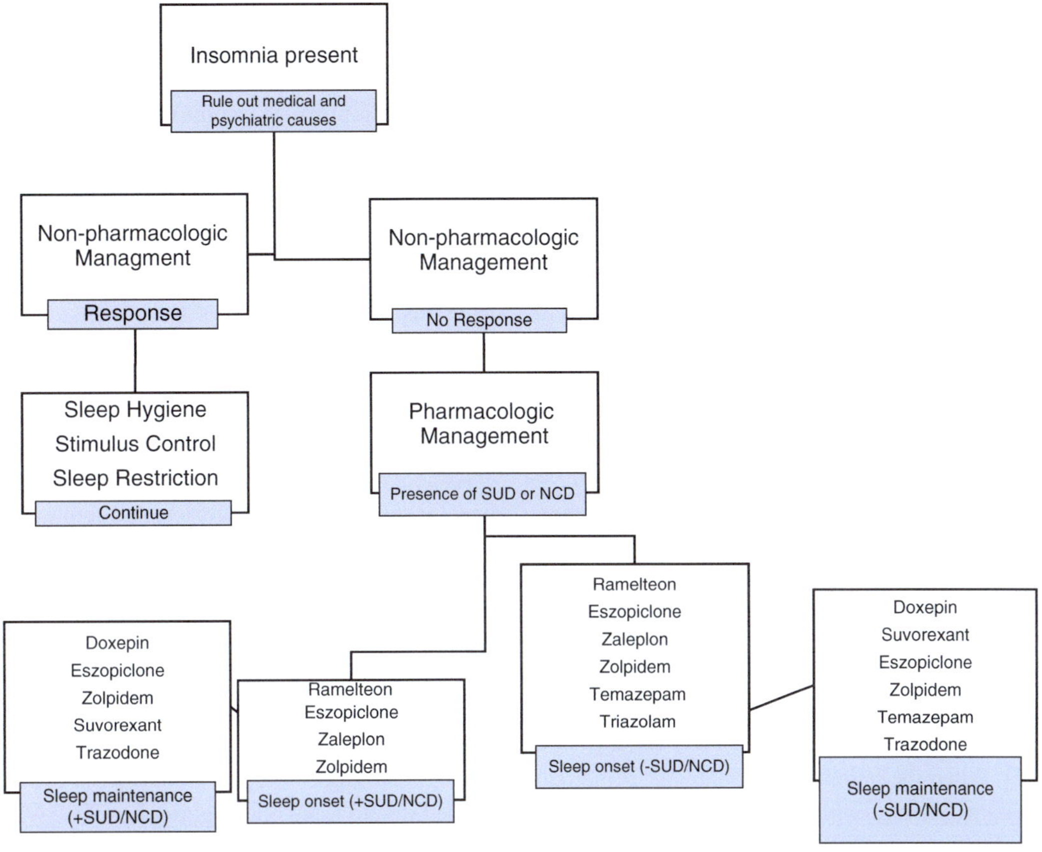

Fig. 11.2 Management flow diagram *SUD* substance use disorder, *NCD* neurocognitive disorder; "+/−" present/not present

eszopiclone, lemborexant, zolpidem, and zolpidem were superior to placebo [99]. For long-term treatment of insomnia, eszopiclone and lemborexant were superior to placebo. After 4 weeks of treatment, short-acting benzodiazepines were superior to daridorexant, lemborexant, and zaleplon; eszopiclone and zolpidem were superior to zaleplon. Suvorexant was found to be better tolerated than lemborexant. The authors concluded that lemborexant and eszopiclone had the best profiles in terms of efficacy, acceptability, and tolerability, with the caveat that eszopiclone caused substantial adverse events and lemborexant safety data was inconclusive. They also concluded that benzodiazepines were effective in acute treatment, with a preference for those with intermediate half-lives like temazepam and lormetazepam; it was also noted that their tolerability and safety profiles are not favorable and that there is a lack of data with regard to long-term use.

In a quantitative comparison by Zheng et al., the authors found that eszopiclone reduced SL by 16 min, increased TST by 34 min, and reduced WASO by 17 min compared to placebo; doxepin reduced SL by 5 min, increased TST by 25 min, and reduced WASO by 20 min compared to placebo; suvorexant reduced SL by 10 min, increased

TST by 20 min, and reduced WASO by 27 min compared to placebo; ramelteon reduced SL by 10 min and increased TST by 9 min compared to placebo [100]. The difference in performance among temazepam, zolpidem, zaleplon, triazolam, zolpidem extended release, and eszopiclone in the reduction of WASO was not clinically significant. The results also showed that doxepin performed on par with zolpidem, zolpidem ER, temazepam, quazepam, and triazolam in terms of the effect on TST and WASO.

As the evaluation of insomnia begins with a consideration of comorbid diagnoses and medications that affect sleep, the treatment should also begin with consideration to optimizing these factors. There is growing evidence that non-pharmacological treatments are not only effective for the treatment of chronic insomnia, but the improvements may also be maintained for up to 10 years after the end of the treatment. As recommended by the AASM and the ACP, initial treatment of insomnia should utilize psychological and behavioral interventions (i.e., CBT-I) [44, 45]. When the initial CBT-I treatment is ineffective, or when an individual is determined to be unable to engage in CBT-I program, the addition of medications can be considered. The choice of which specific medication to start with should be guided by the pattern of insomnia – difficulty with sleep onset vs. reduced total sleep time vs. multiple awakenings – the cost and availability of the medication, presence of comorbid conditions, risk of medication interaction, and side effect profile of each agent [44, 45]. Some medications become higher risk in people with renal or hepatic impairment and in those with compromised respiratory function (COPD) or cardiovascular function (bradycardia and/or hypotension).

While the AASM guidelines (last updated in 2017) currently do not recommend the use of melatonin as the treatment for insomnia due to the lack of data supporting efficacy at the time of writing, melatonin has shown some small benefit for treatment of insomnia in certain populations (those with probable AD and/or Parkinson's) and has a rather benign side effect profile [96]. In contrast to that, the AASM does recommend the use of ramelteon (a melatonin receptor agonist)

for initial treatment of sleep-onset insomnia. While tasimelteon has a similar mechanism of action to ramelteon, it is currently not FDA approved for primary insomnia and is lacking studies showing efficacy for this population.

Doxepin, while being a TCA and therefore having activity at histamine and muscarinic receptors, has shown some efficacy in treating primary insomnia. The AASM does recommend using this for the treatment of sleep-maintenance insomnia [45]. The AGS recommendation is to avoid doses higher than 6 mg (antidepressant doses), which is within its role for treatment of insomnia while minimizing side effects (which were more prevalent at higher doses) [94]. Orexin receptor antagonists (suvorexant and lemborexant) have shown efficacy in the treatment of primary insomnia. The AASM recommends using this for the treatment of sleep-maintenance insomnia. One consideration is that these medications are newer agents that have only recently obtained FDA approval. Long-term side effects are still being investigated.

Benzodiazepine receptor agonists should be avoided due to risks outweighing benefits (AGS supports this in updated criteria) [94]. The research has demonstrated that this class of medication has some benefit in the treatment of acute insomnia (short, limited treatment course) but that due to tolerance will have decreased/little effect beyond 1 month.

Second-generation antipsychotics (olanzapine and quetiapine) should not be prescribed for the treatment of primary insomnia – the risks outweigh the benefits in cases without psychosis and/or affective episodes. Quetiapine also carries a risk for orthostatic hypotension, and therefore usage in older adults may increase the risk for falls.

Mirtazapine is not recommended for the treatment of primary insomnia. Current evidence does not show benefit outside of insomnia as part of the symptom profile of depression. Trazodone is not recommended for the treatment of primary insomnia. Current evidence does not show benefit outside of insomnia secondary to depression. Due to higher cholinergic activity at the doses recommended to treat insomnia, the AGS also recommends avoiding this medication in older adults. Diphenhydramine is not recommended for the treatment of sleep-onset or sleep-maintenance insomnia by the AASM guidelines. The AGS also recommends avoiding this medication class in older adults due to the risks associated with high anticholinergic activity.

Conclusion

Insomnia is a sleep disorder that is clinically diagnosed and affects various aspects of the sleep cycle. The disruption of the sleep cycle can be affected by many factors, including biological, psychological, and/or social factors. Thus, to diagnose a sleep disorder, the assessment will need to consider a multitude of influences. Non-pharmacologic interventions such as CBT-I are always preferred as first-line management especially in older adults given the evidence for its efficacy and lack of adverse effects. Pharmacologic interventions range from FDA-approved to off-label medications. Caution should be taken especially with medications that have antihistaminic, anticholinergic, or GABAergic side effects as these can lead to negative side effects in older adults. Although there are no specific guidelines for the use of hypnotic agents among older adults, it is important to refer to multiple guidelines and use the best clinical judgment for each individual case. Determining the reasons for insomnia and the medication side effect profile are the most important considerations when choosing a hypnotic agent.

References

1. Morin CM, Jarrin DC, Ivers H, Mérette C, LeBlanc M, Savard J. Incidence, persistence, and remission rates of insomnia over 5 years. JAMA Netw Open. 2020;3(11):e2018782. https://doi.org/10.1001/jamanetworkopen.2020.18782.
2. American Psychiatric Association. Diagnostic and statistical manual of mental disorders. 5th ed. Arlington, VA: American Psychiatric Publishing; 2013.
3. Barbar SI, Enright PL, Boyle P, et al. Sleep disturbances and their correlates in elderly Japanese American men residing in Hawaii. J Gerontol A Biol Sci Med Sci. 2000;55(7):M406–11. https://doi.org/10.1093/harac/55.7.m406.
4. Dzierzewski JM, Dautovich N, Ravyts S. Sleep and cognition in older adults. Sleep Med Clin. 2018;13(1):93–106. https://doi.org/10.1016/j.jsmc.2017.09.009.
5. Yaffe K, Falvey CM, Hoang T. Connections between sleep and cognition in older adults. Lancet Neurol. 2014;13(10):1017–28. https://doi.org/10.1016/S1474-4422(14)70172-3.
6. Brassington GS, King AC, Bliwise DL. Sleep problems as a risk factor for falls in a sample of community-dwelling adults aged 64–99 years. J Am Geriatr Soc. 2000;48(10):1234–40. https://doi.org/10.1111/j.1532-5415.2000.tb02596.x.
7. Cole MG, Dendukuri N. Risk factors for depression among elderly community subjects: a systematic review and meta-analysis. Am J Psychiatry. 2003;160(6):1147–56. https://doi.org/10.1176/appi.ajp.160.6.1147.
8. Jaussent I, Bouyer J, Ancelin ML, et al. Insomnia and daytime sleepiness are risk factors for depressive symptoms in the elderly. Sleep. 2011;34(8):1103–10. https://doi.org/10.5665/SLEEP.1170.
9. Perlis ML, Smith LJ, Lyness JM, et al. Insomnia as a risk factor for onset of depression in the elderly. Behav Sleep Med. 2006;4(2):104–13. https://doi.org/10.1207/s15402010bsm0402_3.
10. Pigeon WR, Hegel M, Unützer J, et al. Is insomnia a perpetuating factor for late-life depression in the IMPACT cohort. Sleep. 2008;31(4):481–8. https://doi.org/10.1093/sleep/31.4.481.
11. Javaheri S, Redline S. Insomnia and risk of cardiovascular disease. Chest. 2017;152(2):435–44. https://doi.org/10.1016/j.chest.2017.01.026.
12. Johnson KA, Gordon CJ, Chapman JL, et al. The association of insomnia disorder characterized by objective short sleep duration with hypertension, diabetes and body mass index: a systematic review and meta-analysis. Sleep Med Rev 2021; 59:101456. doi: https://doi.org/10.1016/j.smrv.2021.101456
13. Khan MS, Aouad R. The effects of insomnia and sleep loss on cardiovascular disease. Sleep Med Clin. 2017;12(2):167–77. https://doi.org/10.1016/j.jsmc.2017.01.005.
14. Hepburn M, Bollu PC, French B, Sahota P. Sleep medicine: stroke and sleep. Mo Med. 2018;115(6):527–32.
15. McDermott M, Brown DL, Chervin RD. Sleep disorders and the risk of stroke. Expert Rev Neurother. 2018;18(7):523–31. https://doi.org/10.1080/14737175.2018.1489239.
16. Ogilvie RP, Patel SR. The epidemiology of sleep and diabetes. Curr Diab Rep. 2018;18(10):82. https://doi.org/10.1007/s11892-018-1055-8.
17. Palagini L, Bruno RM, Gemignani A, Baglioni C, Ghiadoni L, Riemann D. Sleep loss and hypertension: a systematic review. Curr Pharm Des.

2013;19(13):2409–19. https://doi.org/10.2174/1381 612811319130009.

18. Dew MA, Hoch CC, Buysse DJ, et al. Healthy older adults' sleep predicts all-cause mortality at 4 to 19 years of follow-up [published correction appears in Psychosom Med. 2003;65(2):210]. Psychosom Med. 2003;65(1):63–73. https://doi.org/10.1097/01. psy.0000039756.23250.7c.

19. American Academy of Sleep Medicine. AASM Sleep Prioritization Survey. 2022. https://aasm.org/ wp-content/uploads/2022/09/sleep-prioritization-survey-losing-sleep-to-finance-worries.pdf (accessed Nov 29, 2022).

20. Crowley K. Sleep and sleep disorders in older adults. Neuropsychol Rev. 2011;21(1):41–53. https://doi. org/10.1007/s11065-010-9154-6.

21. Stores G. Basic aspects of sleep-wake disorders. In: Gelder MG, Andreasen NC, Lopez-Ibor J, Geddes J, editors. New Oxford textbook of psychiatry. 2nd ed. Oxford University Press; 2009. p. 925–6.

22. Moser D, Anderer P, Gruber G, Parapatics S, Loretz E, Boeck M, Kloesch G, Heller E, Schmidt A, Danker-Hopfe H, Saletu B, Zeitlhofer J, Dorffner G. Sleep classification according to AASM and Rechtschaffen & Kales: effects on sleep scoring parameters. Sleep. 2009;32(2):139–49. https://doi. org/10.1093/sleep/32.2.139.

23. Feinsilver SH. Normal and abnormal sleep in the elderly. Clin Geriatr Med. 2021;37(3):377–86. https://doi.org/10.1016/j.cger.2021.04.001.

24. Hastings MH, Maywood ES, Brancaccio M. Generation of circadian rhythms in the suprachiasmatic nucleus. Nat Rev Neurosci. 2018;19(8):453–69. https://doi.org/10.1038/s41583-018-0026-z.

25. Higgins ES, George MS. Chapter 15: Sleep. In: The neuroscience of clinical psychiatry: the pathophysiology of behavior and mental illness. Philadelphia: Wolters Kluwer; 2019. p. 191–200.

26. Pace-Schott EF, Hobson JA. The neurobiology of sleep: genetics, cellular physiology and subcortical networks. Nat Rev Neurosci. 2002;3(8):591–605. https://doi.org/10.1038/nrn895.

27. España RA, Scammell TE. Sleep neurobiology from a clinical perspective. Sleep. 2011;34(7):845–58. https://doi.org/10.5665/SLEEP.1112.

28. Saper CB, Scammell TE, Lu J. Hypothalamic regulation of sleep and circadian rhythms. Nature. 2005;437(7063):1257–63. https://doi.org/10.1038/ nature04284.

29. Scammell TE. Overview of sleep: the neurologic processes of the sleep-wake cycle. J Clin Psychiatry. 2015;76(5):e13. https://doi.org/10.4088/ JCP.14046tx1c.

30. Ohayon MM, Carskadon MA, Guilleminault C, et al. Meta-analysis of quantitative sleep parameters from childhood to old age in healthy individuals: developing normative sleep values across the human lifespan. Sleep. 2004;27(7):1255–73.

31. Redline S, Kirchner HL, Quan SF, et al. The effects of age, ethnicity, and sleep disordered breathing on sleep architecture. Arch Int Med. 2004;164:406–18.

32. Gooneratne NS, Vitiello MV. Sleep in older adults: normative changes, sleep disorders, and treatment options. Clin Geriatr Med. 2014;30(3):591–627. https://doi.org/10.1016/j.cger.2014.04.007.

33. Patel D, Steinberg J, Patel P. Insomnia in the elderly: a review. J Clin Sleep Med. 2018;14(6):1017–24.

34. Spielman AJ. Assessment of insomnia. Clin Psychol Rev. 1986;6(1):11–25.

35. van de Laar M, Verbeek I, Pevernagie D, Aldenkamp A, Overeem S. The role of personality traits in insomnia. Sleep Med Rev. 2010;14(1):61–8. https:// doi.org/10.1016/j.smrv.2009.07.007.

36. Ellis JG, Perlis ML, Espie CA, et al. The natural history of insomnia: predisposing, precipitating, coping, and perpetuating factors over the early developmental course of insomnia. Sleep. 2021;44(9):zsab095. https://doi.org/10.1093/sleep/zsab095.

37. Lou BX, Oks M. Insomnia: pharmacologic treatment. Clin Geriatr Med. 2021;37(3):401–15. https:// doi.org/10.1016/j.cger.2021.04.003.

38. Winkelman JW. Clinical practice. Insomnia disorder. N Engl J Med. 2015;373(15):1437–44. https://doi. org/10.1056/NEJMcp1412740.

39. Spielman AJ, Caruso LS, Glovinsky PB. A behavioral perspective on insomnia treatment. Psychiatr Clin North Am. 1987;10(4):541–53.

40. Sidani S, Ibrahim S, Lok J, O'Rourke H, Collins L, Fox M. Comparing the experience of and factors perpetuating chronic insomnia severity among young, middle-aged, and older adults. Clin Nurs Res. 2021;30(1):12–22. https://doi. org/10.1177/1054773818806164.

41. Schutte-Rodin S, Broch L, Buysse D, Dorsey C, Sateia M. Clinical guideline for the evaluation and management of chronic insomnia in adults. J Clin Sleep Med. 2008;4(5):487–504.

42. Edinger JD, Arnedt JT, Bertisch SM, et al. Behavioral and psychological treatments for chronic insomnia disorder in adults: an American Academy of Sleep Medicine systematic review, meta-analysis, and GRADE assessment. J Clin Sleep Med. 2021;17(2):263–98. https://doi.org/10.5664/ jcsm.8988.

43. Fabbri M, Beracci A, Martoni M, Meneo D, Tonetti L, Natale V. Measuring subjective sleep quality: a review. Int J Environ Res Public Health. 2021;18(3):1082. https://doi.org/10.3390/ ijerph18031082.

44. Qaseem A, Kansagara D, Forciea MA, Cooke M, Denberg TD. Management of chronic insomnia disorder in adults: a clinical practice guideline from the American College of Physicians. Ann Intern Med. 2016;165:125–33.

45. Sateia MJ, Buysse DJ, Krystal AD, Neubauer DN, Heald JL. Clinical practice guideline for the pharma-

cologic treatment of chronic insomnia in adults: an American Academy of Sleep Medicine clinical practice guideline. J Clin Sleep Med. 2017;13:307–49.

46. Beaulieu-Bonneau S, Ivers H, Guay B, Morin CM. Long-term maintenance of therapeutic gains associated with cognitive-behavioral therapy for insomnia delivered alone or combined with Zolpidem. Sleep. 2017;40(3):zsx002.

47. Castronovo V, Galbiati A, Sforza M, et al. Long-term clinical effect of group cognitive behavioral therapy for insomnia: a case series study. Sleep Med. 2018;47:54–9.

48. Chan NY, Chan JWY, Li SX, Wing YK. Non-pharmacological approaches for management of insomnia. Neurotherapeutics. 2021;18(1):32–43. https://doi.org/10.1007/s13311-021-01029-2.

49. Sutton EL. Insomnia. Ann Intern Med. 2021;174(3):ITC33–48. https://doi.org/10.7326/AITC202103160.

50. Chung KF, Lee CT, Yeung WF, Chan MS, Chung EW, Lin WL. Sleep hygiene education as a treatment of insomnia: a systematic review and meta-analysis. Fam Pract. 2018;35(4):365–75. https://doi.org/10.1093/fampra/cmx122.

51. Perlis ML, Posner D, Riemann D, Bastien CH, Teel J, Thase M. Insomnia. Lancet. 2022;400(10357):1047–60. https://doi.org/10.1016/S0140-6736(22)00879-0.

52. Suvorexant (Belsomra) for insomnia. Med Lett Drugs Ther. 2015;57(1463):29–31.

53. Herring WJ, Connor KM, Ivgy-May N, et al. Suvorexant in patients with insomnia: results from two 3-month randomized controlled clinical trials. Biol Psychiatry. 2016;79(2):136–48.

54. Lemborexant (Dayvigo) for insomnia. Med Lett Drugs Ther. 2020;62(1601):97–100.

55. Murphy P, Moline M, Mayleben D, et al. Lemborexant, a dual orexin receptor antagonist (DORA) for the treatment of insomnia disorder: results from a Bayesian, adaptive, randomized, double-blind, placebo-controlled study. J Clin Sleep Med. 2017;13(11):1289–99. https://doi.org/10.5664/jcsm.6800.

56. Rosenberg R, Murphy P, Zammit G, et al. Comparison of lemborexant with placebo and zolpidem tartrate extended release for the treatment of older adults with insomnia disorder: a phase 3 randomized clinical trial published correction appears in JAMA Netw Open. 2020 Apr 1;3(4):e206497 published correction appears in JAMA Netw Open. 2021;4(8):e2127643. JAMA Netw Open. 2019;2(12):e1918254.

57. Michelson D, Snyder E, Paradis E, et al. Safety and efficacy of suvorexant during 1-year treatment of insomnia with subsequent abrupt treatment discontinuation: a phase 3 randomised, double-blind, placebo-controlled trial. Lancet Neurol. 2014;13(5):461–71. https://doi.org/10.1016/S1474-4422(14)70053-5.

58. Center for Drug Evaluation and Research. "Sleep Disorder (Sedative-Hypnotic) drug information." U.S. Food and Drug Administration, FDA, 19 Apr. 2019, https://www.fda.gov/drugs/postmarket-drug-safety-information-patients-and-providers/sleep-disorder-sedative-hypnotic-drug-information.

59. Wang L, Pan Y, Ye C, et al. A network meta-analysis of the long- and short-term efficacy of sleep medicines in adults and older adults. Neurosci Biobehav Rev. 2021;131:489–96. https://doi.org/10.1016/j.neubiorev.2021.09.035.

60. Rösner S, Englbrecht C, Wehrle R, Hajak G, Soyka M. Eszopiclone for insomnia. Cochrane Database Syst Rev. 2018;10(10):CD010703. https://doi.org/10.1002/14651858.CD010703.pub2.

61. Scharner V, Hasieber L, Sönnichsen A, et al. Efficacy and safety of Z-substances in the management of insomnia in older adults: a systematic review for the development of recommendations to reduce potentially inappropriate prescribing. BMC Geriatr. 2022;22:87. https://doi.org/10.1186/s12877-022-02757-6.

62. Hernandez I, He M, Brooks MM, Zhang Y. Exposure-response association between concurrent opioid and benzodiazepine use and risk of opioid-related overdose in medicare Part D beneficiaries. JAMA Netw Open. 2018;1(2):e180919. https://doi.org/10.1001/jamanetworkopen.2018.0919.

63. Boon M, van Dorp E, Broens S, Overdyk F. Combining opioids and benzodiazepines: effects on mortality and severe adverse respiratory events. Ann Palliat Med. 2020;9(2):542–57. https://doi.org/10.21037/apm.2019.12.09.

64. Lucchetta RC, da Mata BPM, Mastroianni PC. Association between development of dementia and use of benzodiazepines: a systematic review and meta-analysis. Pharmacotherapy. 2018;38(10):1010–20. https://doi.org/10.1002/phar.2170.

65. Soyka M. Treatment of benzodiazepine dependence. N Engl J Med. 2017;376(12):1147–57. https://doi.org/10.1056/NEJMra1611832.

66. Ramelteon (Rozerem) for insomnia. Med Lett Drugs Ther. 2005;47(1221):89–91.

67. Kuriyama A, Honda M, Hayashino Y. Ramelteon for the treatment of insomnia in adults: a systematic review and meta-analysis. Sleep Med. 2014;15(4):385–92. https://doi.org/10.1016/j.sleep.2013.11.788.

68. Edmonds C, Swanoski M. A review of Suvorexant, Doxepin, Ramelteon, and Tasimelteon for the treatment of insomnia in geriatric patients. Consult Pharm. 2017;32(3):156–60. https://doi.org/10.4140/TCP.n.2017.156.

69. Tasimelteon (Hetlioz) for non-24-hour sleep-wake disorder. Med Lett Drugs Ther. 2014;56(1441):34–5.

70. Lankford DA. Tasimelteon for insomnia. Expert Opin Investig Drugs. 2011;20(7):987–93. https://doi.org/10.1517/13543784.2011.583235.

71. Silenor [package insert].

72. Yeung WF, Chung KF, Yung KP, Ng TH. Doxepin for insomnia: a systematic review of randomized placebo-controlled trials. Sleep Med Rev. 2015;19:75–83. https://doi.org/10.1016/j.smrv.2014.06.001.

73. Trazodone [package insert].

74. Yi XY, Ni SF, Ghadami MR, et al. Trazodone for the treatment of insomnia: a meta-analysis of randomized placebo-controlled trials. Sleep Med. 2018;45:25–32. https://doi.org/10.1016/j.sleep.2018.01.010.

75. Camargos EF, Louzada LL, Quintas JL, Naves JO, Louzada FM, Nóbrega OT. Trazodone improves sleep parameters in Alzheimer disease patients: a randomized, double-blind, and placebo-controlled study. Am J Geriatr Psychiatry. 2014;22(12):1565–74. https://doi.org/10.1016/j.jagp.2013.12.174.

76. Roth T, Wright KP Jr, Walsh J. Effect of tiagabine on sleep in elderly subjects with primary insomnia: a randomized, double-blind, placebo-controlled study. Sleep. 2006;29(3):335–41. https://doi.org/10.1093/sleep/29.3.335.

77. Mathias S, Wetter TC, Steiger A, Lancel M. The GABA uptake inhibitor tiagabine promotes slow wave sleep in normal elderly subjects. Neurobiol Aging. 2001;22(2):247–53. https://doi.org/10.1016/s0197-4580(00)00232-3.

78. Walsh JK, Randazzo AC, Frankowski S, Shannon K, Schweitzer PK, Roth T. Dose-response effects of tiagabine on the sleep of older adults. Sleep. 2005;28(6):673–6. https://doi.org/10.1093/sleep/28.6.673.

79. Zyprexa [package insert].

80. Sharpley AL, Vassallo CM, Cowen PJ. Olanzapine increases slow-wave sleep: evidence for blockade of central 5-HT(2C) receptors in vivo. Biol Psychiatry. 2000;47(5):468–70. https://doi.org/10.1016/s0006-3223(99)00273-5.

81. Staner L, Haba J, Granier L, Vandenhende F, Macher J-P, Luthringer R. Comparison of the effects on sleep EEG of morning versus evening administration of olanzapine: A placebo controlled study in healthy volunteers. Eur Neuropsychopharmacol. 2002;12:326–6. https://doi.org/10.1016/S0924-977X(02)80497-7.

82. Seroquel [package insert].

83. Cohrs S, Rodenbeck A, Guan Z, et al. Sleep-promoting properties of quetiapine in healthy subjects. Psychopharmacology (Berl). 2004;174(3):421–9. https://doi.org/10.1007/s00213-003-1759-5.

84. Rock PL, Goodwin GM, Wulff K, McTavish SF, Harmer CJ. Effects of short-term quetiapine treatment on emotional processing, sleep and circadian rhythms. J Psychopharmacol. 2016;30(3):273–82. https://doi.org/10.1177/0269881115626336.

85. Karsten J, Hagenauw LA, Kamphuis J, Lancel M. Low doses of mirtazapine or quetiapine for transient insomnia: a randomised, double-blind, cross-over, placebo-controlled trial. J Psychopharmacol. 2017;31(3):327–37. https://doi.org/10.1177/0269881116681399.

86. Rognoni C, Bertolani A, Jommi C. Second-generation antipsychotic drugs for patients with schizophrenia: systematic literature review and meta-analysis of metabolic and cardiovascular side effects. Clin Drug Investig. 2021;41(4):303–19. https://doi.org/10.1007/s40261-021-01000-1.

87. Cates ME, Jackson CW, Feldman JM, Stimmel AE, Woolley TW. Metabolic consequences of using low-dose quetiapine for insomnia in psychiatric patients. Community Ment Health J. 2009;45(4):251–4. https://doi.org/10.1007/s10597-009-9200-0.

88. Monahan K, Cuzens-Sutton J, Siskind D, Kisely S. Quetiapine withdrawal: a systematic review. Aust N Z J Psychiatry. 2021;55(8):772–83. https://doi.org/10.1177/0004867420965693.

89. Aslan S, Isik E, Cosar B. The effects of mirtazapine on sleep: a placebo controlled, double-blind study in young healthy volunteers. Sleep. 2002;25(6):677–9.

90. Kent JM. SNaRIs, NaSSAs, and NaRIs: new agents for the treatment of depression published correction appears in Lancet 2000;355(9219):2000. Lancet. 2000;355(9207):911–8. https://doi.org/10.1016/S0140-6736(99)11381-3.

91. Kolla BP, Mansukhani MP, Bostwick JM. The influence of antidepressants on restless legs syndrome and periodic limb movements: a systematic review. Sleep Med Rev. 2018;38:131–40.

92. Glass JR, Sproule BA, Herrmann N, Busto UE. Effects of 2-week treatment with temazepam and diphenhydramine in elderly insomniacs: a randomized, placebo-controlled trial. J Clin Psychopharmacol. 2008;28(2):182–8. https://doi.org/10.1097/JCP.0b013e31816a9e4f.

93. Vande Griend JP, Anderson SL. Histamine-1 receptor antagonism for treatment of insomnia. J Am Pharm Assoc (2003). 2012;52(6):e210-e219. doi:https://doi.org/10.1331/JAPhA.2012.12051

94. By the 2019 American Geriatrics Society Beers Criteria® Update Expert Panel. American Geriatrics Society 2019 Updated AGS Beers Criteria® for potentially inappropriate medication use in older adults. J Am Geriatr Soc. 2019;67(4):674–94. https://doi.org/10.1111/jgs.15767.

95. Ferracioli-Oda E, Qawasmi A, Bloch MH. Meta-analysis: melatonin for the treatment of primary sleep disorders. PLoS ONE. 2013;8(5):e63773. https://doi.org/10.1371/journal.pone.0063773.

96. Besag FMC, Vasey MJ, Lao KSJ, et al. Adverse events associated with melatonin for the treatment of primary or secondary sleep disorders: a systematic

review. CNS Drugs. 2019;33:1167–86. https://doi.org/10.1007/s40263-019-00680-w.

97. Chiu HY, Lee HC, Liu JW, et al. Comparative efficacy and safety of hypnotics for insomnia in older adults: a systematic review and network meta-analysis. Sleep. 2021;44(5):zsaa260. https://doi.org/10.1093/sleep/zsaa260.

98. Samara MT, Huhn M, Chiocchia V, et al. Efficacy, acceptability, and tolerability of all available treatments for insomnia in the elderly: a systematic review and network meta-analysis. Acta Psychiatr Scand. 2020;142(1):6–17. https://doi.org/10.1111/acps.13201.

99. De Crescenzo F, D'Alò GL, Ostinelli EG, et al. Comparative effects of pharmacological interventions for the acute and long-term management of insomnia disorder in adults: a systematic review and network meta-analysis. Lancet. 2022;400(10347):170–84. https://doi.org/10.1016/S0140-6736(22)00878-9.

100. Zheng X, He Y, Yin F, et al. Pharmacological interventions for the treatment of insomnia: quantitative comparison of drug efficacy. Sleep Med. 2020;72:41–9. https://doi.org/10.1016/j.sleep.2020.03.022.

Senthil Vel Rajan Rajaram Manoharan, Jessy Walia,
and Mack Bozman

Epidemiology

For RLS, a prevalence of 5–10% is reported in various population-based studies that use a full standard diagnostic criterion [1]. Synthesis of the literature reveals that the prevalence rates vary depending on how RLS is evaluated. Studies that look at only one item tend to provide higher prevalence rates as compared to studies using all the four minimal criteria described by the International Restless Legs Syndrome Study Group (IRLSSG). In this last case, the prevalence of RLS in the general adult population ranges between 5% and 8.8%. However, infrequent and/or mild RLS is present in at least half of these cases [2]. More than 50 epidemiologic studies around the world have investigated the prevalence, mostly in North America and Europe. The highest prevalence is in North America and Europe ranging from 5.5% to 11.6% and is lower in Asia with ranges of 1.0–7.5%. These differences across regions may be explained by cultural, environmental, and genetic factors [3]. The prevalence also seems to vary with age and gender. RLS is twice as common in women than in men, and this difference is more prominent above age 35 [4]. The onset of symptoms can occur at any age and is possible in childhood. There may be an association with attention deficit disorders or "growing pains," though prevalence does increase with age [5]. The mean age of onset is around the third or the fourth decade [2]. When symptoms occur at least twice per week with moderate distress, it is clinically significant and affects 3–5% of those over the age of 60 years [1, 2]. The onset of symptoms is often mild and infrequent and slowly progresses, thereby delaying most diagnoses until the fourth–sixth decades of life.

S. V. R. Rajaram Manoharan (✉)
Department of Psychiatry, Huntsville Hospital,
Huntsville, AL, USA

UAB Heersink School of Medicine,
Birmingham, AL, USA

J. Walia
Huntsville Hospital, Huntsville, AL, USA

M. Bozman
UAB Heersink School of Medicine,
Birmingham, AL, USA
e-mail: bozman@uab.edu

Genetics

The significant genetic contribution to the development of RLS is inferred from the inheritance patterns of RLS, genetic anticipation, a positive family history, twin studies, linkage studies in familial RLS, genome-wide association studies (GWAS), exome sequencing studies, and case–control association studies on candidate genes in RLS [6]. So far, no causative genes have been definitively identified. However, variants of sev-

© The Author(s), under exclusive license to Springer Nature Switzerland AG 2024
R. R. Tampi, D. J. Tampi (eds.), *Treatment of Psychiatric Disorders Among Older Adults*,
https://doi.org/10.1007/978-3-031-55711-8_12

eral genes that are associated with RLS risk have been identified through GWAS. The strongest association has been found with the variants of *PTPRD*, *BTBD9*, and *MEIS1* genes. There are higher concordance rates in monozygotic twins (50–80%) when compared with dizygotic twins. Autosomal dominant patterns of transmission have also been noted [7]. Genetic anticipation, which is defined by the earlier age of onset of symptoms from one generation to successive generations, sometimes with an increase in severity, has also been described extensively in families with RLS.

Risk Factors

Female sex and older age are the strongest risk factors for RLS. Associations with other disorders including hypertension, migraine, diabetes mellitus, Parkinson's disease, multiple sclerosis, polyneuropathy, and chronic inflammatory states have been investigated [8]:

– Iron deficiency with or without anemia in the elderly is strongly associated with restless legs syndrome [9].
– Chronic kidney disease is strongly associated with the development of RLS. The prevalence of RLS ranges between 15% and 68% across various studies. Intake of calcium antagonists, lower baseline parathyroid hormone, duration of dialysis, lower serum transferrin saturation, lower educational levels, and conventional hemodialysis (vs. short-term daily hemodialysis) are some of the factors associated with the development of RLS [8].
– About one-third of pregnant women are affected by RLS, and the prevalence peaks during the third trimester [10].
– A close association between RLS and Parkinson's disease (PD) has been noted with increased prevalence of RLS in PD patients [11].
– Migraine: In patients with migraine headaches, comorbidity with RLS ranged between 8% and 39% [12].
– A higher frequency of RLS in multiple sclerosis (MS) is described across various studies. RLS frequency of up to 65% has been described among individuals with MS [8].
– RLS is much more frequent in diabetes mellitus (DM) patients even after excluding polyneuropathy, and the duration of diabetes and insulin use is related to RLS [13].
– RLS is also comorbid with psychiatric disorders like depression and anxiety, which are more common in women [14].
– Poststroke patients may have an increased prevalence of RLS [15].

When diagnosing RLS, it is important to determine if it is due to a primary (idiopathic) or a secondary cause (Fig. 12.1). Primary (idiopathic) causes are less obvious and do not usually

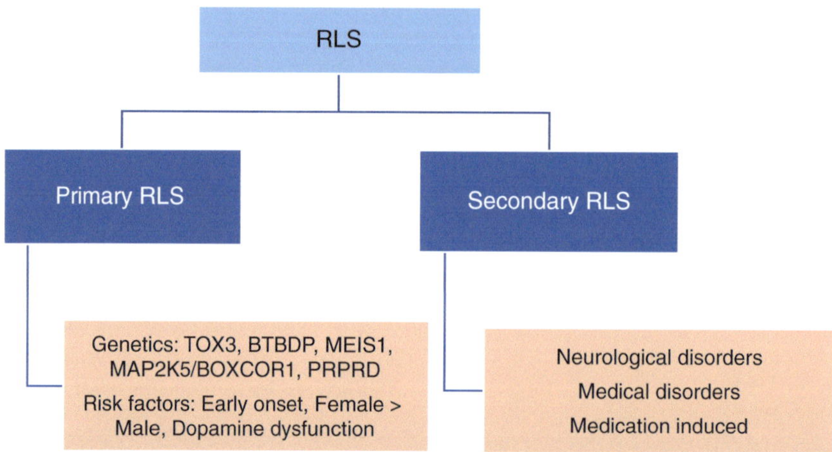

Fig. 12.1 Classification of RLS

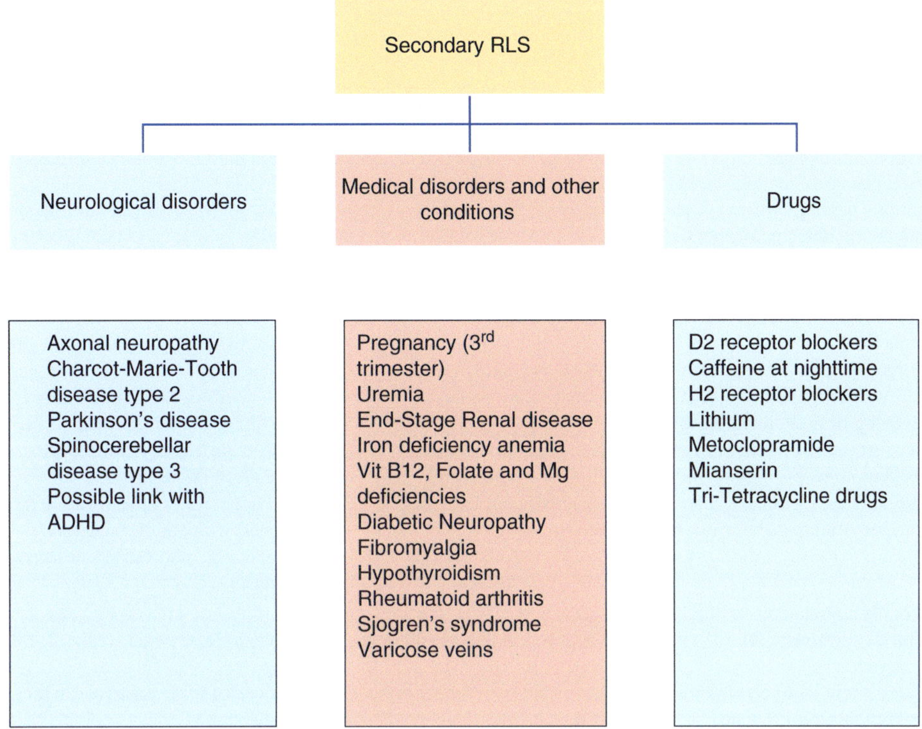

Fig. 12.2 Secondary causes of RLS

resolve. If it is secondary RLS, resolution of the underlying medical condition should typically lead to improvement in symptoms over time [16]. Identify secondary RLS (Fig. 12.2) promptly as this may lead to a reduction in symptoms and possible remission.

Assessment

Restless legs syndrome is characterized by an irresistible urge to move the legs with worsening symptoms at rest and the occurrence or exacerbation of symptoms in the evening or night. RLS is also associated with jerking movements of the legs during sleep, known as periodic limb movements of sleep (PLMS). The term periodic limb movement disorder (PLMD) is used when significant sleep disturbances or impaired daytime functioning occur secondary to PLMS in the absence of RLS or other associated disorders. Although a typical clinical course is usually chronic progressive with periodic exacerbations, some patients may have symptoms that occur in paroxysms or clusters. Dr. Ekbom, who originally described the disorder, believed that the uncomfortable and painful sensation, or dysesthesia, caused the irresistible urge to move. The urge to move can also occur without dysesthesia [17].

Diagnostic Criteria

In 1685, Thomas Willis first described the symptoms of RLS [18]. But it was not until 1945 that the first formal diagnostic criteria were put together by Karl-Axel Ekbom in the seminal monograph "Restless Legs" [19]. The essential features of RLS have not changed since the original description by Dr. Ekbom. The clinical hallmark feature of RLS is the urge to move the legs, which is usually but not always accompanied by an uncomfortable and unpleasant sensation (which patients often have trouble describing) [17]. The remaining four essential criteria are necessary for diagnoses (Table 12.1), with the fifth criterion added to exclude mimickers in

Table 12.1 International Restless Legs Syndrome Study Group (IRLSSG) consensus diagnostic criteria for restless legs syndrome [17, 21]

Essential diagnostic criteria (all must be met)	Additional features
1. An urge to move the legs usually but not always accompanied by, or felt to be caused by, uncomfortable and unpleasant sensations in the legs[a] 2. The urge to move the legs and any accompanying unpleasant sensations begin or worsen during periods of rest or inactivity such as lying down or sitting 3. The urge to move the legs and any accompanying unpleasant sensations are partially or totally relieved by movement, such as walking or stretching, at least as long as the activity continues[b] 4. The urge to move the legs and any accompanying unpleasant sensations during rest or inactivity only occur or are worse in the evening or night than during the day[c] 5. The occurrence of the above features is not solely accounted for as symptoms primary to another medical or a behavioral condition (e.g., myalgia, venous stasis, leg edema, arthritis, leg cramps, positional discomfort, habitual foot tapping)[d]	Supportive features: – Dopaminergic treatment response – Periodic limb movements with arousal (PMLA) – Periodic limb movements during sleep (PMLS) – Positive family history among first-degree relatives Associated features: – Chronic progressive course with periodic exacerbations – Benign neurological examination (except neuropathy) – <u>Lack</u> of expected daytime sleepiness despite sleep disturbance – Age of onset (later onset is more likely associated with another medical condition, e.g., neuropathy or iron deficiency)

Specifiers for clinical course of RLS[e]:
  A. Chronic persistent RLS: Symptoms when not treated would occur on average at least twice weekly for the past year
  B. Intermittent RLS: Symptoms when not treated would occur on average <2/week for the past year, with at least five lifetime events
Specifier for clinical significance of RLS:
  The symptoms of RLS cause significant distress or impairment in social, occupational, educational, or other important areas of functioning by their impact on sleep, energy/vitality, daily activities, behavior, cognition, or mood

[a] Sometimes the urge to move the legs is present without the uncomfortable sensations and sometimes the arms or other parts of the body are involved in addition to the legs
[b] When symptoms are very severe, relief by activity may not be noticeable but must have been previously present
[c] When symptoms are very severe, the worsening in the evening or night may not be noticeable but must have been previously present
[d] These conditions, often referred to as "RLS mimics," have been commonly confused with RLS particularly in surveys because they produce symptoms that meet or at least come very close to meeting criteria 1–4. RLS may also occur with other conditions, but the RLS symptoms will then be more in degree, conditions of expression, or character than those usually occurring as part of the other condition
[e] The clinical course criteria do not apply for pediatric cases nor for some special cases of provoked RLS such as pregnancy or drug-induced RLS where the frequency may be high but limited to duration of the provocative condition

2014 [20]. Specifiers (A) and (B) for the clinical course of symptoms for RLS may be chronic persistent or intermittent. The patient may or may not be experiencing symptoms at the time of the interview. There are no universal screening guidelines for RLS. The diagnosis of RLS is made clinically based on the IRLSSG criteria (Table 12.1). Clinicians should familiarize themselves with these criteria and inquire about symptoms, especially when additional risk factors are present. Table 12.2 identifies the recommended laboratory investigations for RLS.

Table 12.2 Recommended laboratory investigations [23]

Iron studies—Serum ferritin level is essential
Complete blood count
Vitamin B12 and folic acid levels
Serum glucose and HbA1C
Serum creatinine, urea, and serum electrolytes
Albumin (optional)
Thyroid function tests (optional)

Diagnosis can be remembered using the acronym "RESTeD"

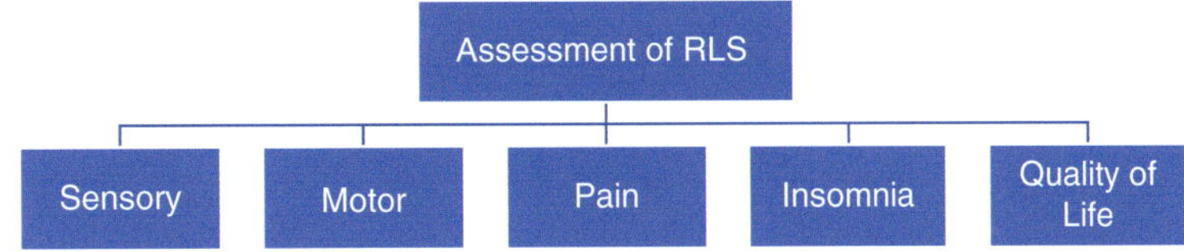

Fig. 12.3 Assessment of RLS symptoms

R = Rest induces symptoms

E = Evening and nighttime worsening

S = Sensations (unpleasant) associated with an urge to move

Te = Tends to get better with activity

D = Does not occur because an RLS mimics such leg cramps

The IRLSSG rating scale (IRLS) consists of 10 questions which are scored into one of five severity categories (from 0 to 4) with a total score of 40 [24]. RLS symptom severity scores are as follows: 1–10 (mild), 11–20 (moderate), 21–30 (severe), and 31–40 (very severe). This score can help decide whether pharmacological treatment would be beneficial [23]. RLS can be screened with a single question that has 100% sensitivity and 96.8% specificity for the diagnosis of RLS. It is, "When you try to relax in the evening or sleep at night, do you ever have unpleasant, restless feelings in your legs that can be relieved by walking or movement?" [25].

Assessment of Symptoms and Quality of Life

RLS patients can experience disabling symptoms that interfere with sleep and social functioning and may cause diminished quality of life [26]. The symptoms typically begin in quiet wakefulness or early sleep as sensory, motor, or pain symptoms (Fig. 12.3). RLS can also present with depressive symptoms, fatigue, poor concentration, and fidgetiness. Clinical presentation is often heterogeneous, with pain, insomnia, and daytime sleepiness as common presentations [27].

Sensory Symptoms

The essential feature of the urge to move the limbs may be considered either a sensory or a motor symptom, as the urge to move may be associated with "dysesthesia," which is more clearly a sensory symptom [28]. RLS symptoms arise from deep in the limb, rather than superficially, and feel like movement within the leg [29]. The sensory symptoms in RLS can vary and can be described as general discomfort, cramps, or even pain. The description of these sensory experiences is often influenced by cultural expressions. This varied description of symptoms among patients can often lead to misdiagnosis and sometimes is even being labeled as "psychogenic" [30]. The broad and unusual spectrum of reported sensations has led to a long list of the words used by the patients (Table 12.3).

Motor Symptoms

Motor restlessness is a characteristic symptom of RLS and is often described as the urge to move the limbs and doing so resolves (partially or completely) the accompanying unpleasant sensations [1]. Periodic limb movements, which can occur during sleep or while awake, develop in approximately 80–85% of RLS patients. PLM disorder is characterized by repetitive stereotype movements of the limbs occurring every 5–90 s resembling flexor withdrawal reflex. The movements often lead to sleep disturbances, awakening the patient or sleep partner [32].

Table 12.3 Common description of sensory symptoms [29, 31]

Elvis legs	Creepy-crawly sensations
Coca cola in veins	Pulling feeling
Itching bones	Electric shock burning legs
Aching calves	Hot poker stabbing legs
Throbbing pain	Deep throbbing pain
Leg cramps	Ants crawling
Worms moving	Bubbling
Tingling	Prickling
Twitching	Grabbing
Squeezing	

Pain in RLS

RLS may manifest predominantly with pain symptoms, causing diagnostic challenges as the pain could also be due to comorbid peripheral neuropathy, osteoarthritis, or rheumatoid disease. Pain can also involve the upper limb, chin, and posterior neck, mimicking radicular pain [33]. A diurnal pattern is typically observed and is usually relieved by medications (gabapentin and dopamine agonists) for RLS. Other therapeutic approaches, like the use of sensory feedback through massage, hot compress, and tight bandage, may also relieve the pain of RLS. The presence of pain in PD patients is worsened by RLS, and vice versa in RLS patients that develop PD [34]. Pain is typically felt deep inside the muscles in the middle portions of the lower limbs, especially the calves. Exclusive or predominant involvement of the feet or joints is rare [35].

RLS and Quality of Life

The Restless Legs Syndrome Foundation commissioned the "Patient Odyssey" survey to assess the day-to-day impact of RLS on patients and their spouses/partners. 1622 adult patients (70% female), and 676 adult spouses/partners (65% men and 35% women), completed the survey online or by mail. This survey highlighted the practical quality-of-life problems caused by RLS and was noted to significantly impact these patients, with 85% reporting inability "to have a restful night," 53% reporting sleep disruption of four or more nights per week, and 58% reporting that they lose three or more hours per affected night. RLS was shown to markedly affect patients' sleep as well as limit travel, work, and mood. About one-third (34%) of patients and spouses/partners reported sleeping in separate beds due to restless legs syndrome (RLS). Patients frequently report feeling that their condition was "trivialized" and are frustrated by a perceived lack of empathy and understanding from loved ones and society [36].

In the REST study (RLS epidemiology, symptom, and treatment survey), 16,202 people were surveyed, and the generic quality-of-life instrument, SF-36, was used. In the study, 7% screened positively for RLS. A strong correlation was noted between the severity of RLS and physical and mental health-related quality of life in patients (HRQol), both from the United States and Europe. Two main issues affecting HRQol were identified: pain and discomfort (88%) and sleep disturbance (76%); in fact, the most common complaints in the REST study were pain and poor sleep. Studies have also suggested that a mixture of anxiety disorders, suicidal thoughts, and depression is common in RLS. Many patients with RLS who have intermittent symptoms suffer from specific fears of traveling and socializing, which can severely impair the quality of life [27]. A two- to fourfold risk of depressive disorder in patients with RLS when compared with healthy controls was reported [37]. As the RLS severity worsens, there is an increased risk of depression [38]. RLS has also been shown to affect cognition, particularly memory [39]. The restless legs syndrome quality-of-life scale (Abetz) is the only scale recommended for use in cross-sectional assessment and treatment-related changes. Daily diaries do hold promise without the need for retrospective recall [40]. Figure 12.4 illustrates the impact of sleep deprivation among individuals with RLS.

Diagnosis for Cognitively Impaired Seniors

Diagnosis of RLS in cognitively impaired seniors is more difficult due to symptom distortion issues in communication. There are no current valid assessment methods for diagnosis of RLS/WED in this patient population [41].

Differential Diagnosis

1. RLS must be differentiated from positional discomfort, akathisia, and other diagnoses that mimic RLS and often lead to misdiagnosis with self-reported patient surveys. These conditions should be individually evaluated to ensure an accurate RLS diagnosis, although it

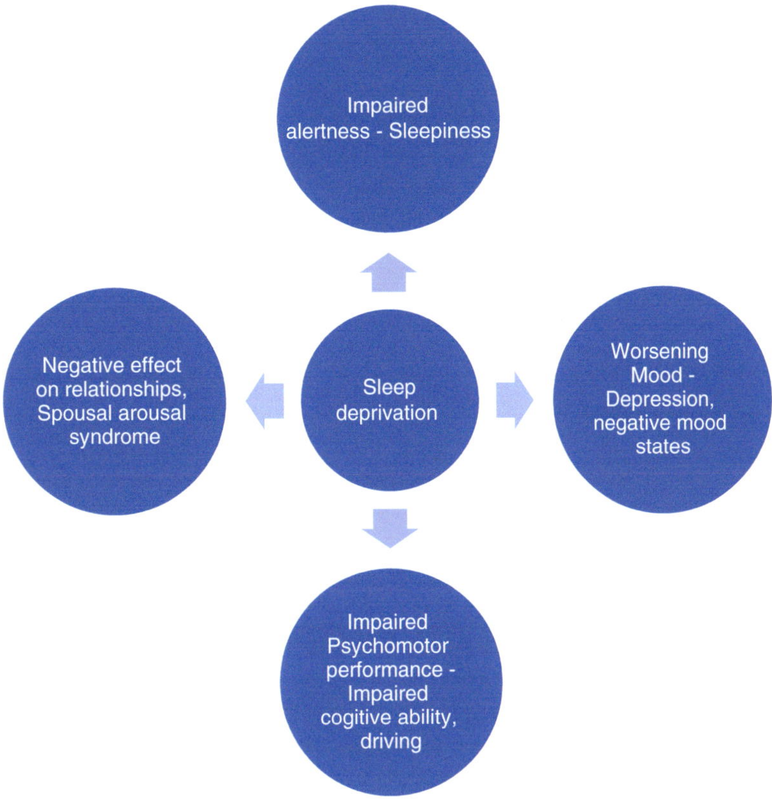

Fig. 12.4 Impact of sleep deprivation

is possible to have RLS with one or more of the other conditions [17]. They are differentiated from RLS as follows *Positional discomfort* is differentiated from RLS by the aching sensations with no motor restlessness, movements, or visible muscle contractions. The distribution is typically symmetrical in the lower limbs and may be relieved by massaging.

2. *Cramps* are characterized by intense muscle contractions that may be visible and usually noted in the calf muscle. As compared to RLS, there are no motor restlessness.

3. *Akathisia* is characterized by motor restlessness that is present all the time and usually is caused by neuroleptics. The movements seen are fast and choreiform (unlike RLS where the movements are slow and repetitive). This may involve the face, tongue, and upper and lower limbs. There is relief with movements. There may be visible muscle contractions (unlike RLS).

Treatments

Nonpharmacological

Nonpharmacological approaches are the foundation of RLS treatment and may obviate the need for medications. Treatment should begin with a careful exploration into both iatrogenic and lifestyle factors that may lead to an exacerbation [42]. Sleep hygiene is useful for the management of sleep disorders and can be adapted for RLS [43]. It is important to investigate patient medications as some common medications will make RLS worse. It is important to discuss good sleep hygiene habits as those changes can enhance the overall quality of sleep. These sleep hygiene measures include sleeping at a constant time, using the bed for only sleep or sexual activity and not for reading or television, and avoiding naps, tea, coffee, or diuretics before bedtime [21]. The presence of other comorbid sleep disorders like

Table 12.4 Drugs that worsen restless legs syndrome [21, 45]

Drugs worsening restless legs syndrome
1. Metoclopramide
2. Prochlorperazine
3. Chlordiazepoxide
4. Traditional antipsychotics (phenothiazines)
5. Atypical neuroleptics (olanzapine and risperidone)
6. Antidepressants[a] (especially norepinephrine or selective serotonin reuptake inhibitors)
7. Anticonvulsants (zonisamide, phenytoin, methsuximide)
8. Antihistamines (diphenhydramine and other over-the-counter cold remedies)
9. Calcium channel-blocking antihypertensives
10. Lithium
11. Antiemetics (except domperidone)
12. Excessive consumption of caffeine in coffee, tea, chocolate, or soda

[a] Bupropion is an exception in the antidepressant category [46]

sleep apnea should be evaluated and pursued if necessary. Sleep apnea treatment may result in improvements in RLS and eliminate the need for medications. Other conditions worsening sleep should be assessed, like depression and anxiety [44]. Table 12.4 lists the drugs that worsen RLS.

Pharmacological

Once an accurate diagnosis is made, reassurance and support are often sufficient treatments for most RLS patients. However, approximately 20% of patients have severe symptoms and require pharmacological intervention [21, 47] (see Table 12.6 for a summary of pharmacological treatment options).

The following needs to be considered before initiating pharmacological treatment for RLS [21]:

- Symptom severity: This can be assessed using the RLS severity scale; a score of 15 out of 40 indicates moderate to severe RLS.
- Age of the patient: There is increased risk of side effects with benzodiazepines and dopamine agonists. Postural hypotension associated with aging may be aggravated by these agents.

- Frequency of symptoms: Most patients have intermittent RLS and need only targeted/timed treatment.
- Presence of other comorbid issues: Cardiac disease, pregnancy, etc.

Medication Classes

Dopaminergic Agonists

It is hypothesized that RLS is due to a "hyperdopaminergic state." The efficacy of dopaminergic agonists that bind to the inhibitory D3 receptor (D3R) supports this claim. The long-term use of these medications leads to the upregulation of the excitatory D1 receptor (D1R), leading to the side effect of RLS augmentation [48, 49].

Oral ropinirole, pramipexole, and transdermal rotigotine are the three non-ergot dopaminergic agonists approved by the US FDA for the treatment of moderate–severe primary RLS [22].

Pramipexole

Pramipexole is effective and well tolerated for RLS and related sleep disturbances [50]. A 6-week, multicenter, randomized, double-blind multinational study (effect-RLS study) that included 345 patients with moderate to severe RLS demonstrated significant improvements in RLS severity in pramipexole-treated patients as compared to placebo. Changes on the IRLS, a validated, disease-specific scale for the evaluation of RLS, and the CGI-I were the primary endpoints. The proportion of patients reporting more than a 50% reduction of their baseline IRLS score was significantly higher in the pramipexole group than in the placebo group. Similarly, the proportion of patients who rated their condition on the Patient Global Impression (PGI) as "much better" and "very much better" at week 6 was significantly higher in the pramipexole group. The alleviating effect of pramipexole occurred rapidly and at the lowest dose [51].

Ropinirole

The European trial called the TREAT-RLS study confirmed the superiority of ropinirole over placebo [52]. It involved 284 patients in a 12-week, randomized, double-blind trial, and RLS patients were randomized to receive either ropinirole at 0.25–4.0 mg/day or placebo. Ropinirole produced significant improvements in patients' RLS severity and clinical global impression (CGI) scores after both 1 and 12 weeks. Furthermore, ropinirole was associated with significantly greater improvements in sleep and parameters measuring the quality of life. TREAT RLS 2 is a 12-week, double-blind, randomized, parallel-group, placebo-controlled study. It showed that ropinirole was well tolerated, and significant improvements in IRLS score at week 12 compared with placebo (−11.2 versus −8.7, respectively) were reported with ropinirole in 267 patients with moderate to severe RLS [53]. In this study, ropinirole (0.25–4.0 mg/day) significantly improved all key secondary endpoints, sleep, and parameters (measured by clinical global impression, the MOS (Medical outcomes study) sleep scale, SF-36 Health Survey, and RLS quality of life scale), in patients with RLS.

Rotigotine

Trenkwalder and colleagues [54] have reported the results from a randomized, double-blind, placebo-controlled trial in 458 patients with moderate to severe RLS using a transdermal rotigotine patch versus placebo. Patients received 1 mg/24 h rotigotine patch ($n = 115$), 2 mg/24 h ($n = 112$), 3 mg/24 h ($n = 114$), or placebo ($n = 117$), with a 6-month maintenance phase followed by a taper phase for 1 week and safety follow-up for 4 weeks. International restless legs syndrome study group severity rating scale (IRLS) and clinical global impression (CGI) were used as primary efficacy outcome measures. Both showed significant improvements from baseline to end of maintenance in each dosage when compared to placebo ($p < 0.0001$, for treatment difference versus placebo with each dose). Mild to moderate skin reaction was noted with the rotigotine skin patch and in only six cases was the application site reaction deemed as serious, which resolved after removal of the patch. Typical dopaminergic side effects were low, and in the study period, there were no signs of augmentation noted. Rotigotine transdermal patch, therefore, is efficacious at doses between 1 and 3 mg for the treatment of moderate to severe RLS with low rates of augmentation. Rotigotine is administered once a day and initiated at 1 mg/24 h. The dosage may be increased depending on the individual patient response to a maximal dosage of 3 mg/24 h.

Ergot Dopamine Agonists

Ergot-derived dopamine agonists, though previously used widely, are no longer recommended as a first-line RLS treatment due to the risk of possible valvulopathy and pulmonary fibrosis [55].

Cabergoline is a long-acting ergot dopamine agonist with a long half-life that allows once-daily dosing, which addresses both day- and nighttime symptoms. In a multicentric, double-blind, randomized, active-controlled, parallel-group study, 361 patients with moderate to severe primary RLS were studied in a head-to-head comparison of fixed daily doses of cabergoline 2–3 mg and levodopa 200 or 300 mg. Cabergoline was better than levodopa in terms of improvement in total IRLS score ($p < 0.0001$) and time to discontinuation due to augmentation ($p = 0.0412$) and loss of efficacy ($p = 0.0029$) [56]. However, compared with cabergoline, levodopa was better tolerated and associated with fewer adverse events (83.1% vs. 77.6%). Pergolide has been withdrawn from the US market, while safety guidelines have been issued in relation to cabergoline. Lisuride is also an ergot dopamine agonist but may have an antagonistic action at the serotonin 5-HT2b receptors, which is believed to negate the tendency to produce cardiac valvulopathies. A proof-of-principle study, which used a combined, open-label, and double-blind design, evaluated a transdermal form of lisuride in ten patients with primary RLS and reported a positive effect on RLS [57].

Levodopa

In a small randomized, double-blind, placebo-controlled, multicenter, crossover trial of 32 patients with primary RLS, levodopa plus benserazide (co-beneldopa) given as a single bedtime dose (110/25) was found to be superior to placebo in reducing the number of PLMS per hour ($p < 0.0001$), in increasing the time in bed without limb movements ($p < 0.0001$), and in improving subjective quality of sleep ($p = 0.0004$) [58]. In patients with unclear diagnosis, the L-DOPA test for helping the diagnosis of RLS has been proposed for diagnostic decision-making [59]. Patients are assessed after the application of one single oral dose of L-DOPA (plus decarboxylase inhibitor) and a subsequent observation period of 2 h. Before and in 15-min intervals after drug intake, the patients are rated on the severity of the "symptoms in the legs" and the "urge to move the legs" using a 100 mm visual analogue scale. Using a 50% improvement as a positive test result, sensitivity values of 88% ("symptoms in the legs") and 80% ("urge to move the legs") with a specificity of 100% for both test items have been noted. Using this test, 83–90% of individuals with RLS could be correctly diagnosed.

Non-dopaminergic Treatments

Alpha-2-Delta Calcium Channel Ligands

Pregabalin, gabapentin, and gabapentin enacarbil (a controlled-release prodrug of gabapentin) belong to this class of medications. They bind at the α-2-δ subunit of the voltage-gated calcium channel, leading to reduction in excitatory neurotransmitters. Since these medications are renally excreted, the dose should be adjusted in older adults and in patients with renal failure or insufficiency who have reductions in glomerular filtration rate [22]. Gabapentin can be used off-label and is effective for the treatment of RLS/WED. There are four studies of gabapentin with a wide dose range (800–1855 mg) that showed efficacy over 12 weeks, especially in patients requiring hemodialysis [60].

The extended-release prodrug, gabapentin enacarbil, is approved in the USA (Horizant®). Patients with moderate to severe symptoms of RLS had significant improvement when treated with gabapentin enacarbil at 600 mg/day for 12 weeks [61]. Two distinct therapeutic doses may exist for treating RLS: 600 mg/day or lower doses are sufficient to treat subjective RLS symptoms, while 1200 mg/day or higher doses may be required to treat both subjective symptoms and associated sleep disturbances [62]. Only the 600 mg dose has been approved by the US Food and Drug Administration, as higher doses provided no additional benefits and had higher rates of side effects, like somnolence and dizziness. However, the data from post hoc analysis showed that 1200 mg once-daily dosing was the most validated intervention targeting both subjective symptoms and sleep disturbances [62].

The increasing awareness of medication-induced worsening of RLS symptoms (augmentation and development of impulse control disorders) associated with dopaminergic agonists has led to the use of alpha-2-delta ligands as a first-line treatment when not contraindicated [44].

Benzodiazepines and Z-Drugs

Benzodiazepines can be used as a co-adjuvant therapy based on a systematic review by the American Academy of Sleep Medicine [63]. Main side effects of this drug group include respiratory depression, falls, dependence, somnolence, and disruption of sleep architecture. Careful monitoring is recommended when patients use benzodiazepines as they can cause cognitive impairment. In RLS with sleep-onset insomnia, short-acting agents, such as zolpidem (5–10 mg) or zaleplon (5–10 mg), may be helpful. When a patient has middle insomnia, intermediate-acting agents may be helpful, such as temazepam (15–30 mg) or eszopiclone (1–3 mg). Lower doses of benzodiazepines should be used in elderly patients [44].

Opioids

When symptom controlling is not achieved with other medications, opioids can be considered. The opioid dose used to treat RLS is typically much lower than what is used for treatment of chronic pain. In a large study of over 300 patients, a combination of naloxone and oxycodone was used for the treatment of RLS and was found to be efficacious over the 12-week trial period [64]. The safety of long-term use of opioids to treat RLS in older adults has not been established. The American Geriatric Society (AGS) issued strong recommendation against combining benzodiazepines or gabapentinoids as the drug-drug interactions can lead to respiratory depressant effects, worsening underlying obstructive sleep apnea, and more severe hypoxia [65].

Antiepileptics

Carbamazepine reduced the frequency and the severity of symptoms in RLS patients in a large but much older 5-week randomized, double-blind, placebo-controlled trial of 174 patients. However, a significant therapeutic effect was reported for both carbamazepine and placebo [66]. Recently, lamotrigine has been tried for RLS with some benefits [67, 68].

Iron Therapy

A state of brain iron deficiency has been associated with RLS. Iron status should be evaluated in all patients presenting with RLS, even when typical causes of iron deficiency are absent. Currently, there are no accepted methods to assess brain iron stores. Assessment includes looking at serum iron, ferritin, and total iron-binding capacity/transferrin saturation, typically in the early morning after an overnight fast [44]. Based on recent guidelines, oral iron supplementation could be beneficial and is considered when serum ferritin is <75 µg/dL or transferrin saturation index is <20% [69]. Serum ferritin is an acute-phase reactant that may be misleadingly high in acute or chronic inflammation, and when this occurs, transferrin saturation of <20% may be more accurate.

A typical oral iron regimen is 325 mg of ferrous sulfate (65 mg elemental iron) combined with vitamin C (100–200 mg) to enhance absorption to be taken on an empty stomach once daily or every other day. It can be taken with food (avoiding foods with high calcium content) if gastrointestinal symptoms develop. Periodic assessment of ferritin levels should be done, at least every 3–4 months until it is greater than 100 mg/L.

Intravenous iron therapy is used when rapid response is desired in severe RLS patients or there is a failed response/contraindication of oral iron therapy. When ferritin levels are <100 µg/dL, along with transferrin saturation less than 45%, intravenous iron therapy can be safely administered without the risk of iron overload [69]. The best evidence exists for ferric carboxymaltose and low-molecular-weight (LMW) iron dextran. The response rates range between 50% and 60% following a 1 g infusion of either formulation with a delay of 2–8 weeks before noticing clinical benefits [22, 69]. Table 12.5 provides information on dosing recommendations and adverse effects of frequently prescribed pharmacological agents in chronic RLS for older adults. Table 12.6 outlines the details of commonly used pharmacological agents used to treat RLS, including time to full effect of therapeutic dose, half-life, and possible side effects.

Table 12.5 Dosing and adverse effects of pharmacological agents for the treatment of chronic restless legs syndrome in older adults [22]

Medication	Starting dose in older (>65 years) patients (mg)	Usually effective daily dose (mg)	Common adverse effects
α-2-δ ligands			
Gabapentin	100	900–2400	Dizziness, weight gain, leg edema, sedation
Pregabalin	75	150–450	
Gabapentin enacarbil	300	600–1200	
Dopaminergic			
Pramipexole	0.125	0.25–0.5	Sedation, hypotension, insomnia, impulse control disorder, augmentation
Ropinirole	0.25	0.5–4	
Rotigotine patch			Rash, sedation, hypotension, insomnia, impulse control disorder, augmentation
Opioids			
Oxycodone	5	10–30	Sedation, constipation, nausea, sleep apnea
Tramadol	25–50	50–200	Sedation, constipation, nausea, sleep apnea, risk of seizures (potentiated by SSRIs)
Methadone	2.5	5–20	Sedation, constipation, nausea, sleep apnea, prolonged QT interval (hence ECG recommended)

Table 12.6 Pharmacological treatment of RLS; recommended dose, time to full therapeutic effect, half-life, and possible side effects [45]

Medication	Minimal starting dose/maximal recommended dose	Time to full effect of the therapeutic dose	Half-life	Side effects
Levodopa	50 mg/200 mg	At first dose	1.5–2 h	High rates of augmentation and loss of efficacy with rebound phenomena
Ropinirole	0.25 mg/4 mg	4–10 days	6 h	Augmentation, impulse control disorder, nausea, low blood pressure, dizziness, headache, nasal congestion, sleepiness in susceptible patients
Pramipexole	0.125 mg/0.54 mg	At first dose	8–12 h	Augmentation, impulse control disorder, nausea, low blood pressure, dizziness, headache, nasal congestion, sleepiness in susceptible patients
Rotigotine	1 mg/3 mg	1 week	5–7 h	Skin irritation, low risk of augmentation, nausea, low blood pressure, dizziness, headache, nasal congestion, sleepiness in susceptible patients. Risk of impulse control disorder (ICD) may be lower
Pregabalin	25 mg/300 mg	3–6 days	10 h	Sleepiness, dizziness, headache, fluid retention

Table 12.6 (continued)

Medication	Minimal starting dose/ maximal recommended dose	Time to full effect of the therapeutic dose	Half-life	Side effects
Clonazepam	0.50 mg/2.0 mg	First dose: effect mainly on sleep	30–40 h	High risk of sleepiness, dizziness, morning drug hangover
Gabapentin	300 mg/2700 mg	3–6 days	5–7 h	Sleepiness, dizziness, fluid retention
Tramadol	25 mg/100 mg	N/A	5–8 h	Dizziness, sleepiness, constipation, dry mouth
Oxycodone	2.5 mg/25 mg	N/A	2–4 h	Dizziness, fatigue, constipation, nausea
Methadone	2.5 mg/20 mg	N/A	15–60 h	Sedation, nausea, constipation, sleep apnea, prolonged QT interval. ECG recommended

The Movement Disorder Society (MDS) commissioned review looked at 40 new studies for efficacy. The results of this review are summarized as follows [60]:

- Pregabalin, gabapentin enacarbil, and oxycodone/naloxone are considered "efficacious."
- There is a change in evidence base on "likely efficacious" to "efficacious" for rotigotine based on new data.
- Intravenous ferric carboxymaltose and pneumatic compression devices—"likely efficacious."
- Bupropion and clonidine—insufficient evidence for efficacy.
- Dopaminergic agonists and gabapentin continue to be considered efficacious as in 2008.
- Bromocriptine, oxycodone, carbamazepine, and valproic acid—"likely efficacious."
- Oral iron is non-efficacious in iron-sufficient subjects.
- Dopaminergic medications and tramadol require special monitoring for augmentation.
- Drugs that require safety monitoring: cabergoline, pergolide, oxycodone, methadone, tramadol, carbamazepine, and valproic acid.

Alternative and Investigational Therapies

There is limited evidence for pneumatic compression devices [70]. The injection of botulinum toxin into the leg muscles has been studied but has not produced convincing evidence of long-term benefits [71]. Patients have anecdotally claimed possible benefits of cannabis use on RLS; however, this has not been established through controlled clinical trials. Additionally, cannabis can interact with several RLS medications [44]. Partial benefit from spinal cord stimulation has been reported for chronic pain and RLS. Transcutaneous spinal cord stimulation, transcranial and local leg electrical stimulation, deep brain stimulation, and transcranial magnetic stimulation have produced varying results on RLS symptoms with no established efficacy [72]. There is no evidence to support the use of magnesium supplementation. A single controlled trial suggested vitamin C and E's benefits in uremic RLS patients [44]. Figure 12.5 describes the management of RLS based on severity and treatment options. Figure 12.6 lists the treatment complications for RLS.

The management of RLS is considered under the following headings: general considerations, intermittent RLS, chronic persistent RLS, and refractory RLS [44].

Early Morning Rebound

The reappearance of RLS symptoms in the early morning as the medication effect wears off is known as early morning rebound. If no medications are taken, the symptoms worsen but disappear several hours later. Early morning rebound occurs more frequently with those that have a

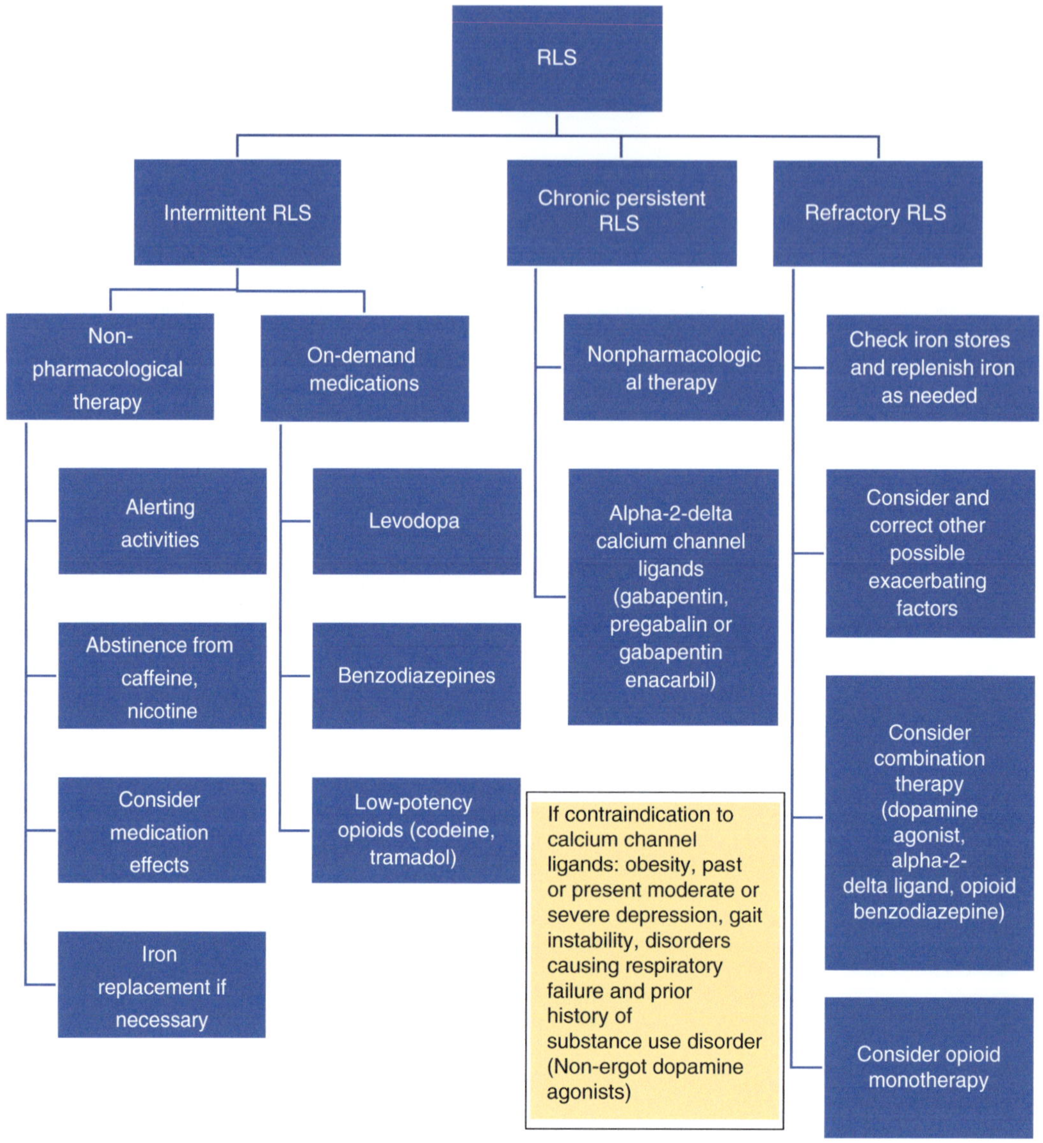

Fig. 12.5 Management of RLS based on severity and treatment options

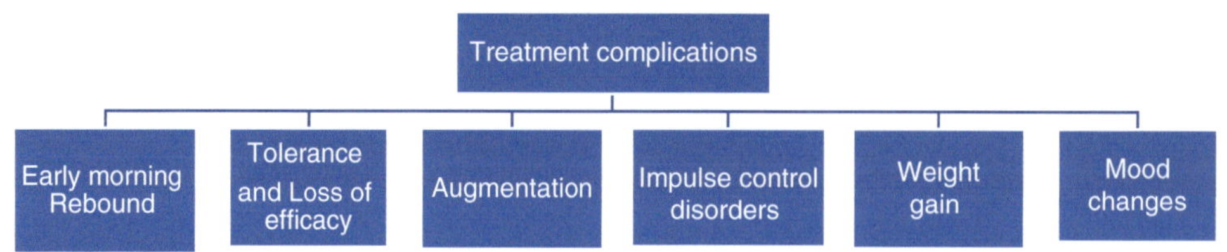

Fig. 12.6 Treatment complications for RLS

short half-life, such as levodopa. Concurrent conditions, such as depression or sleep apnea, should be excluded. Rebound is managed by increasing the dose or changing the time of administration or switching to another dopaminergic drug with a longer half-life [73].

Augmentation

Augmentation is a phenomenon that occurs with chronic daily use of dopaminergic agents and is characterized by onset of symptoms earlier in the day. This is one of the most common reasons for the discontinuation of these agents. There may be an extension of the symptoms to the upper limbs, increase in overall severity, shorter latency to symptom onset, and medication effects lasting for a shorter amount of time. This problem is addressed by gradually increasing the dose of the medication, which can lead to vicious cycle of worsening augmentation. Pramipexole has an annual augmentation rate of 8% [22] and can be as high as 50% with 5 years of use [74].

Levodopa has the greatest rate of augmentation. Among dopaminergic agonists, pramipexole has the highest, and rotigotine has the lowest, with an incidence of approximately 2–3% per year [75]. Low ferritin levels, previous augmentation episodes, and prior tolerance to these medications are predictors of augmentation [75, 76]. Augmentation can be prevented by choosing the lowest effective dose of the dopaminergic medication, choosing long-acting medications like rotigotine, and avoiding medications associated with higher rates of augmentation like levodopa. Dividing the dose with the first dose given in the afternoon before symptoms and the second given at symptom onset may also help; however, this strategy has not been approved [73].

Tolerance and Loss of Efficacy

Tolerance is defined as a decrease in response to a drug over time and requires increased doses to achieve the same response. This must be distinguished from worsening of symptoms due to natural course of the illness, where higher doses would be required. However, with tolerance and loss of efficacy, the symptoms are not worse with treatment initiation, unlike rebound or augmentation [73].

Impulse Control Disorders

Dopaminergic agents can lead to impulse control disorders (ICDs), especially in Parkinson's disease—even though these patients require lower doses of dopaminergic medications [77]. It is estimated to occur in 3% and 17% of patients treated for RLS. Obsessive-compulsive behavior, hypersexuality, and pathologic gambling are some associated symptoms, as well as binge eating, compulsive shopping, and punding (compulsive performance of repetitive, mechanical tasks, such as assembling and disassembling, collecting, or sorting household object) [78]. It is a dose-dependent phenomenon and ceases completely when the dopaminergic agent is stopped. When symptoms are severe, attempts to decrease the dose must be made. If impulse control disturbances continue to persist, switching to another medication is recommended [23].

Weight Gain

Weight gain and obesity are frequently co-occurring problems with sleep disturbances [79]. Approximately 20% and 30% of patients with RLS report eating during nighttime. Alpha-2-delta ligands are associated with weight gain, and the use of dopaminergic agents can cause water retention [23].

Mood Changes

Patients taking alpha-2-delta ligands are at risk of developing depression and suicidal ideations [80]. Furthermore, augmentation is a common trigger of anxiety. Selective serotonin reuptake inhibitors (SSRIs) and serotonin norepinephrine reuptake inhibitors (SNRIs) should be avoided given the risk of worsening RLS symptoms. Depression is preferably treated with medications like bupropion, lamotrigine, trazodone, and desipramine that have a safer adverse effect profile. Cognitive behavior therapy can also be used among these individuals [23].

Conclusion

RLS is a common condition and can have a significant impact on the quality of life due to disturbances of sleep quality and daytime somnolence. Despite being widely prevalent, it is often underrated and trivialized. RLS is associated with a substantial physical and psychological burden; thus, prompt diagnosis and appropriate treatment are critical. Clinicians must be vigilant in recognizing the symptoms and be aware of the effect of RLS on the lives of patients and caregivers. Both nonpharmacological and pharmacological treatments must be used appropriately based on the frequency and severity of symptoms. Mild RLS may be managed with reassurance and lifestyle changes. Secondary causes and exacerbating factors should be identified and treated. Moderate to severe cases require pharmacological treatment. When symptoms are not adequately addressed, significant morbidity can arise and may include anxiety and possible depression. With the advancement in the management of RLS in recent years, there are more options for treatment, resulting in greater relief to patients having this distressing disorder.

References

1. Allen RP, Walters AS, Montplaisir J, Hening W, Myers A, Bell TJ, et al. Restless legs syndrome prevalence and impact: REST general population study. Arch Intern Med. 2005;165(11):1286.
2. Ohayon MM, O'Hara R, Vitiello MV. Epidemiology of restless legs syndrome: a synthesis of the literature. Sleep Med Rev. 2012;16:283.
3. Koo BB. Restless leg syndrome across the globe: epidemiology of the restless legs syndrome/Willis-Ekbom disease. Sleep Med Clin. 2015;10:189.
4. Manconi M, Ulfberg J, Berger K, Ghorayeb I, Wesström J, Fulda S, et al. When gender matters: restless legs syndrome. Report of the 'RLS and woman' workshop endorsed by the European RLS Study Group. Sleep Med Rev. 2012;16:297.
5. Rothdach AJ, Trenkwalder C, Haberstock J, Keil U, Berger K. Prevalence and risk factors of RLS in an elderly population: the MEMO study. Memory and morbidity in Augsburg elderly. Neurology. 2000;54(5):1064.
6. Winkelmann J, Polo O, Provini F, Nevsimalova S, Kemlink D, Sonka K, et al. Genetics of restless legs syndrome (RLS): state-of-the-art and future directions. Mov Disord. 2007;22:S449.
7. Jiménez-Jiménez FJ, Alonso-Navarro H, García-Martín E, Agúndez JAG. Genetics of restless legs syndrome: an update. Sleep Med Rev. 2018;39:108.
8. Trenkwalder C, Allen R, Högl B, Paulus W, Winkelmann J. Restless legs syndrome associated with major diseases: a systematic review and new concept. Neurology. 2016;86(14):1336.
9. O'Keeffe ST, Gavin K, Lavan JN. Iron status and restless legs syndrome in the elderly. Age Ageing. 1994;23(3):200.
10. Darvishi N, Daneshkhah A, Khaledi-Paveh B, Vaisi-Raygani A, Mohammadi M, Salari N, et al. The prevalence of restless legs syndrome/Willis-Ekbom disease (RLS/WED) in the third trimester of pregnancy: a systematic review. BMC Neurol. 2020;20:132.
11. Möller JC, Unger M, Stiasny-Kolster K, Oertel WH. Restless legs syndrome (RLS) and Parkinson's disease (PD)-related disorders or different entities? J Neurol Sci. 2010;289(1–2):135.
12. Schürks M, Winter AC, Berger K, Buring JE, Kurth T. Migraine and restless legs syndrome in women. Cephalalgia. 2012;32(5):382.
13. Akın S, Bölük C, Türk Börü Ü, Taşdemir M, Gezer T, Şahbaz FG, et al. Restless legs syndrome in type 2 diabetes mellitus. Prim Care Diabetes. 2019;13(1):87.
14. Seeman MV. Why are women prone to restless legs syndrome? Int J Environ Res Public Health. 2020;17(1):368.
15. Winter AC, Schürks M, Glynn RJ, Buring JE, Gaziano JM, Berger K, et al. Vascular risk factors, cardiovascular disease, and restless legs syndrome in women. Am J Med. 2013;126(3):220.
16. Clemens S. Restless legs syndrome. In: Zigmond MJ, Wiley CA, Chesselet M-F, editors. Neurobiology of brain disorders. 2nd ed. Academic Press; 2023. p. 659–70 [cited 2022 Sep 20]. Available from: https://linkinghub.elsevier.com/retrieve/pii/B9780323856546000023X.
17. Allen RP, Picchietti DL, Garcia-Borreguero D, Ondo WG, Walters AS, Winkelman JW, et al. Restless legs

syndrome/Willis-Ekbom disease diagnostic criteria: updated International Restless Legs Syndrome Study Group (IRLSSG) consensus criteria—history, rationale, description, and significance. Sleep Med. 2014;15(8):860.

18. Willis T. The London practice of physick. London: Bassett & Cooke; 1685.

19. Ekbom KA. Restless legs: a clinical study of a hitherto overlooked disease in the legs, characterized by peculiar paresthesia. Acta Medica Scand Suppl. 1945;158:1–6.

20. Trenkwalder C, Allen R, Högl B, Paulus W, Winkelmann J. Restless legs syndrome associated with major diseases. Neurology. 2016;86:1336.

21. Byrne R, Sinha S, Chaudhuri KR. Restless legs syndrome: diagnosis and review of management options. Neuropsychiatr Dis Treat. 2006;2:155.

22. During EH, Winkelman JW. Drug treatment of restless legs syndrome in older adults. Drugs Aging. 2019;36:939.

23. Klingelhoefer L, Cova I, Gupta S, Chaudhuri KR. A review of current treatment strategies for restless legs syndrome (Willis-Ekbom disease). Clin Med J R Coll Physicians Lond. 2014;14(5):520.

24. Walters AS, LeBrocq C, Dhar A, Hening W, Rosen R, Allen RP, et al. Validation of the International Restless Legs Syndrome Study Group rating scale for restless legs syndrome. Sleep Med. 2003;4(2):121.

25. Ferri R, Lanuzza B, Cosentino FII, Iero I, Tripodi M, Spada RS, et al. A single question for the rapid screening of restless legs syndrome in the neurological clinical practice. Eur J Neurol. 2007;14(9):1016.

26. Abetz L, Allen R, Follet A, Washburn T, Early C, Kirsch J, et al. Evaluating the quality of life of patients with restless legs syndrome. Clin Ther. 2004;26(6):925.

27. Hening W, Walters AS, Allen RP, Montplaisir J, Myers A, Ferini-Strambi L. Impact, diagnosis and treatment of restless legs syndrome (RLS) in a primary care population: the REST (RLS epidemiology, symptoms, and treatment) primary care study. Sleep Med. 2004;5(3):237.

28. Winkelman JW, Gagnon A, Clair AG. Sensory symptoms in restless legs syndrome: the enigma of pain. Sleep Med. 2013;14:934.

29. Allen RP, Picchietti D, Hening WA, Trenkwalder C, Walters AS, Montplaisi J, et al. Restless legs syndrome: diagnostic criteria, special considerations, and epidemiology. A report from the restless legs syndrome diagnosis and epidemiology workshop at the National Institutes of Health. Sleep Med. 2003;4(2):101.

30. Garcia-Borreguero D, Odin P, Schwarz C. Restless legs syndrome: an overview of the current understanding and management. Acta Neurol Scand. 2004;109:303.

31. Meilak C, Dhawan V, Chaudhuri K. Clinical features. In: Restless legs syndrome. 1st ed. Taylor and Francis Group; 2004.

32. Coleman Phd RM, Pollak CP, Weitzman ED. Periodic movements in sleep (nocturnal myoclonus): relation to sleep disorders. Ann Neurol. 1980;8(4):416.

33. Holmes R, Tluk S, Metta V, Patel P, Rao R, Williams A, et al. Nature and variants of idiopathic restless legs syndrome: observations from 152 patients referred to secondary care in the UK. J Neural Transm. 2007;114(7):929.

34. Rana AQ, Siddiqui I, Mosabbir A, Athar A, Syed O, Jesudasan M, et al. Association of pain, Parkinson's disease, and restless legs syndrome. J Neurol Sci. 2013;327(1–2):32.

35. Karroum EG, Leu-Semenescu S, Arnulf I. Topography of the sensations in primary restless legs syndrome. J Neurol Sci. 2012;320(1–2):26.

36. Ondo W. Restless legs syndrome "patient odyssey" survey of disease burden on patient and spouses/partners. Sleep Med. 2018;47:51.

37. Hornyak M. Depressive disorders in restless legs syndrome: epidemiology, pathophysiology and management. CNS Drugs. 2010;24:89.

38. Koo BB, Blackwell T, Lee HB, Stone KL, Louis ED, Redline S. Restless legs syndrome and depression: effect mediation by disturbed sleep and periodic limb movements. Am J Geriatr Psychiatr. 2016;24(11):1105.

39. Pearson VE, Allen RP, Dean T, Gamaldo CE, Lesage SR, Earley CJ. Cognitive deficits associated with restless legs syndrome (RLS). Sleep Med. 2006;7(1):25.

40. Walters AS, Frauscher B, Allen R, Benes H, Chaudhuri KR, Garcia-Borreguero D, et al. Review of quality of life instruments for the restless legs syndrome/Willis-Ekbom disease (RLS/WED): critique and recommendations. J Clin Sleep Med. 2014;10:1351.

41. Pennestri MH, Whittom S, Adam B, Petit D, Carrier J, Montplaisir J. PLMS and PLMW in healthy subjects as a function of age: prevalence and interval distribution. Sleep. 2006;29(9):1183.

42. Managing patients with restless legs. Drug Ther Bull. 2003;41:91.

43. Chaudhuri KR. The restless legs syndrome: time to recognize a very common movement disorder. Pract Neurol. 2003;3:204.

44. Silber MH, Buchfuhrer MJ, Earley CJ, Koo BB, Manconi M, Winkelman JW, et al. The management of restless legs syndrome: an updated algorithm. Mayo Clin Proc. 2021;96(7):1921–37.

45. Garcia-Borreguero D, Stillman P, Benes H, Buschmann H, Chaudhuri KR, Gonzalez Rodríguez VM, et al. Algorithms for the diagnosis and treatment of restless legs syndrome in primary care. BMC Neurol. 2011;11:28.

46. Bayard M, Bailey B, Acharya D, Ambreen F, Duggal S, Kaur T, et al. Bupropion and restless legs syndrome: a randomized controlled trial. J Am Board Fam Med. 2011;24(4):422.

47. Benamer H. Restless legs syndrome: the underrecognised condition. Libyan J Med. 2006;1(2):172

[cited 2022 Oct 5]. Available from: /pmc/articles/PMC3081357/.

48. Rivera-Oliver M. The modulatory role of caffeine and other adenosine receptor antagonists onto spinal locomotor circuits: evidence for its dependence on adenosine A1-dopamine D1 receptor heteromers in spinal motoneurons. ProQuest Dissertations and Theses. 2017.

49. Ferré S, Quiroz C, Guitart X, Rea W, Seyedian A, Moreno E, et al. Pivotal role of adenosine neurotransmission in restless legs syndrome. Front Neurosci. 2018;11:722.

50. Ferini-Strambi L, Aarskog D, Partinen M, Chaudhuri KR, Sohr M, Verri D, et al. Effect of pramipexole on RLS symptoms and sleep: a randomized, double-blind, placebo-controlled trial. Sleep Med. 2008;9(8):874–81.

51. Oertel WH, Stiasny-Kolster K, Bergtholdt B, Hallström Y, Albo J, Leissner L, et al. Efficacy of pramipexole in restless legs syndrome: a six-week, multicenter, randomized, double-blind study (effect-RLS study). Mov Disord. 2007;22(2):213.

52. Trenkwalder C, Garcia-Borreguero D, Montagna P, Lainey E, de Weerd AW, Tidswell P, et al. Ropinirole in the treatment of restless legs syndrome: results from the TREAT RLS 1 study, a 12 week, randomised, placebo controlled study in 10 European countries. J Neurol Neurosurg Psychiatry. 2004;75(1):92.

53. Walters AS, Ondo WG, Dreykluft T, Grunstein R, Lee D, Sethi K, et al. Ropinirole is effective in the treatment of restless legs syndrome. TREAT RLS 2: a 12-week, double-blind, randomized, parallel-group, placebo-controlled study. Mov Disord. 2004;19(12):1414.

54. Trenkwalder C, Beneš H, Poewe W, Oertel WH, Garcia-Borreguero D, de Weerd AW, et al. Efficacy of rotigotine for treatment of moderate-to-severe restless legs syndrome: a randomised, double-blind, placebo-controlled trial. Lancet Neurol. 2008;7(7):595.

55. Zanettini R, Antonini A, Gatto G, Gentile R, Tesei S, Pezzoli G. Valvular heart disease and the use of dopamine agonists for Parkinson's disease. N Engl J Med. 2007;356(1):39.

56. Trenkwalder C, Benes H, Grote L, Happe S, Högl B, Mathis J, et al. Cabergoline compared to levodopa in the treatment of patients with severe restless legs syndrome: results from a multi-center, randomized, active controlled trial. Mov Disord. 2007;22(5):696.

57. Benes H. Transdermal lisuride: short-term efficacy and tolerability study in patients with severe restless legs syndrome. Sleep Med. 2006;7(1):31.

58. Beneš H, Kurella B, Kummer J, Kazenwadel J, Selzer R, Kohnen R. Rapid onset of action of levodopa in restless legs syndrome: a double-blind, randomized, multicenter, crossover trial. Sleep. 1999;22(8):1073.

59. Stiasny-Kolster K, Kohnen R, Möller JC, Trenkwalder C, Oertel WH. Validation of the 'L-DOPA test' for diagnosis of restless legs syndrome. Mov Disord. 2006;21(9):1333.

60. Winkelmann J, Allen RP, Högl B, Inoue Y, Oertel W, Salminen AV, et al. Treatment of restless legs syndrome: evidence-based review and implications for clinical practice (revised 2017). Mov Disord. 2018;33:1077.

61. Kim ES, Deeks ED. Gabapentin enacarbil: a review in restless legs syndrome. Drugs. 2016;76:879.

62. Kume A. Gabapentin enacarbil for the treatment of moderate to severe primary restless legs syndrome (Willis-Ekbom disease): 600 or 1,200 mg dose? Neuropsychiatr Dis Treat. 2014;10:249.

63. Aurora RN, Kristo DA, Bista SR, Rowley JA, Zak RS, Casey KR, et al. The treatment of restless legs syndrome and periodic limb movement disorder in adults—an update for 2012: practice parameters with an evidence-based systematic review and meta-analyses. Sleep. 2012;35:1037.

64. Trenkwalder C, Beneš H, Grote L, García-Borreguero D, Högl B, Hopp M, et al. Prolonged release oxycodone-naloxone for treatment of severe restless legs syndrome after failure of previous treatment: a double-blind, randomised, placebo-controlled trial with an open-label extension. Lancet Neurol. 2013;12(12):1141.

65. Fick DM, Semla TP, Steinman M, Beizer J, Brandt N, Dombrowski R, et al. American Geriatrics Society 2019 Updated AGS Beers Criteria® for potentially inappropriate medication use in older adults. J Am Geriatr Soc. 2019;67(4):674.

66. Telstad W, Sørensen O, Larsen S, Lillevold PE, Stensrud P, Nyberg-Hansen R. Treatment of the restless legs syndrome with carbamazepine: a double blind study. Br Med J. 1984;288(6415):444.

67. Youssef EA, Wagner ML, Martinez JO, Hening W. Pilot trial of lamotrigine in the restless legs syndrome. Sleep Med. 2005;6:89.

68. Rinaldi F, Galbiati A, Marelli S, Ferini Strambi L, Zucconi M. Treatment Options in Intractable Restless Legs Syndrome/Willis-Ekbom Disease (RLS/WED). Curr Treat Options Neurol. 2016;18(2):7.

69. Allen RP, Picchietti DL, Auerbach M, Cho YW, Connor JR, Earley CJ, et al. Evidence-based and consensus clinical practice guidelines for the iron treatment of restless legs syndrome/Willis-Ekbom disease in adults and children: an IRLSSG task force report. Sleep Med. 2018;41:27–44.

70. Lettieri CJ, Eliasson AH. Pneumatic compression devices are an effective therapy for restless legs syndrome: a prospective, randomized, double-blinded, sham-controlled trial. Chest. 2009;135(1):74.

71. Mittal SO, Machado D, Richardson D, Dubey D, Jabbari B. Botulinum toxin in restless legs syndrome—a randomized double-blind placebo-controlled cross-over study. Toxins (Basel). 2018;10(10):401.

72. Silber MH, Buchfuhrer MJ, Earley CJ, Koo BB, Manconi M, Winkelman JW, et al. The management of restless legs syndrome: an updated algorithm. Mayo Clin Proc. 2021;96(7):1921–37 [cited 2022 Sep

20]. Available from: http://www.mayoclinicproceedings.org/article/S0025619620314890/fulltext.

73. Klingelhoefer L, Cova I, Gupta S, Chaudhuri KR. A review of current treatment strategies for restless legs syndrome (Willis-Ekbom disease). Clin Med (Lond). 2014;14(5):520–4 [cited 2023 Jan 14]. Available from: https://pubmed.ncbi.nlm.nih.gov/25301914/.

74. Silver N, Allen RP, Senerth J, Earley CJ. A 10-year, longitudinal assessment of dopamine agonists and methadone in the treatment of restless legs syndrome. Sleep Med. 2011;12(5):440.

75. García-Borreguero D, Williams AM. Dopaminergic augmentation of restless legs syndrome. Sleep Med Rev. 2010;14:339.

76. Trenkwalder C, Högl B, Benes H, Kohnen R. Augmentation in restless legs syndrome is associated with low ferritin. Sleep Med. 2008;9(5):572.

77. Antonini A, Cilia R. Behavioural adverse effects of dopaminergic treatments in Parkinsons disease: incidence, neurobiological basis, management and prevention. Drug Saf. 2009;32:475.

78. Cornelius JR, Tippmann-Peikert M, Slocumb NL, Frerichs CF, Silber MH. Impulse control disorders with the use of dopaminergic agents in restless legs syndrome: a case-control study. Sleep. 2010;33(1):81.

79. Chaput JP, Després JP, Bouchard C, Tremblay A. The association between sleep duration and weight gain in adults: a 6-year prospective study from the Quebec family study. Sleep. 2008;31(4):517.

80. King MA. Pregabalin and gabapentin associated with depression and suicidal ideation. BMJ. 2018;363:k4979.

Schizophrenia Spectrum and Other Psychotic Disorders

Schizophrenia

13

Alison Liss and Seetha Chandrasekhara

Epidemiology

Schizophrenia is defined by the Diagnostic and Statistical Manual of Mental Disorders, Fifth Edition (DSM-5), as a disorder characterized by the presence of five different symptoms: delusions, hallucinations, disorganized speech, disorganized or catatonic behavior, and negative symptoms such as flat affect or avolition [1]. At least two symptoms must be present over a 1-month period with at least one of the symptoms being either delusions, hallucinations, or disorganized speech. People with schizophrenia have a significantly increased risk of premature mortality when compared to those without schizophrenia; however, people with schizophrenia are now living longer [2]. By 2025, it is estimated that over 25% of those living with schizophrenia will be over the age of 55 years [3, 4]. Since the average life span of people with schizophrenia is 20–25 years shorter than age-matched controls, studies examining older adults with schizophrenia often include individuals who are ≥50 years

[5, 6]. The prevalence of schizophrenia in persons aged 45–60 years is approximately 0.6–1% and for those aged ≥65 years is approximately 0.1–0.5% [3, 7].

While most persons with schizophrenia develop the disorder before the age of 40 years, it is estimated that between 14.8% and 36.4% of individuals can develop this disorder later in life [7]. By consensus, schizophrenia onset before the age of 40 is generally referred to as early-onset schizophrenia (EOS), onset between the ages of 40 and 60 years as late-onset schizophrenia (LOS), and after age 60 as very-late-onset schizophrenia (VLOSP), although newer nomenclature terms the latter as very-late-onset schizophrenia-like psychosis (VLOSLP) [8]. It is not yet clear whether LOS and VLOSLP are the same disorder as EOS that developed later in life, or if they constitute totally separate disorders [9]. Compared to patients with EOS, patients with LOS are more likely to be women and less likely to have relatives with schizophrenia [10, 11]. Patients with LOS are also more likely to have symptoms such as tactile or visual hallucinations, auditory hallucinations with running commentary, and persecutory delusions. Some studies have also shown that LOS patients have fewer negative symptoms, although this has not been consistently replicated [6, 9, 10]. Differences between EOS, LOS, and VLOSLP are organized in Table 13.1.

A. Liss (✉)
Temple University Hospital, Philadelphia, PA, USA
e-mail: alison.liss@tuhs.temple.edu

S. Chandrasekhara
Department of Psychiatry, Lewis Katz School of Medicine at Temple University,
Philadelphia, PA, USA
e-mail: tuc32963@temple.edu

Table 13.1 Differences between schizophrenia categories

Types	Age of onset	Symptom features	Epidemiology and risk factors	Social features
Early-onset schizophrenia (EOS)	Before age 40 years (<40 years)	– Negative symptoms definitely present – Learning/ retention preserved – Cognitive decline	– Family history of schizophrenia/cluster A personality disorder – Substance use	– Lower educational achievement – More social difficulties in childhood
Late-onset schizophrenia (LOS)	Age 40–60 years	– Learning/ retention preserved – Cognitive decline – More positive symptoms	– Family history of schizophrenia/cluster A personality disorder – More in women – Sensory impairment – Less substance use exposure	– Higher educational achievement – Low socioeconomic status – Immigration status – Unemployment
Very late-onset schizophrenia-like psychosis (VLOSLP)	After age 60 years (>60 years)	– Learning/ retention impaired – Progressive cognitive decline very high – More positive symptoms	– More in women – Brain structure aberrations – Sensory impairment – Less substance use exposure	– Higher educational achievement – Low socioeconomic status – Immigration status – Unemployment

Risk Factors

The etiology of schizophrenia is not yet known, although it is thought to be caused by genetic, environmental, and psychosocial factors in what is known as the "two-hit" theory of development of schizophrenia [12]. This theory describes a person with an underlying susceptibility to schizophrenia experiencing a later insult, which leads to the development of the illness. The heritability of schizophrenia is estimated to be approximately 79% with a variety of candidate genes that are currently under investigation [13]. Environmental and psychosocial risk factors for the development of schizophrenia include exposure to urban environments, identity as a first- or second-generation immigrant, maternal exposure to *Toxoplasma gondii*, and adolescent cannabis use [14–17]. Advanced paternal age has also been implicated, although it is not clear if this is due to genetic factors, environmental factors, or a combination of the two [18].

Patients with LOS and VLOSLP have a different set of risk factors compared to those with EOS. Chen et al. found that, when compared to patients with EOS, patients with LOS were less likely to have a positive family history of schizophrenia, less likely to have early psychosocial struggles, more likely to have achieved a higher level of education, and were less likely to have a recent or lifetime substance use history. LOS was associated with significantly higher rates of unemployment [19]. Another study found that baseline visual impairment was a risk factor for LOS [20].

There have been numerous studies investigating the genetic influence on the age of onset in schizophrenia, although to our knowledge only one study has specifically examined the genotype of patients with age of onset of symptoms after 40 years [21–24]. In that study by Rasmussen et al., they focused on the gene encoding the chemokine receptor CCR5, which has been associated with immune-mediated diseases. They compared patients with EOS and LOS and healthy controls and found that people with two copies of a specific deletion allele were overrepresented among the LOS group. The authors proposed two potential mechanisms for this finding: it could be that the deletion allele is a protective factor that delays the onset of illness in those already predisposed towards it, or it could be that the deletion allele is a susceptibility factor itself for LOS [25].

LOS and VLOSLP are relatively more common in women when compared to men, and one hypothesis for this finding is that estrogen is a protective factor against psychosis. It is theorized that declining levels of estrogen after menopause may lead to an unmasking of psychosis [10]. There are a variety of proposed mechanisms of why estrogen can protect against psychosis. These include that estrogen may directly affect brain structure through neurogenesis and neuronal plasticity; that estrogen is neuroprotective against oxidative stress and inflammation; and that estrogen modulates dopaminergic, serotonergic, and glutamatergic activity in the CNS [26].

Assessment

In people presenting with symptoms of psychosis for the first time in later life, the workup should first rule out other medical causes. Common medical causes of psychosis are presented in Table 13.2.

Workup commonly includes a complete blood count (CBC), comprehensive metabolic panel (CMP), thyroid-stimulating hormone (TSH), vitamin B12, folate, rapid plasma reagin (RPR), erythrocyte sedimentation rate (ESR), HIV, and toxicology as well as brain imaging either by magnetic resonance imaging (MRI) or by computerized tomography (CT) scans [3]. The patient's medication list should be examined carefully, as a variety of medications can induce psychosis including glucocorticoids, anticholinergic medications, levodopa, and interferon [27–30]. Additionally, a good psychiatric history

Table 13.2 Psychosis—medical considerations

Classification	Causes
Endocrinologic	Adrenal Pancreas Parathyroid Thyroid
Infectious	Encephalitis Immunodeficiency Meningitis Neurosyphilis Pneumonia
Metabolic	Electrolyte disturbance Encephalopathy Enzyme deficiency Hypoxia/hypercapnia Vitamin/nutritional deficiency
Neurologic	Cerebrovascular event Epilepsy Genetic disorder Inflammatory Neurodegeneration Sleep disorder Tumor

should be taken to differentiate schizophrenia from schizoaffective disorder, bipolar disorder, and major depressive disorder with psychotic features, all of which can present with psychosis.

A major difficulty in the diagnosis of schizophrenia in later life is to differentiate it from dementias such as Alzheimer's disease (AD), dementia with Lewy bodies (DLB), frontotemporal dementia (FTD), vascular dementia (VaD), and Parkinson's disease (PD). Psychosis is present in 75% of patients with DLB, 50% of patients with PD, 30% of patients with AD, 15% of patients with VaD, and 10% of patients with FTD [31]. These symptoms can be present in the early stages of the illness [32, 33]. A study by Woolley et al. found that 28.2% of patients with a neurodegenerative disease initially received a diagnosis of a primary psychiatric disorder [34].

Van Assche et al. described the different phenomenology typically seen in VLOSLP compared to AD and DLB [35]. They found that people with VLOSLP more commonly had paranoid delusions and partition delusions (the belief that things that would normally be considered a barrier can be breached by people, substances, or objects) as well as multimodal hallucinations (auditory, visual, tactile, gustatory, and olfactory). They heard human voices more frequently than those with DLB or AD. Individuals with DLB had prominent visual hallucinations, typically of people or animals, and less frequent delusions when compared to those with AD and VLOSLP. All the patients with AD in the study experienced delusions, the majority of which were paranoid, and many also experienced hallucinations, most frequently visual [35]. Cooper and Ovsiew described the overlapping presentation of FTD and schizophrenia and found that a significant lack of empathy as well as hyperorality or compulsive eating could be used to differentiate FTD from schizophrenia [36].

It is important to carefully differentiate between LOS and VLOSLP and neurocognitive disorders because treatment with atypical antipsychotics in patients with dementia is associated with an increased risk of death compared to placebo [37]. One study in the United States found that there are racial disparities in the diagnosis of schizophrenia in nursing home residents. Specifically, Black schizophrenia nursing home residents with Alzheimer's disease and related dementias (ADRD) are more likely to receive a diagnosis of schizophrenia than white nursing home residents with ADRD [38].

Treatments

Non-pharmacological

Psychosocial Interventions

Robust psychosocial interventions for older adults with schizophrenia are an important part of treatment. Isolation and poor psychosocial functioning are especially problems for older adults who developed EOS, who are less likely to have been employed, pursued long-lasting relationships, or completed their education [19]. They are often cared for by family members who, as they age, are no longer able to provide care [10]. Interventions that target social skills and cognitive remediation are useful in improving the quality of life and functional status of older people with schizophrenia. Three such manualized interventions have shown positive results: Cognitive Behavioral Social Skills Training (CBSST), an intervention designed for older adults with schizophrenia which incorporates techniques from both CBT and social skills training; Functional Adaptation Skill Training (FAST), which emphasizes living skills such as money management; and Helping Older People Experience Success (HOPES), which combines skill training with monthly preventative health care visits [39–42]. Other studies have shown that social clubs, aerobic exercise, and group video game play improve social functioning and decrease isolation [43–45].

Neuromodulation

Electroconvulsive therapy (ECT) has been shown to reduce psychotic symptoms in treatment-resistant patients with schizophrenia [46, 47]. ECT has been extensively studied for use in geriatric depression as well as for the behavioral and psychological symptoms of dementia, where it has been found to be safe and efficacious, but there are limited data about the use of ECT for geriatric schizophrenia in particular [48, 49]. One study by Shelef et al. examined the use of ECT in older adults with serious mental illness, half of whom had schizophrenia [50]. They found that maintenance ECT—that is, ECT continued after the completion of the initial acute treatment which is intended to prevent relapse—led to a reduction in both number of hospitalizations and length of hospitalization. In one case report, a patient with VLOSLP experienced remission of psychotic symptoms after ten sessions of ECT after having failed six atypical antipsychotic trials [51]. Similarly, while deep brain stimulation (DBS) and transcranial magnetic stimulation (TMS) have been shown to be efficacious in schizophrenia, there is no data regarding the treatment efficacy of either treatment modality among older adults [52, 53].

Pharmacological

Medication Classes

Antipsychotics are the psychopharmacological treatments of choice for older adults with schizophrenia, as they are with younger adults [8, 10]. Although the 2019 updated Beers Criteria label antipsychotics as a class of medication to avoid, they note an exception for patients with schizophrenia or bipolar disorder [54]. The majority of studies examining the treatment of both older adults with EOS and patients with LOS and VLOSLP focus on second-generation antipsychotics (SGAs). First-generation antipsychotics (FGAs) are more likely to cause extrapyramidal symptoms (EPS) and tardive dyskinesia, both of which older adults are more sensitive to, and thus are typically avoided. They may still be used in patients with EOS who have been stabilized on a certain drug for a number of years.

Most studies on the use of antipsychotics to treat psychotic disorders focus on people who develop these disorders in early life, but there have been some studies focused on the treatment of LOS and VLOSLP. One study examined that the use of SGAs in both inpatients and outpatients with VLOSLP found that 38% of outpatients and 77% of inpatients had a positive response to treatment with an SGA [55].

Certain antipsychotics are available in long-acting injectable formulations, eliminating the need to take a daily pill. Long-acting injectables can also be used in older adult patients. Lin et al. evaluated rehospitalization rates in older patients with schizophrenia over 1 year following hospital discharge for patients treated with oral antipsychotics compared to long-acting injectables [56]. They found that patients treated with long-acting injectables had significantly lower rehospitalization rates and significantly longer time to rehospitalization compared to patients treated with an oral antipsychotic.

Medication Dosages and Levels

Older individuals typically require lower doses of antipsychotic medication than their younger counterparts. There are a variety of reasons why these patients may be more sensitive to antipsychotics: the blood-brain barrier becomes more permeable with aging, leading to increased penetration of the drug into the brain; there is a decrease in the activity of the dopaminergic system and the synthesis of dopamine enzymes; and the catabolism of dopamine increases and dopamine reuptake decreases [57].

Because there is a paucity of recent data on the efficacy of FGAs in older adults, this subsection will focus on SGAs, which are now the first-line treatment for schizophrenia in older adults.

Amisulpride

Three recent studies have examined the use of amisulpride, an SGA, in VLOSLP. The first, a randomized double-blinded control trial, compared patients in three different treatment arms: the first were given amisulpride 100 mg daily for 36 weeks, the second took amisulpride 100 mg daily for 12 weeks followed by placebo for 24 weeks, and the third placebo for 12 weeks followed by amisulpride 100 mg for 24 weeks [58]. The participants were then assessed for efficacy using the 126-point Brief Psychiatric Rating Scale (BPRS scale). The investigators found a mean improvement of 12 points in the treatment group when compared to 4 points in the placebo group. The most common serious adverse events were infection and extrapyramidal symptoms. This study was also noteworthy for using a significantly lower dose of the drug than the typical dose for people with EOS, which is 400–800 mg. The second study found similar results using doses of amisulpride of 50–200 mg/day; they did not find any changes in abnormal movement scales before and after amisulpride treatment [59]. A final study looked at efficacy as well as blood serum concentration of the drug and D2/D3 receptor occupancy. They similarly found that doses as low as 50 mg daily were efficacious, with correspondingly lower blood drug concentrations. The D2/D3 receptors had occupancy of up to 40%, which is similar to those in younger adults treated with higher doses [60]. Of note, amisulpride is not approved by the Food and Drug Administration (FDA) in the United States for treatment of schizophrenia.

Aripiprazole

Aripiprazole has a more favorable side effect profile compared to many other antipsychotics and thus may be preferred when there are concerns about side effect profile [61]. It is also less likely to cause metabolic disorders and additionally has a lower risk of QTc prolongation compared to other first- and second-generation antipsychotics. There is no controlled data on the use of aripiprazole specifically in older adults, but one study which included subjects up to age 77 years found that aripiprazole 15 mg/day was an effective and tolerable dose in the older adult population [61]. The recommended starting dose of aripiprazole in older adults is 2.5–5 mg/day [10]. One small naturalistic study of using SGAs to treat VLOSLP which used a variety of SGAs, including aripiprazole, found that doses from 5 to 15 mg were efficacious and well tolerated [55]. Aripiprazole is also available as a long-acting injectable medication, although we are not aware of any data evaluating its use in older adults.

Clozapine

Clozapine is often considered to be the gold standard drug for treatment-resistant schizophrenia [62]. However, its use is limited by its serious side effect profile. The clearance of clozapine and its metabolite, norclozapine, decreases with age leading older adults with an increased risk of adverse effects, although some adverse effects such as agranulocytosis do not appear to be related to plasma concentration [63, 64]. Agranulocytosis is the most well-known side effect of clozapine, and several studies have suggested that older adults are more likely to develop agranulocytosis and more likely to die from it. Other adverse side effects include the potential for myocarditis, seizures, severe constipation, as well as significant metabolic syndrome [64]. Due to these serious potential side effects, clozapine is not a first-line choice for the treatment of schizophrenia in older adults but may be considered when other medications have failed or when a patient has been stable on clozapine for several years. When starting clozapine in older adults, the recommended starting dose is as low as 6.25 mg/day, with a target dose of approximately 50–100 mg/day, significantly lower than the target total daily dose for younger adults [10].

Olanzapine

Olanzapine was found by the landmark CATIE study to be the most efficacious antipsychotic in the study as measured by time to discontinuation of the drug as a stand-in for efficacy and tolerability [62]. That study included patients aged 18–65 years, but it has also been studied in older adults, primarily in head-to-head trials with risperidone. One study examined patients over the age of 60 years who switched from an FGA to either olanzapine or risperidone [65]. Drug dosage was at the discretion of the treating physician; the mean daily dose for olanzapine at the close of the trial was 12.4 mg. Olanzapine was associated with a significant decrease in BPRS scores, and there was a significant reduction in parkinsonism between baseline and 6-month follow-up. The investigators also conducted quality-of-life assessments and found that when compared to risperidone, patients treated with olanzapine reported better overall quality of life as well as being more satisfied with their health; they reported being in better physical health and had better social relationships [65]. Another study of patients aged ≥60 years compared treatment with olanzapine to treatment with risperidone and found that olanzapine was associated with a significant reduction in the Positive and Negative Syndrome Scale (PANSS) scores with a mean dose of 10 mg daily [66]. This study found that extrapyramidal symptoms (EPSs) were present in 15.9% of patients treated with olanzapine and that while clinically significant weight gain was found in both groups, it was greater in the cohort treated with olanzapine. Olanzapine is also available as a long-acting injectable formulation; there are no studies that we are aware of on the use of olanzapine long-acting injectable specifically in older adults. However, studies have been conducted with patients up to age 75 years which showed similar safety and efficacy profiles as with oral olanzapine [67].

Olanzapine has also been studied in the VLOSLP population. In this small naturalistic study, a variety of SGAs were used in an effort to determine their efficacy; olanzapine was found to be efficacious with some patients in doses from 5 to 12.5 mg [55].

Quetiapine

Mazeh et al. studied the use of quetiapine in a small group of older adults with schizophrenia with average age of 72.2 years [68]. All patients had been on a different SGA prior to being switched to quetiapine. The investigators found a significant reduction in BPRS score from baseline to the end of the study. Additionally, they found no worsening of movement side effects, and in fact there was an improvement in the Abnormal Involuntary Movement Scale (AIMS) score from baseline. Patients in the study were treated with 50–800 mg quetiapine, with a mean dose of 391 mg. There is limited data on the use of quetiapine in VLOSLP. A small naturalistic study followed patients on a variety of SGAs and found quetiapine to be efficacious at doses of 75–150 mg [55].

Risperidone

As described above, there is data comparing the use of risperidone in older adults with schizophrenia to the use of olanzapine. One study examined patients over the age of 60 who switched from an FGA to either olanzapine or risperidone [65]. Drug dosage was at the discretion of the treating physician; the mean daily dose for risperidone at the close of the trial was 1.97 mg/day. Risperidone was associated with a significant decrease in BPRS scores, and there was a significant reduction in parkinsonism between baseline and 6-month follow-up. Unlike olanzapine, risperidone was not associated with improved quality of life [65]. Another study that was mentioned earlier, which compared treatment with olanzapine to treatment with risperidone, found that risperidone was associated with a significant reduction in PANSS scores, with a mean dose of 2 mg/day [66]. This study found that EPS-related adverse events were reported in 9.2% of patients in the risperidone group and 15.9% in the olanzapine group, but this treatment difference was not statistically significant. While clinically significant weight gain was found in both groups, it was less pronounced in the risperidone group when compared to those individuals treated with olanzapine [66]. There is a long-acting injectable formulation of risperidone which has been studied in older adults. In a study of patients aged ≥65 years, risperidone in doses of 25, 50, or 75 mg using the long-acting injectable formulation all achieved significant reduction in their total PANSS scores [69]. In this study, severity of movement disorders was also significantly reduced with the use of risperidone [69].

Adverse Effects and Their Treatments

Adverse effects of antipsychotics are more common in older adults, including cardiovascular effects, hematologic changes, metabolic changes, hyponatremia, motor symptoms, anticholinergic side effects, and antihistaminic side effects [70, 71].

The most serious adverse event related to antipsychotic drug use in older adults is the risk of sudden death in patients with dementia, which led the FDA to issue a black box warning for all antipsychotics in 2008 [72]. One study that evaluated the risk of sudden death in older adults with dementia newly initiated on SGAs compared them to those individuals not on antipsychotic medications, as well as the risk of sudden death in patients treated with SGAs when compared to those treated with FGAs [73]. New use of SGAs was associated with increased mortality at both 30 and 180 days for both community-dwelling individuals and those individuals in long-term care facilities. The investigators also found that the risk of sudden death in those treated with FGAs was even greater than the risk of those treated with SGAs [73]. Another study compared the risk of death of FGAs to SGAs in older adults with or without dementia. In this study, both groups had increased 180-day mortality, with a 14.1% risk of death in the FGA group and a 9.6% risk of death in the SGA group [74].

Numerous studies have also found an increased risk of cerebrovascular accidents in elderly patients treated with antipsychotics [75]. One study found that current or recent older adult users of antipsychotic medication had an increased risk of cerebrovascular adverse events, with an odds ratio of 1.7 [76]. They found that the risk of these adverse events was highest in the first week after initiation of medication and that by 3 months the risk of cerebrovascular adverse events in users of antipsychotics was comparable to nonusers. There was no increased risk associated with cumulative exposure.

It has long been known that drug-induced parkinsonism secondary to antipsychotic use is more common among older adults, even when controlling for spontaneous PD. This is true for both FGAs and SGAs, even though SGAs are generally understood to have a lower risk of EPS [77]. One study found that 46% of older adults treated with low doses of haloperidol developed parkinsonism; they did not find that this effect was dependent on dosage, duration of use, or plasma concentration of the drug [78]. Another study compared the risk of parkinsonism with the use of risperidone, olanzapine, or quetiapine [79]. They found that, while all of the medications could lead to parkinsonism, the risk was higher with the use of risperidone or olanzapine compared to quetiapine. Other extrapyramidal symptoms, however, are not more likely to occur among older adults; akathisia occurs at similar rates regardless of age, and dystonia is rare [76]. Most studies also show that older adults develop tardive dyskinesia at higher rates and more quickly than younger patients [77]. This risk is lower, however, among patients receiving SGAs; one systematic review found that 23% of older patients treated with FGAs had developed tardive dyskinesia at 1 year, compared to 7% of patients treated with SGAs [80]. Another study compared the risk of tardive dyskinesia among antipsychotic naïve patients aged ≥55 years who were treated with either risperidone or olanzapine [81]. In this study, among patients treated with risperidone, rates of tardive dyskinesia were 5.3% after 1 year and 7.2% after 2 years; among those treated with olanzapine, the rates were 6.7% and 11.1%, respectively. Risk factors for developing

tardive dyskinesia were female sex, African-American race, and co-treatment with FGAs.

Drug-induced parkinsonism can be treated with anticholinergic medications such as benztropine or trihexyphenidyl [82]. However, the risks of using these agents must be weighed carefully, as they can precipitate delirium in older adults as well as other side effects such as memory impairment, urinary retention, and constipation [82]. Drug-induced parkinsonism does not need to be treated, unless it is bothersome to the patient and an alternative to adding a second medication for side effect management could be lowering the dose of the offending agent [82]. In contrast to drug-induced parkinsonism, tardive dyskinesia is not improved by lowering the dose of the offending drug and in fact may be worsened [83]. Vesicular monoamine transporter type 2 (VMAT-2) inhibitors such as deutetrabenazine or valbenazine can be used to treat tardive dyskinesia. Both medications have been shown to be safe and efficacious in older adults [83, 84].

While motor side effects are more common with treatment using FGAs, metabolic side effects are more common using SGAs [85]. However, among older adults, there is limited data about the metabolic risks of second-generation antipsychotic use. One case-control study compared HgbA1c, fasting glucose, total cholesterol, low-density lipoproteins (LDL), ratio, and fasting triglyceride levels over 3 months of users of SGAs compared to controls not on SGAs. The only significant difference found in the metabolic parameters was a small increase in the cholesterol ratio of cases when compared to controls [85]. A review article, which primarily examined studies on the use of SGAs in patients with dementia, found that there was limited evidence for adverse changes in weight, glucose metabolism, or lipids in this population, in contrast to the side effect profile in younger patients [86]. However, the risk of metabolic disturbances as a side effect of SGAs should not be ignored given the fact that metabolic syndrome affects half of the older adults with schizophrenia [87]. There is data that metformin can be used adjunctly to mitigate the risk of antipsychotic-associated

Table 13.3 Medications—dosing for schizophrenia in older adults

Medication	Half-life	Starting daily dose (mg)	Maximum daily dose (mg)
Amisulpride[a]	12 h	50	200
Aripiprazole	75 h Metabolite (94 h)	2.5	20
Clozapine	8 h (4–12 h, single dose) 12 h (4–66 h, steady state)	6.25	100
Olanzapine	30 h (21–54 h)	2.5	15
Quetiapine	6 h	25	300
Risperidone	3–20 h Metabolite (21–30 h)	0.5	3

[a] Not approved for treatment of schizophrenia in the United States by the Food and Drug Administration

weight gain, hyperlipidemia, and insulin resistance though to our knowledge no studies have looked at metformin for antipsychotic-associated metabolic disturbances specifically in older adults [88, 89]. In some practices, it is now standard of practice to begin metformin when initiating olanzapine or clozapine, the antipsychotics with highest risk of metabolic disorders [90].

Other risks of antipsychotic use have been found. One study found that there was a dose-dependent increased risk for community-acquired pneumonia among older adults during treatment with either FGAs or SGAs [91]. Studies have also shown that antipsychotic treatment carries an increased risk of hip fracture, and this risk is particularly elevated among older adults [92]. Medications with their half-life, starting, and maximum doses are listed in Table 13.3.

Evidence-Based Treatment Algorithms

Expert consensus guidelines on the use of antipsychotics in older patients were published in 2004 [93]. Those guidelines favored the use of SGAs over FGAs for schizophrenia, with the majority of experts rating risperidone as the first-line treatment. Quetiapine, olanzapine, and aripiprazole were also recommended. Medical comorbidities lead to additional considerations, particularly in an older population with many comorbidities. Experts recommended avoiding low- and mid-potency FGAs such as loxapine and chlorpromazine, as well as ziprasidone and

clozapine in patients with prolonged QTc interval or congestive heart failure. They also recommended avoiding low- and mid-potency FGAs as well as clozapine and olanzapine in patients with obesity, dyslipidemias, or diabetes mellitus. Finally, in patients with PD, quetiapine was the first-line recommendation; risperidone was not recommended in these patients due to risk of worsening extrapyramidal symptoms [93].

The evidence reviewed here shows that second-generation antipsychotics are an efficacious way to treat the symptoms of schizophrenia in older adults, although there is a relative paucity of data on the use of SGAs in older adults and the studies that do exist are primarily small and not randomized or blinded. Additionally, the data shows that SGAs exert only a modest effect on symptoms of psychosis; for instance, amisulpride treatment was found to produce only a 12-point reduction on the 126-point BPRS scale and this is similar to other studies [58].

The use of SGAs must be carefully considered given the risk of significant adverse effects including cerebrovascular events and sudden cardiac death. In addition to those devastating potential events, SGAs are associated with movement side effects such as drug-induced parkinsonism and tardive dyskinesia, metabolic side effects such as obesity, dyslipidemia, and diabetes mellitus, among other potential side effects. There is evidence, too, that older adults are more sensitive to the side effects of these medications than are younger adults.

For these reasons, non-pharmacological interventions are an important tool in the treatment of

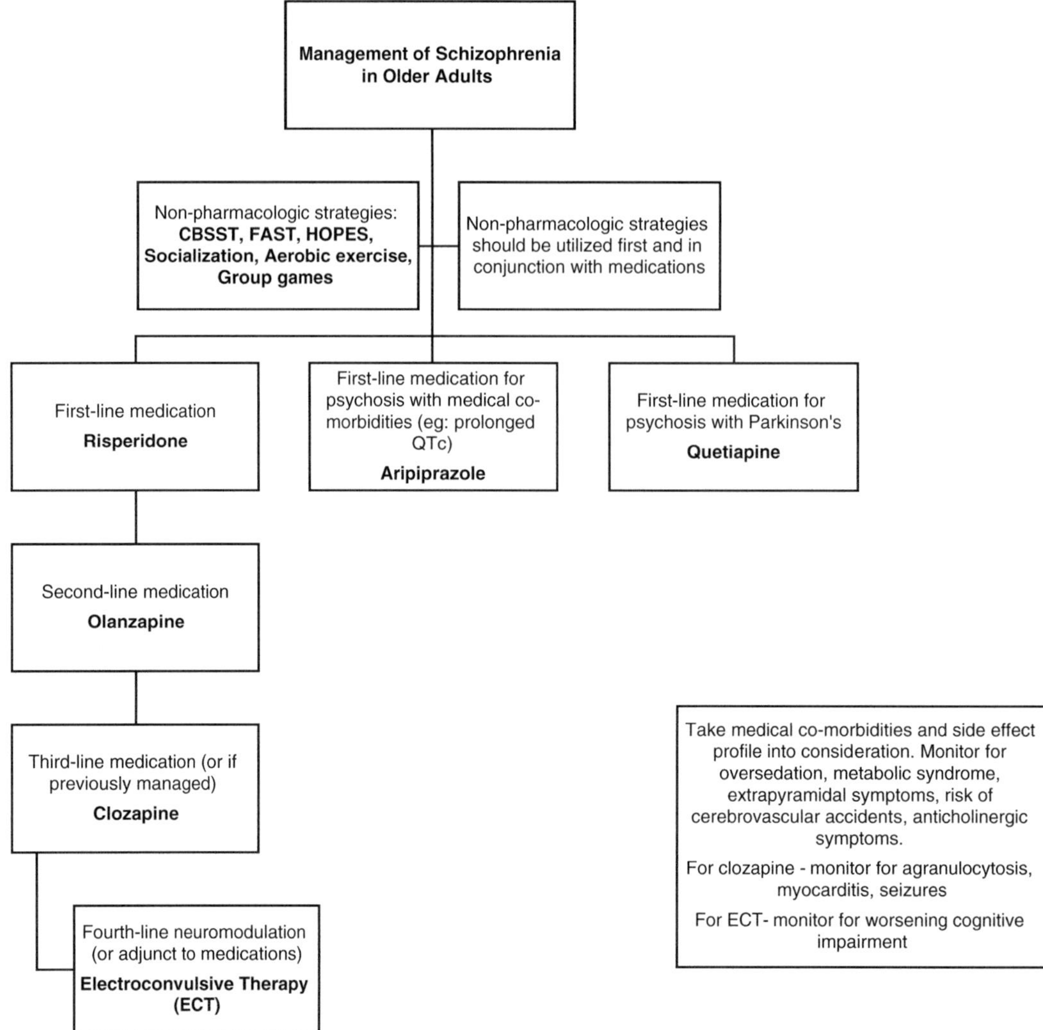

Fig. 13.1 Treatment flow diagram

schizophrenia in older adults. There are a variety of psychosocial interventions designed for older adults with schizophrenia, and neuromodulation is also an option, though to our knowledge, only ECT has been studied in older adults. These interventions may be used in addition to antipsychotics or in lieu of them when antipsychotics are not tolerated. Please refer to Fig. 13.1 for the treatment flow diagram.

Conclusion

Schizophrenia is a mental illness characterized by both positive symptoms such as hallucinations and delusions and negative symptoms such as flat affect or avolition. Although most patients develop symptoms of schizophrenia in young adulthood, a significant number of individuals develop schizophrenia later in life. Patients with early-onset schizophrenia have shorter life spans than their counterparts without schizophrenia, due to a variety of factors, but are now increasingly living longer. Assessment of older adults with schizophrenia should first rule out psychosis due to other medical factors, as this is the most common etiology for new onset of psychosis in older adults. If the psychosis is determined to be from a primary psychiatric disorder, assessment should then focus on differentiating between schizophrenia and other psychiatric illnesses, which can have a similar presentation including schizoaffective disorder, bipolar disorder, and major depressive disorder with psychotic features. The treatment of choice for schizophrenia in older adults is SGAs. The choice of which SGA to use is primarily driven by the side effect profile of the particular medication, as these agents have similar efficacy. Finally, non-pharmacological treatments may be considered in patients for whom SGAs are not sufficient to treat their symptoms or among those individuals who cannot tolerate SGAs.

References

1. American Psychiatric Association. Diagnostic and statistical manual of mental disorders. 5th ed. American Psychiatric Association Publishing; 2013.
2. Olfson M, et al. Premature mortality among adults with schizophrenia in the United States. JAMA Psychiatry. 2015;72(12):1172–81.
3. Reinhardt M, Cohen CI. Late-life psychosis: diagnosis and treatment. Curr Psychiatry Rep. 2015;17(1):1–13.
4. Cohen CI, et al. Schizophrenia in later life: clinical symptoms and social well-being. Psychiatr Serv. 2008;59(3):232–4.
5. Jeste DV, et al. Divergent trajectories of physical, cognitive, and psychosocial aging in schizophrenia. Schizophr Bull. 2011;37(3):451–5.
6. Cohen CI. Advances in the conceptualization and study of schizophrenia in later life: 2020 update. Clin Geriatr Med. 2020;36(2):221–36.
7. Coljin MA, et al. Psychosis in later life: a review and update. Harv Rev Psychiatry. 2015;23(5):354–67.
8. Howard R, et al. Late-onset schizophrenia and very-late-onset schizophrenia-like psychosis: an international consensus. Am J Psychiatry. 2000;157(2):172–8.
9. Maglione JE, et al. Late-onset schizophrenia: do recent studies support categorizing LOS as a subtype of schizophrenia? Curr Opin Psychiatry. 2014;27(3):173–8.
10. Khan A, et al. Current concepts in the diagnosis and treatment of schizophrenia in later life. Curr Geriatr Rep. 2015;4(4):290–300.
11. Van Assche L, et al. The neuropsychology and neurobiology of late-onset schizophrenia and very-late-onset schizophrenia-like psychosis: a critical review. Neurosci Behav Rev. 2017;2017(83):604–21.
12. Bayer TA, et al. Genetic and non-genetic vulnerability factors in schizophrenia: the basis of the "two hit hypothesis". J Psychiatr Res. 1999;33(6):543–8.
13. Hilker R, et al. Heritability of schizophrenia and schizophrenia spectrum based on the Nationwide Danish Twin Register. Biol Psychiatry. 2018;83:492–8.
14. Vassos E, et al. Meta-analysis of the association of urbanicity with schizophrenia. Schizophr Bull. 2012;38(6):1118–23.
15. Henssler J, et al. Migration and schizophrenia: meta-analysis and explanatory framework. Eur Arch Psychiatry Clin Neurosci. 2020;270:325–35.
16. Cheslack-Postava K, Brown AS. Prenatal infection and schizophrenia: a decade of further progress. Schizophr Res. 2022;247:7–15.
17. Shahzade C, et al. Patterns in adolescent cannabis use predict the onset and symptom structure of schizophrenia-spectrum disorder. Schizophr Res. 2018;197:539–43.
18. Khachadourian V, et al. Advanced paternal age and risk of schizophrenia in offspring—review of epidemiological findings and potential mechanisms. Schizophr Res. 2021;233:72–9.
19. Chen L, et al. Risk factors in early and late onset schizophrenia. Compr Psychiatry. 2018;80:155–62.
20. Brunelle S, et al. Risk factors for the late-onset psychoses: a systematic review of cohort studies. Int J Geriatr Psychiatry. 2012;27:240–53.
21. Vares M, et al. Association between methylenetetrahydrofolate reductase (MTHFR) C677T polymorphism and age of onset in schizophrenia. Am J Med Genet. 2009;153B(2):610–8.
22. Saetre P, et al. Methylenetetrahydrofolate reductase (MTHFR) C677T and A1298C polymorphisms and age of onset in schizophrenia: a combined analysis of independent samples. Am J Med Genet. 2011;156(2):215–24.
23. Hamshere ML, et al. Phenotype evaluation and genome-wide linkage study of clinical variables in schizophrenia. Am J Med Genet. 2011;156B(8):929–40.
24. Xiu M, et al. The TNF-alpha gene—1031T>C polymorphism is associated with onset age but not with risk of schizophrenia in a Chinese population. Neuropsychology. 2019;33(4):482–9.
25. Rasmussen HB. Association between the CCR5 32-bp deletion allele and late onset schizophrenia. Am J Psychiatry. 2006;163(3):507–11.
26. Gogas A, et al. A role for estrogen in schizophrenia: clinical and preclinical findings. Int J Endocrinol. 2015;2015:1–16.

27. Dubovsky AN, et al. The neuropsychiatric complications of glucocorticoid use: steroid psychosis revisited. Psychosomatics. 2012;53:103–15.

28. Cancelli I, et al. Drugs with anticholinergic properties as a risk factor for psychosis in patients affected by Alzheimer's disease. Clin Pharmacol Ther. 2008;84(1):63–8.

29. Beaulieu-Boire I, Lang AE. Behavioral effects of levodopa. Mov Disord. 2015;30(1):90–102.

30. Silverman BC, et al. Interferon-induced psychosis as a "psychiatric contraindication" to hepatitis C treatment: a review and case-based discussion. Psychosomatics. 2011;51(1):1–7.

31. Cummings J. Pimavanserin: potential treatment for dementia-related psychosis. J Prev Alzheimers Dis. 2018;5(4):253–8.

32. Monastero R, et al. A systematic review of neuropsychiatric symptoms in mild cognitive impairment. J Alzheimers Dis. 2009;18:11–30.

33. Pachi I, et al. Late life psychotic features in prodromal Parkinson's disease. Parkinsonism Relat Disord. 2021;86:67–73.

34. Woolley JD, et al. The diagnostic challenge of psychiatric symptoms in neurodegenerative disease: rates of and risk factors for prior psychiatric diagnosis in patients with early neurodegenerative disease. J Clin Psychiatry. 2011;72(2):126–33.

35. Van Assche L, et al. The neuropsychological profile and phenomenology of late onset psychosis: a cross-sectional study on the differential diagnosis of very-late-onset schizophrenia-like psychosis, dementia with Lewy bodies and Alzheimer's type dementia with psychosis. Arch Clin Neuropsychol. 2019;34:183–99.

36. Cooper JJ, Ovsiew F. The relationship between schizophrenia and frontotemporal dementia. J Geriatr Psychiatry Neurol. 2013;26(3):131–7.

37. Schneider LS. Risk of death with atypical antipsychotic drug treatment for dementia. JAMA. 2005;294(15):1934–43.

38. Cai S, et al. The diagnosis of schizophrenia among nursing home residents with ADRD: does race matter? Am J Geriatr Psychiatr. 2022;30(5):636–46.

39. Granholm E, et al. A randomized, controlled trial of cognitive behavioral social skills training for middle-aged and older outpatients with chronic schizophrenia. Am J Psychiatry. 2005;162(3):520–9.

40. Rajji TK, et al. Cognitive-behavioral social skills training for patients with late-life schizophrenia and the moderating effect of executive dysfunction. Schizophr Res. 2022;239:160–7.

41. Patterson TL, et al. Functional adaptation skills training (FAST): a randomized trial of a psychosocial intervention for middle-aged and older patients with chronic psychotic disorders. Schizophr Res. 2006;86:291–9.

42. Bartels SJ, et al. Long-term outcomes of a randomized trial of integrated skills training and preventive healthcare for older adults with serious mental illness. Am J Geriatr Psychiatry. 2014;22(11):1251–61.

43. Meesterd PD. Promoting personal and social recovery in older persons with schizophrenia: the case of the new club, a novel Dutch facility offering social contact and activities. Community Ment Health J. 2019;55:994–1003.

44. Kern RS. Effects of aerobic exercise on cardiorespiratory fitness and social functioning in veterans 40 to 65 years old with schizophrenia. Psychiatry Res. 2020;291:113258.

45. Dobbins S. Play provides social connection for older adults with serious mental illness: a grounded theory analysis of a 10-week exergame intervention. Aging Ment Health. 2020;24(4):596–603.

46. Chan CYW, et al. Clinical effectiveness and speed of response of electroconvulsive therapy in treatment-resistant schizophrenia. Psychiatry Clin Neurosci. 2019;73:416–22.

47. Petrides G, et al. Electroconvulsive therapy augmentation in clozapine-resistant schizophrenia: a prospective, randomized study. Am J Psychiatry. 2015;172(1):52–8.

48. Kellner CH, et al. Right unilateral ultrabrief pulse ECT in geriatric depression: phase 1 of the PRIDE study. Am J Psychiatry. 2016;173(11):1101–9.

49. Hermida AP, et al. Efficacy and safety of ECT for behavioral and psychological symptoms of dementia (BPSD): a retrospective chart review. Am J Geriatr Psychiatr. 2020;28(2):157–63.

50. Shelef A, et al. Acute electroconvulsive therapy followed by maintenance electroconvulsive therapy decreases hospital re-admission rates of older patients with severe mental illness. J ECT. 2015;31(2):125–8.

51. Satake Y, et al. Clinical utility of electroconvulsive therapy for the treatment of multidrug-resistant psychosis emerging in older adults: a case report. Psychogeriatrics. 2022;22:757–61.

52. Gault JM, et al. Approaches to neuromodulation for schizophrenia. J Neurol Neurosurg Psychiatry. 2018;89(7):777–87.

53. Jin Y, et al. Alpha EEG guided TMS in schizophrenia. Brain Stimul. 2012;5(4):560–8.

54. 2019 American Geriatrics Society Beers Criteria Update Expert Panel. American Geriatrics Society 2019 Updated AGS Beers Criteria for potentially inappropriate medication use in older adults. J Am Geriatr Soc. 2019;67:674–94.

55. Scott J, et al. Atypical (second generation) antipsychotic treatment response in very-late onset schizophrenia-like psychosis. Int Psychogeriatr. 2011;23(5):742–8.

56. Lin C, et al. A comparison of long-acting injectable antipsychotics with oral antipsychotics on time to rehospitalization within 1 year of discharge in elderly patients with schizophrenia. Am J Geriatr Psychiatr. 2019;28(1):23–30.

57. Stepien-Wyrobiec O. Crossroad between current knowledge and new perspective of diagnostic and therapy of late-onset schizophrenia and very late-onset schizophrenia-like psychosis: an update. Front Psych. 2022;13:1025414.

58. Howard R, et al. Antipsychotic treatment of very late-onset schizophrenia-like psychosis (ATLAS): a randomized, controlled, double-blind trial. Lancet Psychiatry. 2018;5:553–63.
59. Psarros C, et al. Amisulpride for the treatment of very-late-onset schizophrenia-like psychosis. Int J Geriatr Psychiatry. 2009;24:518–22.
60. Reeves S, et al. Therapeutic D2/D3 receptor occupancies and response with low amisulpride blood concentration in very late-onset schizophrenia-like psychosis. Int J Geriatr Psychiatry. 2018;33:396–404.
61. Pigott TA, et al. Aripiprazole for the prevention of relapse in stabilized patients with chronic schizophrenia: a placebo-controlled 26 week study. J Clin Psychiatry. 2003;64(9):1048–56.
62. Lieberman JA, et al. Effectiveness of antipsychotic drugs in patients with chronic schizophrenia. N Engl J Med. 2005;353:1209–23.
63. Ismail Z, et al. Age and sex impact clozapine plasma concentrations in inpatients and outpatients with schizophrenia. Am J Geriatr Psychiatr. 2011;20(1):53–60.
64. Bishara D, Taylor D. Adverse effects of clozapine in older patients: epidemiology, prevention and management. Drugs Aging. 2014;31:11–20.
65. Ritchie CW, et al. A comparison of the efficacy and safety of olanzapine and risperidone in the treatment of elderly patients with schizophrenia: an open study of six months duration. Int J Geriatr Psychiatry. 2006;21:171–9.
66. Jeste DV, et al. International multisite double-blind trial of the atypical antipsychotics risperidone and olanzapine in 175 elderly patients with chronic schizophrenia. Am J Geriatr Psychiatr. 2003;11(6):638–47.
67. Kane JM, et al. Olanzapine long-acting injection: a 24-week, randomized, double-blind trial of maintenance treatment in patients with schizophrenia. Am J Psychiatry. 2010;167(2):181–9.
68. Mazeh D, et al. Quetiapine for elderly non-responsive schizophrenia patients. Psychiatry Res. 2008;157:265–7.
69. Lasser RA, et al. Efficacy and safety of long-acting risperidone in elderly patients with schizophrenia and schizoaffective disorder. Int J Geriatr Psychiatry. 2004;19:898–905.
70. Sajatovic M, et al. Prescribing antipsychotics in geriatric patients: focus on schizophrenia and bipolar disorder. Curr Psychiatr Ther. 2017;16(10):20–8.
71. Tampi RR, et al. Psychotic disorders in late life: a narrative review. Therap Adv Psychopharmacol. 2019;9:2045125319882798.
72. American Psychiatric Association. FDA extends black-box warning to all antipsychotics. Psychiatric News. 2008. https://psychnews.psychiatryonline.org/doi/full/10.1176/pn.43.14.0001. Accessed 16 Dec 2022.
73. Gill SS, et al. Antipsychotic drug use and mortality in older adults with dementia. Ann Intern Med. 2007;146(11):775–86.
74. Schneeweiss S, et al. Risk of death associated with the use of conventional versus atypical antipsychotic drugs among elderly patients. CMAJ. 2007;176(5):627–32.
75. Sacchetti E. Cerebrovascular accidents in elderly people treated with antipsychotics: a systematic review. Drug Saf. 2010;33(4):273–88.
76. Kleijer BC. Risk of cerebrovascular events in elderly users of antipsychotics. J Psychopharmacol. 2009;23(8):909–14.
77. Uchida H, et al. Increased antipsychotic sensitivity in elderly patients: evidence and mechanisms. J Clin Psychiatry. 2009;70(3):397–405.
78. Knol W, et al. Parkinsonism in elderly users of haloperidol. J Clin Psychopharmacol. 2012;32(5):688–93.
79. Chyou T, et al. Comparative risk of parkinsonism with olanzapine, risperidone, and quetiapine in older adults: a propensity score matched cohort study. Pharmacoepidemiol Drug Saf. 2020;29(6):692–700.
80. O'Brien A. Comparing the risk of tardive dyskinesia in older adults with first-generation and second-generation antipsychotics: a systematic review and meta-analysis. Int J Geriatr Psychiatry. 2016;31:683–93.
81. Woerner MG, et al. Incidence of tardive dyskinesia with risperidone or olanzapine in the elderly: results from a 2-year, prospective study in antipsychotic naïve patients. Neuropsychopharmacology. 2011;36:1738–46.
82. Lopez-Sendon JL, et al. Drug-induced parkinsonism in the elderly: incidence, management and prevention. Drugs Aging. 2012;29(2):105–18.
83. Sajatovic M, et al. Long-term safety and efficacy of deutetrabenazine in younger and older patients with tardive dyskinesia. Am J Geriatr Psychiatr. 2022;30(3):360–71.
84. Sajatovic M, et al. One-daily valbenazine is effective for tardive dyskinesia in elderly patients (>=65 years). Am J Geriatr Psychiatr. 2022;30(4S):S67–8.
85. Chacko E, et al. Metabolic side effects of atypical antipsychotics in older adults. Int Psychogeriatr. 2018;30(10):1557–66.
86. Guenette MD, et al. Atypical antipsychotic-induced metabolic disturbances in the elderly. Drugs Aging. 2014;31:159–84.
87. Kassm SA, et al. Metabolic syndrome among older adults with schizophrenia spectrum disorder: prevalence and associated factors in a multicenter study. Psychiatry Res. 2019;275:238–46.
88. Wu RR, et al. Metformin treatment of antipsychotic-induced dyslipidemia: an analysis of two randomized, placebo-controlled trials. Mol Psychiatry. 2016;21:1537–44.
89. de Silva VA, et al. Metformin in prevention and treatment of antipsychotic induced weight gain: a systematic review and meta-analysis. BMC Psychiatry. 2016;16:341.
90. Stahl SM, et al. How and when to treat the most common adverse effects of antipsychotics: expert review from research to clinical practice. Acta Psychiatr Scand. 2020;143:172–80.

91. Trifiro G. Association of community-acquired pneumonia with antipsychotic drug use in elderly patients. Ann Intern Med. 2010;152:418–25.
92. Lee SH, et al. Use of antipsychotics increases risk of fractures: a systematic review and meta-analysis. Osteoporos Int. 2017;28(4):1167–78.
93. Alexopoulos GS. Expert consensus guidelines for using antipsychotic agents in older patients. J Clin Psychiatry. 2004;65(Suppl 2):100–2.

Schizoaffective Disorder

Adiel Carlo and Marianne Klugheit

Introduction

Schizoaffective disorder has been a controversial diagnosis since it was first observed in patients. The concept of schizoaffective psychosis was introduced in 1933 where it was described to have psychotic features associated with schizophrenia and affective symptoms characteristic of bipolar disorder [1]. It was previously considered a subtype of schizophrenia and was described as "good prognosis schizophrenia" [1]. This was because long-term functions like cognitive ability were better when compared to schizophrenia, but worse than bipolar disorder [1]. It was not until 1980s where schizoaffective disorder was first recognized as its own diagnosis under the Diagnostic and Statistical Manual of Mental Disorders, Third Edition (DSMIII) [1].

The Diagnostic and Statistical Manual of Mental Disorders, Fifth Edition Text Revision (DSM 5-TR) characterizes schizoaffective disorder as an uninterrupted period of illness during which there is a major mood episode (major depressive or manic) concurrent with criterion A for schizophrenia; the major depressive episode must include depressed mood [2]. Further diagnostic criteria for schizoaffective disorder are noted in Table 14.1.

Schizoaffective disorder is situated somewhere in between schizophrenia and bipolar disorder. However, there are important differences in symptomatology and functioning between these disorders. Patients with schizoaffective disorder have similar thought disorders as with patients who have schizophrenia [1]. Their depressive symptoms are more severe when compared to schizophrenia and similar in intensity to those with bipolar disorder [1]. Cognitive functioning is better than schizophrenia, but worse than with bipolar disorder [1]. Individuals with schizoaffective disorder perform similarly to bipolar disorder patients in independent skills [1]. They have more hospital admissions and longer hospital stays than those with schizophrenia [1]. Individuals with schizoaffective disorder also show poorer subjective physical and mental health functions [1]. They are also less likely to live independently, be married, and drive [3]. It was previously believed that psychotic illnesses "burn out" as the individual ages. However, there has been no relationship found between age and the presence of negative symptoms [4].

In the DSM V-TR, it is noted that schizoaffective disorder is about one-third as common as schizophrenia [2]. The lifetime prevalence of schizoaffective disorder is 0.3%. In a study by Meesters et al., the one-year prevalence for schizoaffective disorder was 0.14% in patients

A. Carlo (✉) · M. Klugheit
Department of Psychiatry, University of Arizona School of Medicine, Tucson, AZ, USA
e-mail: adielcarlo@arizona.edu;
Marianne.Klugheit@va.gov

© The Author(s), under exclusive license to Springer Nature Switzerland AG 2024
R. R. Tampi, D. J. Tampi (eds.), *Treatment of Psychiatric Disorders Among Older Adults*,
https://doi.org/10.1007/978-3-031-55711-8_14

Table 14.1 DSM-5 TR criterion for schizoaffective disorder [2]

Diagnostic criteria for schizoaffective d/o
A. An uninterrupted period of illness during which there is a major mood episode (major depressive or manic) concurrent with criterion A of schizophrenia
B. Delusions or hallucinations for 2 or more weeks in the absence of a major mood episode (depressive or manic) during the lifetime duration of the illness
C. Symptoms that meet criteria for a major mood episode are present for the majority of the total duration of the active and residual portions of the illness
D. The disturbance is not attributable to the effects of a substance (e.g., a drug of abuse, a medication) or another medical condition

Criterion A for schizophrenia
Two (or more) of the following, each present for a significant portion of time during a 1-month period (or less if successfully treated). At least one of these must be (1), (2), or (3):
1. Delusions
2. Hallucinations
3. Disorganized speech (e.g., frequent derailment or incoherence)
4. Grossly disorganized or catatonic behavior
5. Negative symptoms (i.e., diminished emotional expression or avolition)

Table 14.2 Prevalence of schizoaffective disorder among adults [5]

Age	One-year prevalence (%)
60–69	0.17
70–79	0.17
>80	0.03
Age of onset	Prevalence (%)
<40	0.09
40–59	0.04
>60	0.004

older than 60 (Table 14.2) [5]. The prevalence decreased as age increased. Women are often times overrepresented in studies. In women, it is thought that estradiol levels impact psychotic symptoms as psychotic symptoms are often exacerbated when levels are low as seen in the follicular phase of the menstrual cycle, post-partum, and in menopause [6].

Schizoaffective disorder in the older adult is a field where little research has been done as most research focuses on the younger adult. This poses a problem as there is a known increase in the geriatric population in the coming years. In 2010, 4% of adults over age 55 were designated as having Severe Mental Illness (SMI), this number is expected to double by the year 2050 [7]. There have been several barriers to conducting research in the older adults such as getting consent in the older adult. Older adults are not analyzed separately as a group in most research studies [8]. The terminology that is used in research also varies. Studies combine schizoaffective disorder research with schizophrenia spectrum disorders or psychotic disorders research where only a very small subset of patients carry a schizoaffective disorder diagnosis.

Risk Factors

In comparison to the general population, individuals with schizoaffective disorder have higher levels of lifetime trauma. This higher lifetime trauma was associated with non-remission of positive symptoms [9]. The lifetime trauma has not been associated with non-remission of negative symptoms or presence of depression or anxiety [9].

Consequences

Quality of life is affected in individuals with schizoaffective disorder and changes throughout the disease process. Quality of Life is defined by the World Health Organization as an "individual's perception of their position in life in the context of culture and value system in which they live, and in relation to their goals, expectations, standards, and concerns" [10].

Studies looking at the younger adult show that quality of life can serve as a predictor of symptomatic and functional improvement [10]. Factors such as anxiety, depression, and psychotic symptoms have been shown to reduce quality of life

[10]. Lower quality of life was found to predict increased social anxiety and symptom instability in one study [10]. One study by Cohen et al. looked at different factors impacting quality of life in the older adult and found that higher religiousness, higher perceived well-being versus others/past selves, and lower scores on Center for Epidemiologic Studies Depression scale (CES-D) predicted higher quality of life [10]. Both depression and perceived well-being vs others/past selves were seen to have bidirectional relationship with quality of life [10]. Religiousness had a unidirectional relationship in which it predicts subsequent quality of life [10].

Other studies show that having fewer positive symptoms and anxiety symptoms related to higher subjective quality of life [11]. It is also important to note that an individual with a larger network size, presence of a confidant, regular social participation, and higher level of social functioning was associated with higher subjective quality of life [11].

Individuals with psychotic illnesses are known to have increased mortality at a younger age than those without psychotic illness [12]. The National Association of State Mental Health Program Directors show that individuals with serious mental illness (SMI) have up to 25 years of decreased life span. This is likely due to poor management of preventable medical causes of death. Coronary artery disease was the primary cause of death for individuals with schizoaffective disorder [12]. Other studies have shown that the primary causes of death in these individuals are cardiovascular, neoplastic, and pulmonary disease [12].

When looking at unnatural causes of death such as suicide, elderly suicide completers had greater physical health burdens and more functional disabilities when compared to those who did not commit suicide. The quality of life was significantly worse in individuals completing suicide [13].

In a Finnish study, it was noted that the most common causes of death matched that of individuals in the general population, but the standardized mortality ratio was increased in those with schizoaffective disorder [14]. In looking at unnatural causes of death, accidental falls were the most common cause of death followed by suicide and choking on food [14]. Mortality was almost three times higher than the age matched and sex matched individuals in the general population. The most common cause of death was circulatory disease which was believed to be because of unhealthy living habits and exposure to antipsychotic medications [14].

Individuals with SMI have lower rates of preventive care and inadequate medical care [15]. This leads to higher comorbid risks and greater risk of elderly adults having more nursing homes placements, increased hospitalizations, and early mortality. Compared to those without SMI, individuals had worse communication with their provider and reported that their medical visits were too short [15]. This may be due to providers not knowing how to communicate with individuals with SMI. Older adults felt that their healthcare providers did not explain clinical information in a comprehensible way. Many factors can contribute to this miscommunication as older age is associated with lower health literacy rates [15]. There also exists cognitive limitations impacting information processing and ability to understand sequential instructions. The use of peer specialists may be of some benefit for older adults with SMI in their medical and psychiatric management [15].

Prognosis

Older adulthood is not necessarily a quiescent period for persons with schizoaffective disorder, as there are fluctuations in remission status over time [16]. Remission is defined as the absence or low intensity of symptoms over a 6-month period. When remission is not attained, symptomatic control is considered the second-best concept to recovery which includes satisfying social functioning and quality of life. A diagnosis of schizoaffective disorder is associated with greater remission when compared to other psychotic illnesses such as schizophrenia [17]. Other components associated with increased remission rates were lower Positive Scale, Negative Scale, and

General Psychopathology Scale (PANSS) score at baseline, lower positive and negative PANSS symptom subscale scores, having a partner, and having a larger social network [17]. Other studies show that variables including female gender, younger age, later age of onset, taking antipsychotic medication, rapid onset, baseline social functioning, better cognitive functioning, fewer severe negative symptoms, and employment status are associated with increased remission rates [16]. Providing supported employment has been shown to be beneficial for individuals to attain competitive employment, increase number of weeks worked, and wages earned [18].

Assessment of Schizoaffective Disorder in the Older Adult

Schizoaffective disorder typically presents in early adulthood [2]. As first-time psychotic illnesses are rare in older adults, one must distinguish if the individual's psychotic symptoms are caused by a medical etiology and therefore considered a secondary psychotic illness rather than a primary psychotic disorder like schizoaffective disorder [19]. Initial assessment of the older adult with psychosis should include a detailed history and physical [19]. Collateral information should be obtained from individuals close to the patient for a complete history [19]. Following the history and physical examination, laboratory testing is done to rule out underlying medical illnesses.

Common laboratory work-up includes complete blood count (CBP), comprehensive metabolic panel (CMP), thyroid stimulating hormone (TSH), folate, vitamin B12, toxicology screen, UA, rapid plasma reagin (RPR), and HIV when indicated [19]. Other tests can include EEG and polysomnography if indicated by patient history [19].

Neuroimaging like CT head or MRI can be utilized to rule out structural abnormalities that can cause psychosis, especially when there is a neurological deficit present on physical exam [19].

Studies to track symptoms of schizoaffective disorder often rely on scales for schizophrenia and mood disorders. These include PANSS, Hamilton Rating Scale for Depression (HAM-D), Montgomery-Asberg Depression Rating Scale (MADRS), and the Young Mania Rating Scale (YMRS) among others [20]. These have not been validated specifically for schizoaffective disorder [20]. The Clinical Global Impression for Schizoaffective disorder Scale (CGI-SCA) was developed in 2012 that addresses several domains and can assess severity and change in the disease; however, it has low generalizability [20]. This was modified from the Clinical Global Impression Scale for psychosis [20].

Treatments

Treatment guidelines for schizoaffective disorder are not well established in the elderly due to scarce research in this group of individuals [21]. Treatment is increasingly difficult as the older adult is notorious for having comorbid physical illness, polypharmacy, cognitive impairments, poor compliance/adherence to treatment, and sensitivity to developing side effects [22].

When selecting treatment options, one must look at the patient's medical comorbidities and the patient's medications to select a treatment that is effective and safe [23]. We will explore the different pharmacological and nonpharmacological treatments for individuals with schizoaffective disorder.

Pharmacotherapy

Treatment should start by ruling out medical or medication causes to presentation [24]. Once completed, the patient's adherence should be reviewed [24]. Schizoaffective disorder can be managed with second generation antipsychotics (SGA) as these are well tolerated in the elderly. When switching from a first-generation antipsychotic (FGA), there is a decrease in anticholinergic and extrapyramidal symptoms (EPS) in this population [22]. Therefore, the individual should be switched to an atypical antipsychotic, if not taking one already [24]. The dose should be

Table 14.3 Treatment for schizoaffective disorder among older adults

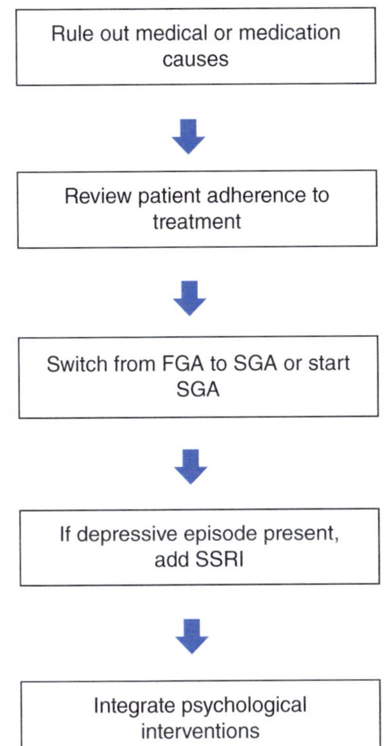

adjusted to target depressive symptoms, positive symptoms, and negative symptoms [24]. If depressive symptoms persist, adding a selective serotonin reuptake inhibitor (SSRI) agent is reasonable [24] (Table 14.3). The starting dose should be low and slowly increased to reduce symptoms. An acute episode should be treated at least 6–9 months and longer treatments should be considered for those with residual symptoms, very severe or high comorbid major depressive episodes, ongoing stressors, or recurrent episodes [24]. The incorporation of psychosocial interventions aimed at improving adherence, hope, and quality of life and function is also recommended.

Olanzapine has been shown to decrease positive, negative symptoms, and depressive symptoms among individuals with schizoaffective disorder [25]. Olanzapine in younger adults shows an increase in weight and lipid levels. In the older adult, weight gain and increase in lipid

levels do not appear to happen [25]. Risperidone has been shown to decrease positive and negative symptoms, disorganized thoughts, and uncontrolled hostility and excitement [26]. Risperidone was the first second-generation antipsychotic to have a long-acting injectable formulation (LAI). This is helpful for patients where adherence is an issue. Side effects associated with this LAI include insomnia, constipation, bronchitis, rhinitis, and psychosis [26]. These side effects were not found to be dose related. There has been a reduction of movement disorders when using an LAI [26]. Changes noted with laboratory data, EKG and vital signs were not clinically significant [26]. Quetiapine and aripiprazole have shown good response in older adults. Clozapine is reserved for patients who are treatment resistant or those who suffer from significant extrapyramidal symptoms (EPS). Clozapine has not had enough research to determine if the same outcomes for decrease in suicidal behaviors seen in the young adult are present in the older adult [8]. Little is known about its effect on function, quality of life, ability to live independent, and caregiver burden. The older adults are more susceptible to agranulocytosis, postural hypotension, anticholinergic effects, sedation, cognitive dysfunction, and delirium [8].

In individuals with EPS, treatment with quetiapine should be started first. Olanzapine or aripiprazole can be used as second-line agents [21]. Those with prolactin-related disorders such as galactorrhea or gynecomastia should be trialed on quetiapine or olanzapine rather than risperidone. In individuals with congestive heart failure, avoid using agents like clozapine, ziprasidone, and first-generation antipsychotics [21].

The use of SSRIs has been shown to aid with symptoms of depression in schizoaffective disorder. Citalopram results in some improvements in social functioning and mental health related functioning [27].

The use of mood stabilizers has been largely studied in younger adults and are regularly used among individuals with schizoaffective disorder [21]. There is paucity of research regarding mood stabilizers in older adults with schizoaffective disorder. Most of the research on mood stabilizers in older adults have been in the treatment of bipolar disorder.

There are some studies looking at estrogen as a potential treatment for women with treatment resistant psychosis [6]. In animal studies, estradiol has been seen to enhance serotonin concentrations in the brain, stimulate metabotropic glutamate receptor signaling, reduce inflammation, and stimulate dopamine activity in the cortical and striatal regions [6]. More research is needed to determine its safety given its effect on breast tissue and endometrium [6]. Table 14.3 describes the treatment for schizoaffective disorder among older adults.

Nonpharmacological Treatments

Nonpharmacological treatment approaches are integral to the care of older adults. Individuals with schizoaffective disorder are at high risk for early placement in facilities and early morbidity/ mortality [7, 28]. The use of nonpharmacological treatments can aid individuals utilize community resources to delay these outcomes.

Individuals with SMI are known to have increased morbidity, earlier mortality, and increased healthcare utilization and cost [7]. Therefore, it is important to utilize interventions to aid individuals navigate their community. Psychosocial skills training and preventive healthcare intervention (Helping Older People Experience Success- HOPES) were designed to improve independent functioning and community living [7]. This manualized group intervention teaches older adults to develop social skills, community living skills, and healthy living skills in the community [7]. It focuses on integration of preventive health with the help of nurse coordination. HOPES improved community living skills, showed greater self-efficacy, and decreased overall severity of psychiatric and negative symptoms [7]. With incorporation of integrated preventive health care, older adults engaged in this modality showed greater preventive health screenings and completion of advanced directives [7]. There is a version of HOPES intervention that is individu-

ally tailored to the individual's needs instead engaging in group sessions. With individual sessions, participants are provided with immediate training and reinforcement as needed [29].

Cognitive Behavioral Social Skills Training (CBSST) is a psychosocial intervention to help improve social functioning that combines social skills and cognitive behavioral therapy [30]. CBSST was developed for younger patients and consisted of manualized group therapy with 3 modules. In the elderly, the modules are tailored to age needs such as addressing cognitive impairment, identifying, and challenging ageist beliefs, and age relevant role-playing situations, and age specific problem solving [30]. This intervention may be utilized to prevent decline in social functioning [30].

Functional Adaptation Skills Training (FAST) is a manualized intervention that targets areas of everyday functioning (medication management, social skills, communication skills, organization and planning, transportation, and financial management) [31]. The use of FAST resulted in improvements in a person's ability to manage daily tasks including finances, transportation, shopping, and communicating with others [31].

Electroconvulsive Therapy

Electroconvulsive therapy (ECT) has been used for the treatment of individuals with psychosis. In the elderly, a big concern is ECT's impact on cognition and overall safety of treatment [32]. There is little research dedicated to the use of ECT among older adults with schizoaffective disorder, and there is a lack of consensus in treatment guidelines [32]. In a literature review, ECT has been shown to improve psychosis and catatonia in nearly all elderly patients with a primary psychotic condition [32]. Some of these individuals were treatment resistant or severally ill. No ECT-related fatalities were seen in the literature review [32]. Those with schizophrenia were less likely to have cognitive impairment when compared to those with depression [32]. There is a lack of consensus regarding predictors of ECT efficacy. Prior positive response to ECT, suicidality, violent behavior, and catatonia were associated with more favorable response to ECT treatment while anticonvulsant medication use and psychotropic treatment resistance cases had poorer response [32]. In adult literature, positive psychotic symptoms have been associated with better response to ECT while evidence regarding the duration of psychotic illness and psychotic exacerbation with ECT use remains conflicting [32].

Conclusion

Schizoaffective disorder has been largely understudied among older adults. There are currently no consensus guideline treatments for schizoaffective disorder among older adults. Treatment for schizoaffective disorder among older adults uses antipsychotic medications and SSRIs. The use of mood stabilizers is largely studied under individuals with bipolar disorder. ECT has been effective for treatment, but guidelines for this treatment modality are lacking. It is important to maintain social functioning of patients with schizoaffective disorder and there are interventions which have been found to be beneficial.

References

1. Rolin SA, Aschbrenner KA, Whiteman KL, Scherer E, Bartels SJ. Characteristics and service use of older adults with schizoaffective disorder versus older adults with schizophrenia and bipolar disorder. Am J Geriatr Psychiatry. 2017;25(9):941–50. https://doi.org/10.1016/j.jagp.2017.03.014.
2. Diagnostic and statistical manual of mental disorders. 5th ed. Text revision. Washington, DC: American Psychiatric Association Publishing; 2022.
3. Gupta S, Steinmeyer CH, Lockwood K, Lentz B, Schultz K. Comparison of older patients with bipolar disorder and schizophrenia/schizoaffective disorder. Am J Geriatr Psychiatry. 2007;15(7):627–33. https://doi.org/10.1097/JGP.0b013e318065b06b.
4. Cohen CI, Natarajan N, Araujo M, Solanki D. Prevalence of negative symptoms and associated factors in older adults with schizophrenia spectrum disorder. Am J Geriatr Psychiatry. 2013;21(2):100–7. https://doi.org/10.1016/j.jagp.2012.10.009.
5. Meesters PD, de Haan L, Comijs HC, Stek ML, Smeets-Janssen MM, Weeda MR, et al. Schizophrenia spectrum disorders in later life: prevalence and distribution of age at onset and sex in a dutch catchment area. Am J Geriatr Psychiatry. 2012;20(1):18–28. https://doi.org/10.1097/JGP.0b013e3182011b7f.
6. Kulkarni J, Gavrilidis E, Gwini SM, Worsley R, Grigg J, Warren A, et al. Effect of adjunctive raloxifene therapy on severity of refractory schizophrenia in women: a randomized clinical trial. JAMA Psychiatry. 2016;73(9):947–54. https://doi.org/10.1001/jamapsychiatry.2016.1383.
7. Bartels SJ, Pratt SI, Mueser KT, Forester BP, Wolfe R, Cather C, et al. Long-term outcomes of a randomized trial of integrated skills training and preventive healthcare for older adults with serious mental illness. Am J Geriatr Psychiatry. 2014;22(11):1251–61. https://doi.org/10.1016/j.jagp.2013.04.013.
8. Renzenbrink M, Wand APF. A systematic review of clozapine's effectiveness for primary psychotic and bipolar disorders in older adults. Int Psychogeriatr. 2022;34(10):875–87. https://doi.org/10.1017/s1041610220004172.
9. Cohen CI, Palekar N, Barker J, Ramirez PM. The relationship between trauma and clinical outcome variables among older adults with schizophrenia spectrum disorders. Am J Geriatr Psychiatry. 2012;20(5):408–15. https://doi.org/10.1097/JGP.0b013e318211817e.
10. Cohen CI, Vengassery A, Garcia Aracena EF. A longitudinal analysis of quality of life and associated factors in older adults with schizophrenia spectrum disorder. Am J Geriatr Psychiatry. 2017;25(7):755–65. https://doi.org/10.1016/j.jagp.2017.01.013.
11. Meesters PD, Comijs HC, de Haan L, Smit JH, Eikelenboom P, Beekman AT, et al. Subjective quality of life and its determinants in a catchment area based population of elderly schizophrenia patients. Schizophr Res. 2013;147(2–3):275–80. https://doi.org/10.1016/j.schres.2013.04.030.
12. Capasso RM, Lineberry TW, Bostwick JM, Decker PA, St. Sauver J. Mortality in schizophrenia and schizoaffective disorder: an Olmsted County, Minnesota cohort: 1950–2005. Schizophrenia Res. 2008;98(1–3):287–94. https://doi.org/10.1016/j.schres.2007.10.005.
13. Kasckow J, Montross L, Golshan S, Mohamed S, Patterson T, Sollanzano E, et al. Suicidality in middle aged and older patients with schizophrenia and depressive symptoms: relationship to functioning and quality of life. Int J Geriatr Psychiatry. 2007;22(12):1223–8. https://doi.org/10.1002/gps.1817.
14. Talaslahti T, Alanen HM, Hakko H, Isohanni M, Häkkinen U, Leinonen E. Mortality and causes of death in older patients with schizophrenia. Int J Geriatr Psychiatry. 2012;27(11):1131–7. https://doi.org/10.1002/gps.2833.
15. Fortuna KL, Lohman MC, Batsis JA, DiNapoli EA, DiMilia PR, Bruce ML, et al. Patient experience with healthcare services among older adults with serious

mental illness compared to the general older population. Int J Psychiatry Med. 2017;52(4–6):381–98. https://doi.org/10.1177/0091217417738936.

16. Cohen CI, Iqbal M. Longitudinal study of remission among older adults with schizophrenia spectrum disorder. Am J Geriatr Psychiatry. 2014;22(5):450–8. https://doi.org/10.1016/j.jagp.2013.09.004.

17. Lange SMM, Meesters PD, Stek ML, Wunderink L, Penninx BWJH, Rhebergen D. Course and predictors of symptomatic remission in late-life schizophrenia: a 5-year follow-up study in a Dutch psychiatric catchment area. Schizophrenia Res. 2019;209:179–84. https://doi.org/10.1016/j.schres.2019.04.025.

18. Twamley EW, Vella L, Burton CZ, Becker DR, Bell MD, Jeste DV. The efficacy of supported employment for middle-aged and older people with schizophrenia. Schizophr Res. 2012;135(1–3):100–4. https://doi.org/10.1016/j.schres.2011.11.036.

19. Reinhardt MMC, C.I. Late-life psychosis: diagnosis and treatment. Curr Psychiatry Rep. 2015;17 https://doi.org/10.1007/s11920-014-0542-0.

20. Allen MH, Daniel DG, Revicki DA, Canuso CM, Turkoz I, Fu DJ, Alphs L, Ishak KJ, Bartko JJ, Lindenmayer JP. Development and psychometric evaluation of a clinical global impression for schizoaffective disorder scale. Innov Clin Neurosci. 2012;9(1):15–24.

21. Felmet K, Zisook S, Kasckow JW. Elderly patients with schizophrenia and depression: diagnosis and treatment. Clin Schizophr Relat Psychoses. 2011;4(4):239–50. https://doi.org/10.3371/csrp.4.4.4.

22. Barak Y, Shamir E, Mirecki I, Weizman R, Aizenberg D. Switching elderly chronic psychotic patients to olanzapine. Int J Neuropsychopharmacol. 2004;7(2):165–9. https://doi.org/10.1017/s1461145703004048.

23. Jeste DV, Barak Y, Madhusoodanan S, Grossman F, Gharabawi G. International multisite double-blind trial of the atypical antipsychotics risperidone and olanzapine in 175 elderly patients with chronic schizophrenia. Am J Geriatr Psychiatry. 2003;11(6):638–47. https://doi.org/10.1176/appi.ajgp.11.6.638.

24. Kasckow JW, Zisook S. Co-occurring depressive symptoms in the older patient with schizophrenia. Drugs Aging. 2008;25(8):631–47. https://doi.org/10.2165/00002512-200825080-00002.

25. Barak Y, Aizenberg D. Effects of olanzapine on lipid abnormalities in elderly psychotic patients. Drugs Aging. 2003;20(12):893–6. https://doi.org/10.2165/00002512-200320120-00003.

26. Lasser RA, Bossie CA, Zhu Y, Gharabawi G, Eerdekens M, Davidson M. Efficacy and safety of long-acting risperidone in elderly patients with schizophrenia and schizoaffective disorder. Int J Geriatr Psychiatry. 2004;19(9):898–905. https://doi.org/10.1002/gps.1184.

27. Kasckow J, Lanouette N, Patterson T, Fellows I, Golshan S, Solorzano E, et al. Treatment of subsyndromal depressive symptoms in middle-aged and older adults with schizophrenia: effect on functioning. Int J Geriatr Psychiatry. 2010;25(2):183–90. https://doi.org/10.1002/gps.2318.

28. Mueser KT, Pratt SI, Bartels SJ, Swain K, Forester B, Cather C, et al. Randomized trial of social rehabilitation and integrated health care for older people with severe mental illness. J Consult Clin Psychol. 2010;78(4):561–73. https://doi.org/10.1037/a0019629.

29. Pratt SI, Mueser KT, Wolfe R, Santos MM, Bartels SJ. One size doesn't fit all: a trial of individually tailored skills training. Psychiatr Rehabil J. 2017;40(4):380–6. https://doi.org/10.1037/prj0000261.

30. Rajji TK, Mamo DC, Holden J, Granholm E, Mulsant BH. Cognitive-behavioral social skills training for patients with late-life schizophrenia and the moderating effect of executive dysfunction. Schizophr Res. 2022;239:160–7. https://doi.org/10.1016/j.schres.2021.11.051.

31. Patterson TL, Mausbach BT, McKibbin C, Goldman S, Bucardo J, Jeste DV. Functional adaptation skills training (FAST): a randomized trial of a psychosocial intervention for middle-aged and older patients with chronic psychotic disorders. Schizophrenia Res. 2006;86(1–3):291–9. https://doi.org/10.1016/j.schres.2006.05.017.

32. Kumagaya D, Halliday G. Acute electroconvulsive therapy in the elderly with schizophrenia and schizoaffective disorder: a literature review. Australas Psychiatry. 2019;27(5):472–6. https://doi.org/10.1177/1039856219839470.

Substance-Related and Addictive Disorders

Alcohol Use Disorder

15

Christina Spoleti, Gibson George,
and Padmapriya Marpuri

Introduction

Alcohol use disorder is described in the Diagnostic and Statistical Manual of Mental Disorders, Fifth Edition (DSM-5), as a condition that is characterized as mild (2–3 symptoms), moderate (4–5 symptoms), or severe (6 or more symptoms) and is defined by a maladaptive pattern of substance use leading to clinically significant impairment or distress, as manifested by 2 or more of the following occurring at any time in the same 12-month period [1]:

- Alcohol is often taken in larger amounts or over a longer period than was intended.
- There is a persistent desire or unsuccessful efforts to cut down or control alcohol use.
- A great deal of time is spent in activities necessary to obtain alcohol, use alcohol, or recover from its effects.
- Craving or strong desire or urge to use alcohol.

- Recurrent alcohol use resulting in a failure to fulfill major role obligations at work, school, or home.
- Continued alcohol use despite having persistent or recurrent social or interpersonal problems caused or exacerbated by the effects of alcohol.
- Important social, occupational, or recreational activities are given up or reduced because of alcohol use.
- Recurrent alcohol use in situations in which it is physically hazardous.
- Alcohol use is continued despite knowledge of having a persistent or recurrent physical or psychological problem that is likely to have been caused or exacerbated by alcohol.
- Tolerance, as defined by either of the following:
  - A need for markedly increased amount of alcohol to achieve intoxication or desired effect.
  - A markedly diminished effect with continued use of the same amount of alcohol.
- Withdrawal, as manifested by either of the following:
  - The characteristic withdrawal syndrome for alcohol.
  - Alcohol (or closely related substance, such as benzodiazepine) is taken to relieve or avoid withdrawal symptoms.

C. Spoleti · P. Marpuri (✉)
Department of Psychiatry, St. Luke's University Health Network, Easton, PA, USA
e-mail: christina.spoleti@sluhn.org;
padmapriya.marpuri@sluhn.org

G. George
St. Luke's Penn Foundation, Department of Psychiatry, St. Luke's University Health Network, Easton, PA, USA
e-mail: gibson.george@sluhn.org

© The Author(s), under exclusive license to Springer Nature Switzerland AG 2024
R. R. Tampi, D. J. Tampi (eds.), *Treatment of Psychiatric Disorders Among Older Adults*,
https://doi.org/10.1007/978-3-031-55711-8_15

The National Institute of Alcohol Abuse and Alcoholism (NIAA) recommends older adults greater than 65 years of age consume no more than one drink per day for women and no more than two drinks per day for men [2]. The NIAA defines one drink as 1–1.5 ounces of hard liquor [2].

It is estimated that AUD affects 1–3% of the elderly population [3]. According to the 2019 National Survey on Drug Use and Health (NSDUH), the lifetime prevalence of alcohol use in adults aged 65 years or older was 81.9%, and the yearly prevalence of use was 56.1% [4]. The World Health Organization (WHO) reported the age range with the highest percentage of total deaths attributable to alcohol was between ages 60 and 64 years of age at a rate of 17% [5].

Within the older adult community, AUD is often underdiagnosed and underreported as the social and occupational impairments due to alcohol use may go unnoticed or unreported secondary to retirement and decreased social activities [6]. Compounding the difficulty assessing functional impairment, AUD in older adults may mimic other diagnoses such as cognitive impairment or depression [6].

Risk Factors and Neurobiology

Demographic risk factors for developing AUD prior to age 60 years old include male sex, young age at first use, and family history of substance use disorders. Demographic risk factors for developing AUD after age 60 years old include female sex, high socioeconomic class, and family history of substance use disorders [3].

Physiological changes in the older adults lead to higher blood-alcohol levels related to decrease in body water and body mass with age leading to a smaller volume of distribution, increased sensitivity, and decreased metabolism of alcohol [3].

Consequences

Alcohol use can lead to intoxication, and prolonged use can lead to withdrawal. Intoxication is defined as behavioral and psychological changes which impair functioning, including impaired gait, coordination, speech, and attention which can lead to stupor or coma [7]. Alcohol withdrawal occurs in stages. The first stage occurs on average 6–12 h after abstinence from substance with symptoms of autonomic instability including change in blood pressure, heart rate, and respiratory rate, as well as tremors, nausea, and vomiting [8]. The second stage typically begins after 12 h after last use and is characterized by transient alterations in perception including visual, tactile, or auditory hallucinations [8]. The third stage occurs on an average of 24–48 h after alcohol cessation and may include seizures. Delirium tremens is a potentially life-threatening sequelae of alcohol withdrawal which occurs 48–72 h after last use and is characterized by rapid fluctuations of perception and consciousness, autonomic instability, and agitation [8]. Due to the seriousness of alcohol withdrawal complications, multiple protocols exist to monitor and manage withdrawal symptoms including the Clinical Institute Withdrawal Assessment for Alcohol Scale Revised (CIWA-Ar) and the Severity of Ethanol Withdrawal Scale (SEWS).

Alcohol use leads to chronic health conditions including but not limited to alcohol-associated liver disease including cirrhosis, heart disease, cardiac dysrhythmias, colorectal, hepatic, and esophageal cancers, gastrointestinal hemorrhage, vitamin deficiencies, pancreatitis, and hypertension [8]. Alcohol contributes to approximately 20–25% of cases of cirrhosis and approximately 50% of hospital admissions among individuals with cirrhosis in the United States [9]. Chronic use also leads to pancreatic cell injury resulting in atrophy and scarring of the pancreas seen in alcoholic chronic pancreatitis [9]. Alcohol-induced pancreatitis accounts for 30% of pancreatitis admissions, which is the most common gastrointestinal cause of hospitalization in the United States [10, 11]. Regarding cardiovascular changes, alcohol use is a preventable and modifiable cause contributing to hypertension, cardiomyopathy, heart failure, arrhythmias, and stroke [12, 13].

Alcohol also has significant effects on the nervous system. Alcohol use disorder is associated with cognitive impairment, cerebellar ataxia, confusion, and peripheral neuropathy [8]. Abrupt cessation of alcohol in the setting of chronic use can lead to alcohol withdrawal as outlined above. Additionally, Wernicke encephalopathy, an acute neurologic condition characterized by nystagmus, ataxia, and condition secondary to thiamine deficiency can occur [8]. In addition to Wernicke encephalopathy, Korsakoff's syndrome may develop. Korsakoff's syndrome involves progression of the encephalopathy and results in permanent damage to the brain thalamus and hypothalamus [7].

Vitamin deficiencies seen in alcohol use include thiamine (B1), pyridoxine (B6), and cobalamin (B12) which are associated with peripheral neuropathies. Thiamine deficiency is also associated with encephalopathy and long-term neurological complications as mentioned above [8]. Peripheral neuropathies increase the risk of fall which is compounded in the setting of alcohol use in the geriatric age-group as this population is also at an increased risk of low bone mass, osteopenia, and osteoporosis [8].

Overall, alcohol affects the geriatric population differently compared to younger adults due to age-related physiological changes including decreased lean body mass, decreased total body water, decreased liver metabolism, and increased blood–brain barrier permeability and neuronal sensitivity to alcohol [6].

In addition to physiological effects, AUD has a significant effect on psychosocial aspects of afflicted individuals. AUD is associated with motor vehicle accidents, poor academic performance, increased risk of suicide, increased criminal activity including intimate partner violence perpetration, and increased risk of death by overdose [14].

Assessment

In the elderly population, AUD has an atypical presentation leading to underdiagnosis [3]. This is compounded by the lack of awareness and sensitization of AUD among physicians, hesitancy by providers to screen older adults for AUD, failure to link coexisting medical problems with AUD, and increased prescription medication use in older adults hinders detection of AUD [3].

The American Psychiatric Association (APA) recommends the initial psychiatric evaluation of all stable individuals with suspected alcohol use disorder include a thorough substance use history including assessment of current and past alcohol, tobacco, and other substance use—including prescribed and over-the-counter supplements [14]. The APA recommends further assessment for co-occurring conditions including other psychiatric and medical disorders which may influence treatment [14]. Clinicians should also complete a full psychiatric, medical, family, and social history as well as a comprehensive physical exam when evaluating individuals for AUD [6].

The American Society of Addiction Medicine (ASAM) recommends incorporating universal screening for unhealthy alcohol use into medical settings using a validated scale [15]. Screening tools specific to the geriatric population have been developed and include:

- Michigan Alcohol Screening Test-Geriatric Version (MAST-G) which is a 24-item questionnaire. Five or more yes responses indicate a problematic relationship with alcohol. The sensitivity for detecting problematic alcohol use for MAST-G is 0.86 [8].
- Short Michigan Alcohol Screening Test-Geriatric Version (SMAT-G) which is a 10-item questionnaire condensed from the MAST-G. Two or more yes responses indicate possible AUD. The sensitivity for detecting problematic alcohol use for SMAT-G is 0.75 [8, 16].

Two commonly used screening tools not specific to the geriatric population are the CAGE Alcohol Questionnaire (CAGE) and the Alcohol use Disorders Identification Test (AUDIT). The CAGE screening is a 4-question screening (Fig. 15.1).

The AUDIT is a ten-question tool which separates responses on a scale of 0–4 for each question [18]. A score of 8 or more indicates hazardous drinking; 13 or more indicates problem with alcohol in women; and 15 or more indicates problem with alcohol in men [18]. In studies

CAGE Questionnaire:
Have you ever felt you needed to cut down on your drinking?
Have people annoyed you by criticizing your drinking?
Have you ever felt guilt about drinking?
Have you ever felt you needed a drink first thing in the morning (eye-opener) to steady your nerves or to get rid of a hangover?
Two or more positive responses are indicative of problematic alcohol use

Fig. 15.1 CAGE questionnaire [17]

assessing effectiveness of the tools in the elderly population, the AUDIT had superior sensitivity to identify AUD, and the CAGE had superior sensitivity in identifying alcohol dependence symptoms [19]. When compared against specific geriatric screening tools, studies have demonstrated the MAST-G and SMAT-G identified hazardous drinking in geriatric individuals not detected by CAGE questionnaire [8] (Fig. 15.1).

The ASAM also recommends regular screening for alcohol withdrawal in individuals known to be using alcohol recently, regularly, and heavily even in the absence of withdrawal signs and symptoms. In individuals with signs and symptoms of withdrawal, it is recommended to assess the quantity, frequency, and time of day alcohol was last consumed to determine whether the individual is experiencing or is at risk of developing alcohol withdrawal syndrome [15].

During evaluations, it may be beneficial to incorporate a blood, breath, or urine test for alcohol levels. This is especially true in emergent situations during which an individual is unable to communicate or give a complete alcohol use history [15].

Treatments

Treatments for AUD, like many substance use disorders, are often a combination of non-pharmacological and pharmacological therapies.

Non-pharmacological

Multiple psychotherapy modalities have evidence for the treatment of AUD. Cognitive behavioral therapy (CBT) has been studied in the geriatric population, including The Geriatric Evaluation Team: Substance Misuse/Abuse Recognition and Treatment (GET SMART) study, for the treatment of AUD. In the GET SMART trial, which enrolled veterans aged 53–82 years, 55% of participants who completed at least 13 of the 16 GET SMART sessions were significantly more likely to remain abstinent from alcohol use [20]. In addition to CBT, adaptive interventions, including brief intervention, motivational interviewing, and behavioral self-control therapy (BSCT) have been shown to improve outcomes in alcohol abstinence and reduced use [8].

Community and self-help groups, such as Alcoholics Anonymous (AA), utilize peer-to-peer support, meetings, and may include sponsors for sobriety [8]. A Cochrane review in 2020 assessed studies comparing AA and other 12 step programs with CBT, which demonstrated that AA and 12 step programs were more effective in increasing abstinence and producing substantial health care cost benefits for individuals with AUD in a general adult population ages 34–51 years old [21]. Studies examining the geriatric population, ages 55–77 years old, demonstrated that older adults have longer retention in treatment, and noted that better treatment outcomes may be associated with smaller groups for therapy and/or groups focusing on issues specific to the older adult population [22].

Individuals can receive psychosocial treatment in multiple settings, which include inpatient rehabilitation facilities, outpatient rehabilitation facilities, intensive outpatient programs (IOP), and within community and self-help group sessions.

Pharmacological

The three medications approved by the Food and Drug Administration (FDA) for AUD in the United States are naltrexone, acamprosate, and disulfiram.

1. Opioid antagonist.

    Naltrexone is an opioid antagonist which binds and blocks μ-opioid and K-opioid receptors [23]. Its mechanism of action for promoting abstinence from alcohol is thought to be by reducing the euphoric effects of alcohol use, which decrease heavy drinking and curbs cravings [8]. Studies assessing the efficacy of naltrexone in the older adult population are limited, while data from the general adult population demonstrates effectiveness [24]. Naltrexone oral formulation is initiated at 25–50 mg daily and maintenance dose is typically 50 mg daily [8]. The extended release (ER) injectable naltrexone is dosed at 380 mg every 4 weeks [8]. Adverse effects of naltrexone include nausea, headache, sleep disturbance, anxiety, and depression [8, 25]. The injectable form is associated with injection site reactions. Naltrexone can increase liver enzymes and creatinine phosphokinase, which should be of careful consideration in individuals with AUD as chronic alcohol use can lead to liver dysfunction and disease [26]. Naltrexone is contraindicated in individuals with moderate to severe hepatic impairment and acute hepatitis [25]. Naltrexone is also contraindicated in individuals who are on opioids or who have an anticipated need for opioids [14].

2. N-Methyl D-Aspartic Acid (NMDA) and Gamma Aminobutyric Acid (GABA) receptor modulator.

    Acamprosate is a NMDA and GABA receptor modulator [27]. The approved dose for acamprosate is 1998 mg daily, typically dosed at 666 mg three times daily [28].

    Acamprosate is renally metabolized and requires dose adjustments in those with renal impairment. For creatinine clearance between 30 and 50 mL/min, acamprosate dosing should be reduced to 333 mg three times daily [28]. Acamprosate is contraindicated in individuals with renal failure [14]. As decline in renal function is found in aging, it is recommended to monitor kidney function regularly for geriatric individuals who are prescribed acamprosate.

3. Aldehyde dehydrogenase inhibitor.

    Disulfiram inhibits aldehyde dehydrogenase which creates a buildup of acetaldehyde when an individual consumes alcohol. This causes nausea, vomiting, dizziness, flushing, and blood pressure changes when alcohol and disulfiram are used in conjunction [6, 29]. Disulfiram is available in oral administration and is typically dosed between 250 and 500 mg daily [29]. Tablets can be crushed and mixed with liquids. Disulfiram should not be taken until an individual has abstained from alcohol use for at least 12 h. The most common adverse effects are headache, sleepiness, and halitosis or metallic taste in the mouth [29]. However, serious side adverse effects such as hypotension, arrhythmia, hepatitis, hepatotoxicity, psychosis, seizure, and drug–drug interactions with medications utilizing the P450 enzyme system have limited disulfiram use in the geriatric population [8, 29].

4. Off-label medications.

    Two medications used off-label for alcohol use disorder are gabapentin and topiramate. Gabapentin binds the alpha-2-delta subunit of presynaptic voltage-sensitive calcium channels and blocks the release of excitatory neurotransmitters, such as glutamate [30]. Studies have found gabapentin to help with mild alcohol withdrawal syndrome and neuropathic pain, which may be present in the setting of thiamine deficiency and other comorbidities in individuals with chronic alcohol use [6, 14, 30]. Gabapentin was typically dosed between 900 and 1800 mg daily and was associated with an increased rate of abstinence and a reduction in heavy drinking days [14]. Most commonly reported side effects are fatigue, insomnia, and headache [14].

    The second medication, topiramate, is an anticonvulsant with FDA indications for migraine prevention and seizures. The mechanism of action is believed to be antagonism of excitatory neurotransmitters, such as glutamate, and decreased dopamine release in the reward pathway [6]. It is used off-label in AUD for cravings and withdrawal symptoms [6, 14]. In trials for use in AUD, topiramate was dosed at 200–300 mg daily [14]. Topiramate is associated with cognitive impairment, weight reduction, paresthesia, and dizziness which makes it a medication to be used with caution in the geriatric population [6, 14].

Alcohol Withdrawal Management

The first-line treatment of alcohol withdrawal to help prevent seizures and delirium tremens is benzodiazepines, as well as phenobarbital in settings where the providers are experienced with its use [15]. For individuals with contraindications for benzodiazepine use, phenobarbital, gabapentin, and carbamazepine may be used [15]. Short acting benzodiazepines such as lorazepam and oxazepam are recommended in the elderly population as well as in the presence of liver dysfunction and disease, while diazepam and chlordiazepoxide should be avoided in this age group due to their long half-life and liver metabolism [15]. Careful consideration should be made when determining the level of care for alcohol detoxification and withdrawal management in the older adult population as they are at higher risk for developing delirium, having protracted withdrawal, and worsening of medical conditions when compared to the younger adult population [6].

Important to note is the efficacy and safety of the above pharmacological treatments have not been specifically studied in individuals 65 years and older [8].

Evidence-Based Treatment Algorithms

Current evidence demonstrates that a combination of pharmacologic and non-pharmacologic treatments is most effective in treatment of AUD. Improved treatment outcomes are seen when shared decision-making with the individual is utilized and when individuals are incorporated in treatment programs where other members are of similar age and functional status [6].

Individuals with AUD of any severity should begin treatment with screening and assessment. Elderly individuals should be screened yearly with a validated screening tool such as AUDIT, MAST-G, SMAT-G, or CAGE.

1. For individuals who drink </= 1 drink/day.

    Provide psychoeducation and reinforce the recommended daily drinking limit, assess for functioning and for co-occurring psychiatric diagnoses, and rescreen annually [6].
2. For individuals who drink > 1 drink/day.

    Complete a comprehensive substance use evaluation and assess readiness to quit drinking or cutting down.

    (a) If the individual is prepared to cut down—assess history of use, withdrawal, and longest recovery time. Give consideration for history of complicated withdrawal symptoms including delirium tremens, seizures, and multiple medical comorbidities [6].

    (b) If the individual is not prepared to cut down or quit, provide a brief intervention and information on available non-pharmacologic resources [6].
3. In an individual with potential high-risk drinking who is prepared to decrease consumption or quit, evaluate the need for inpatient detoxification or outpatient detoxification followed by a rehabilitation program.

    (a) Refer individuals to services as appropriate, including addiction medicine and addiction psychiatry [6].

    (b) Once the detoxification process is completed, consider initiation of maintenance treatment with both pharmacologic and non-pharmacologic options [6].

    (i) Pharmacologic options: Naltrexone, acamprosate, and other options to consider are gabapentin and topiramate. Recommend avoidance of disulfiram in the elderly population due to its adverse effects.

(ii) Non-pharmacologic options: Recovery support groups, peer support groups, and psychotherapy.

Conclusions

Substance use disorders in general are increasing in older adults, and alcohol is the most commonly used substance in this age-group. Long-term adverse effects of problematic drinking and AUD are seen in the geriatric population. AUD often goes underdiagnosed or undiagnosed in these individuals due to their atypical presentation as compared to the general adult population, and providers' lack of awareness and sensitization of AUD in the geriatric population. This results in under screening of elderly individuals for AUD. Screening should be regularly completed with tools specific to the geriatric population, and assessment should include comprehensive substance use history. Evaluation should also include a thorough evaluation of psychosocial supports and limitations to aid in development of treatment plan. Approved medications for the treatment of AUD include naltrexone, acamprosate, and disulfiram with the latter being seldom used in the elderly due to its adverse effects. Pharmacologic treatments should be combined with psychotherapy and social supports which promote recovery and focus on individuals in a similar age-group for improved effectiveness.

References

1. Substance Related and Addictive Disorders, American Psychiatric Association. Desk reference to the diagnostic criteria from DSM −5. Washington DC: American Psychiatric Publishing; 2013. p. 93–114.
2. National Institute of alcohol abuse and alcoholism. Older adults. Bethesda, MD: Access at: https://www.niaaa.nih.gov/alcohol-health/special-populations-co-occurring-disorders/older-adults. NIAAA: 2017.
3. Fagbemi M. How do you effectively evaluate the elderly for alcohol use disorder? Cleve Clin J Med. 2021;88(8):434–9. https://doi.org/10.3949/ccjm.88a.20123.
4. Substance Abuse and Mental Health Services Administration. 2019. Key substance use and mental health indicators in the United States: results from the 2019 National Survey on drug use and health. Rockville, MD: Center for Behavioral health statistics and quality, Substance Abuse and Mental Health Services Administration. Retrieved from https://www.samhsa.gov/data/
5. Global status report on alcohol and health 2018. World Health Organization. Access at: https://appswhoint/iris/handle/10665/274603 License: CC BY- NC-SA 30 IGO; May 02, 2023.
6. Joshi P, Duong KT, Trevisan LA, Wilkins KM. Evaluation and management of alcohol use disorder among older adults. Curr Geriatr Rep. 2021;10(3):82–90. https://doi.org/10.1007/s13670-021-00359-5.
7. Jesse S, Bråthen G, Ferrara M, Keindl M, Ben-Menachem E, Tanasescu R, Brodtkorb E, Hillbom M, Leone MA, Ludolph AC. Alcohol withdrawal syndrome: mechanisms, manifestations, and management. Acta Neurol Scand. 2017;135(1):4–16. https://doi.org/10.1111/ane.12671.
8. Fenollal-Maldonado G, Brown D, Hoffman H, Kahlon C, Grossberg G. Alcohol use disorder in older adults. Clin Geriatr Med. 2022;38(1):1–22. https://doi.org/10.1016/j.cger.2021.07.006.
9. Rocco A, Compare D, Angrisani D, Sanduzzi Zamparelli M, Nardone G. Alcoholic disease: liver and beyond. World J Gastroenterol. 2014;20(40):14652–9. https://doi.org/10.3748/wjg.v20.i40.14652.
10. Singal AK, Anand BS. Recent trends in the epidemiology of alcoholic liver disease. Clin Liver Dis (Hoboken). 2013;2(2):53–6. https://doi.org/10.1002/cld.168.
11. Peery AF, Dellon ES, Lund J, Crockett SD, McGowan CE, Bulsiewicz WJ, Gangarosa LM, Thiny MT, Stizenberg K, Morgan DR, Ringel Y, Kim HP, DiBonaventura MD, Carroll CF, Allen JK, Cook SF, Sandler RS, Kappelman MD, Shaheen NJ. Burden of gastrointestinal disease in the United States: 2012 update. Gastroenterology. 2012;143(5):1179–1187.e3. https://doi.org/10.1053/j.gastro.2012.08.002.
12. Kalla A, Figueredo VM. Alcohol and cardiovascular disease in the geriatric population. Clin Cardiol. 2017;40(7):444–9. https://doi.org/10.1002/clc.22681.
13. Jaubert MP, Jin Z, Russo C, Schwartz JE, Homma S, Elkind MS, Rundek T, Sacco RL, Di Tullio MR. Alcohol consumption and ambulatory blood pressure: a community-based study in an elderly cohort. Am J Hypertens. 2014;27(5):688–94. https://doi.org/10.1093/ajh/hpt235.
14. Reus VI, Fochtmann LJ, Bukstein O, Eyler AE, Hilty DM, Horvitz-Lennon M, Mahoney J, Pasic J, Weaver M, Wills CD, McIntyre J, Kidd J, Yager J, Hong SH. The American Psychiatric Association practice guideline for the pharmacological treatment of individuals with alcohol use disorder. Am J Psychiatry. 2018;175(1):86–90. https://doi.org/10.1176/appi.ajp.2017.1750101.

15. Alvanzo A, Kleinschmidt K, Kmiec JA. The ASAM clinical practice guideline on alcohol withdrawal management. J Addict Med. 2020;14(3S Suppl. 1):1–72. https://doi.org/10.1097/ADM.0000000000000668.

16. Johnson-Greene D, McCaul ME, Roger P. Screening for hazardous drinking using the Michigan alcohol screening test-geriatric version (MAST-G) in elderly persons with acute cerebrovascular accidents. Alcohol Clin Exp Res. 2009;33(9):1555–61. https://doi.org/10.1111/j.1530-0277.2009.00987.x.

17. Ewing JA. Detecting alcoholism. The CAGE questionnaire. JAMA. 1984;252(14):1905–7. https://doi.org/10.1001/jama.252.14.1905.

18. Williams N. The AUDIT questionnaire. Occup Med (Lond). 2014;64(4):308. https://doi.org/10.1093/occmed/kqu011.

19. Hays RD, Hill L, Gillogly JJ, Lewis MW, Bell RM, Nicholas R. Response times for the CAGE, short-MAST, AUDIT, and JELLINEK alcohol scales. Behav Res Methods Instrum Comput. 1993;25(2):304–7. https://doi.org/10.3758/BF03204515.

20. Schonfeld L, Dupree LW, Dickson-Euhrmann E, Royer CM, McDermott CH, Rosansky JS, Taylor S, Jarvik LF. Cognitive-behavioral treatment of older veterans with substance abuse problems. J Geriatr Psychiatry Neurol. 2000;13(3):124–9. https://doi.org/10.1177/089198870001300305.

21. Kelly JF, Humphreys K, Ferri M. Alcoholics anonymous and other 12-step programs for alcohol use disorder. Cochrane Database Syst Rev. 2020;3(3):CD012880. https://doi.org/10.1002/14651858.CD012880.pub2.

22. Satre DD, Mertens JR, Areán PA, Weisner C. Five-year alcohol and drug treatment outcomes of older adults versus middle-aged and younger adults in a managed care program. Addiction. 2004;99(10):1286–97. https://doi.org/10.1111/j.1360-0443.2004.00831.x.

23. Strang J, Volkow ND, Degenhardt L, Hickman M, Johnson K, Koob GF, Marshall BDL, Tyndall M, Walsh SL. Opioid use disorder. Nat Rev Dis Primers. 2020;6(1):3. https://doi.org/10.1038/s41572-019-0137-5.

24. Jonas DE, Amick HR, Feltner C, Bobashev G, Thomas K, Wines R, Kim MM, Shanahan E, Gass CE, Rowe CJ, Garbutt JC. Pharmacotherapy for adults with alcohol use disorders in outpatient settings: a systematic review and meta-analysis. JAMA. 2014;311(18):1889–900. https://doi.org/10.1001/jama.2014.3628.

25. Dufort A, Samaan Z. Problematic opioid use among older adults: epidemiology, adverse outcomes and treatment considerations. Drugs Aging. 2021;38(12):1043–53. https://doi.org/10.1007/s40266-021-00893-z.

26. Coffa D, Snyder H. Opioid use disorder: medical treatment options. Am Fam Physician. 2019;100(7):416–25.

27. Kalk NJ, Lingford-Hughes AR. The clinical pharmacology of acamprosate. Br J Clin Pharmacol. 2014;77(2):315–23. https://doi.org/10.1111/bcp.12070.

28. FDA Label Acamprosate. Access at: https://www.accessdata.fda.gov/drugsatfda_docs/label/2010/021431s013lbl.pdf; May 28, 2023.

29. Stokes M, Abdijadid S. Disulfiram 2022 Oct 24. In: StatPearls. Treasure Island, FL: StatPearls Publishing. p. 2023.

30. Mason BJ, Quello S, Goodell V, Shadan F, Kyle M, Begovic A. Gabapentin treatment for alcohol dependence: a randomized clinical trial. JAMA Intern Med. 2014;174(1):70–7. https://doi.org/10.1001/jamainternmed.2013.11950.

Nicotine Use Disorder

Amber Khan, Rajesh R. Tampi, and Deena J. Tampi

Introduction

Nicotine use disorder, also called tobacco use disorder, is defined within the Diagnostic and Statistical Manual of Mental Disorders (Fifth edition-text revision) as the problematic use of tobacco causing impairment or distress [1]. Individuals meet criteria for this disorder by demonstrating 2 of 11 criteria within a 12-month period. The criteria are "(1) tobacco taken over a longer period of time or in a larger amount than intended, (2) there is a persistent desire or unsuccessful efforts to cut down or control tobacco use, (3) a great deal of time is spent in activities necessary to obtain or use tobacco, (4) craving, or a strong desire or urge to use tobacco, (5) recurrent tobacco use resulting in a failure to fulfill major role obligations at work, school or home, (6) continued tobacco use despite having persistent or recurrent social or interpersonal problems caused or exacerbated by the effects of tobacco, (7) important social, occupation or recreational activities are given up or reduced because of tobacco use, (8) recurrent tobacco use in situations in which it is physically hazardous, (9) tobacco use is continued despite knowledge of having a persistent or recurrent physical or psychological problem that is likely to have been caused or exacerbated by tobacco, (10) tolerance defined as either a need for markedly increased amounts of tobacco to achieve the desired effect or a markedly diminished effect with continued use of the same amount of tobacco, and (11) withdrawal manifesting as either the characteristic withdrawal syndrome for tobacco or the use of tobacco (or a closely related substance such as nicotine) is taken to relieve or avoid withdrawal symptoms" [1].

Tobacco products include cigarettes, cigars (including little cigars and cigarillos), dissolvable, hookah, nicotine gels, pipe tobacco, roll-your-own tobacco, smokeless tobacco (dip, snuff, snus and chewing tobacco), vapes, e-cigarettes, and other electronic nicotine delivery systems. Smoking refers to inhaling and exhaling of smoke produced by cigarettes, cigars, and pipes. Vaping refers to inhaling and exhaling of aerosols produced by e-cigarettes [2].

A. Khan
Department of Psychiatry, Yale School of Medicine, New Haven, CT, USA

R. R. Tampi (✉)
Department of Psychiatry, Yale School of Medicine, New Haven, CT, USA

Department of Psychiatry, Creighton University School of Medicine, Omaha, NE, USA

D. J. Tampi
Behavioral Health Advisory Group, Princeton, NJ, USA

R. R. Tampi, D. J. Tampi (eds.), *Treatment of Psychiatric Disorders Among Older Adults*, https://doi.org/10.1007/978-3-031-55711-8_16

Epidemiology

Cigarette smoking is the leading preventable cause of death in the United States, and smoking related mortality has a significant impact in older adults. In 1990, approximately 70% of smoking attributable deaths occurred in adults age 65 and older [3]. Between 1965 and 1994, even as the prevalence of smoking among older adults decreased, the total number of smokers over the age of 65 increased by 20%. In addition, older adults had a decreased rate of decline in smoking compared to younger adults [4]. Among older adults in the United States, the prevalence of smoking is estimated to be 9–14% [5–8]. The population of older adults is projected to increase as is the population of older smokers.

Risk Factors

Nicotine dependence is highly heritable [9]. Studies also demonstrate that there is shared susceptibility to nicotine addiction with alcohol use and depression [9, 10]. Smoking in older age is associated with male gender, African American and Hispanic race, low education, and low income [11, 12]. It is also associated with binge drinking, illicit/nonmedical drug use, and depressive symptoms [11, 13, 14]. While studies demonstrate comorbidity of smoking and psychiatric disorders in younger populations, more studies are needed to evaluate the overlap of tobacco use disorder and psychiatric disorders in older adults.

Consequences

Smoking is causally related with several medical conditions. Smoking is the biggest risk factor for lung cancer and chronic obstructive pulmonary disease (COPD). One half of lung cancers occur among older adults [15]. Smoking is associated with head and neck cancers, gastrointestinal and genitourinary cancers, stroke, cardiovascular disease, heart failure, peripheral vascular disease, type 2 diabetes, nonobstructive lung disease,

osteoporosis, age-related macular degeneration, skin wrinkling, chronic rhinosinusitis, and delayed wound healing [14–22].

Smoking among older adults is associated with a two-fold increased risk for cardiovascular mortality and all-cause mortality. Excess risk increases with increased smoking and declines with time after cessation [23–25].

Smoking is related to cognitive decline in older adults. Smoking is associated with disproportionate loss of gray matter in the brain and progression of white matter hyperintensities [26, 27]. Neuroimaging studies show decreased brain connectivity, structural decreases in several brain regions, and cortical thinning in smokers compared to nonsmokers [28]. Among older adults, current smokers have an increased risk of Alzheimer's disease compared to former smokers and an increased risk for any dementia compared to nonsmokers [29].

Smoking is the primary cause of residential fires, and residential fires are a leading cause of accidental death among older adults [30, 31]. The risk of a residential fire related injury is significantly higher in households in which one or more members smoke compared to nonsmoking households [32].

In addition to numerous medical and safety consequences, there is a significant economic cost to smoking. Healthcare costs due to smoking amount to hundreds of billions of dollars. In 1993, Medicare spent approximately 9–10% of its budget on smoking-related illnesses [33].

Neurobiology and Nicotine Addiction

Nicotine inhaled from smoke quickly reaches the brain where it binds to nicotinic cholinergic receptors (nAChRs). These ligand gated ion channels are widely distributed throughout the brain. When nicotine binds to nAChRs, dopamine is released. In addition to dopamine, nicotine's effects are mediated by other neurotransmitters including norepinephrine, γ-aminobutyric acid (GABA), glutamate, serotonin, and endorphins. Nicotine-mediated dopamine release affects the frontal cortex, amygdala, nucleus accumbens, and ventral tegmental area, which are involved in cognition and the reward pathway [34, 35].

Acutely, nicotine increases brain reward function through brief enhanced cognition, increased arousal, and decreased anxiety. This is mediated by dopamine release. Nicotine withdrawal occurs within hours after smoking. Withdrawal symptoms include depressed mood, irritability, anxiety, insomnia, increased appetite, concentration difficulties, restlessness, and feeling little reward from previously satisfying activities [1]. Chronic nicotine use is perpetuated by the desire for the brief, reinforcing effects of nicotine use, and avoidance of withdrawal symptoms. Nicotine use is conditioned to psychological and environmental cues and the reinforcing aspects of nicotine. Chronic nicotine use leads to tolerance, whereby more nicotine is needed over time to produce the same reinforcing effects [34, 35]. Withdrawal and tolerance pose two challenges to sustained abstinence.

Metabolism

Through inhalation, nicotine rapidly enters circulation and bypasses first pass metabolism. Nicotine is primarily metabolized in the liver by CYP2A6 enzymes, and to a lesser degree by CYP2B6 and CYP2E1 enzymes [34]. Nicotine has a short half-life of approximately 2 h. Cotine is the major metabolite generated via the liver enzyme CYP2A6 and the most widely used biomarker of nicotine intake in clinical trials using biochemical testing. The half-life of cotine can last from 8 to 30 h [36]. In older adults, there is decreased clearance and decreased volume of distribution of cotine, though clinical correlates have not been found [37].

Nicotine can alter the metabolism of other medications, primarily through induction of cytochrome P450 enzymes in the liver. Nicotine causes increased clearance of caffeine, theophylline, tacrine, clozapine, olanzapine, and fluvoxamine by CYP1A2 induction, thus increased doses may be required in adults who smoke. Nicotine use is also associated with decreased sedation from benzodiazepines, decreased effectiveness of beta-blockers on heart rate and blood pressure, increased clearance of heparin, decreased insulin absorption, and decreased analgesic effects from opioids [38].

Assessment

Tobacco use should be assessed for every patient at every clinic visit [2, 39]. A detailed smoking history should be obtained along with other components of the general psychiatric evaluation. A smoking history includes asking about current and past smoking. Older adults should be asked about the brand and form of tobacco used [40]. Older adults should be asked when they started smoking and number of cigarettes smoked daily. Multiplying the number of packs of cigarettes smoked per day by the number of years smoked yields the pack-year smoking history, which allows clinicians to measure how much the older adult has smoked over a long period of time. Assessment further includes asking whether smoking occurs alone or with others, the location of smoking, and whether family members or other members of the household smoke. Older adults should be asked about sleeping patterns, including whether they wake from sleep to smoke and the timing of the first cigarette of the day. Older adults should be asked about triggers for smoking and how long they can abstain from smoking before experiencing cravings. Finally, it is important to ask about past cessation attempts, including the number of attempts, any pharmacologic or non-pharmacologic aids used, the length of time of cessation, and factors leading to return to use [15, 41].

Evidence-based guidelines for clinicians and healthcare systems recommend that clinicians offer tobacco users counseling on cessation. Thus, an assessment of nicotine use in older adults should also include an assessment of the older adult's motivation to quit smoking [39].

The United States Preventative Services Task Force (USPSTF) describes the 5A's approach as a brief strategy to assess and treat tobacco use. The 5A's include ask, advise, assess, assist, and arrange. They refer to the following steps: *ask* about tobacco use, *advise* cessation, *assess* willingness to quit, *assist* the patient in quitting by providing counseling, medication, and a quit plan, and *arrange* follow-up contact [39].

Benefits and Challenges of Smoking Cessation

There are several benefits for older adults who quit smoking. Studies show that smoking cessation after the age of 60 is associated with increased life expectancy and decreased risk of cardiovascular disease, coronary heart disease, and cardiovascular mortality [25, 42, 43]. Older adults who quit smoking experience less cognitive decline and brain atrophy than older adults who smoke [44].

There may also be unique challenges to smoking cessation in older adults. Current evidence demonstrates a benefit to cessation in older age; however, older adults are less likely to be offered cessation advice than younger adults [45, 46]. They may have less access to quit lines and online resources [47]. Older adults may have smoked longer with high levels of addiction. They may have had multiple past quit attempts and hold beliefs that they are too old to benefit from quitting or that they cannot quit [46–48]. Older adults may have misunderstandings about nicotine replacement therapy [49]. Older adults may associate smoking with stress reduction and habitual use, and they may express concerns associated with quitting including cravings, weight gain, irritability, anxiety, insomnia, trouble with concentration, and boredom [46, 49]. Age-related executive function deficits have been associated with decreased cessation [44]. These factors must be considered in assessment and counseling.

As with any addictive behavior, relapse prevention is an important component of treatment. There is insufficient evidence among older adults to support the use of behavioral interventions for relapse prevention [50]. Limited data suggests extended treatment with varenicline may reduce relapse and that extended treatment with bupropion is unlikely to be beneficial. Extended treatment with NRT and additional behavioral interventions for relapse prevention requires further study [50, 51]. Thus, clinicians should use evidence-based cessation strategies and closely follow up after a successful quit attempt to identify withdrawal symptoms, cravings, and triggers for relapse. If a relapse occurs, clinicians should continue to follow closely with the patient, encourage cessation, and identify motivation to quit. The next quit attempt may benefit from identifying reasons for relapse after the prior quit attempt, changing medications if the prior medication was used for a full trial at an appropriate dose, or increasing the intensity of the intervention [52]. This may include enhancing behavioral and social support. Within the general adult population, factors associated with relapse are triggers associated with smoking, availability of cigarettes, alcohol use, being around other smokers, negative affect, weight gain, younger age at cessation, shorter duration of abstinence, stress, and withdrawal symptoms [39, 53, 54]. However, studies on relapse risk factors among older adults are specifically needed.

Treatment

Predictors of Treatment Success

More studies on smoking cessation interventions tailored to diverse populations of older adults are needed. Most studies of older adults do not reflect the racial and ethnic diversity of the general population, and many existing studies in older adults include adults aged 50 and over [55, 56]. Thus, the oldest older adults may not be as well represented in current studies.

Qualitative research shows that motivating factors for older adults to quit smoking are knowledge of consequential medical problems, clear and specific messages, and materials inclusive of older people that also consider lifestyles and limitations of older adults [57, 58]. Predictors of smoking cessation among older adults include social support, high motivation, a new health diagnosis, hospitalization at time of consultation, short duration of smoking, no alcohol use, smoking more cigarettes per day, and a prior quit attempt of either less than one day or longer than 1 month [59–62]. One study in adults aged 75–94 found that increased cognitive dysfunction and more medications were associated with increased rates of smoking cessation, in contrast to other studies. However, the associations in this study may be proxy for increased caregiver support and limited ability to procure cigarettes [63].

Motivational interviewing is the recommended intervention for adults who are not ready to quit smoking, and it has been shown to increase quit attempts among current smokers who are not ready to quit [39]. Motivational interviewing includes the 5Rs model for smoking cessation: help the patient identify the *relevance* of quitting, *risks* of smoking, *rewards* of cessation, *roadblocks* to quitting, and this intervention should be *repeated* at each visit [64, 65]. In addition, studies show that behavioral and pharmacologic interventions for smokers not ready to quit can be as effective as they are for smokers who are motivated to quit [66]. Thus, older adults who are not ready to quit smoking may benefit from FDA approved pharmacotherapy to reduce smoking and increase motivation to quit. However, more data is needed on motivational interviewing within the population of older adult smokers who are not ready to quit smoking.

Tobacco dependence is a chronic and relapsing condition, often requiring multiple interventions and repeated attempts to quit [67]. Current data show that the combination of behavioral counseling and pharmacotherapy is most effective in older adults [55, 56, 68]. They also demonstrate that face-to-face interventions are more effective than phone interventions for increasing cessation rates, and studies using biochemical verification showed higher cessation rates [56].

Non-pharmacological

Non-pharmacologic treatment methods include self-help programs, phone counseling, cognitive behavioral approaches, individual and group counseling, and healthcare provider interventions [67]. Systematic reviews demonstrate the efficacy of these interventions in adults of all ages. Counseling and physician interventions are particularly effective [69–71]. However, there is a need for more randomized controlled trials in older adults and data is limited to few studies in this population. Current evidence shows that self-help interventions are more effective if tailored to older adults [57, 72]. In older adults, there is increased uptake of a telephone hotline compared to younger adults [73, 74]. Office-based physician counseling, counseling from other healthcare clinicians, and extended treatment with cognitive behavioral therapy are associated with increased cessation rates and longer duration of abstinence in older adults [58, 74–76].

Pharmacological

Medication Classes

There are three medication classes that are approved by the Food and Drug Administration (FDA) for smoking cessation: nicotine replacement therapy (NRT), varenicline (Chantix), and bupropion (Zyban). Clonidine and nortriptyline are considered second-line agents whose efficacy has been demonstrated in clinical trials.

NRT includes nicotine patches, gum, inhaler, nasal spray, and lozenges. They act on nAChRs to mimic the effects of nicotine. Bupropion increases dopamine levels in the brain by blocking dopamine reuptake [77]. Varenicline is a high-affinity, highly selective partial agonist of the primary nAChR receptor in the brain. It provides dopaminergic effects, though to a lesser degree than nicotine, and it blocks effects of added nicotine [78]. The goal of these medications is to reduce cravings and withdrawal symptoms.

Medication Dosages and Levels

Current evidence shows that age alone does not impact the pharmacokinetics of varenicline and bupropion [79, 80]. However, there are other considerations. Decreased renal function must be considered in dosing varenicline [80, 81]. In addition, older adults may have increased sensitivity to adverse effects of bupropion [82].

A 24-h nicotine patch comes in strengths of 7 mg, 14 mg, and 21 mg. The dose of the patch should correspond to the number of cigarettes smoked daily. The nicotine patch can be applied once daily to a clean, dry, and hairless site, and the site of application should rotate with each application. The dose of the patch can be tapered by 7 mg every 2 weeks as withdrawal symptoms and cravings decrease. Nicotine lozenges and nicotine gum come in 2 mg and 4 mg doses and can be dosed every 1–2 h. The strength of the dose is based on cigarettes per day or time to first cigarette of the day. Nicotine nasal sprays can be used 1–2 times per hour delivering 1 spray in each nostril. Typically, 12–15 doses are used daily. Nicotine inhalers can be dosed 6–16 cartridges per day and can be used for up to 6 months. All NRTs can be tapered as tolerated. While the patch, gum and lozenge can be obtained over the counter, nicotine sprays and nicotine inhalers require a prescription [39].

It is recommended to take varenicline 0.5 mg once daily for three days, followed by 0.5 mg twice daily for four days, then 1 mg twice daily for 12 weeks. It is recommended that each dose of varenicline be taken with a full glass of water to decrease gastrointestinal upset. Varenicline is excreted through the kidney; therefore, renal impairment must be considered in dosing [80, 83]. In adults with decreased renal clearance [creatinine clearance (CrCl < 30)], a maximum dose of 0.5 mg twice daily is recommended. In adults with end-stage renal disease on hemodialysis, a maximum dose of 0.5 mg once daily is recommended [84]. Treatment should be initiated one week prior to the intended quit date and continue for 3–6 months [39].

It is recommended to take bupropion 150 mg sustained release (SR) daily for 3 days, then to increase to 150 mg SR twice daily if tolerated. These doses are recommended to be taken at least 8 h apart. Treatment should be initiated 1–2 weeks prior to the intended quit date. Treatment typically lasts for 7–12 weeks; however, therapy can be prescribed for up to 6 months [39, 85].

Data in adult smokers over age 18 demonstrate that each of these treatments is more effective than placebo. Studies show that combination NRT (nicotine patch plus a fast-acting, oral NRT) is associated with higher cessation rates than a single form of NRT [86]. Additionally, varenicline is associated with greater cessation rates than NRT and bupropion SR, and there is insufficient data to determine if bupropion SR is superior to NRT [87, 88]. There is limited data on the use of pharmacologic treatments in older adults with nicotine use disorder. In older adults specifically, smaller scale studies demonstrate the effectiveness of NRT, varenicline, and bupropion [83, 89]. Additional considerations are that varenicline may be more effective for patients with comorbid psychiatric disease, and bupropion may attenuate post cessation weight gain. Finally, polypharmacy must be considered in older adults, and varenicline has fewer drug–drug interactions.

While clonidine and nortriptyline are considered second-line agents in the general population, they should be used with caution in older adults due to their side effects, particularly effects on cardiac function and the central nervous system. To date, there are no studies of these medications for smoking cessation in older adults.

Adverse Effects

Side effects associated with NRTs include palpitations and chest pain, nausea, vomiting, gastrointestinal upset, and insomnia. Nicotine patches may cause skin irritation, and oral NRTs are associated with coughing, mouth ulcers, and mouth and throat soreness [90].

Side effects commonly associated with bupropion, seen in >5% of participants in clinical trials, include insomnia, nervous disturbance, dry mouth, dizziness, nausea, arthralgia, rhinitis, constipation, and anxiety [91]. Angle closure glaucoma and increases in blood pressure may occur. Agitation may be associated with discontinuation, and while rare, bupropion induced mania has been described [92]. Older adults who plan to stop drinking alcohol or stop using sedatives should not be prescribed bupropion. Concurrent use of a monoamine oxidase inhibitor and bupropion is contraindicated. Bupropion-induced seizures are associated with a history of prior seizures, organic brain disease, or eating disorder. Thus, these conditions are contraindications for use and seizure incidence is a reason for discontinuation. Seizures are also associated with rapid dose escalation and high plasma levels of bupropion or its metabolites. However, bupropion peak plasma levels are 50% lower with the sustained release (SR) formulation used for smoking cessation than with the immediate release (IR) formulation. The incidence of seizures with the SR formulation of bupropion is also lower [92].

The most common side effects associated with varenicline, seen in >5% of participants in clinical trials, include nausea, constipation, vomiting, flatulence, and abnormal or vivid dreams [84, 93, 94]. Rare adverse effects include hypersensitivity and angioedema as well as skin reactions which are reasons for discontinuation. Accidental injury when driving or operating machinery has also been reported. While varenicline and bupropion historically have had a warning of severe neuropsychiatric effects, data from a large RCT of over 8000 people showed that both did not have significantly more of these effects than the nicotine patch or placebo in adults up to age 75 with and without psychiatric disorders [93, 95]. In addition, an RCT of over 8000 people showed that varenicline, bupropion, and nicotine patch did not cause an increase in adverse cardiovascular events in adults age 18–75 years old [96].

Evidence-Based Treatment Algorithms

Figure 16.1 describes the process of screening for nicotine use and the possible interventions for nicotine use. Table 16.1 describes the first-line medications that can be used for smoking cessation. Table 16.2 describes the treatment approaches for nicotine use disorders. Table 16.3 describes the relapse risk factors and relapse strategies. Table 16.4 describes the two methods of asking about tobacco use.

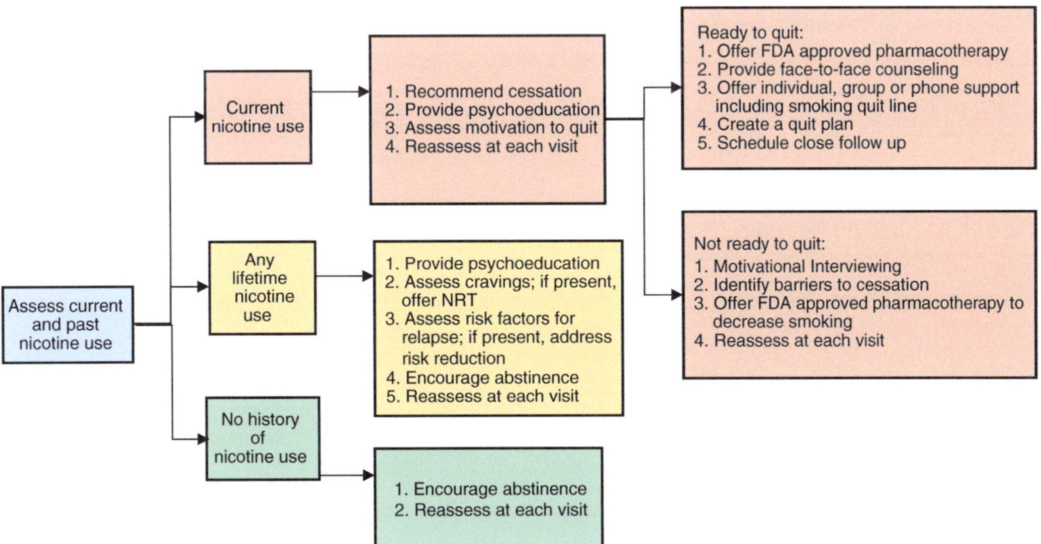

Fig. 16.1 Nicotine use screening and intervention

Table 16.1 First-line medications for smoking cessation

Medication	Dose	Treatment duration and taper	Adverse effects
Nicotine patch	>10 cpd = 21 mg patch <10 cpd = 14 mg patch	Use initial dose for 6 weeks, then taper by 7 mg every 2 weeks	Patch only: Skin irritation Oral only: Cough, ulcers, mouth, and throat soreness
Nicotine lozenge	>30 min after waking = 2 mg <30 min after waking = 4 mg	Use 1 piece every 1–2 h for 6 weeks, then 1 piece every 2–4 h for 2 weeks, then 1 piece every 4–8 h for 2 weeks	All NRT: chest pain, GI upset, palpitations, nausea, vomiting, insomnia
Nicotine gum	>30 min after waking = 2 mg <30 min after waking = 4 mg	Use 1 piece every 1–2 h for 6 weeks, then 1 piece every 2–4 h for 2 weeks, then 1 piece every 4–8 h for 2 weeks	
Nicotine inhaler	6–16 cartridges daily	Taper after 12 weeks. No tapering schedule shown to be optimal	
Nicotine spray	1–2 doses per hour, maximum 5 doses per hour or 40 doses per day	Maximum treatment duration is 3 months. No tapering may be needed, and no tapering schedule shown to be optimal	
Varenicline	0.5 mg daily/3 days, 0.5 mg twice daily/4 days, 1 mg twice daily/12 weeks If CrCL < 30: 0.5 mg twice daily maximum If ESRD on HD: 0.5 mg daily maximum	No taper needed. Start 1 week prior to quit date, treatment duration is 3–6 months	Nausea, constipation, vomiting, flatulence, abnormal/vivid dreams
Bupropion	150 mg SR daily/3 days, 150 mg SR twice daily	No taper needed. Start 1–2 weeks prior to quit date, treatment duration is 7–12 weeks but can last 6 months	Seizures (contraindicated in organic brain disease, seizure history and eating disorder); insomnia, dry mouth, dizziness, nausea, constipation, anxiety, arthralgia, rhinitis

*cpd cigarettes per day

Table 16.2 Treatment approaches for nicotine use disorders

Treatment factor	Recommended approach
Evidence-based pharmacotherapy	Varenicline > single NRT or bupropion Combination NRT > single NRT Combination NRT = varenicline Pharmacotherapy should be combined with behavioral interventions
Behavioral support adjunct to pharmacotherapy	Psychosocial support: phone, individual, group counseling Effective counseling: Social support, skills training and problem solving National smoking quit line: 1-800-QUIT-NOW Spanish smoking quit line: 1-855-DEJELO-YA Veterans smoking quit line 1-855-QUIT-VET
After relapse	Consider alternative pharmacotherapy Increase psychosocial support

Table 16.3 Relapse risk factors and prevention

Risk factors for relapse	Approach to relapse prevention
Triggers Availability of cigarettes Alcohol use Proximity to other smokers Negative affect Weight gain Younger age at cessation Shorter duration of abstinence Stress Nicotine withdrawal symptoms	Use effective smoking cessation intervention Schedule close follow-up Assess and address risk factors for relapse Identify motivation for abstinence Encourage continued abstinence

Table 16.4 Asking about tobacco use

Tobacco use assessment, 1
Number of cigarettes smoked daily
Time passed since last cigarette
Form of smoking (cigarettes, cigars, e-cigarettes, pipes, hookah, gels, vapes, snuff, chewing tobacco, dip, dissolvable)
Brand of smoking product
Onset of cigarette use, age, and circumstances
Smoking alone or with others
Locations of smoking
Presence of other smokers at home
Quality of sleep and whether adult wakes up from sleep to smoke
Time from waking to first cigarette
Triggers to smoke
Presence of cravings
Frequency of smoking
Past quit attempts, aids used, length of time of cessation
Past relapses and circumstances and triggers for relapse
Beliefs about smoking including benefits and consequences
Motivation to quit

Tobacco use assessment, 2
How many cigarettes do you smoke daily? Have you previously smoked more or less?
When was your last cigarette?
What forms of smoking do you use? (Cigarettes, cigars, e-cigarettes, pipes, hookah, gels, vapes, snuff, chewing tobacco, dip, dissolvable)
What brand of smoking products are you currently using?

Table 16.4 (continued)

Tobacco use assessment, 2
When did you start smoking? What were the circumstances?
Do you smoke by yourself or with others?
Where do you smoke?
Do other people at home smoke?
Do you wake up from sleep to smoke?
How long after you wake up do you have your first cigarette?
What triggers you to smoke?
Do you get cravings?
How much time passes between your last cigarette and cravings?
How often do you smoke?
Have you ever attempted to quit smoking in the past? How many times? If so, did you use any medications or other resources (physician counseling, hotline, group support)? How long did you quit for?
What led to you smoking after a prior quit attempt?
What benefits do you get from smoking? What consequences do you believe result from smoking?
Do you want to quit smoking?

Conclusions

With the growing population of older adults, the population of older smokers is expected to increase. Nicotine use disorder among older adults negatively impacts health and cognition and increases safety risks and societal costs. However, this disorder is highly preventable and treatable. Therefore, assessment of nicotine use must be routine in the psychiatric assessment of older adults. Assessment includes determining the presence of current and past nicotine use, form and frequency of use, triggers for use, past quit attempts and relapses, and assessment of motivation to quit. Clinicians should be prepared to offer cessation counseling and assist with cessation by providing pharmacologic and non-pharmacologic interventions and close follow-up. Current evidence supports the use of a combination of FDA approved pharmacotherapy and behavioral interventions. Available evidence has not supported the efficacy of relapse prevention. After a successful quit attempt, clinicians should monitor for risk factors for relapse, encourage

236 A. Khan et al.

abstinence, and consider changes to smoking cessation treatment in a subsequent quit attempt. Older adults have unique considerations in evaluation, such as multiple past quit attempts and relapses as well as beliefs about smoking and cessation. They may have unique barriers to treatment that must be considered. There is a need for additional randomized controlled trials to assess the efficacy smoking cessation interventions and relapse prevention in older adults specifically.

References

1. Substance-Related and Addictive Disorders. Diagnostic and statistical manual of mental disorders.
2. Force UPST. Interventions for tobacco smoking cessation in adults, including pregnant persons: US Preventive Services Task Force Recommendation Statement. JAMA. 2021;325(3):265–79. https://doi.org/10.1001/jama.2020.25019.
3. Ossip-Klein DJ, Pearson TA, McIntosh S, Orleans CT. Smoking is a geriatric health issue. Nicotine Tobacco Res. 1999;1(4):299–300. https://doi.org/10.1080/14622299050011421.
4. Husten CG, Shelton DM, Chrismon JH, Lin YC, Mowery P, Powell FA. Cigarette smoking and smoking cessation among older adults: United States, 1965–94. Tob Control. 1997;6(3):175–80. https://doi.org/10.1136/tc.6.3.175.
5. Cornelius ME, Loretan CG, Wang TW, Jamal A, Homa DM. Tobacco product use among adults—United States, 2020. MMWR Morb Mortal Wkly Rep. 2022;71(11):397–405. https://doi.org/10.15585/mmwr.mm7111a1.
6. Office on Smoking and Health NCfCDPaHP, Centers for Disease Control and Prevention. Burden of Cigarette Use in the U.S. 2022 [updated August 3, 2022October 22, 2022]. Available from: https://www.cdc.gov/tobacco/campaign/tips/resources/data/cigarette-smoking-in-united-states.html#references.
7. Moore AA, Karno MP, Grella CE, Lin JC, Warda U, Liao DH, et al. Alcohol, tobacco, and nonmedical drug use in older U.S. Adults: data from the 2001/02 national epidemiologic survey of alcohol and related conditions. J Am Geriatr Soc. 2009;57(12):2275–81. https://doi.org/10.1111/j.1532-5415.2009.02554.x.
8. CfBHSa Q. Results from the 2019 National Survey on Drug Use and Health: detailed tables. Rockville, MD: Substance Abuse and Mental Health Services Administration; 2020. November 18,2022). Available from: https://www.samhsa.gov/data/sites/default/files/reports/rpt29394/NSDUHDetailedTabs2019/NSDUHDetailedTabs2019.pdf
9. Lessov-Schlaggar CN, Pergadia ML, Khroyan TV, Swan GE. Genetics of nicotine dependence and pharmacotherapy. Biochem Pharmacol. 2008;75(1):178–95. https://doi.org/10.1016/j.bcp.2007.08.018.
10. Kendler KS, Neale MC, MacLean CJ, Heath AC, Eaves LJ, Kessler RC. Smoking and major depression. A causal analysis. Arch Gen Psychiatry. 1993;50(1):36–43. https://doi.org/10.1001/archpsyc.1993.01820130038007.
11. Blazer DG, Wu LT. Patterns of tobacco use and tobacco-related psychiatric morbidity and substance use among middle-aged and older adults in the United States. Aging Ment Health. 2012;16(3):296–304. https://doi.org/10.1080/13607863.2011.615739.
12. Sachs-Ericsson N, Collins N, Schmidt B, Zvolensky M. Older adults and smoking: characteristics, nicotine dependence and prevalence of DSM-IV 12-month disorders. Aging Ment Health. 2011;15(1):132–41. https://doi.org/10.1080/13607863.2010.505230.
13. Lam TH, Li ZB, Ho SY, Chan WM, Ho KS, Li MP, et al. Smoking and depressive symptoms in Chinese elderly in Hong Kong. Acta Psychiatr Scand. 2004;110(3):195–200. https://doi.org/10.1111/j.1600-0447.2004.00342.x.
14. Bassil NK, Ohanian MLK, Bou Saba TG. Nicotine use disorder in older adults. Clin Geriatr Med. 2022;38(1):119–31. https://doi.org/10.1016/j.cger.2021.07.008.
15. Appel DW, Aldrich TK. Smoking cessation in the elderly. Clin Geriatr Med. 2003;19(1):77–100. https://doi.org/10.1016/s0749-0690(02)00053-8.
16. Nadruz W, Claggett B, Gonçalves A, Querejeta-Roca G, Fernandes-Silva MM, Shah AM, et al. Smoking and cardiac structure and function in the elderly. Circulation: Cardiovasc Imaging. 2016;9(9):e004950. https://doi.org/10.1161/CIRCIMAGING.116.004950.
17. Ambrose JA, Barua RS. The pathophysiology of cigarette smoking and cardiovascular disease: an update. J Am Coll Cardiol. 2004;43(10):1731–7. https://doi.org/10.1016/j.jacc.2003.12.047.
18. Hernigou J, Schuind F. Tobacco and bone fractures: a review of the facts and issues that every orthopaedic surgeon should know. Bone Joint Res. 2019;8(6):255–65. https://doi.org/10.1302/2046-3758.86.Bjr-2018-0344.R1.
19. Reh DD, Higgins TS, Smith TL. Impact of tobacco smoke on chronic rhinosinusitis: a review of the literature. Int Forum Allergy Rhinol. 2012;2(5):362–9. https://doi.org/10.1002/alr.21054.
20. Velilla S, García-Medina JJ, García-Layana A, Dolz-Marco R, Pons-Vázquez S, Pinazo-Durán MD, et al. Smoking and age-related macular degeneration: review and update. J Ophthalmol. 2013;2013:895147. https://doi.org/10.1155/2013/895147.
21. Pan B, Jin X, Jun L, Qiu S, Zheng Q, Pan M. The relationship between smoking and stroke: a meta-analysis. Medicine. 2019;98(12):e14872. https://doi.org/10.1097/md.0000000000014872.
22. Sairenchi T, Iso H, Nishimura A, Hosoda T, Irie F, Saito Y, et al. Cigarette smoking and risk of Type 2 diabe-

tes mellitus among middle-aged and elderly Japanese men and women. Am J Epidemiol. 2004;160(2):158–62. https://doi.org/10.1093/aje/kwh183.

23. Gellert C, Schöttker B, Brenner H. Smoking and all-cause mortality in older people: systematic review and meta-analysis. Arch Internal Med. 2012;172(11):837–44. https://doi.org/10.1001/archinternmed.2012.1397.

24. Mons U, Müezzinler A, Gellert C, Schöttker B, Abnet CC, Bobak M, et al. Impact of smoking and smoking cessation on cardiovascular events and mortality among older adults: meta-analysis of individual participant data from prospective cohort studies of the CHANCES consortium. BMJ. 2015;350:h1551. https://doi.org/10.1136/bmj.h1551.

25. LaCroix AZ, Lang J, Scherr P, Wallace RB, Cornoni-Huntley J, Berkman L, et al. Smoking and mortality among older men and women in three communities. N Engl J Med. 1991;324(23):1619–25. https://doi.org/10.1056/nejm199106063242303.

26. Almeida OP, Garrido GJ, Alfonso H, Hulse G, Lautenschlager NT, Hankey GJ, et al. 24-month effect of smoking cessation on cognitive function and brain structure in later life. Neuroimage. 2011;55(4):1480–9. https://doi.org/10.1016/j.neuroimage.2011.01.063.

27. Power MC, Deal JA, Sharrett AR, Jack CR Jr, Knopman D, Mosley TH, et al. Smoking and white matter hyperintensity progression: the ARIC-MRI study. Neurology. 2015;84(8):841–8. https://doi.org/10.1212/wnl.0000000000001283.

28. Boksa P. Smoking, psychiatric illness and the brain. J Psychiatry Neurosci. 2017;42(3):147–9. https://doi.org/10.1503/jpn.170060.

29. Anstey KJ, von Sanden C, Salim A, O'Kearney R. Smoking as a risk factor for dementia and cognitive decline: a meta-analysis of prospective studies. Am J Epidemiol. 2007;166(4):367–78. https://doi.org/10.1093/aje/kwm116.

30. Leistikow BN, Martin DC, Milano CE. Fire injuries, disasters, and costs from cigarettes and cigarette lights: a global overview. Prev Med. 2000;31(2 Pt 1):91–9. https://doi.org/10.1006/pmed.2000.0680.

31. Marshall SW, Runyan CW, Bangdiwala SI, Linzer MA, Sacks JJ, Butts JD. Fatal residential fires: who dies and who survives? JAMA. 1998;279(20):1633–7. https://doi.org/10.1001/jama.279.20.1633.

32. Ballard JE, Koepsell TD, Rivara F. Association of smoking and alcohol drinking with residential fire injuries. Am J Epidemiol. 1992;135(1):26–34. https://doi.org/10.1093/oxfordjournals.aje.a116198.

33. Zhang X, Miller L, Max W, Rice DP. Cost of smoking to the Medicare program, 1993. Health Care Financ Rev. 1999;20(4):179–96.

34. Benowitz NL. Pharmacology of nicotine: addiction, smoking-induced disease, and therapeutics. Annu Rev Pharmacol Toxicol. 2009;49:57–71. https://doi.org/10.1146/annurev.pharmtox.48.113006.094742.

35. Markou A. Review: neurobiology of nicotine dependence. Philos Trans R Soc Lond B Biol Sci. 2008;363(1507):3159–68. https://doi.org/10.1098/rstb.2008.0095.

36. Benowitz NL, Bernert JT, Foulds J, Hecht SS, Jacob P, Jarvis MJ, et al. Biochemical verification of tobacco use and abstinence: 2019 update. Nicotine Tob Res. 2020;22(7):1086–97. https://doi.org/10.1093/ntr/ntz132.

37. Molander L, Hansson A, Lunell E. Pharmacokinetics of nicotine in healthy elderly people. Clin Pharmacol Ther. 2001;69(1):57–65. https://doi.org/10.1067/mcp.2001.113181.

38. Zevin S, Benowitz NL. Drug interactions with tobacco smoking. An update. Clin Pharmacokinet. 1999;36(6):425–38. https://doi.org/10.2165/00003088-199936060-00004.

39. Clinical Practice Guideline Treating Tobacco Use and Dependence 2008 Update Panel, Liaisons, and Staff. A clinical practice guideline for treating tobacco use and dependence: 2008 update. A U.S. Public Health Service report. Am J Prev Med. 2008;35(2):158–76. https://doi.org/10.1016/j.amepre.2008.04.009.

40. Cornelius ME, Wang TW, Jamal A, Loretan CG, Neff LJ. Tobacco product use among adults—United States, 2019. MMWR Morb Mortal Wkly Rep. 2020;69(46):1736–42. https://doi.org/10.15585/mmwr.mm6946a4.

41. Center TUoTMAC. Tobacco Cessation-Adult 2021 [cited 2022 December 18, 2022]. Available from: https://www.mdanderson.org/content/dam/mdanderson/documents/for-physicians/algorithms/screening/risk-reduction-tobacco-cessation-web-algorithm.pdf.

42. Iso H, Date C, Yamamoto A, Toyoshima H, Watanabe Y, Kikuchi S, et al. Smoking cessation and mortality from cardiovascular disease among Japanese men and women: the JACC Study. Am J Epidemiol. 2005;161(2):170–9. https://doi.org/10.1093/aje/kwi027.

43. Doll R, Peto R, Boreham J, Sutherland I. Mortality in relation to smoking: 50 years' observations on male British doctors. BMJ. 2004;328(7455):1519. https://doi.org/10.1136/bmj.38142.554479.AE.

44. Kleykamp BA, Heishman SJ. The older smoker. JAMA. 2011;306(8):876–7. https://doi.org/10.1001/jama.2011.1221.

45. Maguire CP, Ryan J, Kelly A, O'Neill D, Coakley D, Walsh JB. Do patient age and medical condition influence medical advice to stop smoking? Age Ageing. 2000;29(3):264–6. https://doi.org/10.1093/ageing/29.3.264.

46. Rimer BK, Orleans CT, Keintz MK, Cristinzio S, Fleisher L. The older smoker: status, challenges and opportunities for intervention. Chest. 1990;97(3):547–53. https://doi.org/10.1378/chest.97.3.547.

47. Kulak JA, LaValley S. Cigarette use and smoking beliefs among older Americans: findings from a nationally representative survey. J Addict Dis. 2018;37(1–2):46–54. https://doi.org/10.1080/10550887.2018.1521255.

48. Orleans CT, Rimer BK, Cristinzio S, Keintz MK, Fleisher L. A national survey of older smokers: treatment needs of a growing population.

Health Psychol. 1991;10(5):343–51. https://doi.org/10.1037//0278-6133.10.5.343.

49. Kerr S, Watson H, Tolson D, Lough M, Brown M. Smoking after the age of 65 years: a qualitative exploration of older current and former smokers' views on smoking, stopping smoking, and smoking cessation resources and services. Health Soc Care Community. 2006;14(6):572–82. https://doi.org/10.1111/j.1365-2524.2006.00659.x.

50. Livingston G, Johnston K, Katona C, Paton J, Lyketsos CG, Old Age Task Force of the World Federation of Biological Psychiatry. Systematic review of psychological approaches to the management of neuropsychiatric symptoms of dementia. Am J Psychiatry. 2005;162(11):1996–2021. https://doi.org/10.1176/appi.ajp.162.11.1996.

51. Hajek P, Stead LF, West R, Jarvis M, Hartmann-Boyce J, Lancaster T. Relapse prevention interventions for smoking cessation. Cochrane Database Syst Rev. 2013;(8):Cd003999. https://doi.org/10.1002/14651858.CD003999.pub4.

52. Hughes J. An algorithm for choosing among smoking cessation treatments. J Subst Abuse Treat. 2008;34(4):426–32. https://doi.org/10.1016/j.jsat.2007.07.007.

53. Shimada S, Komiyama M, Wada H, Yamakage H, Shimatsu A, Takahashi Y, et al. Analysis of factors associated with smoking relapse. Eur Cardiol. 2017;12(2):111. https://doi.org/10.15420/ecr.2017:23:20.

54. García-Rodríguez O, Secades-Villa R, Flórez-Salamanca L, Okuda M, Liu SM, Blanco C. Probability and predictors of relapse to smoking: results of the National Epidemiologic Survey on Alcohol and Related Conditions (NESARC). Drug Alcohol Depend. 2013;132(3):479–85. https://doi.org/10.1016/j.drugalcdep.2013.03.008.

55. Zbikowski SM, Magnusson B, Pockey JR, Tindle HA, Weaver KE. A review of smoking cessation interventions for smokers aged 50 and older. Maturitas. 2012;71(2):131–41. https://doi.org/10.1016/j.maturitas.2011.11.019.

56. Chen D, Wu LT. Smoking cessation interventions for adults aged 50 or older: a systematic review and meta-analysis. Drug Alcohol Depend. 2015;154:14–24. https://doi.org/10.1016/j.drugalcdep.2015.06.004.

57. Rimer BK, Orleans CT. Tailoring smoking cessation for older adults. Cancer. 1994;74(S7):2051–4. https://doi.org/10.1002/1097-0142(19941001)74:7+<2051::AID-CNCR2820741711>3.0.CO;2-4.

58. Morgan GD, Noll EL, Orleans CT, Rimer BK, Amfoh K, Bonney G. Reaching midlife and older smokers: tailored interventions for routine medical care. Prev Med. 1996;25(3):346–54. https://doi.org/10.1006/pmed.1996.0065.

59. Abdullah AS, Ho LM, Kwan YH, Cheung WL, McGhee SM, Chan WH. Promoting smoking cessation among the elderly: what are the predictors of intention to quit and successful quitting? J Aging Health. 2006;18(4):552–64. https://doi.org/10.1177/0898264305281104.

60. Dale LC, Olsen DA, Patten CA, Schroeder DR, Croghan IT, Hurt RD, et al. Predictors of smoking cessation among elderly smokers treated for nicotine dependence. Tob Control. 1997;6(3):181–7. https://doi.org/10.1136/tc.6.3.181.

61. Rigotti NA, Regan S, Levy DE, Japuntich S, Chang Y, Park ER, et al. Sustained care intervention and postdischarge smoking cessation among hospitalized adults: a randomized clinical trial. JAMA. 2014;312(7):719–28. https://doi.org/10.1001/jama.2014.9237.

62. Keenan PS. Smoking and weight change after new health diagnoses in older adults. Arch Intern Med. 2009;169(3):237–42. https://doi.org/10.1001/archinternmed.2008.557.

63. Cohen-Mansfield J. Predictors of smoking cessation in old-old age. Nicotine Tob Res. 2016;18(7):1675–9. https://doi.org/10.1093/ntr/ntw011.

64. Lindson N, Thompson TP, Ferrey A, Lambert JD, Aveyard P. Motivational interviewing for smoking cessation. Cochrane Database Syst Rev. 2019;7(7):Cd006936. https://doi.org/10.1002/14651858.CD006936.pub4.

65. Quality AfHRa. Patients not ready to make a quit attempt now (The "5 R's") Rockville, MD; 2012 [updated December 2012; cited 2022 December 18, 2022]. Available from: https://www.ahrq.gov/prevention/guidelines/tobacco/5rs.html.

66. Ali A, Kaplan CM, Derefinko KJ, Klesges RC. Smoking Cessation for smokers not ready to quit: meta-analysis and cost-effectiveness analysis. Am J Prev Med. 2018;55(2):253–62. https://doi.org/10.1016/j.amepre.2018.04.021.

67. Niaura R. Nonpharmacologic therapy for smoking cessation: characteristics and efficacy of current approaches. Am J Med. 2008;121(4 Suppl. 1):S11–9. https://doi.org/10.1016/j.amjmed.2008.01.021.

68. Stead LF, Lancaster T. Combined pharmacotherapy and behavioural interventions for smoking cessation. Cochrane Database Syst Rev. 2012;10:Cd008286. https://doi.org/10.1002/14651858.CD008286.pub2.

69. Lancaster T, Stead LF. Individual behavioural counselling for smoking cessation. Cochrane Database Syst Rev. 2017;3(3):Cd001292. https://doi.org/10.1002/14651858.CD001292.pub3.

70. Stead LF, Lancaster T. Group behaviour therapy programmes for smoking cessation. Cochrane Database Syst Rev. 2005;(2):Cd001007. https://doi.org/10.1002/14651858.CD001007.pub2.

71. Gorin SS, Heck JE. Meta-analysis of the efficacy of tobacco counseling by health care providers. Cancer Epidemiol Biomarkers Prev. 2004;13(12):2012–22.

72. Lancaster T, Stead LF. Self-help interventions for smoking cessation. Cochrane Database Syst Rev. 2002;(3):Cd001118. https://doi.org/10.1002/14651858.Cd001118.

73. Ossip-Klein DJ, Carosella AM, Krusch DA. Self-help interventions for older smokers. Tob Control. 1997;6(3):188–93. https://doi.org/10.1136/tc.6.3.188.

74. Nancy Aldrich WFB. CDC urges older adults to improve health, increase longevity, through smoking Cessation National Association of Chronic Disease Directors [cited 2022 November 11, 2022]. Available from: https://chronicdisease.org/resource/resmgr/healthy_aging_critical_issues_brief/ha_cib_smoking.pdf.

75. Hall SM, Humfleet GL, Muñoz RF, Reus VI, Robbins JA, Prochaska JJ. Extended treatment of older cigarette smokers. Addiction. 2009;104(6):1043–52. https://doi.org/10.1111/j.1360-0443.2009.02548.x.

76. Vetter NJ, Ford D. Smoking prevention among people aged 60 and over: a randomized controlled trial. Age Ageing. 1990;19(3):164–8. https://doi.org/10.1093/ageing/19.3.164.

77. Paterson NE, Balfour DJ, Markou A. Chronic bupropion attenuated the anhedonic component of nicotine withdrawal in rats via inhibition of dopamine reuptake in the nucleus accumbens shell. Eur J Neurosci. 2007;25(10):3099–108. https://doi.org/10.1111/j.1460-9568.2007.05546.x.

78. Coe JW, Brooks PR, Vetelino MG, Wirtz MC, Arnold EP, Huang J, et al. Varenicline: an alpha4beta2 nicotinic receptor partial agonist for smoking cessation. J Med Chem. 2005;48(10):3474–7. https://doi.org/10.1021/jm050069n.

79. Wellbutrin [package insert]. Research Triangle Park, NC: GlaxoSmithKline; 2009.

80. Ravva P, Gastonguay MR, Tensfeldt TG, Faessel HM. Population pharmacokinetic analysis of varenicline in adult smokers. Br J Clin Pharmacol. 2009;68(5):669–81. https://doi.org/10.1111/j.1365-2125.2009.03520.x.

81. Burstein AH, Fullerton T, Clark DJ, Faessel HM. Pharmacokinetics, safety, and tolerability after single and multiple oral doses of varenicline in elderly smokers. J Clin Pharmacol. 2006;46(11):1234–40. https://doi.org/10.1177/0091270006291837.

82. Sweet RA, Pollock BG, Kirshner M, Wright B, Altieri LP, DeVane CL. Pharmacokinetics of single- and multiple-dose bupropion in elderly patients with depression. J Clin Pharmacol. 1995;35(9):876–84. https://doi.org/10.1002/j.1552-4604.1995.tb04132.x.

83. Scholz J, Santos PC, Buzo CG, Lopes NH, Abe TO, Gaya PV, et al. Effects of aging on the effectiveness of smoking cessation medication. Oncotarget. 2016;7(21):30032–6. https://doi.org/10.18632/oncotarget.9090.

84. Chantix [package insert]. New York, NY: Pfizer, Inc.; 2012.

85. Wilkes S. The use of bupropion SR in cigarette smoking cessation. Int J Chron Obstruct Pulmon Dis. 2008;3(1):45–53. https://doi.org/10.2147/copd.s1121.

86. Lindson N, Chepkin SC, Ye W, Fanshawe TR, Bullen C, Hartmann-Boyce J. Different doses, durations and modes of delivery of nicotine replacement therapy for smoking cessation. Cochrane Database Syst Rev. 2019;4(4):Cd013308. https://doi.org/10.1002/14651858.Cd013308.

87. Howes S, Hartmann-Boyce J, Livingstone-Banks J, Hong B, Lindson N. Antidepressants for smoking cessation. Cochrane Database Syst Rev. 2020;4(4):Cd000031. https://doi.org/10.1002/14651858.CD000031.pub5.

88. Cahill K, Lindson-Hawley N, Thomas KH, Fanshawe TR, Lancaster T. Nicotine receptor partial agonists for smoking cessation. Cochrane Database Syst Rev. 2016;2016(5):Cd006103. https://doi.org/10.1002/14651858.CD006103.pub7.

89. Chang CP, Huang WH, You CH, Hwang LC, Lu IJ, Chan HL. Factors correlated with smoking cessation success in older adults: a retrospective cohort study in Taiwan. Int J Environ Res Public Health. 2019;16(18) https://doi.org/10.3390/ijerph16183462.

90. Mills EJ, Wu P, Lockhart I, Wilson K, Ebbert JO. Adverse events associated with nicotine replacement therapy (NRT) for smoking cessation. A systematic review and meta-analysis of one hundred and twenty studies involving 177,390 individuals. Tob Induc Dis. 2010;8(1):8. https://doi.org/10.1186/1617-9625-8-8.

91. Zyban [package insert]. Research Triangle Park, NC: GlaxoSmithKline; 2016.

92. William T, Howard M, Warnock JK. The efficacy and toxicity of Bupropion in the elderly. Jefferson J Psychiatry. 2000;15(1) https://doi.org/10.29046/JJP.015.1.004.

93. Thomas KH, Martin RM, Knipe DW, Higgins JPT, Gunnell D. Risk of neuropsychiatric adverse events associated with varenicline: systematic review and meta-analysis. BMJ. 2015;350:h1109. https://doi.org/10.1136/bmj.h1109.

94. Ebbert JO, Wyatt KD, Hays JT, Klee EW, Hurt RD. Varenicline for smoking cessation: efficacy, safety, and treatment recommendations. Patient Prefer Adher. 2010;4:355–62. https://doi.org/10.2147/ppa.s10620.

95. Anthenelli RM, Benowitz NL, West R, St Aubin L, McRae T, Lawrence D, et al. Neuropsychiatric safety and efficacy of varenicline, bupropion, and nicotine patch in smokers with and without psychiatric disorders (EAGLES): a double-blind, randomised, placebo-controlled clinical trial. Lancet. 2016;387(10037):2507–20. https://doi.org/10.1016/s0140-6736(16)30272-0.

96. Benowitz NL, Pipe A, West R, Hays JT, Tonstad S, McRae T, et al. Cardiovascular safety of varenicline, bupropion, and nicotine patch in smokers: a randomized clinical trial. JAMA Internal Med. 2018;178(5):622–31. https://doi.org/10.1001/jamainternmed.2018.0397.

Cannabis Use Disorder

Amanda L. Campbell, Gibson George,
and Padmapriya Marpuri

Introduction

Cannabis use disorder, as defined by the DSM-5-TR, is problematic cannabis use leading to significant impairment or distress as defined by meeting at least two of 11 criteria [1]. These criteria include using cannabis in larger amounts or for longer periods of time than intended, persistent desire to cut down on use, cravings to use cannabis, spending significant time to obtain cannabis or to recover from the effects of intoxication by cannabis, recurrent use that leads to impairment in fulfilling obligations, persistent use despite social consequences, having to give up important social, occupational, or recreational activities due to cannabis use, the use of cannabis in physically hazardous situations, continued use despite knowledge of the physical or psychological consequences it is causing, as well as symptoms of tolerance or withdrawal. Severity of the cannabis use disorder depends on the number of symptoms present, with mild having 2–3 of the above criteria met, moderate with 4–5, and severe with 6 or more of the afore-mentioned symptoms [1].

Cannabis is the most frequently used illicit substance among the older adult population [2, 3]. Cannabis use continues to increase in frequency among the older individuals throughout the years [2, 4]. In data collected between 2015 and 2016, 9.0% of adults aged 50–64 and 2.9% of adults aged 65 or older used marijuana in the past year [5]. Between 2015 and 2018, there was a 75% relative increase in the prevalence of cannabis use in those aged 65 and older [2]. This increase in cannabis use is more apparent among women, racial and ethnic minorities, individuals with higher incomes, and those with co-occurring mental illnesses [4]. Though the prevalence of cannabis use itself is greater, the prevalence of cannabis use disorder among adults 65 or older ranges from less than 1% to 4.5% [6, 7].

According to data collected between 2015 and 2018, approximately 1.7 million individuals of all ages receiving Medicare benefits met the DSM-IV criteria for substance use disorder (SUD) annually [8]. The most prevalent subsets of SUD were alcohol use disorder at 77.2%, opioid use disorder at 14.0%, and cannabis use disorder at 10% [8]. Individuals aged over 65 with the diagnosis of SUD were over three times as likely to endorse serious psychological distress when compared to those without SUD [8]. Of note, only 6% of individuals receiving Medicare

A. L. Campbell · P. Marpuri (✉)
Department of Psychiatry, St. Luke's University
Health Network, Easton, PA, USA
e-mail: amanda.campbell@sluhn.org;
padmapriya.marpuri@sluhn.org

G. George
St. Luke's Penn Foundation, Department of
Psychiatry, St. Luke's University Health Network,
Easton, PA, USA
e-mail: gibson.george@sluhn.org

© The Author(s), under exclusive license to Springer Nature Switzerland AG 2024
R. R. Tampi, D. J. Tampi (eds.), *Treatment of Psychiatric Disorders Among Older Adults*,
https://doi.org/10.1007/978-3-031-55711-8_17

benefits who met the criteria for SUD received treatment [8]. Cannabis use increases the risk of comorbid alcohol and tobacco use disorder, among other psychiatric diagnoses [3, 9]. From 2006 to 2013, a 63.4% increase in alcohol use and 55.8% increase in tobacco use were identified among older cannabis users [3].

Among cannabis users, most of them initiated the use of marijuana before the age of 18 [3]. Cannabis users were more likely to have college education according to several of the studies that were examined in one literature review. However, some studies reported this was different based on the age stratification, with those between 50 and 64 years old having completed some college, but those 65 and older had less education [3]. Several studies found that older cannabis users were more likely to be self-reported as non-Hispanic Black, multiracial, or American-Indian compared to nonusers, while one study found those aged between 50 and 64 were more likely to be non-Hispanic White, and those aged 65 and older were more likely to be African-American [3].

In an epidemiological database study comparing the demographics among current older adult users and past older adult users, it was found that 3.9% of individuals were past-year cannabis users, and 21.7% were former cannabis users [9]. Those that used cannabis in the last year had higher risk of other substance use in the past year, as well as increased risk of alcohol and nicotine use disorders. This population also had the highest rate of major depressive disorders, anxiety disorders, PTSD, and bipolar disorders, at a rate of 33.2% for any or multiple of these illnesses. Notably, heavier use during peak periods of use correlated with increased likelihood of substance use disorder diagnosis. Among those with former cannabis use, the quantity of use during the period of peak use was also associated with mental illness and substance use disorder, including CUD. Personality disorders occurred at a much higher rate among past-year users at 34.8%, compared to 18.7% in former users and 9% of never users of cannabis [9].

Risk Factors and Neurobiology

Examining the neurobiology of CUD allows for a more in-depth understanding of the pathophysiology of the disease process. As with other SUDs, the development of CUD is likely due to a combination of the neurobiological effects including alternations in memory and reward pathways, as well as psychological and social influences [10, 11]. The human central nervous system contains an endogenous endocannabinoid system, which consists of endocannabinoids, enzymes for their synthesis and regulation, and cannabinoid receptor types 1 and 2 (CB1 and CB2). This system contributes to the regulation of several behavioral aspects, including memory, stress response, anxiety, and pain [10]. The primary psychoactive component of cannabis, delta-9-tetrahydrocannabinol, binds with CB1 with high affinity, and contributes to the euphoric and reinforcing effects of cannabis use [10, 11]. The CB1 receptor is expressed in multiple areas of the brain such as the amygdala, hippocampus, cerebellum, cerebral cortex, basal ganglia, hypothalamus, and the brainstem. The stimulation of these areas of the brain contributes to the reinforcing effects of cannabis, which may be implicated in the development of CUD [11].

Among the older adult population, the highest rates of cannabis use disorder occur in those with co-occurring psychiatric illnesses, and in those with co-occurring SUDs [9]. Specifically, the psychiatric illnesses that are most common include mood disorders, anxiety disorders, PTSD, and personality disorders [6, 9]. Males have the highest risk of CUD among both older adults and among the general population [7, 12]. Older individuals with two or more chronic health conditions, a history of depression within the last year, and those who received mental health treatment have a higher prevalence of past-year cannabis use, indicating potential increased risk for development of CUD among these populations [12].

Although not specific to the geriatric population, among the general adult population, earlier onset of first use of cannabis is also related to highest risk of CUD [7]. The odds of developing CUD within the last year were higher in Native American and Black individuals and lower in Asian/Pacific Islander and Hispanic individuals. Those who were never married and those with lowest income were found to have higher risk of CUD [6].

Consequences

Research directly related to the consequences of CUD specific to older adults is limited. As humans age, it has been noted that there are changes to the endocannabinoid system, including a decrease in binding of specific agonists to the CB1 receptor in areas such as the cerebral cortex, limbic system, and the hypothalamic structures. The direct translation of these findings may indicate that the physiological effects of cannabis use in geriatric patients may differ from those in younger adult populations [13]. The meaningful clinical consequences of CUD have limited research, though the correlations in the afore-mentioned risk factors may speak to possible consequences of CUD in this population. Special considerations in this population include interactions with drugs, falls and injury, effects on cognitive impairment, and the association between cannabis and cognition, all of which has limited evidence in the existing literature [14].

Assessment

There is no consensus regarding the utility of universal screening for cannabis use. However, literature suggests that clinicians should be screening every patient for cannabis use at least once, and more frequent screening should be considered for higher risk populations, such as those with comorbid substance use or psychiatric disorders [15, 16]. If patients indicate cannabis use, further questions should inquire into frequency and amount, as well as social impact of use, and difficulties at work or school due to use [15, 16]. If there are concerns for problematic cannabis use, there should then be further questioning to fit the DSM criteria for CUD, which will be discussed in more detail below. Another option is to utilize available screening and assessment tools [16]. All assessments should also include evaluating for comorbid psychiatric disorder or substance use disorders [15].

Questions common for evaluating substance use include time of last use, frequency and quantity of use, route of administration, age of first use, history of past treatment including detoxification, rehabilitation, or outpatient treatments, and duration of use including the extent of any periods of abstinence [15]. To evaluate for active cannabis intoxication, physical symptoms can manifest as conjunctival erythema and injection, increased appetite, dry mouth, and tachycardia [15].

The most cited screening tools for cannabis use are The Cannabis Use Disorders Identification Test (CUDIT), Cannabis Use Disorders Identification Test-Revised (CUDIT-R), and the Cannabis Use Disorders Identification Test-Short Form (CUDIT-SF). The CUDIT and CUDIT-R were both originally designed for validity with the DSM-IV; however, the more recent CUDIT-R was later established to have concurrent validity with DSM-5 criteria [17, 18].

The CUDIT-R contains 8 items and has been shown not only to be an effective screening tool, but also effective at distinguishing severity of cannabis use and stage of change, giving it clinical utility in determining appropriateness of treatment [17]. At a cutoff score of 13, the CUDIT-R was found to have a positive predictive value of 96% and negative predictive value of 80% [17]. The short form, CUDIT-SF is a shortened version with three questions designed for a busy clinic setting and has sensitivity of 78.26 and a specificity of 76.7 in participants sampled from the United States [19].

According to the DSM-5-TR, individuals must meet at least 2 out of 11 listed criteria to be diagnosed with CUD. Examples of these criteria include but are not limited to consuming cannabis in larger amounts than intended, unsuccessful efforts to control use, spending significant time

Table 17.1 DSM-5-TR criteria

DSM-5-TR Criteria for CUD. Must meet 2 or more of the following 11 criteria, within a 12-month period: (1)
1. Cannabis is consumed in larger amounts or over a longer period than intended
2. There are unsuccessful efforts of, or ongoing desire to cut back on use of cannabis
3. A considerable amount of time is spent in either obtaining cannabis, using cannabis, or recovering from the effects of cannabis
4. Experiencing cravings to use cannabis
5. Cannabis use resulting in impacted performance in work, school, or home
6. Continuing to use cannabis despite having social or interpersonal problems resulting from the use of cannabis
7. Having given up or reduced important social, work, or recreational activities due to cannabis use
8. The use of cannabis in physically hazardous situations
9. Continuing to use cannabis despite having had persistent or recurrent physical or psychological problems caused or worsened by cannabis use
10. Tolerance of cannabis in the form of either requiring more cannabis for desired physiological effects or having had notably diminished effects while using the same amount of cannabis consistently
11. Having experienced withdrawal symptoms from not using cannabis, or using cannabis to avoid the withdrawal symptoms

obtaining, using, or recovering from cannabis use, having cravings, interference with functioning at work, home, or school, tolerance, and withdrawal. See Table 17.1 for full DSM-5-TR criteria [1].

Urine drug screening may be used to screen for current use or to assess for continued abstinence during treatment. Urine drug screens do have limitations, such as not detecting synthetic cannabinoids, and of the possibility of continued positive test results for up to 4 weeks after cessation of use, therefore should be utilized cautiously [16].

Treatments

The mainstay of treatment for cannabis use disorder is largely psychotherapeutic in nature, including cognitive behavioral therapy, motivation enhancement therapy, and contingency management. There are currently no United States Food and Drug Administration (USFDA) approved pharmacological treatment options for treatment of CUD. Limited studies have been conducted on various antidepressants, mood stabilizers, and cannabinoids for treatment of cannabis use disorder [20–32].

Psychotherapy

Numerous psychosocial interventions have shown promise in management of cannabis use disorder. The most prominently studied psychotherapeutic modalities for treatment of CUD are cognitive behavioral therapy (CBT), motivational enhancement therapy (MET), and contingency management (CM) [20, 21, 22]. Available research focuses on the general adult population, with a dearth of research examining the treatments for CUD among the older adult population. Therefore, the following paragraphs will discuss evidence for treatment options for adults in general, with limitations of lack of specificity for the geriatric population. Given this lack of availability of older adult specific literature, research into treatment of CUD specifically in the geriatric population is a potential area for future research.

The goal of cognitive behavior therapy (CBT) is to reduce or stop substance use by focusing on the development of coping skills, reduction/cessation skills, and relapse prevention skills via counseling sessions and assigned practice between sessions. The session frequency in the literature varies from 6 to 14 sessions and duration varies from 45 to 60 min [21]. Chatters et al analyzed 33 randomized trials across several countries and found that CBT significantly improved outcomes compared to wait list, which was maintained at 9 months in one included study [24]. Another review found that individuals who received CBT used cannabis for fewer days of the month compared to the control group [16].

The goal of motivational enhancement therapy (MET) is to increase the patient's motivation and commitment to reduce or abstain from use of substances utilizing empathy, reflective listening, and affirmation [16, 21]. MET can be delivered in both individual and group therapy settings. A review of the existing literature utilizing MET as a treatment for CUD indicates that the number of sessions vary typically between 1 and 4 with a duration of 45–90 min for each [21]. Motivational interviewing (MI) is similarly based on examining and addressing a patient's motivation for continuing the use of the substance or with difficulty quitting the substance use [23]. In a meta-analysis by Chatters et al, findings on MI and MET were mixed, with some included studies demonstrating modest improvements, and others describing nonsignificant findings [24]. Specifically, MET has been noted to reduce the number of cannabis use days during a month, reducing cannabis-related problems, and severity of CUD, with no significant difference between overall abstinence in MET versus control groups [16].

The practice of contingency management (CM) utilizes principles of reinforcement to support treatment adherence. Specifically, when treating CUD, a CM style of treatment may utilize monetary-based incentives for attendance at appointments or for frequency of clean urine specimens [21]. In a literature review conducted by Davis et al, available evidence supported the use of CM in SUDs in the general adult population, though only two of the included articles were specific to cannabis [25]. Utilizing CM to augment MET, CBT, or a combination of the two increases the number of abstinent days compared to the use of these interventions alone [16].

Utilizing any of the above therapeutic techniques individually has been demonstrated to provide benefits over placebo [16, 21, 26, 27]. However, the combination of multiple or all three of these treatment methods provides the most robust benefit based on the existing literature. Combining CBT, MET, and CM has demonstrated superior short-term effects on treatment of CUD [16, 21, 26]. CBT with MET can increase the likelihood of reducing the frequency of cannabis use and longer term abstinence, with one study finding significant improvement over CBT or MET alone at up to 14 months follow-up [26, 27]. A meta-analysis examining 33 randomized trials across several countries found that CBT significantly improved outcomes compared to

wait list, which was maintained at up to 9 months in one included study. However, this article also noted that the intensity of treatment impacted the benefits, meaning that interventions over multiple sessions had improved outcomes compared to brief interventions. Additionally, most studies did not demonstrate long-lasting remission, and relapse within 1 month was common among most studies examining long-term outcomes [24]. The combination of CBT with CM has been shown to increase readiness to change by cannabis users [28].

Pharmacotherapy

Pharmacological treatment options for cannabis use disorder are limited. In the United States, there are currently no FDA-approved pharmacological treatments for CUD [20]. Limited research has been conducted on various pharmacological options in the general population and has yielded mixed results [22, 29, 30]. There was no specific research found which exclusively examined the older adult population, therefore the following paragraphs will discuss research that has been conducted on adults of all ages. Given this dearth of research, this would be another important area of future study.

A recent meta-analysis examined available research conducted on a variety of classes of medications that have been used experimentally for treatment of CUD [30]. In studies of antidepressants comparing escitalopram, bupropion, and nefazodone to placebo, there was no difference in abstinence rates. One trial found that those who were given venlafaxine may have had a lower rate of abstinence compared to placebo. In studies with mood stabilizers, divalproex and lithium, there was no significant difference between either medication or placebo in terms of abstinence rates or frequency of cannabis use. One trial examined N-acetylcysteine (NAC) versus placebo in the general adult population and found no difference in reduction of cannabis use [30].

Anticonvulsants such as gabapentin and topiramate were also discussed in the meta-analysis by Kondo et al [30]. Whereas topiramate was found to have no effect on cannabis use compared to placebo, gabapentin demonstrated significant decrease in cannabis use, depressive symptoms, and greater neurocognitive performance, along with improvement in withdrawal symptoms [30, 31]. There has also been some consideration of utilizing pharmacologic substitutes for cannabis to treat CUD, akin to the use of methadone or buprenorphine for medication-assisted treatment for opioid use disorder. Dronabinol, a pharmaceutically prepared synthetic THC, nabilone, an FDA-approved synthetic cannabinoid, and nabiximols, a pharmaceutically prepared nasal spray of 27 mg/ml of THC and 25mg of cannabidiol (CBD) were examined for their effect on abstinence, reduction of use, and craving, with no observed difference [30, 32]. Dronabinol had no effect on abstinence, but had mixed effects on withdrawal and treatment retention [32]. Overall, there was low strength evidence that cannabinoids had no difference on reducing cannabis use compared to placebo [30].

Evidence-Based Treatment Algorithm

Given the lack of approved pharmacological treatments and limited research in the area as detailed above, pharmaceutical options cannot currently be part of an evidence-based treatment algorithm. When considering an evidence-based algorithm for treatment of cannabis use disorder in the geriatric population, we must consider that much of the available research has been done in the general adult population and is generalized to the geriatric population.

Evidence-based treatment should consist of non-pharmacological treatment options including various psychotherapy modalities such as CBT, MET, and CM. The most effective treatment utilizes a combination of two or more of these modalities. Combining CBT and MET has the most robust evidence for longer term efficacy, and as such should be considered as the first-line management for cannabis use disorder in the geriatric population. However, utilizing CM in addition to either MET or CBT can be a viable option, with demonstrated superiority over each individual treatment option alone.

Conclusions

Cannabis use disorder should be considered in the older adult population, especially in the presence of risk factors or high-risk comorbidities, such as co-occurring SUD or psychiatric illness. Screening can consist of a series of questions during any medical or psychosocial evaluation regarding cannabis use, tailoring questions to DSM-5-TR criteria, or by administration of validated measures such as the CUDIT-R. Treatment options are limited, with no approved pharmacological options, leaving non-pharmacological treatment as the most appropriate first-line treatment option. Non-pharmacological treatment options include various therapeutic techniques such as CBT, CM, and MET, with the most effective treatment being a combination of two or more of these modalities, such as CBT and MET.

References

1. Substance-Related and Addictive Disorders, American Psychiatric Association. Diagnostic and statistical manual of mental disorders: DSM-5-TR. Washington DC: American Psychiatric Publishing; 2022.
2. Khoury R, Maliha P, Ibrahim R. Cannabis use and misuse in older adults. Clin Geriatr Med. 2022;38(1):67–83.
3. Lloyd SL, Striley CW. Marijuana use among adults 50 years or older in the 21st century. Gerontol Geriatr Med. 2018;4:2333721418781668.
4. Han BH, Palamar JJ. Trends in Cannabis use among older adults in the United States, 2015–2018. JAMA Intern Med. 2020;180(4):609–11.
5. Han BH, Palamar JJ. Marijuana use by middle-aged and older adults in the United States, 2015–2016. Drug Alcohol Depend. 2018;191:374–81. https://doi.org/10.1016/j.drugalcdep.2018.07.006.
6. Hasin DS, Kerridge BT, Saha TD, Huang B, Pickering R, Smith SM, Jung J, Zhang H, Grant BF. Prevalence and correlates of DSM-5 cannabis use disorder, 2012–2013: findings from the National Epidemiologic Survey on Alcohol and Related Conditions-III. Am J Psychiatry. 2016;173(6):588–99.

7. Leung J, Chan GCK, Hides L, Hall WD. What is the prevalence and risk of cannabis use disorders among people who use cannabis? a systematic review and meta-analysis. Addict Behav. 2020;109:106479.

8. Parish WJ, Mark TL, Weber EM, Steinberg DG. Substance use disorders among medicare beneficiaries: prevalence, mental and physical comorbidities, and treatment barriers. Am J Prev Med. 2022;63(2):225–32.

9. Choi NG, DiNitto DM, Marti CN. Older-adult marijuana users and ex-users: comparisons of sociodemographic characteristics and mental and substance use disorders. Drug Alcohol Depend. 2016 Aug;1(165):94–102.

10. Haney M. Cannabis use and the endocannabinoid system: a clinical perspective. Am J Psychiatry. 2022;179(1):21–5.

11. Ferland JN, Hurd YL. Deconstructing the neurobiology of cannabis use disorder. Nat Neurosci. 2020;23(5):600–10.

12. Han BH, Sherman S, Mauro PM, Martins SS, Rotenberg J, Palamar JJ. Demographic trends among older cannabis users in the United States, 2006–13. Addiction. 2017;112(3):516–25.

13. Weinstein G, Sznitman SR. The implications of late-life cannabis use on brain health: A mapping review and implications for future research. Ageing Res Rev. 2020;59:101041.

14. Greenstein A, DeLisi L, Solomon H. Cannabis use in the age of legalization: Implications for the geriatric population. Am J Geriatr Psychiatry. 2020;28(4):S36–7.

15. Connor JP, Stjepanović D, Le Foll B, Hoch E, Budney AJ, Hall WD. Cannabis use and cannabis use disorder. Nat Rev Dis Primers. 2021;7(1):16.

16. Lévesque A, Le Foll B. When and how to treat possible Cannabis use disorder. Med Clin North Am. 2018;102(4):667–81.

17. Adamson SJ, Kay-Lambkin FJ, Baker AL, Lewin TJ, Thornton L, Kelly BJ, Sellman JD. An improved brief measure of cannabis misuse: the Cannabis use disorders identification test-revised (CUDIT-R). Drug Alcohol Depend. 2010;110(1–2):137–43.

18. Schultz NR, Bassett DT, Messina BG, Correia CJ. Evaluation of the psychometric properties of the cannabis use disorders identification test-revised among college students. Addict Behav. 2019;95:11–5.

19. Bonn-Miller MO, Heinz AJ, Smith EV, Bruno R, Adamson S. Preliminary development of a brief Cannabis use disorder screening tool: the Cannabis use disorder identification test short-form. Cannabis Cannabinoid Res. 2016;1(1):252–61.

20. Available treatments for marijuana use disorders. National Institutes of Health. U.S. Department of Health and Human Services; 2021 [cited 2022 Nov 26]. Available from: https://nida.nih.gov/publications/research-reports/marijuana/available-treatments-marijuana-use-disorders

21. Winters KC, Mader J, Budney AJ, Stanger C, Knapp AA, Walker DD. Interventions for cannabis use disorder. Curr Opin Psychol. 2021;38:67–74.

22. Sabioni P, Le Foll B. Psychosocial and pharmacological interventions for the treatment of cannabis use disorder. Focus (Am Psychiatr Publ). 2019;17(2):163–8.

23. Smedslund G, Berg RC, Hammerstrøm KT, Steiro A, Leiknes KA, Dahl HM, Karlsen K. Motivational interviewing for substance abuse. Cochrane Database Syst Rev. 2011;2011(5):CD008063.

24. Chatters R, Cooper K, Day E, Knight M, Lagundoye O, Wong R, et al. Psychological and psychosocial interventions for cannabis cessation in adults: a systematic review. Addict Res Theory. 2015;24(2):93–110.

25. Davis DR, Kurti AN, Skelly JM, Redner R, White TJ, Higgins ST. A review of the literature on contingency management in the treatment of substance use disorders, 2009–2014. Prev Med. 2016;92:36–46.

26. Gates PJ, Sabioni P, Copeland J, Le Foll B, Gowing L. Psychosocial interventions for cannabis use disorder. Cochrane Database Syst Rev. 2016;2016(5):CD005336

27. Lees R, Hines LA, D'Souza DC, Stothart G, Di Forti M, Hoch E, Freeman TP. Psychosocial and pharmacological treatments for cannabis use disorder and mental health comorbidities: a narrative review. Psychol Med. 2021;51(3):353–64.

28. Peters EN, Petry NM, Lapaglia DM, Reynolds B, Carroll KM. Delay discounting in adults receiving treatment for marijuana dependence. Exp Clin Psychopharmacol. 2013;21(1):46–54.

29. Sherman BJ, McRae-Clark AL. Treatment of Cannabis use disorder: current science and future outlook. Pharmacotherapy. 2016;36(5):511–35.

30. Kondo KK, Morasco BJ, Nugent SM, Ayers CK, O'Neil ME, Freeman M, Kansagara D. Pharmacotherapy for the treatment of Cannabis use disorder: a systematic review. Ann Intern Med. 2020;172(6):398–412.

31. Mason BJ, Crean R, Goodell V, Light JM, Quello S, Shadan F, Buffkins K, Kyle M, Adusumalli M, Begovic A, Rao S. A proof-of-concept randomized controlled study of gabapentin: effects on cannabis use, withdrawal and executive function deficits in cannabis-dependent adults. Neuropsychopharmacology. 2012;37(7):1689–98.

32. Levin FR, Mariani JJ, Brooks DJ, Pavlicova M, Cheng W, Nunes EV. Dronabinol for the treatment of cannabis dependence: a randomized, double-blind, placebo-controlled trial. Drug Alcohol Depend. 2011;116(1–3):142–50.

Stimulant Use Disorder

18

Michael Duerden, Marianne Klugheit,
and Mathew Erisman

Epidemiology

Gathering precise epidemiological data on stimulant use disorder in older adults is difficult. Most of the evidence comes from large-scale data sets collected at regional and national levels, and these often select different upper-end cut-offs on age without a precise definition of an "older adult." With no precise definition of an "older adult" with a substance use disorder, many data sets include 50 or 55 and up, with others as low as 40 years [1–3]. Weber and Lynch (2022) looked at Substance Abuse and Mental Health Services Administration (SAMSHA) data from 2008 to 2018 for first time admissions to substance use treatment programs for patients 55+ and found that cocaine and methamphetamine comprised 14.8% and 5.8%, respectively, of the individual substances mentioned in the cohort. They also found that methamphetamine admissions grew by 0.61 percentage points each year in older populations [2].

General rates of cocaine use disorder are higher in younger populations than older populations, but in data sets looking at 2001 to 2002 and 2012 to 2013, increases in cocaine use were seen among older populations (12-month prevalence increasing from 0.14% to 0.49% and 0.07% to 0.19%, respectively) [1]. Another study found that older substance using individuals prefer cocaine use more than younger counterparts (35.14% vs. 15.70%) [3]. Using data from the 2015 to 2018 *National Survey on Drug Use and Health (NSDUH)*, Ghantous, Ahmed et al. (2022) estimated that the prevalence rate for past-year methamphetamine use was 3.2/1000 (95% confidence interval [CI], 2.8–3.9) among those participants 50 years and older [1].

In a recent retrospective study at a Level 1 trauma center in the US involving 5278 patients aged 55 years and older, 2% had positive methamphetamine drug screens in 2009 compared with 8% in 2018 [4]. Finally, in looking at NSDUH data, there appears to be a cohort effect showing increasing age of methamphetamine users, with most users in the early 2000s being aged 18–25 and more recent data showing that a large proportion are in the 35+ age group—possibly showing a trend with aging that will be important to continue to follow [1].

M. Duerden (✉) · M. Klugheit · M. Erisman
Department of Psychiatry,
University of Arizona School of Medicine,
Tucson, AZ, USA
e-mail: mduerden@arizona.edu;
Marianne.Klugheit@va.gov;
Mathew.Erisman@bannerhealth.com

R. R. Tampi, D. J. Tampi (eds.), *Treatment of Psychiatric Disorders Among Older Adults*,
https://doi.org/10.1007/978-3-031-55711-8_18

Neurobiology and Health Consequences

Stimulants are a broad class of psychoactive substances that include compounds derived from the coca plant (cocaine hydrochloride), amphetamine, and amphetamine-like substances (including those produced synthetically for prescription or illicit use and naturally occurring from plants such as khat) [5, 6]. What has been primarily studied in the literature and is most relevant because of worldwide prevalence of use has been cocaine and amphetamines (usually as methamphetamine). These are what we will primarily reference while discussing stimulant use disorder and treatment in older patients throughout this chapter [6].

While the effects of stimulants as a class of psychoactive substance are grossly similar, their direct mechanisms of action vary between amphetamine/amphetamine-like substances and cocaine/cocaine derivatives [5]. Broadly speaking, stimulants work in the central nervous system primarily through their effects on the monoamine system (including dopaminergic, serotonergic, and adrenergic mechanisms). This can either be through direct interactions on syn-apses in the nervous system or through interaction with neurotransmitter transports systems [7]. While cocaine's mechanism of action is primarily through blocking the reuptake of monoamines in the synaptic cleft, amphetamines have a multi-modal effect leading to direct release of mono-amines along with altering reuptake and breakdown in the synaptic cleft [8].

Acute stimulant intoxication can cause a variety of effects, including euphoria, grandiosity, increased energy, appetite suppression, anxiety, agitation, restlessness, impaired judgment, and stereotypic movements and behaviors[7] (Table 18.1). Their impact on the central and peripheral monoamine systems can lead to autonomic hyperactivity, including high blood pressure, rapid heart rate, hyperthermia, diaphoresis, and dilated pupils. Heavy stimulant use can induce psychosis, vomiting, seizures, and hyperactive delirium [6, 7] (Table 18.1). Supportive care is usually sufficient for management of acute stimulant intoxication, but in more severe cases treatment should include monitoring and management of blood pressure and vital abnormalities, benzodiazepines for acute anxiety or agitation, and antipsychotic medications for psychosis, if indicated [9].

Table 18.1 Examples of health consequences/risks associated with stimulant use [6–8, 11]

Acute use or intoxication	Chronic use
Psychological/behavioral	**Psychological/behavioral**
Euphoria	Persistent paranoia or psychosis
Grandiosity	Apprehension/fear of impending doom
Increased energy	Depression
Appetite suppression	Anxiety
Anxiety	Neurocognitive impairment
Agitation	**Physiological**
Impaired judgment	Chronic hypertension
Stereotypic movements and behaviors	Elevated risk of myocardial infarctions
Paranoia	Arrhythmias
Psychosis	Elevated stroke risk
Physiological	Ventricular hypertrophy
Autonomic hyperactivity	Kidney damage
High blood pressure	Respiratory damage
Rapid heart rate	Myocarditis
Hyperthermia	Heart failure
Diaphoresis	Skin disorder
Dilated pupils	Poor self-care
Insomnia	Seizures
	Choreoathetoid movements
	Extreme weight loss

Chronic or heavy stimulant use followed by acute cessation can cause withdrawal symptoms that include dysphoria, fatigue, sleep disturbances (insomnia, hypersomnia, vivid dreams), increased appetite, and psychomotor disturbances (agitation or hypoactivity) [6, 10] (Table 18.1). Typical pattern follows an early "crash" phase (12–24 h) primarily consisting of fatigue and exhaustion. This can then extend to a more prolonged withdrawal phase (2–4 weeks) with symptoms most severe in the first week. They have also described a more protracted course, including cognitive deficits and mood symptoms [10] (Table 18.1). Given the sequela of stimulant withdrawal symptoms, there has been some investigation into trying to identify effective pharmacotherapy for its treatment outside of general symptom supportive management (i.e., benzodiazepines for agitation or insomnia) [9]. Acheson, Williams et al. (2022) looked at nine randomized controlled trials (RCTs) assessing medication trials for amphetamine/methamphetamine withdrawal with their conclusion being that there is insufficient evidence to support any pharmacotherapy being effective, but that there was also insufficient evidence to confirm that any of the studied medications (including amineptine, mirtazapine, modafinil, and amantadine) were not effective [10].

Over time, chronic stimulant use is associated with increased risk of sudden death, primarily because of cardiac complications or vascular problems [8] (Table 18.1). These risks include hypertension, myocardial infarction, arrhythmias, cerebral infarcts and hemorrhages, ventricular hypertrophy, cerebrovascular atherosclerosis, kidney damage, and pulmonary complications (worse if smoked) [3, 8] (Table 18.1). These effects compound and complicate preexisting cardiovascular and neurological sequela, which older patients are at increased risk for already. Additionally, there is an increased risk of dementia along with impairment in attention, memory, and other neurocognitive domains with chronic use [3]. The annual rate of global gray matter volume loss in cocaine-dependent individuals was found to be almost twice the rate of healthy volunteers (3 mL/y [SD 0.49] vs 1.69 mL [SD 0.41], respectively) in a recent study [1]. Animal and human studies have also shown that the neurotoxic effects of methamphetamines can cause general cortical volume loss and damage to dopaminergic neurons, leading to increased risk of Parkinson's disease [1]. Table 18.1 describes the health consequences/risks associated with stimulant use.

Screening/Assessment/Risk Factors-Barriers

The DSM-5 sets out criteria for stimulant use disorder and is considered the gold standard for diagnostic assessment [1]. Diagnosis involves a thorough evaluation and history of stimulant use in the last year (12 months) that composed of at least 2 of the following expressions (in brief summary) including: stimulants being taken in larger quantities or for longer than intended, cravings, extended amount of time spent in the process of acquiring/recovering from use, inability to control use, the development of tolerance, manifestation of specific withdrawal pattern, continued use despite negative impact on personal relationships, problems from stimulant use leading to negative impact on social/occupational roles, important life experiences are missed/given up, use in physically hazardous scenarios, and continued use despite knowledge of negative physical or psychological consequences. These expressions also need to cause clinically significant distress or impairments within that same one-year period [5].

When working with older patients, we should take some considerations in the screening and application of the DSM-5 criteria. For older patients who also have comorbid neurocognitive concerns, there could be an impact on self-report measures around the amount consumed, cravings, or physical/social/psychological consequences associated with heavy use, and collateral information should be obtained [1]. While younger populations may be more inclined to use methamphetamines or other stimulants for performance enhancement and/or recreational purposes, older patients may be more likely to use in order to "self-medicate" [11]. Also, because of some of the physiological changes with aging, tolerance and withdrawal symptoms may develop at much lower doses than in younger populations. Lastly, older individuals often have different role obligations depending on their stage in life (retirement, caretaking of grandchildren, etc.), and providers should be aware of how impairment or consequences of substance use is being assessed [12].

Screening for substance use is an important part of caring for older patients as they are at increased risk of being under-diagnosed due to a multitude of factors including denial, isolation, shame, ageism within the medical system, and lack of specialty training of healthcare workers; additionally, they may be less likely to seek help on their own when compared to younger patients [1, 13, 14]. The older adult population is diverse and given historical and generational considerations (e.g., Baby Boomer generation), some may be more open to talking to providers about substance use history as well [14]. Also, there can be a misconception in older adults that signs and symptoms of substance use are related to aging or other disease processes, and education and communication from providers are needed [13]. Additional general risk factors would include limited social supports, bereavement, transitions in care/living situations, chronic pain/physical health concerns, history of substance use, and polypharmacy [1, 13].

In looking at specific standardized screening tools for stimulant use disorder, different protocols have been evaluated, and Tiet et al. (2021) recently assessed a modified version of the Screen of Drug Use (SoDU), a two-question screening tool around general substance use and harmful consequences. The SoDU alone has a greater than 92% sensitivity and specificity for detecting any drug use. In a large sample of VA clinic patients in Northern California (1300), they found the modified SoDU was 93% sensitive and 99% specific in identifying stimulant use disorders when an additional question about stimulants was added after a positive screen (asking about intent of use to get high or alter one's

Table 18.2 Screening for substance use in older adults [1, 14, 16]

Considerations for screening in older adults
Individual risk factors
Limited or low perceived social supports
Bereavement
Transitions in care/living situations
Chronic pain/physical health concerns
History of substance use
Polypharmacy
History of psychiatric comorbidities
Less than college education
Risks for underdiagnosis/misdiagnosis
Patient isolation/limited contact with healthcare system
Feelings of shame/guild around substance use
Ageism within the medical system
Lack of specialty training of healthcare workers
Possible comorbid neurocognitive concerns contributing to poor self and situational assessment
Different role obligations than younger adults
Differences in presentation of withdrawal or tolerance

mood) [15]. This is compared to the self-administered version of tobacco, alcohol, prescription medication, and other substance use (TAPS) which they reported as 60% sensitive and 99% specific in identifying cocaine or methamphetamine use disorder and a self-interview version of the Alcohol, Smoking, and Substance Involvement Screening Test (ASSIST) which was reported as 89.7% sensitive and 86.8% specific in identifying cocaine abuse or dependence [15]. Table 18.2 describes the screening for substance use in older adults.

Treatment

Psychotherapies and psychosocial interventions have the most evidence for efficacy in the treatment of stimulant use disorders [6]. The evidence for specific pharmacotherapies is not as clear, as several clinical trials and meta-analysis of available studies have either not shown any strong or significant benefits or find that there is not sufficient evidence to support pharmacotherapy [17–19]. Here we will present some of the available reviewed treatment evidence along with potential treatments that could be beneficial in the setting of further research. These include somatic therapies such as rTMS. Studies evaluating treatment for stimulant use disorder specifically looking at older adults are limited. Much of the evidence below has been taken from the general literature on the treatment of stimulant use disorder.

Psychotherapies and Psychosocial Interventions

Contingency management (CM) is a behavior modification approach that uses tangible rewards and reinforcing consequences to increase progress toward treatment goals and decrease behaviors that would hinder goals [18, 19]. In the treatment of SUD, CM is used for increasing adherence to treatment and promoting abstinence from stimulant use. CM interventions may include the use of vouchers or other rewards for negative drug screens or attendance at treatment sessions [18]. In a recent systematic review Ronsley, Nolan et al. (2020) found a significant benefit with contingency management alone for the outcomes of abstinence at 12 weeks (Odds Ratio [OR] 2.29, 95% Confidence Interval [CI] 1.62, 3.24), abstinence at the end of treatment (OR 2.22, 95% CI 1.59, 3.10), dropout at 12 weeks (OR 1.39, 95% CI 1.09, 1.78), and dropout at the end of treatment (OR 1.41, 95% CI 1.10, 1.82), but the effect was not sustained at longest follow-up (OR 1.10, 95% CI 0.83, 1.46) [19]. Contingency management has also shown an added effect when combined with other psychotherapeutic/psychosocial approaches and even in pharmacological interventions (with NNT between 3 and 8) in all ages [19].

Cognitive-behavioral therapy (CBT) is a psychotherapeutic approach aimed at modifying cognitions and behaviors and has shown effectiveness for treatment of a variety of substance use disorders [18]. In looking specifically at CBT for stimulant use disorders, there is less evidence available for its efficacy when compared to other substance use disorders, showing that additional research in this area is needed [19]. In reviewing the evidence that is available, CBT has shown benefit in outcome of dropout in treatment including at 12 weeks (OR 1.42, 95% CI 1.05, 1.93)

and the end of treatment (OR 1.47, 95% CI 1.08, 2.00) [19]. While the evidence for additive effects with CM is mixed, CM appears to have superiority to CBT in head-to-head comparisons with some consideration that CM benefit may be seen sooner and that CBT benefit may have a more delayed, but prolonged positive effects [18, 19].

Twelve-step programs are modeled after alcoholics anonymous (AA) with an emphasis on acceptance, surrendering to a higher power, and active involvement in meetings and fellowship. They have been shown to be beneficial with the treatment of cocaine use disorder, but there have been limited studies assessing their effectiveness in other stimulants such as methamphetamines [18].

The matrix model is a structured treatment approach which combines CM, CBT, 12 steps along with family interventions, psychoeducation, group work and peer support over a 16-week period. It has been found to be effective in reducing methamphetamine use and cravings along with improving retention and abstinence rates, when compared with other behavioral interventions [18].

Additional Behavioral and Somatic Therapies

reSET is an FDA approved mobile application based on CBT which aims to teach skills to help improve engagement with outpatient treatment and achieve abstinence from substance abuse (including stimulant use), and was found to be effective in reducing methamphetamine use and craving during treatment [18].

Acupuncture has been studied several times, and there appears to be no benefit for the treatment of stimulant use disorder [19].

Recent trials of somatic therapies such as Repetitive Transcranial Magnetic Stimulation (rTMS) and Transcranial Direct Current Stimulations (tDCS) have shown to reduce methamphetamine craving and increase executive functions when compared to controls with effects lasting throughout the treatment and at least up to 1-month post-treatment [18].

Pharmacological Interventions

In a recent systematic review and meta-analysis of pharmacotherapy for stimulant use disorder, Chan et al. (2019) found that there was no strong, consistent evidence for any medication in improving outcomes for patients including abstinence, reduction of use, or improved treatment retention. Below is a consideration of the evidence for class-specific pharmacological interventions.

Antidepressants including selective serotonin reuptake inhibitors (SSRI) and non-SSRI medications have shown no significant benefit on rates of abstinence in stimulant use disorders, although there may be a non-significant trend favoring antidepressants over placebo for sustained abstinence, with low-strength evidence that bupropion is significantly better than placebo [17, 19]. There is some low-quality class evidence of the benefit of antidepressants in the outcomes of lapse and relapse [17].

Antipsychotics are no better than placebo in treating stimulant use disorder (evaluating abstinence, cravings, reduction of use, etc.), but there is some moderate strength evidence of better retention in treatment programs for participants receiving an antipsychotic (with no identified difference between first- or second-generation antipsychotics or for any individual medication) [17, 19].

Psychostimulants may have low-strength evidence as a class (which could include mixed amphetamine salts, methylphenidate, methamphetamine, Lis-dexamphetamine, etc.) as per a recent systematic review by Chan et al. (2019) [17]. Psychostimulants may be better than placebo for sustained abstinence ($N = 1549$; combined RR 1.36 [95% CI 1.05–1.77]), but was specifically noted in the review that low-quality studies hamper the body of literature around psychostimulants for stimulant use disorder treatment, with concerns about incomplete outcome data [17].

Anticonvulsants have not been found to have sufficient evidence for treatment in cocaine or methamphetamine use disorder [17, 19]. In multiple systematic reviews and meta-analysis, there has not been evidence of benefit in any outcome measures including, abstinence, reduction in use, or retention in treatment. The exception to this data is topiramate that has been shown to have some potential benefit in reduction of use and abstinence, but the study data is limited and more trials are needed [19].

Additional Pharmacological interventions

There are no effects noted for baclofen (low strength of evidence) or any other muscle relaxant for stimulant use disorder [17].

No benefit or improvement in dropout, abstinence, or severity of dependence has been noted for dopamine agonists in the treatment of stimulant use disorder [19].

There is low-quality evidence supporting the use of disulfiram for treating cocaine dependence, but disulfiram treatment was associated with lower treatment retention than placebo [17, 19].

A recent systematic review of 6 human and 16 animal studies on the use of N-acetylcysteine had some preliminary results that there may be some benefit in reduction of cravings in cocaine use disorder, but further studies and trials needed [19].

A recent phase III double-blind, placebo-controlled study found that a combination of oral bupropion and injectable naltrexone was safe and successfully reduced methamphetamine use and cravings. There was some slight effect but significant benefit when compared to placebo [18].

Medications for methamphetamine use disorder currently or recently under different stages of clinical trials include oxytocin, doxazocin, lobeline, disulfiram, acamprosate, atomoxetine, and entacapone [18].

In summary, the strongest evidence for effective treatment for stimulant use disorder is contingency management interventions (alone or with other treatment modalities) [6, 8, 19] (Fig. 18.1). There is no strong and consistent evidence for benefit from any pharmacological interventions, with the best evidence available

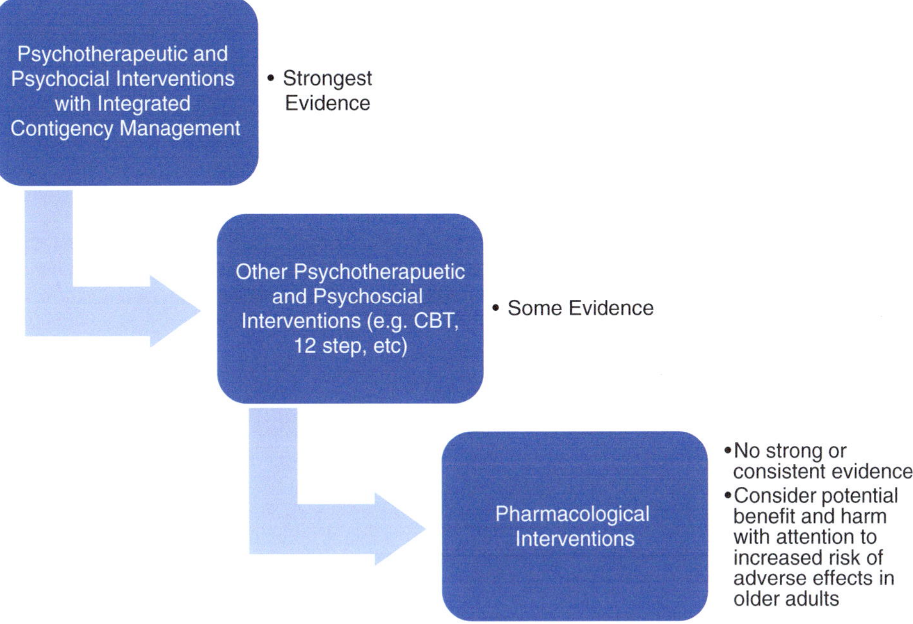

Fig. 18.1 Proposed algorithm for treating stimulant use disorder in older adults [6, 14, 17–21]

being largely negative or without clear efficacy [19]. Any decision to use pharmacotherapy in the treatment of stimulant use disorder needs to consider the potential benefits and harm. While there could be a consideration for the use of medications with lower strength of evidence, but the potential for adverse outcomes with these treatment strategies has not been well-explored in the literature [14, 17, 19].

While there is a lack of clear guidance for treatment of stimulant use disorder in older adults, an emphasis on psychotherapeutic and psychosocial interventions does appear to be the most evidenced based [17, 20] (Fig. 18.1). Additionally, utilizing recommendations/resources from the literature on the treatment for general substance use disorders in older adults should be considered within the appropriate context [14, 19] (Fig. 18.1). With the limited evidence for medications in the treatment of stimulant use disorder, additional pause should be taken when considering the use of psychopharmacological treatment for older patients, given the generally increased risk of adverse effects from medications in this population [14, 21] (Fig. 18.1).

References

1. Ghantous Z, Ahmad V, Khoury R. Illicit drug use in older adults: an invisible epidemic? Clin Geriatr Med. 2022;38(1):39–53. https://doi.org/10.1016/j.cger.2021.07.002.
2. Weber A, Lynch A, Miskle B, Arndt S, Acion L. Older adult substance use treatment first-time admissions between 2008 and 2018. Am J Geriatr Psychiatry. 2022;30(10):1055–63. https://doi.org/10.1016/j.jagp.2022.03.003.
3. Yarnell S, Li L, MacGrory B, Trevisan L, Kirwin P. Substance use disorders in later life: a review and synthesis of the literature of an emerging public health concern. Am J Geriatr Psychiatry. 2020;28(2):226–36. https://doi.org/10.1016/j.jagp.2019.06.005.
4. Benham DA, Rooney AS, Calvo RY, Carr MJ, Diaz JA, Sise CB, et al. The rising tide of methamphetamine use in elderly trauma patients. Am J Surg. 2021;221(6):1246–51. https://doi.org/10.1016/j.amjsurg.2021.02.030.
5. American Psychiatric Association, American Psychiatric Association. DSM-5 Task Force. Diagnostic and statistical manual of mental disorders: DSM-5. 5th ed ed. Washington, D.C.: American Psychiatric Publishing; 2013.
6. Substance Abuse and Mental Health Services Administration (SAMHSA). Treatment for stimulant use disorders. Treatment improvement protocol (TIP) series. Rockville, MD; 2021.

7. Sofuoglu M, DeVito EE, Kosten TR. Neurobiology of stimulants. In: The American Psychiatric Association Publishing textbook of substance use disorder treatment. American Psychiatric Association Publishing; 2021.

8. Docherty JR, Alsufyani HA. Pharmacology of drugs used as stimulants. J Clin Pharmacol. 2021;61(S2):S53–69. https://doi.org/10.1002/jcph.1918.

9. Treatment of Stimulant-Related Disorders. The American Psychiatric Association publishing textbook of substance use disorder treatment.

10. Acheson LS, Williams BH, Farrell M, McKetin R, Ezard N, Siefried KJ. Pharmacological treatment for methamphetamine withdrawal: a systematic review and meta-analysis of randomised controlled trials. Drug Alcohol Rev. 2022; https://doi.org/10.1111/dar.13511.

11. Paulus MP, Stewart JL. Neurobiology, clinical presentation, and treatment of methamphetamine use disorder: a review. JAMA Psychiatry. 2020;77(9):959–66. https://doi.org/10.1001/jamapsychiatry.2020.0246.

12. Han BH, Moore AA. Prevention and screening of unhealthy substance use by older adults. Clin Geriatr Med. 2018;34(1):117–29. https://doi.org/10.1016/j.cger.2017.08.005.

13. Kuerbis A, Sacco P, Blazer DG, Moore AA. Substance abuse among older adults. Clin Geriatr Med. 2014;30(3):629–54. https://doi.org/10.1016/j.cger.2014.04.008.

14. Substance Abuse and Mental Health Services Administration (SAMHSA). Treating substance use disorder in older adults. Treatment improvement protocol (TIP) series. Rockville, MD; 2020.

15. Tiet QQ, Moos RH. Screen of drug use: diagnostic accuracy for stimulant use disorder. Addict Behav. 2021:112. https://doi.org/10.1016/j.addbeh.2020.106614.

16. Kuerbis A. Substance use among older adults: an update on prevalence, etiology, assessment, and intervention. Gerontology. 2020;66(3):249–58. https://doi.org/10.1159/000504363.

17. Chan B, Freeman M, Kondo K, Ayers C, Montgomery J, Paynter R, et al. Pharmacotherapy for methamphetamine/amphetamine use disorder—a systematic review and meta-analysis. Addiction. 2019;114(12):2122–36. https://doi.org/10.1111/add.14755.

18. Moszczynska A. Current and emerging treatments for methamphetamine use disorder. Curr Neuropharmacol. 2021;19(12):2077–91. https://doi.org/10.2174/1570159X19666210803091637.

19. Ronsley C, Nolan S, Knight R, Hayashi K, Klimas J, Walley A, et al. Treatment of stimulant use disorder: a systematic review of reviews. PLoS One. 2020;15(6):e0234809. https://doi.org/10.1371/journal.pone.0234809.

20. Tran MTN, Luong QH, Le Minh G, Dunne MP, Baker P. Psychosocial interventions for amphetamine type stimulant use disorder: an overview of systematic reviews. Front Psychiatry. 2021:12. https://doi.org/10.3389/fpsyt.2021.512076.

21. Pagliaro LA, Pagliaro AM. Drug and substance abuse among older adults: identification, analysis, and synthesis. In: Drug and substance abuse among older adults: identification, analysis, and synthesis. Taylor and Francis Inc.; 2022.

Christina Spoleti, Gibson George,
and Padmapriya Marpuri

Introduction

Opioid use disorder is described in the Diagnostic and Statistical Manual of Mental Disorders, Fifth Edition (DSM-5) [1], as a condition that is characterized as mild (2–3 symptoms), moderate (4–5 symptoms), or severe (6 or more symptoms) involving the following symptoms:

- Opioids are often taken in larger amounts or over a longer period of time than intended.
- There is a persistent desire or unsuccessful efforts to cut down or control opioid use.
- A great deal of time is spent in activities necessary to obtain the opioid, use the opioid, or recover from its effects.
- Craving, or a strong desire to use opioids.
- Recurrent opioid use resulting in failure to fulfill major role obligations at work, school, or home.
- Continued opioid use despite having persistent or recurrent social or interpersonal problems causes or exacerbated by the effects of opioids.
- Important social, occupational, or recreation activities are given up or reduced because of opioid use.
- Recurrent opioid use in situation in which it is physically hazardous.
- Continued use despite knowledge of having a persistent or recurrent physical or psychological problem that is likely to have been caused or exacerbated by opioids.
- Tolerance as defined by either of the following: a needed for markedly increased amounts of opioid to achieve intoxication or desired effect, markedly diminished effect with continued use of the same amount of an opioid.
- Withdrawal as manifested by either of the following: the characteristic opioid withdrawal syndrome, the same (or closely related) substances are taken to relieve or avoid withdrawal symptoms.
- The severity of the disorder is determined by the number of above symptoms that are present concurrently. The disorder is considered mild if 2–3 symptoms are present; moderate if 4–5 symptoms are present; and severe if ≥ 6 symptoms are present.

OUD is a chronic and relapsing disease with personal, economic, and public health consequences [2]. Prescription opioids, heroin, and fentanyl use have been increasing in the United

C. Spoleti · P. Marpuri (✉)
Department of Psychiatry, St. Luke's University Health Network, Easton, PA, USA
e-mail: christina.spoleti@sluhn.org;
padmapriya.marpuri@sluhn.org

G. George
St. Luke's Penn Foundation, Department of Psychiatry, St. Luke's University Health Network, Easton, PA, USA
e-mail: gibson.george@sluhn.org

States (US) since the early 2000s and have led to an opioid epidemic [3]. According to the National Study of Drug Use and Health, in 2020 2.7 million people were living with OUD in the US with their numbers expected to increase soon [4].

As per the Center for Disease Control (CDC), 82.9% of overdose deaths in the US in 2020 were due to opioids [5]. Of those individuals, 24.3% had a documented mental health diagnosis [5]. Within the opioid fatal overdoses, 43.3% were male and 18.1% were female in the US [5]. Patients aged 55 years and older accounted for 46.2% of overall documented fatal opioid overdoses [5]. The CDC also monitors nonfatal opioid overdoses and found, with 35 states reporting, the US saw an increase of 26.45% of nonfatal opioid overdoses in people 55 years and older in 2020 [5]. According to available Medicare data, the prevalence of OUD disorder in older adults has tripled from 2013 to 2018 [6].

According to the CDC, factors contributing to the opioid epidemic are increased prescribing rates, taking increasingly high doses of medications, and patients receiving more than one prescription from multiple providers [5, 7].

Within the older adult community, individuals may develop OUD from recreational experimentation and from taking prescribed medications given by a health-care provider [8]. Per Maree et al, analysis of ambulatory data demonstrated that older adults are at greater risk of non-medical use of prescription opioids due to the increase in clinic visits and chief complaints involving pain [9].

Risk Factors and Neurobiology

Demographic risk factors for developing OUD include younger age, male sex, lower socioeconomic status, non-completion of secondary education, and unemployment [3, 10]. Identifying as Native American, Black, and non-Hispanic White are also risk factors for developing OUD in the United States [10]. Family history of OUD increases risk of developing OUD, as this disorder demonstrates moderate to high heritability [3].

Diagnosis of other substance use disorders, mood disorders, and anxiety disorders is associated with increased risk of developing OUD [2, 10]. Additionally, a history of trauma and adverse childhood events (ACEs) increase the risk of developing OUD [11].

Among older adults, the presence of a co-occurring pain diagnosis increases the risk of developing OUD [8, 12]. The combination of pain diagnoses along with social factors, psychological issues, and the physical limitations commonly seen among older adults makes them a vulnerable group to experience negative consequences of opioid use [9].

In addition to pain, physiological factors which increase the risk of problematic opioid use and rate of adverse events in the elderly are age-related changes in the brain, drug metabolism, and pharmacokinetics. Overall, elderly individuals have an increased percentage of body fat which delays elimination of lipophilic agents, which include opioids such as fentanyl and methadone [6]. Additionally, among the elderly, metabolism of opioids is prolonged [13]. Opioids are metabolized primarily by the hepatic system and excreted primarily by the renal system. Metabolic activity of the liver is reduced in older adults secondary to decreased size of the liver and decreased hepatic blood flow [6]. Renal clearance declines by 1% per year after age 50 and decreased renal clearance can lead to the increase of opioids metabolites, which in turn increases the risk of neurotoxicity in the elderly who have problematic opioid use [6]. Physiologic reserve is decreased in the elderly individuals, which can lead to worsening or acceleration of underlying health conditions [6, 13].

Meta-analyses of imaging studies have revealed gray and white matter changes in individuals with OUD. Gray matter changes include atrophy of the frontotemporal region including the superior frontal gyrus, inferior frontal gyrus, superior temporal gyrus, orbitofrontal gyrus, and the insula [14]. White matter changes include changes to the bilateral frontal subgyral regions extending from the limbic structures to the prefrontal cortex [14]. Overall, impaired neurocognitive function is associated with chronic opioid use including changes in working memory, attention, cognitive impulsivity, and cognitive flexibility [14, 15].

Consequences

Substance use disorders (SUDs) in elderly individuals have been associated with greater risk of falls, cognitive impairments, delirium, and negative effects on comorbid diagnoses [16]. Opioid use in older adults is associated with impaired motor function, risk of falls, constipation, respiratory depression, anorexia, nausea, and impaired cognitive function [6]. Neurocognitive effects of opioid use are of important consideration as they may be more pronounced in the elderly population due to underlying cognitive impairment [6].

Assessment

As per the American Society of Addiction Medicine (ASAM), the first clinical priority of assessment in OUD should be identifying and making appropriate referrals for the management of urgent or emergency medical or psychiatric symptoms [17].

In a stable patient, assessment should begin with a thorough medical and psychiatric history with special attention given to substance use history. Providers should emphasize to the patient that the questions are being asked regarding their substance use history to provide them with better and safer and not to be judgmental [18]. A family and social history should also be obtained. Once history and review of current symptoms is completed, it should be determined whether the patient meets criteria for OUD according to the DSM-5 [1].

Identifying OUD, and other SUDs, is challenging in older adults because of the difficulty of assessing the functional impairment due to confounders including lack of job, loss or decline in functioning due to age, decreased number of legal issues, and reduction in social involvement when compared to younger adults [19, 20]. Assessment should include a multidimensional approach, reviewing social, familial, and environmental factors to aid in identifying facilitators and barriers to treatment and recovery [17, 20].

ASAM recommends completion of a physical examination and laboratory testing including complete blood count, metabolic panel, and liver enzyme tests. Due to the possibility of intravenous route of use in OUD, tests for infectious disease including viral hepatitis, human immunodeficiency virus (HIV), tuberculosis, and sexually transmitted infections must be included in the laboratory panel [17].

Urine drug testing is a recommended part of the assessment process, with continued testing to monitor and assess adherence among patients who are prescribed opioids [17]. Opioids which appear on standard urine drug screens include morphine, codeine, and semisynthetic opioids including heroin, hydrocodone, hydromorphone, and oxycodone [20]. Separate screens are required to test for the presence of synthetic opioids such as methadone, fentanyl, and tramadol [20]. Screening should also be utilized in the unconscious patient, the patient with altered sensorium, and in those with clinical symptoms consistent with opioid intoxication or withdrawal.

During assessment of an individual utilizing opioids whether prescribed, recreational, or both, symptoms of opioid intoxication, opioid overdose, and opioid withdrawal should be identified [6, 10]. Opioid intoxication may present as euphoria, drowsiness, nausea, constipation, and confusion [21]. Opioid overdose presents as a decreased level of consciousness, decreased respiratory rate and miotic pupils, and decreased bowel sounds. Opioids can cause peripheral vasodilation, and patients may present with hypotension that is responsive to fluids. Opioids can lower the seizure threshold, and overdose may result in generalized seizures [21]. Opioid overdose is life-threatening and requires emergent medical attention.

Opioid withdrawal presents with autonomic signs including tachycardia, tachypnea, hypertension or hypotension, mydriasis, piloerection, and hyperglycemia [10]. Symptoms also include lacrimation, rhinorrhea, diaphoresis, yawning, tremor, restlessness, abdominal pain, nausea, vomiting, and diarrhea [10]. Fever, anorexia, and insomnia may also occur [10]. Providers can utilize standardized measures such as the Clinical Opiate Withdrawal Scale (COWS) and the Subjective Opiate Withdrawal Scale (SOWS) to assess the severity of acute withdrawal [11]. The duration of withdrawal is variable and depends on the half-life of the opioid utilized [6]. Opioid withdrawal is typically non-life-threatening although it can cause significant discomfort.

Treatments

Treatments for OUD are often a combination of non-pharmacological and pharmacological modalities.

Non-pharmacological

As per the American Society of Addiction Medicine, counseling is an approved treatment for OUD and is recommended in conjunction with medication-assisted treatment (MAT) [17, 22]. Psychosocial treatment should include a psychosocial needs assessment, supportive counseling, establishing, and maintaining links to social supports and referrals to community services [17].

Therapy can be completed in multiple settings including inpatient and outpatient as well as in multiple formats including individual and group settings [20]. Dugosh et al. outlined how therapy can differ in structure while still maintaining common therapeutic elements which aims to modify the underlying processes that serve to maintain addictive behavior, encourage engagement with pharmacotherapy, and treat psychiatric comorbidities [20]. Patients can receive psychosocial treatment in inpatient rehabilitation units, outpatient rehabilitation facilities, intensive outpatient programs (IOPs), and through community support such as Narcotics Anonymous (NA) or other substance use support organizations. Results from systematic reviews support the efficacy of psychosocial therapy in combination with MAT [22].

Pharmacological

Pharmacological treatment with opioid receptor agonists, partial agonists, and opioid antagonists has been shown to facilitate recovery from OUD. Methadone, buprenorphine, and naltrexone are Food and Drug Administration (FDA) approved for the treatment of opioid use disorder [10]. Dugosh et.al, in their systematic reviews demonstrated that MAT is cost effective and clinically effective at reducing opioid use, opioid cravings, opioid withdrawal, and public health issues related to opioid use such as the incidence of infectious diseases and overdoses [23].

The physiology of aging should be considered when initiating pharmacological treatment of opioids either for pain or as treatment in OUD. Many opioids undergo metabolism by the renal and hepatic systems. Decline in renal function can result in increased opioids and their metabolites in the body. The liver decreases in size and experiences decreased blood flow as individuals age. There is decreased first pass metabolism for drugs in older adults. This can lead to an increase in bioavailability of certain opioids [6]. Decreasing lipophilic stores delays the elimination of some opioids, including methadone, and results in the accumulation of the substance in tissues [6].

Medication Classes

Medications for OUD (MOUDs) work by reducing withdrawal symptoms and opioid cravings. Treatments also decrease the biological response to future drug use [7]. Guidelines for older adults recommend opioid agonist therapy as the first-line treatment for opioid withdrawal and detoxification, with buprenorphine preferred over methadone [6, 24].

Opioid Agonists

Methadone belongs to this class of medications. Methadone is a full μ-opioid receptor agonist and an N-methyl-D-aspartate (NMDA) receptor antagonist [3]. Methadone has been utilized since the 1960s for the treatment of opioid use disorder [7].

Daily dose of methadone typically ranges from 60 to 120 mg [17]. Titration should be individualized and should not be increased by more than 10 mg every 5 days [17]. Methadone can only be provided through opioid treatment programs and acute care settings [17]. Treatment programs which dispense methadone are regulated at both the federal and state levels and are required to provide counseling to patients [23].

Methadone is primarily metabolized by the CYP3A, CYP2D6, and CYP1A2 enzymes and is subject to drug–drug interactions by CYP-450 inhibitors and inducers [3]. Methadone should be used with caution in patients with hepatic impairment. The half-life of methadone increases in renal impairment, and dose reductions should be considered in individuals with a creatinine clearance of <10 [6].

Adverse effects of methadone include sedation, constipation, and in rare cases hypogonadism [11]. Life-threatening adverse effects include overdose at high doses or in combination with other medications [11]. As a full agonist, overdose is possible with methadone administration which can be treated with naloxone.

Especially important to note both the geriatric and psychiatric populations are the risk of prolonged QT interval with methadone [11]. A baseline QT/QTc should be obtained with continued monitoring when utilizing methadone for OUD. Methadone has a long half-life of approximately 24 h, as such, withdrawal is common in discontinuation [3].

Partial Opioid Agonist

Buprenorphine is a partial μ-opioid receptor agonist and a K- and δ- opioid receptor antagonist [3]. Buprenorphine has a ceiling effect, allowing its effects to plateau in the body, thereby reducing the risk of misuse, side effects, and overdose. Buprenorphine was approved for use in the treatment of OUD in 2002 [7]. Buprenorphine can be given as an oral formulation, transdermal patch, or an injectable monoproduct. The extended-release (ER) injectable was approved in 2017 for use in opioid use disorder [7]. Buprenorphine can

also be utilized in combination products with opioid antagonists to discourage diversion.

Initial oral dosing should be 2–4 mg daily and titrated by increments of 2–8 mg once to twice daily [17]. There is limited evidence on the initial dosing in older adults. A set of Canadian guidelines recommend reducing initial dose by 25–50% and lengthening dose escalation by 25–50% [12]. Maintenance dosing is typically 16 mg daily often dosed as 8 mg twice daily [17]. There is limited evidence for the efficacy of doses greater than 16 mg daily, and evidence demonstrates that it increases the risk of diversion [17]. Randomized control trials have demonstrated buprenorphine and methadone to be comparably efficacious and effective at reducing opioid use and treatment retention [3].

Buprenorphine is primarily metabolized by the liver, and dose reductions should be considered in patients with hepatic impairment [6]. A combination of buprenorphine and naloxone products should also be avoided in individuals with hepatic disease. Buprenorphine can be administered in individuals with renal impairment with no necessary dose adjustments [6].

Adverse effects of buprenorphine include headache, nausea, constipation, and insomnia [11]. Buprenorphine may cause precipitated withdrawal in patients who initiate therapy while still experiencing opioid intoxication, therefore objective signs of withdrawal need to be observed prior to initiating of buprenorphine [3].

Combination of Partial Opioid Agonist and Antagonist

This is a combination of buprenorphine/naloxone. These come in sublingual films, tablets, and buccal films. Sublingual dosing is like that of buprenorphine monoproduct, and the initial dosing is 2–4 mg buprenorphine and 0.5–1 mg naloxone daily [25]. Maintenance dosing is typically 8/2 mg once to twice daily and can be increased to 12/3 mg once to twice daily, not to exceed 32 mg of buprenorphine daily [25]. The sublingual tablets induction dosing is recommended to be 1.4/0.36 mg [25]. Maintenance dose is recommended 11.4/2.9 mg once daily and not to exceed

17.2/4.2 mg total daily [25]. The buccal film induction dose is recommended to be 4.2/0.7 mg [25]. Single daily doses can be titrated up to 8.4/1.4 mg [25].

Contrary to methadone, buprenorphine and buprenorphine combination medications can be provided by clinicians in all settings and are not limited to opioid treatment programs and acute care settings [17].

Opioid Receptor Antagonists

In this class of medications are naltrexone and naloxone. These medications bind and block μ-opioid and K-opioid receptors [3].

Naltrexone

Extended-release (ER) injectable naltrexone is approved from use in OUD patients who are no longer physically dependent on opioids [17]. ER injectable naltrexone is 380 mg dosed every 4 weeks [17].

Oral doses of naltrexone are initiated at 25–50 mg, and maintenance dose is typically 50 mg daily [10].

Patients initiating naltrexone therapy must have opioids eliminated completely from their system. If therapy is initiated prior to elimination, immediate opioid withdrawal will occur.

Adverse effects of naltrexone include headache and depression. The injectable form is associated with injection site reactions [11]. Naltrexone can cause increased liver enzymes and increased creatinine phosphokinase [11]. It is contraindicated in patients with moderate to severe hepatic impairment and in acute hepatitis [6].

Naloxone

Naloxone is not utilized as maintenance therapy for opioid use disorder and is used only for preventing or reversing opioid overdoses [17]. The medication comes in intranasal, intramuscular, and intravenous forms. The starting dose is typically 0.4–1 mg intravenously in adults. The medication can be given as a continuous drip through an intravenous route at 4–5 μg/kg/h following an initial 1.5 μg/kg bolus, if required [26]. Intramuscular forms of medication are given at 0.4–2 mg per injection. Intranasal forms of the medication are given at 2–4 mg per spray [26].

Adverse effects of naloxone include precipitated withdrawal which may present as piloerection, vomiting, hypertension, anxiety, and tachycardia. Naloxone may cause aggressive and agitation in patients, when used to reverse opioid-induced sedation [26].

Transitions Between Opioid Agonists, Partial Agonists, and Antagonists

If transitioning a patient from methadone to buprenorphine, it is recommended patients be on lower doses of methadone, 30–40 mg daily or less, to avoid discomfort when transitioning [17].

If transitioning from methadone to naltrexone, patients must be completely weaned from methadone therapy before receiving naltrexone [17].

If transitioning from buprenorphine to naltrexone, it is recommended 7–14 days should separate buprenorphine discontinuation and naltrexone initiation [17].

If transitioning from naltrexone to opioid agonists or partial opioid agonists, there is no risk of precipitated withdrawal, as there is no physical dependence to antagonist therapy [17]. Patients should not be transitioned until 28 days after ER injection or 1 day after oral naltrexone [17].

Opioid Withdrawal Symptom Management

Pharmacological treatment for opioid withdrawal and detoxification includes buprenorphine and methadone as described above, as well as medications aimed at providing symptomatic relief. Alpha-2-adrenergic agonists including FDA approved lofexidine and the off-label use of clonidine have been shown to be effective in providing symptom relief in acute opioid withdrawal [17]. Lofexidine is approved for mitigation of withdrawal symptoms up to 14 days after discontinuation of opioids in adults [26]. Lofexidine has not been studied in patients older than 65 years in age, therefore its use is not formally recommended in this population [27]. Of note, cloni-

Table 19.1 Pharmacologic treatment for OUD and opioid overdose

Medication	Class of medication	Formulations	Dosing
Methadone	Opioid agonist—full μ-opioid receptor agonist NMDA receptor antagonist	Oral	Starting dose: 10–20 mg daily Dose range: 60–120 mg daily
Buprenorphine	Partial opioid agonist–μ-opioid receptor agonist and K- and δ-opioid antagonist	Oral, transdermal patch, extended-release injectable	Oral starting dose: 2–4 mg daily Dose range: 8–24 mg daily Transdermal patch starting dose: 5–10 mcg/h Dose range: 5–20 mcg/h Extended-release injectable starting dose: 100 mg monthly Dose range: 100 mg or 300 mg monthly
Buprenorphine/ naloxone combination	Partial opioid agonist and full opioid antagonist combination	Sublingual tablet, sublingual film, and buccal film	Sublingual tablet starting dose: 1.4/0.36 mg Dose range: 11.4–17.2/2.9–4.2 mg daily Sublingual film starting dose: 2–4 mg buprenorphine and 0.5–1 mg naloxone. Sublingual film dose range: 2/0.5–24/6 mg Buccal film starting dose: 4.2/0.7 mg Dose range: 4.2–8.4/0.7–1.4 mg
Naloxone	Opioid antagonist—full μ- and K-opioid receptor antagonist	Intranasal, intramuscular injection, intravenous	Starting intranasal dose: 2 mg May require titration to 4–8 mg in opioid overdose Starting intramuscular dose: 0.4–2 mg May require repeat administration in opioid overdose Starting intravenous dose: 0.4–1 mg Requires titration, continuous titration dose is 4–5 μg/kg/h
Naltrexone	Opioid antagonist—full μ- and K-opioid receptor antagonist	Oral, extended-release injectable	Starting oral dose: 25–50 mg daily Dose range: 25–50 mg daily Extended-release injectable starting and maintenance dose: 380 mg every 4 weeks

dine is a medication listed on the Beers Criteria for caution in older adults [28].

Analgesics including acetaminophen, non-steroidal anti-inflammatory agents (NSAIDs), and gabapentin can be useful for the treatment of pain during opioid withdrawal. Antidiarrheal agents including loperamide, and antiemetics including ondansetron are also helpful for symptom management.

Table 19.1 lists the pharmacologic treatment for OUD and opioid overdose [7, 17, 25, 26]

Evidence-Based Treatment Algorithms

Available evidence indicates that MAT demonstrates superior efficacy in preventing relapse and maintaining recovery in OUD when compared to detoxification and non-pharmacologic treatments alone. Recommendations for treatment include combining MAT with psychosocial supports, which include a variety of therapy modalities in the inpatient and outpatient setting.

Individuals with OUD of any stage (mild, moderate, severe) should begin treatment with assessment and essential harm reduction which includes overdose risk awareness and education, overdose management training for individual and family including take home naloxone, hepatitis B vaccination, hepatitis, and HIV screening with treatment, if positive results are noted.

1. For patients with mild OUD:

   Outpatient-based therapies and inpatient detoxification/rehabilitations should be discussed with naltrexone offered post-detoxification. If abstinence is not achieved, consider MAT with or without psychosocial support.

2. For patients with moderate and severe OUD:

   Initiate MAT with an opioid agonist, agonist-antagonist combination, or antagonist therapy, with preference for buprenorphine use in older adults. If a good response is achieved, add psychosocial support.

   If MAT is suboptimal or not therapeutic for the patient, correct or adjust dosing or choice of MAT, and increase psychosocial support. If MAT remains suboptimal, discuss residential or inpatient rehabilitation.

   If MAT is not available or declined, consider inpatient or home-based detoxification, inpatient or residential rehabilitation, and review essential harm reduction. Figure 19.1 describes the treatment algorithm for OUD.

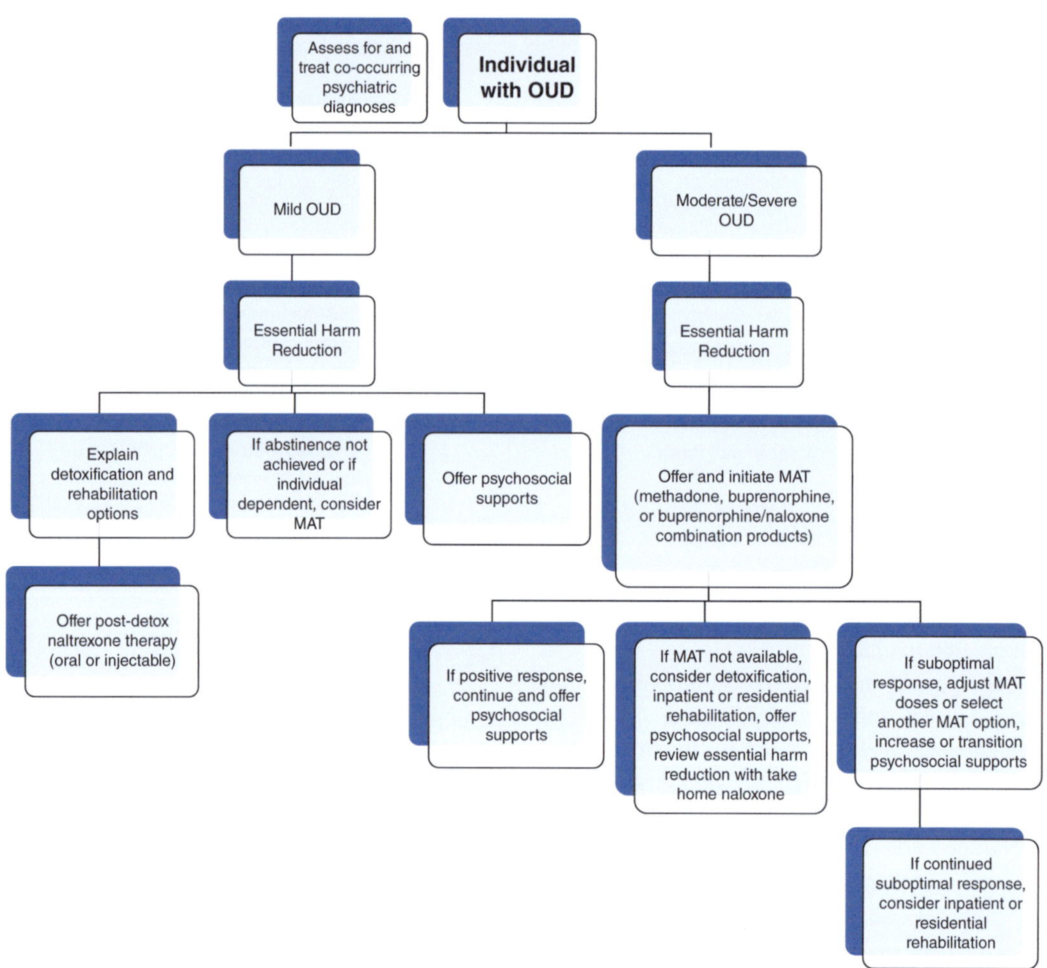

Fig. 19.1 Treatment algorithm for OUD [3]

Conclusions

OUD is a chronic, relapsing disease with increasing prevalence in all age-groups worldwide. Assessment should include complete medical and psychiatric history with a thorough evaluation of family, social, and substance use history. A complete physical evaluation and laboratory testing including complete blood count, liver enzyme tests, tests for infectious disease including viral hepatitis, human immunodeficiency virus (HIV), tuberculosis, and sexually transmitted infections should be performed. Additionally, a thorough evaluation of psychosocial supports and their limitations is an integral part of the assessment. Older adults are a vulnerable population for developing OUD. This population experiences increased prescribing rates of opioids, as they present for care more frequently and have increased amounts of comorbid medical conditions including pain diagnoses. Once OUD is established, pharmacologic treatment with MAT is recommended. Opioid agonists (methadone), partial agonists (buprenorphine), combination of opioid partial agonist-antagonist, and opioid antagonist (naltrexone) therapies are available and approved for patients with OUD. It is recommended to utilize buprenorphine products in older adults, given its preferable side effect profile when compared to other opioid agonists and opioid antagonists. Psychosocial therapies should be adjunct to MAT to aid patients in their recovery process and for relapse prevention.

References

1. Substance Related and Addictive Disorders, American Psychiatric Association. Desk reference to the diagnostic criteria from DSM-5. Washington DC: American Psychiatric Publishing; 2013. p. 93–114.
2. Tsoy-Podosenin M, Thomas A. Opioids. In: Marienfeld C, editor. Absolute addiction psychiatry review. Cham: Springer; 2020. p. 169–84.
3. Strang J, Volkow ND, Degenhardt L, Hickman M, Johnson K, Koob GF, Marshall BDL, Tyndall M, Walsh SL. Opioid use disorder. Nat Rev Dis Primers. 2020;6(1):3. https://doi.org/10.1038/s41572-019-0137-5.
4. Substance Abuse and Mental Health Services Administration. Key substance use and mental health indicators in the United States: results from the 2020 National Survey on Drug Use and Health (HHS Publication No. PEP21-07-01-003, NSDUH Series H-56). Rockville, MD: Center for Behavioral Health Statistics and Quality, Substance Abuse and Mental Health Services Administration; 2021. Retrieved from https://www.samhsa.gov/data/
5. Centers for Disease Control and Prevention. State unintentional drug overdose reporting system (SUDORS). Atlanta, GA: US Department of Health and Human Services, CDC; 2020. Access at: https://www.cdc.gov/drugoverdose/fatal/dashboard
6. Dufort A, Samaan Z. Problematic opioid use among older adults: epidemiology, adverse outcomes and treatment considerations. Drugs Aging. 2021;38(12):1043–53. https://doi.org/10.1007/s40266-021-00893-z.
7. Hoffman KA, Ponce Terashima J, McCarty D. Opioid use disorder and treatment: challenges and opportunities. BMC Health Serv Res. 2019;19(1):884. https://doi.org/10.1186/s12913-019-4751-4.
8. Substance Abuse and Mental Health Services Administration. Medications for opioid use disorder. Treatment Improvement Protocol (TIP) Series 63 Publication No. PEP21-02-01-002. Substance Abuse and Mental Health Services Administration: Rockville, MD; 2021.
9. Maree RD, Marcum ZA, Saghafi E, Weiner DK, Karp JF. A systematic review of opioid and benzodiazepine misuse in older adults. Am J Geriatr Psychiatry. 2016;24(11):949–63. https://doi.org/10.1016/j.jagp.2016.06.003.
10. Blanco C, Volkow ND. Management of opioid use disorder in the USA: present status and future directions. Lancet. 2019;393(10182):1760–72. https://doi.org/10.1016/S0140-6736(18)33078-2.
11. Coffa D, Snyder H. Opioid use disorder: medical treatment options. Am Fam Physician. 2019;100(7):416–25.
12. Rieb LM, Samaan Z, Furlan AD, Rabheru K, Feldman S, Hung L, Budd G, Coleman D. Canadian Guidelines on opioid use disorder among older adults. Can Geriatr J. 2020;23(1):123–34. https://doi.org/10.5770/cgj.23.420.
13. Le Roux C, Tang Y, Drexler K. Alcohol and opioid use disorder in older adults: neglected and treatable illnesses. Curr Psychiatry Rep. 2016;18(9):87. https://doi.org/10.1007/s11920-016-0718-x.1.
14. Herlinger K, Lingford-Hughes A. Opioid use disorder and the brain: a clinical perspective. Addiction. 2022;117(2):495–505. https://doi.org/10.1111/add.15636.
15. Baldacchino A, Balfour DJ, Passetti F, Humphris G, Matthews K. Neuropsychological consequences of chronic opioid use: a quantitative review and meta-analysis. Neurosci Biobehav Rev. 2012;36(9):2056–68. https://doi.org/10.1016/j.neubiorev.2012.06.006.

16. Dombrowski D, Norrell N, Holroyd S. Substance use disorders in elderly admissions to an academic psychiatric inpatient service over a 10-year period. J Addict. 2016;2016:4973018. https://doi.org/10.1155/2016/4973018.

17. Crotty K, Freedman KI, Kampman KM. Executive summary of the focused update of the ASAM National Practice Guideline for the treatment of opioid use disorder. J Addict Med. 2020;14(2):99–112. https://doi.org/10.1097/ADM.0000000000000635.

18. Moran S, Isa J, Steinemann S. Perioperative management in the patient with substance abuse. Surg Clin North Am. 2015;95(2):417–28. https://doi.org/10.1016/j.suc.2014.11.001.

19. Yarnell S, Li L, MacGrory B, Trevisan L, Kirwin P. Substance use disorders in later life: a review and synthesis of the literature of an emerging public health concern. Am J Geriatr Psychiatry. 2020;28(2):226–36. https://doi.org/10.1016/j.jagp.2019.06.005.

20. Schiller EY, Goyal A, Mechanic OJ. Opioid overdose. 2022 Sep 19. In: StatPearls. Treasure Island (FL): StatPearls Publishing; 2023.

21. Haymond S, Nagpal G, Heiman H. Urine drug screens to monitor opioid use for managing chronic pain. JAMA. 2017;318(11):1061–2. https://doi.org/10.1001/jama.2017.10593.

22. Chalk M, Alanis-Hirsch K, Woodworth A, Kemp J, McLellan T. FDA Approved medications for the treatment of opiate dependence: literature reviews on effectiveness & cost- effectiveness, Treatment Research Institute (TRI). In: Advancing access to addiction medications: implications for opioid addiction treatment; 2013. [cited 2022 December 1]. Available from: https://nosorh.org/wp-content/uploads/2017/05/Access-to-MAT-by-state.pdf.

23. Dugosh K, Abraham A, Seymour B, McLoyd K, Chalk M, Festinger D. A systematic review on the use of psychosocial interventions in conjunction with medications for the treatment of opioid addiction. J Addict Med. 2016;10(2):93–103. https://doi.org/10.1097/ADM.0000000000000193.

24. Joshi P, Shah NK, Kirane HD. Medication-assisted treatment for opioid use disorder in older adults: an emerging role for the geriatric psychiatrist. Am J Geriatr Psychiatry. 2019;27(4):455–7. https://doi.org/10.1016/j.jagp.2018.12.026.

25. Coe MA, Lofwall MR, Walsh SL. Buprenorphine pharmacology review: update on transmucosal and long-acting formulations. J Addict Med. 2019;13(2):93–103. https://doi.org/10.1097/ADM.0000000000000457.

26. Rzasa Lynn R, Galinkin JL. Naloxone dosage for opioid reversal: current evidence and clinical implications. Ther Adv Drug Saf. 2018;9(1):63–88. https://doi.org/10.1177/2042098617744161.

27. Bryce C. Lofexidine (Lucemyra) for treatment of opioid withdrawal symptoms. Am Fam Physician. 2019;99(6):392–4.

28. By the 2019 American Geriatrics Society Beers Criteria Update Expert Panel. American Geriatrics Society 2019 updated AGS beers criteria for potentially inappropriate medication use in older adults. J Am Geriatr Soc. 2019;67(4):674–94. https://doi.org/10.1111/jgs.15767.

Benzodiazepine Use Disorder

20

Megan Mazzella, Marisa Fallone,
and Esther Akinyemi

Introduction

Benzodiazepines are commonly used for treatment of anxiety and insomnia. They are effective for short-term treatment of these conditions. There are very few indications for long-term benzodiazepine use, including seizure disorder, REM sleep behavior disorder, or severe anxiety disorders [1]. Their long-term use in older adults for other disorders is not recommended due to potential adverse effects. Specifically, the recommendation from the American Geriatric Society Beers Criteria from 2019 is to avoid these medications among older adults as older adults have increased sensitivity to and decreased metabolism with long-acting agents and increased risk of cognitive impairment, delirium, falls, fractures, and motor vehicle crashes [1]. These adverse effects including increased risks for falls, fractures, and the risk of worsening cognition and the development of dementia are well documented in studies [2–4]. Despite these adverse effects, benzodiazepines remain highly utilized among older adults, with up to 13.5% of older adults using benzodiazepines, with close to 10% of persons older than 65 years of age being prescribed benzodiazepine, and 0.5% misusing the

medication [5]. Few older adult benzodiazepine users receive a clinical mental health diagnosis, and almost none is provided or referred to psychotherapy. Prescribing benzodiazepines to older adults continues despite decades of evidence documenting safety concerns [6]. New benzodiazepine prescription after hospitalization occurs frequently in older adults and may result in chronic use [7]. Older adults are often unaware of the risks of these medications [8]. Educating older adults on the risks of these medications and empowering them to be stronger partners in their health care can lead to deprescribing of these medications, without increasing adverse effects or worsening underlying conditions [8]. Non pharmacologic measures will need to be explored more aggressively to help manage older adults with anxiety, insomnia, and behavioral symptoms of dementia and limit inappropriate use of benzodiazepines in this population [6].

Epidemiology

Benzodiazepine misuse, abuse, and dependence continue to be a concern in the elderly, despite the increased risk of side effects in this population (5). Misuse of substances occur when they are not used in a way that is consistent with prescription instructions or recommended guidelines. Examples include taking increased doses, taking at increased frequency, or using for rea-

M. Mazzella (✉) · M. Fallone · E. Akinyemi
Department of Psychiatry, Henry Ford Health,
Detroit, MI, USA
e-mail: Mmazzel1@hfhs.org; Mfallon1@hfhs.org;
Eakinye2@hfhs.org

R. R. Tampi, D. J. Tampi (eds.), *Treatment of Psychiatric Disorders Among Older Adults*,
https://doi.org/10.1007/978-3-031-55711-8_20

sons other than what they are prescribed for [9]. This differs from abuse which occurs when individuals use the substances to get high or harm themselves [10]. Individuals may also develop a physical or psychological dependence [11]. Full criteria for a benzodiazepine use disorder as defined in the DSM 5 TR refer to persistent problematic use with loss of control, physical dependence, and use despite adverse consequences [12].

A study to describe determinants of current and subsequent benzodiazepine use in an elderly population found a baseline rate of benzodiazepine use in that population to be 31.9% [13]. Benzodiazepines are the second most commonly prescribed class of medications that are implicated in overdose deaths, secondary to opioids [13, 14]. According to Liu et al., more than 75% of benzodiazepine-related deaths also involve opioids [15] and older adults experience the highest rates of co-prescribing of these two classes of medications [16]. Up to 10% of persons older than 65 years of age are being prescribed benzodiazepines and 0.5% are misusing the medication [5]. A study found that the rate for benzodiazepine visits doubled from 2003 to 2015 among primary care physicians [17]. One study found that substance use disorders may be present in as many as 20% of geriatric patients, with 11.4% of those being benzodiazepine dependent [18]. Geriatric patients with substance use disorders have a higher risk for medical and psychiatric morbidity when compared to patients without substance use disorder [18]. Elderly patients have significant changes in the pharmacokinetics and pharmacodynamics of medications, which may put them at higher risk for the side effects of benzodiazepines [19, 20]. These side effects are more prevalent in those with a benzodiazepine use disorder as they are more likely to use the medication chronically [13]. Elderly patients are also at higher risk for medication interactions and polypharmacy given that they are the largest consumers of over-the-counter medications [21, 22]. Significant side effects of benzodiazepines in this population include falls, hip fractures, and cognitive decline [2–4]. They have also been shown to be associated with increased risk of death in those with Alzheimer's disease (AD) [23, 24]. It has been shown that patients who are exposed to benzodiazepines are dying at a 1.2–3.7 times higher rate per year compared to unexposed patients [24].

Risk Factors

Older adults have risk factors for benzodiazepine use disorder and a higher likelihood of experiencing adverse effects from the use of benzodiazepines [19, 25]. These risk factors include age, chronic pain/disability, Caucasian ethnicity, social withdrawal, cognitive impairment, hospitalization, and social isolation [13, 26–29]. A study in homebound older adults found higher levels of controlled medication usage associated with younger-old age, white race, postsurgical status, injuries, referral from inpatient settings, and rural location [29].

Psychiatric comorbidities such as insomnia, suicidal ideation, and current or previous substance use disorder (especially alcohol use) can also predispose to benzodiazepine use disorder [30, 31]. Specifically, patients with depression have greater likelihood of using benzodiazepines [30]. In one study, baseline use of benzodiazepine was associated with female gender, previous psychiatric diagnosis, concomitant antidepressant use, depressive symptomatology, multiple drug use, multiple chronic diseases, and poor self-perceived health. Incident use of benzodiazepines in the following 5-year period was associated with previous psychiatric diseases, poor self-perceived life satisfaction, and multiple comorbidities [13].

Another study found that symptoms of depression, hypertension, pain-related joint complaints, and the perception of poor physical health predicted new-onset chronic use. Persistent use after filling the first prescription was predicted only by pain-related joint complaints. Living alone was however found to be protective against chronic benzodiazepine use in this population [26].

Among older adults, age and cognitive impairment predicted long-term continuous use, but no association was found between the patient's gender, anxiety level; the physician gender or physician specialty status [28]. Although female gender has previously been noted to be a risk factor, the data appears to be mixed on this issue. One study found that women are more likely to report misusing benzodiazepines, but are not actually more likely to have benzodiazepine use disorder [22]. Women are also more likely to receive a prescription for benzodiazepines than men are [32].

Longer prescription duration or chronic use is another risk factor, and it has been shown that elderly patients tend to receive scripts for longer periods of time when compared to non-elderly patients [25, 33, 34]. Use of multiple different benzodiazepines and/or z drugs simultaneously is also more likely lead to dependence [25]. Opioid misuse and abuse or dependence were found to be strongly associated with benzodiazepine misuse [35].

The specific benzodiazepine utilized may increase the risk of misuse. A study by Maust et al. showed that alprazolam was the benzodiazepine most likely to be misused (likely due to high potency and short half-life), followed by lorazepam and diazepam [35]. Clonazepam is another high potency benzodiazepine that has been shown to have high abuse potential [36]. It is important to note that although some benzodiazepines have been associated with higher risk of abuse, none of the benzodiazepines are exempt from misuse or dependence.

Assessment

Benzodiazepine use disorder falls under sedative, hypnotic, or anxiolytic use disorder in the DSM-5. The diagnostic criteria include the following: a problematic pattern of sedative, hypnotic, or anxiolytic use leading to clinically significant impairment or distress as manifested by at least two of the following occurring within a 12-month period: taking in larger than intended amounts, inability to cut down despite wanting to, craving to use and spending a lot of time obtaining the medication, failure to fulfill obligations, use despite problems in social, occupational, or recreational activities, in hazardous situations, or health problems, or evidence of physical dependence [12].

The assessment of benzodiazepine use begins by taking a detailed history. It is important to understand why and where the patient is receiving the benzodiazepine, either by prescription or illicit use, what specific benzodiazepine the patient is taking, the dose of the benzodiazepine, the frequency, the duration of use, and the last use. The severity of the disorder should be defined. Mild use disorder refers to the presence of two to three criteria; for moderate use, there is the presence of four to five criteria, while severe use is classified if there is the presence of six or more criteria [12]. Since patients that meet criteria for benzodiazepine use disorder may initially present in withdrawal, it is important to understand the date and time of last use to help with treatment decisions. Symptoms of withdrawal include autonomic hyperactivity, hand tremor, insomnia, nausea or vomiting, transient visual, tactile or auditory hallucinations or illusions, psychomotor agitation, anxiety, and grand mal seizures [12].

A thorough substance use history should be obtained from all patients. Patients should be screened for other psychiatric comorbidities including mood and anxiety disorders among others. Assessment of cognition is very important and should include the use of validated scales including the Mini Mental Status Examination (MMSE) or the Montreal Cognitive Assessment (MoCA) test, given an increased risk of cognitive dysfunction and AD with benzodiazepine use [36]. Screening for underlying and associated medical comorbidities is necessary as comorbid conditions can increase the risk of adverse effects. Benzodiazepine use in patients with Chronic Obstructive Pulmonary Disease (COPD) has been associated with an increased risk of mortality in a dose–response fashion [37]. Benzodiazepines have a dose–response relationship with an increased risk of overdose death in patients receiving opioid analgesics [38].

Physical examination should pay specific attention to signs of intoxication or withdrawal. Signs of intoxication may include slurred speech, incoordination, unsteady gait, and altered mental status while signs of withdrawal may include tachycardia, hypertension, tremor, nausea, vomiting, anxiety, and agitation [12].

Laboratory studies should be obtained. This should include blood count, metabolic panel, and urine drug screens. It is important to interpret the findings from urine drug screens with caution however as standard urine drug screens may not detect all benzodiazepines including alprazolam, clonazepam, and lorazepam [39]. Other objective data include reviewing the online monitoring system for prescriptions of controlled substances, this is available in many states in the United States and can give insight to the dose, number of clinicians prescribing the medications, and other controlled substances that the patient may be receiving [40]. Where this is not available, efforts should be made to obtain collateral from treating clinicians and family members.

It may be difficult to assess and ultimately diagnose benzodiazepine use disorder in a patient who is prescribed this class of medication. This is often the case with distinguishing between patients with untreated or undertreated anxiety symptoms that are seeking relief versus patients misusing the medication. Some behaviors that may raise red flags for medication misuse or dependence include requesting early refills and frequent dose increases, reporting losing medications often, refusing to discuss other treatment options, withdrawal symptoms including rebound anxiety and insomnia when the drug is stopped, driving while using benzodiazepines, continued use despite significant side effects, use of other substances including other hypnotics, and continued use despite the recommendation to discontinue [41] (Table 20.1).

Table 20.1 Red flags for benzodiazepine misuse or dependence

Continued use despite significant adverse effects
Concurrent use of other substances
Continued use despite recommendations to discontinue the medication
Frequent reports of losing medications
Presence of withdrawal symptoms (including rebound anxiety or insomnia)
Requests for early refills
Requests for frequent dose increases
Refusal to discuss other treatment options
Use of medication in dangerous situations such as driving

Treatments

Treatment of benzodiazepine use disorder consists of assessing the need for continued use of the medication, aggressively treating underlying or comorbid conditions and tapering of the medication when it is no longer clinically indicated [42, 43]. A study found that 80% of older adults who had been on benzodiazepines long term and motivated to discontinue treatment with benzodiazepines were successful in tapering the medication and that this resulted in improved cognitive function [42]. Tapering benzodiazepines is often successful with educational non-pharmacological interventions which have been shown to reduce benzodiazepine use in the elderly population [43], as well as pharmacological interventions. Underlying disorders such as anxiety disorders should be addressed with non-pharmacologic measures such as psychotherapy as well other pharmacologic options such as antidepressants.

Non-pharmacological Treatment

Older adults are often unaware of the risks of these medications and remain on them for significantly prolonged periods beyond recommended time frames [29]. In the EMPOWER study, an educational intervention was implemented to reduce the use of benzodiazepines among older adults [8]. This intervention described the risks of benzodiazepine use, empowered older adults to discuss their medications with their providers, and provided a stepwise tapering protocol. This intervention yielded a benzodiazepine discontinuation rate of 27% when compared with 5% in the control group 6 months after the intervention. An additional 11% of recipients achieved dose reductions. Providing direct consumer education to patients may help reduce inappropriate use of benzodiazepines [8].

The PASSE60 study evaluated what psychological factors predict discontinuation of benzodiazepines [43]. It studied how the intensity of depressive symptoms, social support satisfaction, self-perceived competence in the ability to withdraw, and overall quality of sleep predict discontinuation in long-term older benzodiazepine consumers. Length of use and the dose predicted short-term discontinuation of benzodiazepine in the elderly. Self-perceived competence in the ability to stop benzodiazepines predicts long-term discontinuation. Social support was a reliable predictor of short- and long-term discontinuation. It was also shown in this study that more depressive symptoms predict long-term discontinuation. This study suggested that benzodiazepine use disorder treatment programs should also focus on these psychological factors as they predict long-term discontinuation [44].

Psychotherapeutic interventions such as brief cognitive therapy with psychoeducation and motivational enhancement may be helpful during the tapering process [8, 45–48]. It has also been suggested that osteopathic manipulative treatment to decrease paravertebral muscle tension may be beneficial during the tapering process [47].

Pharmacological

The benzodiazepine taper is the main pharmacological treatment for benzodiazepine use disorder. A gradual reduction and slow taper are recommended for outpatient treatment [45, 49]. Longer duration of use has been associated with a higher likelihood of symptoms during the taper [47]. There is limited evidence to support the use of adjunct therapy to decrease the severity of benzodiazepine withdrawal during a taper [50–52]. Several medications however have been suggested as adjuncts including melatonin, gabapentin, pregabalin, and carbamazepine [52–58].

Medication Classes

Benzodiazepines

There is insufficient evidence to support the use of a particular benzodiazepine for tapering in older adults, but some physicians recommend switching to a long-acting benzodiazepine and then gradually decreasing the dose [59]. No large randomized controlled trials have been done to support this recommendation. As there is no clear evidence suggesting an optimum rate of taper, schedules tend to vary [49]. Many suggest slow tapers as it is thought this would decrease the rebound anxiety associated with benzodiazepine withdrawal [8, 49, 59]. Paquin et al. performed a systematic literature review of 28 studies of older outpatients tapering from long-term benzodiazepine use [60]. Common schedules involved a 25% dose reduction over 1–2 weeks until the patients were drug free [58]. It was found that 60% of the patients became benzodiazepine free with 4-week protocols using this regimen [60]. However, some patients may require longer tapering schedules. Tannenbaum et al. used a 22-week taper protocol during the EMPOWER trial [8], which was also successful.

Carbamazepine

There is some evidence from case reports, case series, and open label studies which suggest that carbamazepine may be helpful for benzodiazepine withdrawal symptoms. Specifically, carbamazepine has shown potential in assisting taper completion and reducing withdrawal severity [49]. There have also been studies that have shown carbamazepine to reduce symptoms of anxiety [56]. However, this body of evidence is weak and no specific clinical recommendations can be drawn from current studies [49–52].

Gabapentin and Pregabalin

There are multiple case reports that have shown positive effects of using gabapentin or pregabalin for withdrawal symptoms during inpatient benzodiazepine tapers [55–57]. A randomized double-blind study found that a nonsignificant higher proportion of patients remained benzodiazepine free when receiving pregabalin when compared with placebo during gradual benzodiazepine taper [56]. Most studies that have evaluated pregabalin as an adjunctive therapy in benzodiazepine discontinuation failed to find a significant difference in discontinuation rates. Many studies have shown improvements in withdrawal symptoms, anxiety symptoms, and cognitive function with pregabalin use in benzodiazepine discontinuation [57].

Melatonin

Melatonin has been proposed as an adjunctive therapy during benzodiazepine withdrawal. One double-blinded placebo-controlled study of 36 participants showed that sleep quality scores were significantly higher in the melatonin therapy group when compared to placebo [53]. Double-blind studies have indicated that melatonin may improve sleep quality, but provide conflicting information on improving benzodiazepine discontinuation rates. Studies have also found no difference in withdrawal symptoms with the use of melatonin when compared to placebo [54].

Anxiolytics and Insomnia Treatment

Some authors have suggested that replacing benzodiazepines with the treatment for anxiety or insomnia may be beneficial [58]. However, no randomized controlled trials have addressed whether substituting one of these agents is beneficial during benzodiazepine taper.

Adverse Effects and Their Treatments

Older adults are at risk of adverse effects from use of benzodiazepine. These risks are associated with changes in the pharmacokinetics of the medications due to aging and include increasing risks of falls, fractures, and risk of worsening cognition including development of dementia [2–4, 61, 62]. Benzodiazepine use has also been shown to increase the risk of suicide in elderly patients and is also frequently used in intentional overdoses [63].

The risk of falls is likely due to benzodiazepines causing decreased reaction time, unsteady gait, sedation, and impaired vision [3, 62, 64]. It has been estimated that exposure to benzodiazepines increases the risk of falling by 50% [3]. Tapering of benzodiazepines decreases the risk of falls [64]. Benzodiazepines have been shown to cause decline in cognitive function including in memory, attention, and visuospatial ability. There is also an association with long-term cognitive decline including dementia with prolonged benzodiazepine use. Studies have shown that in long-term benzodiazepine users, cognitive function may improve after tapering benzodiazepines [37, 38].

Prolonged use of central nervous system depressant (CNSD) medications, which include benzodiazepines, and prolonged use of opioids are both positively associated with pain intensity [65]. These results may have implications for treatment and long-term pain management for older patients [65]. Older patients with prolonged CNSD use reported poorer health-related quality of life (HRQoL). They also had more pain and higher depression scores. Prolonged use of CNSDs was not independently associated with higher HRQoL [66]. It has also been shown that Medicare's expansion of benzodiazepine coverage may have been associated with increases in the rates of overdose among adults ages 65 to 69 years, and in the rates of overdose and fall-related injury among those 80 years or older [63]. Benzodiazepine use is also associated with an increase in mortality. It has been shown that patients that are exposed to benzodiazepines are dying at a 1.2–3.7 times higher rate per year compared to unexposed patients [24].

Evidence-based Treatment Algorithms

There are no clear guidelines for treatment of benzodiazepine use disorder. We propose an approach based on available literature.

Steps:
1. Take a detailed history: How much, how long, last use, where from, what else is going on clinically.
   (a) If use is deemed appropriate:- continue.
   (b) If use is inappropriate: Determine the severity of use including the duration and amount of use. If a patient has a history of serious benzodiazepine withdrawal including seizure, consider inpatient detoxification. For mild to moderate use: consider outpatient treatment.

2. Determine and start to address the relevant comorbid conditions including depression, anxiety, insomnia, and other substance use.
3. Design a treatment plan: inpatient versus outpatient.
4. Discuss the plan with the patient including what to do when things do not go as planned.
5. Treatment setting will determine the speed of the taper.
   (a) In an outpatient setting, tapering should be relatively slow and can be completed over months. The EMPOWER study provides a framework for tapering of benzodiazepines [8].
   (b) Taper can be done more rapidly in an inpatient setting over a period of days.

Open discussion with patients on the risks and benefits of benzodiazepines is very important.

There are educational materials available that have been shown to be helpful with discontinuation of benzodiazepines [8]. Other non-pharmacological treatments including cognitive behavioral therapy should also be considered [45–48, 67]. There is no clear evidence to support an optimal rate of taper during discontinuation. Slow taper is typically recommended with evidence supporting tapers as short as 4 weeks and as long as 22 weeks [8, 49, 59, 60]. A faster taper may be considered during inpatient setting and specific circumstances, such as if a patient is falling and confused. There are no randomized control trials to support switching short-acting to long-acting benzodiazepines during the taper process. There is no strong evidence for adjunct treatment during discontinuation. Please see Fig. 20.1 for evidence-based algorithm for management of benzodiazepine use disorder.

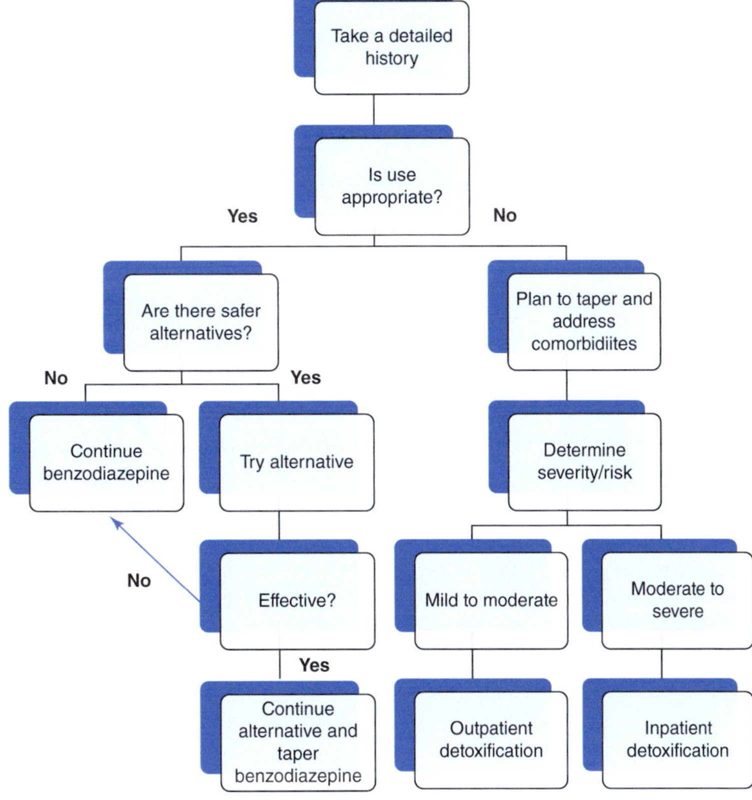

Fig. 20.1 Evidence-based algorithm for management of benzodiazepine use disorder

Conclusion

Benzodiazepines continue to be widely used in the elderly population, despite the recommendation against its use and the risk of serious adverse effects. Clinicians need to be cautious when prescribing benzodiazepines to older adults, carefully weighing the risks of misuse, dependence, and adverse effects. They should ensure that benzodiazepines are utilized for clear and appropriate indications. When indicated, benzodiazepines should be used for the shortest amount of time possible and at the lowest effective doses, and patients should be clearly educated on the risks and expected duration of use. The mainstay of pharmacologic treatment remains a benzodiazepine taper which should be slow and tailored to the individual, with consideration of the use of adjunctive agents when needed. It is important to diagnose and treat any psychiatric comorbidities. Education remains a significant and effective intervention in reducing inappropriate use of benzodiazepine and should be utilized freely to empower patients to meaningfully engage in reducing their risk with use of benzodiazepines.

References

1. By the 2019 American Geriatrics Society Beers Criteria® Update Expert Panel. American Geriatrics Society 2019 Updated AGS Beers Criteria® for Potentially Inappropriate Medication Use in Older Adults. J Am Geriatr Soc. 2019;67(4):674–94.
2. Ryynänen OP, Kivelä SL, Honkanen R, Laippala P, Saano V. Medications and chronic diseases as risk factors for falling injuries in the elderly. Scand J Soc Med. 1993;21(4):264–71.
3. Ray WA, Griffin MR, Schaffner W, Baugh DK, Melton LJ 3rd. Psychotropic drug use and the risk of hip fracture. N Engl J Med. 1987;316(7):363–9.
4. Penninkilampi R, Eslick GD. A systematic review and meta-analysis of the risk of dementia associated with benzodiazepine use, after controlling for protopathic bias. CNS Drugs. 2018;32(6):485–97.
5. Gress T, Miller M, Meadows C 3rd, Neitch SM. Benzodiazepine overuse in elders: defining the problem and potential solutions. Cureus. 2020;12(10):e11042.
6. Maust DT, Kales HC, Wiechers IR, Blow FC, Olfson M. No end in sight: benzodiazepine use in older adults in the United States. J Am Geriatr Soc. 2016;64(12):2546–53.
7. Bell CM, Fischer HD, Gill SS, Zagorski B, Sykora K, Wodchis WP, Herrmann N, Bronskill SE, Lee PE, Anderson GM, Rochon PA. Initiation of benzodiazepines in the elderly after hospitalization. J Gen Intern Med. 2007;22(7):1024–9.
8. Tannenbaum C, Martin P, Tamblyn R, Benedetti A, Ahmed S. Reduction of inappropriate benzodiazepine prescriptions among older adults through direct patient education: the EMPOWER cluster randomized trial. JAMA Intern Med. 2014;174(6):890–8.
9. Votaw VR, Geyer R, Rieselbach MM, McHugh RK. The epidemiology of benzodiazepine misuse: a systematic review. Drug Alcohol Depend. 2019;200:95–114.
10. Schmitz A. Benzodiazepine use, misuse, and abuse: a review. Ment Health Clin. 2016;6(3):120–6.
11. O'brien CP. Benzodiazepine use, abuse, and dependence. J Clin Psychiatry. 2005;66(Suppl 2):28–33.
12. American Psychiatric Association. Diagnostic and statistical manual of mental disorders. 5th. ed, text rev.; 2022.
13. Fourrier A, Letenneur L, Dartigues JF, Moore N, Bégaud B. Benzodiazepine use in an elderly community-dwelling population. Characteristics of users and factors associated with subsequent use. Eur J Clin Pharmacol. 2001;57(5):419–25.
14. Park TW, Saitz R, Ganoczy D, Ilgen MA, Bohnert AS. Benzodiazepine prescribing patterns and deaths from drug overdose among US veterans receiving opioid analgesics: case-cohort study. BMJ. 2015;350:h2698.
15. Liu S, O'Donnell J, Gladden RM, McGlone L, Chowdhury F. Trends in nonfatal and fatal overdoses involving benzodiazepines—38 states and the District of Columbia, 2019-2020. MMWR Morb Mortal Wkly Rep. 2021;70(34):1136–41.
16. Santo L, Rui P, Ashman JJ. Physician office visits at which benzodiazepines were prescribed: findings from 2014-2016 National Ambulatory Medical Care Survey. Natl Health Stat Rep. 2020;137:1–16.
17. Agarwal SD, Landon BE. Patterns in outpatient benzodiazepine prescribing in the United States. JAMA Netw Open. 2019;2(1):e187399.
18. Holroyd S, Duryee JJ. Substance use disorders in a geriatric psychiatry outpatient clinic: prevalence and epidemiologic characteristics. J Nerv Ment Dis. 1997;185(10):627–32.
19. Morse RM. Substance abuse among the elderly. Bull Menn Clin. 1988;52(3):259–68.
20. Kennedy GJ, Efremova I, Frazier A, et al. The emerging problems of alcohol and substance abuse in late life. J Soc Distress Homeless. 1999;8:227–39.
21. Rolita L, Freedman M. Over-the-counter medication use in older adults. J Gerontol Nurs. 2008;34(4):8–17.
22. Kuerbis A, Sacco P, Blazer D, Moore A. Substance abuse among older adults. Geriatr Psychiatry. 2014;30:629–54.
23. Saarelainen L, Tolppanen AM, Koponen M, et al. Risk of death associated with new benzodiaz-

epine use among persons with Alzheimer disease: a matched cohort study. Int J Geriatr Psychiatry. 2017;33(4):583–90.

24. Palmaro A, Dupouy J, Lapeyre-Mestre M. Benzodiazepines and risk of death: results from two large cohort studies in France and UK. Eur Neuropsychopharmacol. 2015;25:1566–77.

25. Victorri-Vigneau C, Laforgue EJ, Grall-Bronnec M, Guillou-Landreat M, Rousselet M, Guerlais M, Feuillet F, Jolliet P, FAN-Network. Are seniors dependent on benzodiazepines? A national clinical survey of substance use disorder. Clin Pharmacol Therap. 2020;109:528–35.

26. Luijendijk HJ, Tiemeier H, Hofman A, Heeringa J, Stricker BH. Determinants of chronic benzodiazepine use in the elderly: a longitudinal study. Br J Clin Pharmacol. 2008;65(4):593–9.

27. Airagnes G, Pelissolo A, Lavallée M, Flament M, Limosin F. Benzodiazepine misuse in the elderly: risk factors, consequences, and management. Curr Psychiatry Rep. 2016;18(10):89.

28. Egan M, Moride Y, Wolfson C, Monette J. Long-term continuous use of benzodiazepines by older adults in Quebec: prevalence, incidence and risk factors. J Am Geriatr Soc. 2000;48(7):811–6.

29. Cotton BP, Lohman MC, Brooks JM, Whiteman KL, Bao Y, Greenberg RL, Bruce ML. Prevalence of and factors related to prescription opioids, benzodiazepines, and hypnotics among Medicare home health recipients. Home Healthcare Now. 2017;35:304–13.

30. Lugoboni F, Mirijello A, Faccini M, Casari R, Cossari A, Musi G, Bissoli G, Quaglio G, Addolorato G. Quality of life in a cohort of high-dose benzodiazepine dependent patients. Drug Alcohol Depend. 2014;142:105–9.

31. Morel A, Grall-Bronnec M, Bulteau S, Chauvin-Grelier P, Gailledrat L, Pinot ML, Jolliet P, Victorri-Vigneau C. Benzodiazepine dependence in subjects with alcohol use disorders: what prevalence? Expert Opin Drug Saf. 2016;15(10):1313–9.

32. McHugh RK, Geyer RB, Chase AR, Griffin ML, Bogunovic O, Weiss RD. Sex differences in benzodiazepine misuse among adults with substance use disorders. Addict Behav. 2021;112:106608.

33. Gerlach LB, Maust DT, Leong SH, Mavandadi S, Oslin DW. Factors associated with long-term benzodiazepine use among older adults. JAMA Intern Med. 2018;178(11):1560–2.

34. Morgan K, Dallosso H, Ebrahim S, Arie T, Fentem PH. Prevalence, frequency, and duration of hypnotic drug use among the elderly living at home. Br Med J (Clin Res Ed). 1988;296(6622):601–2.

35. Maust DT, Lin LA, Blow FC. Benzodiazepine use and misuse among adults in the United States. Psychiatr Serv. 2019;70(2):97–106.

36. Taipale H, Särkilä H, Tanskanen A, Kurko T, Taiminen T, Tiihonen J, Sund R, Tuulio-Henriksson A, Saastamoinen L, Hietala J. Incidence of and characteristics associated with long-term benzodiazepine use in Finland. JAMA Netw Open. 2020;3(10):e2019029.

37. Ekström MP, Bornefalk-Hermansson A, Abernethy AP, Currow DC. Safety of benzodiazepines and opioids in very severe respiratory disease: national prospective study. BMJ. 2014;348:g445.

38. Olfson M, King M, Schoenbaum M. Benzodiazepine use in the United States. JAMA Psychiatry. 2015;72(2):136–42.

39. Moeller KE, Kissack JC, Atayee RS, Lee KC. Clinical interpretation of urine drug tests: what clinicians need to know about urine drug screens. Mayo Clin Proc. 2017;92(5):774–96.

40. Prescription Drug Monitoring Program Training and Technical Assistance Center. Prescription drug monitoring frequently asked questions. 2023.

41. Curran HV, Collins R, Fletcher S, Kee SC, Woods B, Iliffe S. Older adults and withdrawal from benzodiazepine hypnotics in general practice: effects on cognitive function, sleep, mood and quality of life. Psychol Med. 2003;33(7):1223–37.

42. Dou C, Rebane J, Bardal S. Interventions to improve benzodiazepine tapering success in the elderly: a systematic review. Aging Ment Health. 2019;23(4):411–6.

43. Allary A, Proulx-Tremblay V, Bélanger C, Hudon C, Marchand A, O'Connor K, Pérodeau G, Roberge P, Tannenbaum C, Vasiliadis HM, Desrosiers C, Cruz-Santiago D, Grenier S. Psychological predictors of benzodiazepine discontinuation among older adults: results from the PASSE 60. Addict Behav. 2020;102:106195.

44. Lader M, Tylee A, Donoghue J. Withdrawing benzodiazepines in primary care. CNS Drugs. 2009;23:19–34.

45. Ten Wolde GB, Dijkstra A, van Empelen P, van den Hout W, Neven AK, Zitman F. Long-term effectiveness of computer-generated tailored patient education on benzodiazepines: a randomized controlled trial. Addiction. 2008;103(4):662–70.

46. Reeves RR, Kamal A. Complicated withdrawal phenomena during benzodiazepine cessation in older adults. J Am Osteopath Assoc. 2019;119(5):327–31.

47. Mugunthan K, McGuire T, Glasziou P. Minimal interventions to decrease long-term use of benzodiazepines in primary care: a systematic review and meta-analysis. Br J Gen Pract. 2011;61(590):e573–8.

48. Pottie K, Thompson W, Davies S, Grenier J, Sadowski CA, Welch V, Holbrook A, Boyd C, Swenson R, Ma A, Farrell B. Deprescribing benzodiazepine receptor agonists: evidence-based clinical practice guideline. Can Fam Physician. 2018;64(5):339–51.

49. Rowan-Robinson K. Pharmacological interventions for benzodiazepine discontinuation in chronic benzodiazepine users. Int J Evid Based Healthc. 2019;17(2):143–4.

50. Welsh JW, Tretyak V, McHugh RK, Weiss RD, Bogunovic O. Review: adjunctive pharmacologic approaches for benzodiazepine tapers. Drug Alcohol Depend. 2018;189:96–107.

51. Baandrup L, Ebdrup BH, Rasmussen JØ, Lindschou J, Gluud C, Glenthøj BY. Pharmacological interventions for benzodiazepine discontinuation in chronic

benzodiazepine users. Cochrane Database Syst Rev. 2018;3(3):CD011481.

52. Garfinkel D, Zisapel N, Wainstein J, Laudon M. Facilitation of benzodiazepine discontinuation by melatonin. Arch Intern Med. 1999;159:2456.

53. Wright A, Diebold J, Otal J, Stoneman C, Wong J, Wallace C, Duffett M. The effect of melatonin on benzodiazepine discontinuation and sleep quality in adults attempting to discontinue benzodiazepines: a systematic review and meta-analysis. Drugs Aging. 2015;32:1009–18.

54. Leung E, Ngo DH, Espinoza JA Jr, Beal LL, Chang C, Baris DA, Lackey BN, Lane SD, Wu HE. A retrospective study of the adjunctive use of gabapentin with benzodiazepines for the treatment of benzodiazepine withdrawal. J Psychiatr Pract. 2022;28(4):310–8.

55. Hadley SJ, Mandel FS, Schweizer E. Switching from long-term benzodiazepine therapy to pregabalin in patients with generalized anxiety disorder: a double-blind, placebo-controlled trial. J Psychopharmacol. 2011;26:461–70.

56. Caniff K, Telega E, Bostwick JR, Gardner KN. Pregabalin as adjunctive therapy in benzodiazepine discontinuation. Am J Health Syst Pharm. 2018;75(2):67–71.

57. Di Costanzo E, Rovea A. The prophylaxis of benzodiazepine withdrawal syndrome in the elderly: the effectiveness of carbamazepine. Double-blind study vs placebo. Minerva Psichiatr. 1992;33(4):301–4.

58. Morton S, Lader M. Buspirone treatment as an aid to benzodiazepine withdrawal. J Psychopharmacol. 1995;9(4):331–5.

59. Brett J, Murnion B. Management of benzodiazepine misuse and dependence. Aust Prescr. 2015;38(5):152–5.

60. Paquin AM, Zimmerman K, Rudolph JL. Risk versus risk: a review of benzodiazepine reduction in older adults. Expert Opin Drug Saf. 2014;13(7):919–34.

61. Xing D, Ma XL, Ma JX, Wang J, Yang Y, Chen Y. Association between use of benzodiazepines and risk of fractures: a meta-analysis. Osteoporos Int. 2014;25:105–20.

62. Carlsten A, Waern M, Holmgren P, Allebeck P. The role of benzodiazepines in elderly suicides. Scand J Public Health. 2003;31(3):224–8.

63. Bjelkarøy MT, Cheng S, Siddiqui TG, Benth JŠ, Grambaite R, Kristoffersen ES, Lundqvist C. The association between pain and central nervous system depressing medication among hospitalised Norwegian older adults. Scand J Pain. 2021;22(3):483–93.

64. Cumming RG, Le Couteur DG. Benzodiazepines and risk of hip fractures in older people. CNS Drugs. 2003;17(11):825–37.

65. Cheng S, Siddiqui TG, Gossop M, Stavem K, Kristoffersen ES, Lundqvist C. Health-related quality of life in hospitalized older patients with versus without prolonged use of opioid analgesics, benzodiazepines, and Z-hypnotics: a cross-sectional study. BMC Geriatr. 2020;20(1):425.

66. Maust DT, Lin LA, Goldstick JE, Haffajee RL, Brownlee R, Bohnert AS. Association of medicare part D benzodiazepine coverage expansion with changes in fall-related injuries and overdoses among medicare advantage beneficiaries. JAMA Netw Open. 2020;3(4):e202051.

67. Darker CD, Sweeney BP, Barry JM, Farrell MF, Donnelly-Swift E. Psychosocial interventions for benzodiazepine harmful use, abuse or dependence. Cochrane Database Syst Rev. 2015;5:CD009652.

Generalized Anxiety Disorder

Ali M. Molaie, Hans F. von Walter, and Brandon C. Yarns

Introduction

Generalized Anxiety Disorder (GAD) is a prevalent and disabling anxiety disorder characterized by worry across multiple life domains that is perceived as excessive, difficult to control, and associated with significant distress or impairment. As per the Diagnostic and Statistical Manual for Mental Disorders, Fifth Edition (DSM-5; [1]), a diagnosis of GAD requires that the worry has occurred on more days than not for at least 6 months, concomitant with at least three of the following somatic symptoms: restlessness or feeling keyed up or on edge, fatigability, difficulty concentrating or mind going blank, irritability, muscle tension, and sleep disturbance. Older adults exhibit a wide variety of worry content, most prominently about their own and loved ones' health and well-being [2, 3].

Estimated prevalence of GAD among older adults ranges from 1.2% to 7.3%, with studies comparing age-groups generally documenting a decline in prevalence across the lifespan [4]. Reynolds and colleagues reported a past-year prevalence of 2.8% among a nationally representative sample of community-dwelling U.S. adults aged 55 and older [4]. While the age of onset for GAD is variable, a bi-modal distribution has been described with new onset cases typically appearing in early adulthood, followed by a second peak during older adulthood [5]. Earlier onset of symptoms is associated with higher psychiatric comorbidity, whereas patients reporting later-onset GAD are more likely to report functional limitations and poor health-related quality of life [5, 6].

Studies examining sociodemographic associations with GAD often report higher rates among women (e.g., [7]) and significant comorbidity with other anxiety, depressive, and substance use disorders [8]. Research chronicling the co-occurrence of GAD and major depressive disorder report roughly a 30% comorbidity rate between GAD and depression in treatment-seeking older adult samples [9, 10]. Retrospective and longitudinal studies further demonstrate that chronic presentations of GAD often precede and/or overlap with major depressive episodes, the combination of which is associated with long-

A. M. Molaie
Department of Mental Health/Psychiatry, VA Greater Los Angeles Healthcare System,
Los Angeles, CA, USA
e-mail: Ali.Molaie@va.gov

H. F. von Walter · B. C. Yarns (✉)
Department of Mental Health/Psychiatry, VA Greater Los Angeles Healthcare System,
Los Angeles, CA, USA

Department of Psychiatry and Biobehavioral Sciences, David Geffen School of Medicine at University of California, Los Angeles (UCLA),
Los Angeles, CA, USA
e-mail: Hans.VonWalter@va.gov;
byarns@mednet.ucla.edu

standing vulnerability [11, 12]. As one of the most common anxiety disorders among older long-term care residents, GAD is also present in up to 15% of older patients with probable dementia [13].

Risk Factors

Several prospective studies have elucidated psychosocial risk factors for GAD in older adults [12, 14, 15]. Following a cohort of 1711 anxiety-free, non-demented adults ages 65 and older over the course of 12 years, Zhang and colleagues reported female gender, recent adverse life events, chronic physical (respiratory disorders, cardiac illness, cognitive impairment), and mental (depression, phobia, and a history of GAD) health problems as principal predictors of late-onset GAD [15]. Poverty, parental loss or separation, history of parental mental illness, and low emotional support during childhood were also independently associated with incident late-onset GAD [15]. Several gene variants in adrenergic receptors have been hypothesized to moderate the effect of adverse life events on risk of GAD [16].

Specific cognitive functioning impairments have shown to longitudinally predict elevated risk for GAD during middle and older adulthood encompassing both executive (e.g., poor inhibition, set shifting, working memory updating) and non-executive (e.g., inductive reasoning) functions [17]. Older adults with GAD also demonstrate an attentional preference for negative information and avoidance of positive information [18, 19], though findings vary by experimental task [20]. Improvement in executive dysfunction and short-term memory have been observed following treatment [21, 22]. Anxiety may portend risk for dementia [23], with worry in particularly associated with accelerated brain aging [24] along with a host of health-related causes of mortality in late life [25, 26].

Neurobiological correlates of GAD include heightened indiscriminate amygdala activity in response to anticipatory threat [27] and alterations in amygdalar subregional connectivity patterns [28]. In studies of older adults, worry severity has been positively correlated with orbitofrontal cortex volume [29] and decreased activation in the precuneus and prefrontal cortex [30]. Several functional connectivity findings have been proposed to underlie emotion regulation deficits in late-life GAD, including greater insula-orbitofrontal cortex connectivity during worry induction, with failure to engage prefrontal structures during worry reappraisal [31, 32]. Broader physiological changes implicated in late-life GAD suggest hypothalamic–pituitary–adrenal (HPA) axis hyperactivity, characterized by elevated cortisol levels that are reduced by treatment [33–35].

Assessment

Available evidence suggests that many cases of GAD in older adults go undiagnosed, particularly in primary care [36]. Assessing for GAD requires a thorough clinical history, detailed mental status examination, cognitive screening, targeted physical and neurologic examination, laboratory testing, and self-report assessment scales. The examination begins with a clinical history to ascertain presence and severity of anxiety symptoms, as well as psychiatric and medical comorbidities commonly present among older adults. Differential diagnosis with later-onset cognitive (e.g., delirium) and medical (e.g., thyroid disease) conditions that resemble or contribute to anxiety is critical when working with older patients. Inquiring about recent initiation or withdrawal from anxiogenic medications and substances can further rule out disparate etiologies [37]. Common medical conditions and substances that may cause or exacerbate symptoms that overlap with GAD are presented in Table 21.1. Laboratory testing should evaluate for the medical conditions in Table 21.1 and should also include a urine drug screen if indicated by history.

Additional features of clinical assessment include evaluating the impact of anxiety, worry, or physical symptoms on the older adult's quality of life, with a particular emphasis on avoidance

Table 21.1 Common medical conditions and substances/medications that are associated with anxiety

Anxiety due to another medical condition[a]	Anxiety due to substances/medications[b]
Hyperthyroidism	Sympathomimetics (e.g., nasal decongestants)
Hyperparathyroidism	
Hypoxia or ischemia	Amphetamines (e.g., methamphetamine)
Hypoglycemia	
Cardiac arrythmias	Anticholinergics (e.g., diphenhydramine)
Pheochromocytoma	
	Vasopressors
	Caffeine-containing medications
	Alcohol

[a] Usually acute onset and resolves with treatment of the underlying condition
[b] Can be due to either acute intoxication or withdrawal

behaviors. Theoretical frameworks of GAD have variously conceptualized worry as a function of cognitive [38] and experiential [39] avoidance, emotion dysregulation [40], intolerance of uncertainty [41], and maladaptive meta-beliefs about worry (e.g., "worrying helps me to cope"; "worrying is uncontrollable") [42]. Identifying whether problematic worry is a function of one of these factors may be useful from a psychotherapeutic standpoint. In addition, obtaining information on past strategies for managing symptoms pharmacologically and non-pharmacologically can guide targeted recommendations for treatment. Obtaining collateral information from family members, caregivers, or medical providers is additionally useful for gathering etiological and risk factors that can inform an individualized treatment plan.

Clinical interviewing should be supplemented by administration of brief screening instruments found to have treatment utility in older adults. Clinical measures assist with detecting GAD in older adults who often present with somatic symptoms that confound proper diagnosis, and in circumventing potential reluctance or difficulty disclosing mental health experiences to medical professionals [43, 44]. Psychometric validity for older adults has been established for several measures, including the Generalized Anxiety Disorder scale (GAD-7; [45, 46]), Geriatric Anxiety Inventory [47, 48], and the Penn State Worry Questionnaire (PSWQ; [49, 50]). Wild et al. showed that clinical cut-off scores of five for the GAD-7 and two for a briefer format, the GAD-2, yielded high specificity and reasonable sensitivity among a general population of older adults living at home [46]. Structured assessment through self-report instruments can also serve as a form of outcome-based measurement to guide treatment decisions through repeated administration over time [51].

Treatments

Pharmacotherapy and a wide range of non-pharmacologic treatments are evidence based for GAD in older adults. However, far fewer randomized clinical trials (RCTs) of either have been conducted in older adults compared to younger adults [52]. In comparing pharmacologic and non-pharmacologic treatments for anxiety disorders in older adults, one meta-analysis found overall large effects for both types of treatment, but a larger pooled effect size for pharmacologic treatments ($d = 1.76$) versus non-pharmacologic treatments ($d = 0.86$) [52, 53]. Yet the authors noted that effect sizes for control groups were substantially greater in pill-placebo controlled trials of medications ($d = 1.06$) compared to non-pharmacologic controls ($d = 0.10$). Adjusting for nonspecific effects in the control group, effects of both pharmacologic ($d = 0.80$) and non-pharmacologic treatments ($d = 0.83$) were similar and large.

Psychotherapy

Randomized clinical trials have evaluated a wide range of non-pharmacologic interventions for older adults with anxiety disorders and GAD, including relaxation training, meditation, cognitive behavioral therapy (CBT), worry discussion groups, supportive counseling, enhanced community treatment, and exercise training [52, 54, 55]. A 2003 meta-analysis in older adults (mean age = 55 years) with mixed anxiety disorders found a medium effect size ($d = 0.55$) for 20 different non-pharmacologic treatments at post-treatment [56].

CBT for GAD has been tested in RCTs in older adults in synchronous in-person, telephone, and internet-based formats [57–59]. A meta-analysis evaluated results from 14 RCTs of CBT for GAD that included 985 older adults (mean age = 65 years) [55]. This meta-analysis demonstrated that CBT was superior to waitlist control groups or treatment-as-usual both at post-treatment (g = 0.67) and 6-month follow-up (g = 0.83), but was not superior to active controls (e.g., exercise programs) at any time point. CBT was also found to be inferior to relaxation training in another meta-analysis of 10 controlled studies [54]. In this meta-analysis, the pooled effect size for CBT was g = 0.00, whereas the effect size for relaxation training alone was large (g = 0.90). Direct comparisons of CBT to other forms of psychological treatments (e.g., worry discussion groups [60] or supportive counseling [61]) for GAD or anxiety disorders in older adults have shown few or no advantages for CBT over other psychological treatments.

Given the nominal response of CBT for GAD and other anxiety disorders in older adults relative to other active treatments, one research group developed an "enhanced" CBT that included memory and learning aids, such as a greater emphasis on psychoeducation, slower pace, repeated explanations, and reminder phone calls for homework [62]. In two small clinical trials (published together) that directly compared standard CBT to enhanced CBT, effect size advantages and greater response rates were found for enhanced CBT [62].

In sum, despite fewer trials in older adults compared to younger adults, available evidence indicates that non-pharmacologic treatments are effective for GAD in older adults with medium-to-large effect sizes and no particular advantages for CBT—the most studied treatment—over other non-pharmacologic options. Non-pharmacologic treatments may result in smaller effect size benefits than pharmacologic treatments due to substantial additional nonspecific (i.e., placebo) effects for pharmacotherapy.

Pharmacotherapy

In comparison to depressive disorders, far fewer studies have been conducted on pharmacotherapy for GAD in older adults [52]. Nearly all RCTs for the treatment of GAD have excluded older adults; this is partially due to the difficulty inherent in studying pharmacotherapy in this population, as older adults are more susceptible to treatment-resistant anxiety, drug–drug interactions, and multiple chronic medical conditions affecting the pharmacokinetics of the studied agents [63]. Nonetheless, study outcomes from the available body of evidence demonstrate reasonably consistent guidelines for the use of medications in older adults with anxiety [4]. Studied medications include selective serotonin reuptake inhibitors (SSRIs), serotonin-norepinephrine reuptake inhibitors (SNRIs), tricyclic antidepressants (TCAs), benzodiazepines, and buspirone [52, 64, 65].

SSRIs and SNRIs lend themselves as the most favorable choices for treatment of GAD in older adults, owing to their reasonably consistent efficacy in RCTs as well as their favorable side effect profiles in this age-group [66]. Among SSRIs, citalopram, escitalopram, and sertraline have been studied in RCTs that generally showed improvement in older adults with GAD [66]. In two trials, Lenze and colleagues found response rates of 69% and 65% for escitalopram and citalopram, respectively [67, 68]. Sertraline has also been compared to CBT and compared to buspirone in two separate trials [69, 70]. In one trial, sertraline was superior to CBT and placebo for anxiety symptoms, worry in particular, while both sertraline and buspirone demonstrated comparable efficacy to each other in another trial.

Among SNRIs, a pooled analysis of five RCTs found extended-release venlafaxine superior to placebo with a 66% response rate among older adults [71]. Duloxetine showed vastly improved rates in multiple measures of anxiety in one large RCT; however, there was a significantly greater rate of discontinuation due to adverse effects compared to placebo (22 vs. 0%) [72].

Side effects for both SSRIs and SNRIs most commonly include gastrointestinal upset (e.g., nausea, diarrhea), dizziness, headaches, and sleep disturbance, though they are typically tolerable with cautious dosage adjustment [73]. Citalopram also carries a dose-dependent increased concern for prolongation of the QTc-interval, and adults older than 60 years of age are at greater risk for this complication relative to younger cohorts [74]. Attrition rates for duloxetine compared to placebo noted by Davidson et al. additionally lend concern to consideration of duloxetine as a first-line agent for treatment of GAD [72].

Although the adverse effect profile of TCAs renders most of them unfavorable as first-line medications in GAD, one study on the use of nortriptyline in post-stroke older patients diagnosed with GAD and comorbid depression found fairly encouraging response rates across several outcome measures [75]. A notable finding of the study was the resolution of anxiety symptoms that generally occurred prior to remission of depressive symptoms. The side effect profile of TCAs will likely deter further research or recommendation of their primary use for GAD, as older adults are at higher risk for developing dry mouth, visual problems, sedation, cognitive impairment, constipation, and orthostatic hypotension. Additionally, TCAs are much more likely to be lethal in overdose compared to SSRIs and SNRIs, an important consideration with older patients who may have difficulty with medication management [8].

Other antidepressants with established efficacy for GAD in younger adults include the SSRIs fluoxetine and paroxetine, the TCA imipramine, and atypical agents such as mirtazapine, vilazodone, and vortioxetine [76]. To date, no high-quality trials for use of these medications in older adults with GAD have been conducted. Side effect profiles (particularly with fluoxetine, paroxetine, and imipramine), cost, and/or availability generally preclude the use of these agents in older adults with GAD [8].

Benzodiazepines are among the most prescribed medications for GAD in late life, with upwards of 25% of geriatric patients with anxiety reporting being treated at some point with a benzodiazepine [4]. Data on specific benzodiazepines in older adults with GAD are primarily from older studies. Among them, one 4-week clinical multicenter trial found that oxazepam significantly reduced anxiety symptoms, while another 4-week trial showed similar results with alprazolam [77, 78]. Additional data on the efficacy and safety of benzodiazepines for GAD is well-established in the general adult population, with most studies supporting their use for short-term treatment of anxiety symptoms, with potential concerns for long-term use including tolerance, abuse, and withdrawal [76]. Older patients are especially susceptible to further adverse outcomes from long-term benzodiazepine use, including but not limited to increased risk of falls, fractures, drug–drug interactions, and cognitive impairment [79]. Consequently, benzodiazepines should be avoided in general as first-line treatment for GAD in older adults. If an older patient requires the use of a benzodiazepine for treatment of anxiety, lorazepam and oxazepam are generally preferred as they are shorter-acting and bypass phase 1 metabolism in the liver, lowering the risk of potential medication interactions [8].

Buspirone is a partial serotonin agonist with established effectiveness and safety among older adults [52]. In one recent study of 384 older individuals that examined buspirone use within the context of social stressors, buspirone significantly reduced symptoms of generalized anxiety [80]. Buspirone's side effect profile is relatively benign; dizziness and nausea are the most commonly reported side effects, present in up to 12% and 8% of patients, respectively [81]. Despite these favorable attributes, buspirone is less frequently used relative to the agents previously discussed. Reasons for this may include delayed onset of anxiety relief from initiation, frequent comorbidity of GAD with depression (for which buspirone is not effective), and evidence suggesting that prior usage of benzodiazepines may reduce the effectiveness of buspirone [8].

Medications in other pharmacologic classes with RCTs investigating effectiveness in geriatric GAD include the GABA-analogue pregabalin, the anticonvulsant carbamazepine, and the antipsychotic risperidone [52]. All have shown promising results, with pregabalin in particular showing significant improvements across anxiety symptoms in as little as 2 weeks [82]. Other agents used in younger patients such as the antihistamine hydroxyzine have demonstrated superiority in treatment of GAD over placebo, but have not had robust trials in older patients [8]. Common medications used to treat GAD among older adults are detailed in Table 21.2.

Table 21.2 Common medications used to treat GAD among older adults

Medication class/name	Starting dose	Target dose/range	Major side effects/risks
SSRIs			
Citalopram	5 mg/day or 10 mg/day	10–20 mg/day	Nausea, reduced appetite, weight loss, sweating, tremor, flushing, agitation, anxiety, jitteriness, sedation, insomnia, headache, sexual dysfunction, diarrhea, syndrome of inappropriate antidiuretic hormone secretion (SIADH), hyponatremia, dry mouth, prolonged bleeding time, bleeding tendencies, cognitive impairment, serotonin syndrome, weight gain with long-term treatment, QT-interval prolongation
Escitalopram	5 mg/day	10–20 mg/day	Same as above
Sertraline	12.5 mg/day or 25 mg/day	50–150 mg/day	Same as above except for QTc-interval prolongation
SNRIs			
Venlafaxine	37.5 mg/day	75–225 mg/day	Nausea, insomnia, anxiety, nervousness, sedation, sexual dysfunction, headache, tremor, dizziness, constipation, sweating, tachycardia, palpitation, blood pressure elevation
Duloxetine	20 mg/day	30–120 mg/day	Nausea, anxiety, dry mouth, insomnia, sedation, sexual dysfunction, headache, sweating, dizziness
TCAs			
Nortriptyline	10 mg/day	25–150 mg/day Therapeutic plasma level: 50–150 ng/mL	Sedation, orthostatic hypotension, anticholinergic effects (dry mouth, constipation, urinary retention, blurred vision, diminished working memory, dental cavities), cardiac conduction defects, significant weight gain, sexual dysfunction (erectile), cardiotoxicity, seizures, and respiratory arrest in overdose
Benzodiazepines			
Lorazepam	0.5 mg/day	1–2 mg/day; NTE 6 mg/day; target minimally effective dose for short-term relief	Drowsiness, sedation, orthostatic hypotension, confusion, delirium, falls, dizziness, restlessness, hypoventilation
Oxazepam	10 mg/day	Aim for 15–30 mg/day in 2–3 divided doses; target minimally effective dose for short-term relief	Same as above
Alprazolam	0.25–0.5 mg/day or	2–4 mg/day, NTE 4 mg/day in 2–3 divided doses; target minimally effective dose for short-term relief	Same as above

Table 21.2 (continued)

Medication class/name	Starting dose	Target dose/range	Major side effects/risks
Other			
Buspirone	10 mg/day	20–60 mg/day in 2–3 divided doses	Dizziness, nausea, headaches, diarrhea, drowsiness, confusion, chest pain, skin rash, nervousness, insomnia, irritability, blurred vision, tremor
Pregabalin	150 mg/day in 2–3 divided doses	300 mg/day in 2–3 divided doses	Peripheral edema, weight gain, dry mouth, dizziness, drowsiness, fatigue, headache, blurred vision, visual disturbances, chest pain, hypertension, hypotension, nausea, constipation, urinary incontinence, thrombocytopenia, bronchitis, dyspnea, muscle aches

Algorithm

Pharmacologic and non-pharmacologic treatments are supported by clinical trial evidence for older adults with GAD. Therefore, either type of treatment may be used clinically, and patient preference should be considered. However, clinical trials that include direct comparisons have suggested that pharmacotherapy may produce a larger effect size on average compared to non-pharmacologic treatments. One clinical trial aimed to determine whether sequenced treatment combining pharmacotherapy and CBT would lead to improved outcomes among older adults with GAD [83]. In this trial, all patients received 12 weeks of open-label escitalopram and were then randomized to several conditions including combined escitalopram and CBT, escitalopram alone, or placebo. Compared to escitalopram alone, combination treatment with CBT led to improvements on the Penn State Worry Questionnaire, but not the Hamilton Anxiety Rating Scale. Both escitalopram and CBT prevented relapse compared to placebo. Thus, there is some support for combined treatment with an antidepressant and CBT. A treatment algorithm is presented in Table 21.3.

Table 21.3 Evidence-based treatment algorithm for GAD in older adults

First-line treatments that are supported by RCTs with lower side effect and risk burden compared to other treatments	SSRIs (especially sertraline or escitalopram; caution citalopram due to potential QTc-prolongation) SNRIs (venlafaxine ER, duloxetine) Buspirone Benzodiazepines (lorazepam or oxazepam for severe symptoms and ≤4 weeks only) And/or Non-pharmacologic (CBT, relaxation training, supportive psychotherapy)
Second-line treatments that are supported by RCTs but with relatively greater side effect/risk potential compared to first-line treatments	Pregabalin Nortriptyline Carbamazepine (discouraged due to potential drug-drug interactions) Risperidone (discouraged due to potential side effect profile) Alprazolam (discouraged due to potential tolerance)
Maintenance treatment	Escitalopram

Conclusions

GAD is highly prevalent in older adults and comes with a high burden to patients and society, including an increased risk of cognitive impairment and dementia. Yet, fewer treatment studies have been performed for GAD in older adults compared to other conditions in older adults, such as late-life depression, and compared to GAD in younger patients. Nonetheless, available evidence provides support for several pharmacologic and non-pharmacologic treatment approaches, including SSRI and SNRI medications, relaxation training, and CBT. Greater attention to GAD among older adults both in clinical and research settings can lead to improvements in the lives of these patients.

References

1. Anxiety Disorders. Diagnostic and statistical manual of mental disorders. 5th ed (DSM-5). Arlington, VA: American Psychiatric Association; 2013. p. 189–234.
2. Altunoz U, Kokurcan A, Kirici S, Bastug G, Ozel-Kizil ET. Clinical characteristics of generalized anxiety disorder: older vs. young adults. Nord J Psychiatry. 2018;72(2):97–102.
3. Gonçalves DC, Byrne GJ. Who worries most? Worry prevalence and patterns across the lifespan. Int J Geriatr Psychiatry. 2013;28(1):41–9.
4. Wolitzky-Taylor KB, Castriotta N, Lenze EJ, Stanley MA, Craske MG. Anxiety disorders in older adults: a comprehensive review. Depress Anxiety. 2010;27(2):190–211.
5. Le Roux H, Gatz M, Wetherell JL. Age at onset of generalized anxiety disorder in older adults. Am J Geriatr Psychiatry. 2005;13(1):23–30.
6. Chou KL. Age at onset of generalized anxiety disorder in older adults. Am J Geriatr Psychiatry. 2009;17(6):455–64.
7. Mackenzie CS, Reynolds K, Chou KL, Pagura J, Sareen J. Prevalence and correlates of generalized anxiety disorder in a national sample of older adults. Am J Geriatr Psychiatry. 2011;19(4):305–15.
8. Flint AJ. Generalised anxiety disorder in elderly patients : epidemiology, diagnosis and treatment options. Drugs Aging. 2005;22(2):101–14.
9. Lenze EJ, Mulsant BH, Mohlman J, et al. Comorbid anxiety disorders in depressed elderly patients. Am J Psychiatry. 2000;157(5):722–8.
10. Porensky EK, Dew MA, Karp JF, et al. The burden of late-life generalized anxiety disorder: effects on disability, health-related quality of life, and healthcare utilization. Am J Geriatr Psychiatry. 2009;17(6):473–82.
11. Lenze EJ, Mulsant BH, Mohlman J, et al. Generalized anxiety disorder in late life: lifetime course and comorbidity with major depressive disorder. Am J Geriatr Psychiatry. 2005;13(1):77–80.
12. Schoevers RA, Deeg DJ, van Tilburg W, Beekman AT. Depression and generalized anxiety disorder: co-occurrence and longitudinal patterns in elderly patients. Am J Geriatr Psychiatry. 2005;13(1):31–9.
13. Starkstein SE, Jorge R, Petracca G, Robinson RG. The construct of generalized anxiety disorder in Alzheimer disease. Am J Geriatr Psychiatry. 2007;15(1):42–9.
14. Chou KL, Mackenzie CS, Liang K, Sareen J. Three-year incidence and predictors of first-onset of DSM-IV mood, anxiety, and substance use disorders in older adults: results from wave 2 of the National Epidemiologic Survey on Alcohol and Related Conditions. J Clin Psychiatry. 2011;72(2):144–55.
15. Zhang X, Norton J, Carriere I, Ritchie K, Chaudieu I, Ancelin ML. Risk factors for late-onset generalized anxiety disorder: results from a 12-year prospective cohort (the ESPRIT study). Transl Psychiatry. 2015;5(3):e536.
16. Zhang X, Norton J, Carriere I, et al. Preliminary evidence for a role of the adrenergic nervous system in generalized anxiety disorder. Sci Rep. 2017;7:42676.
17. Zainal NH, Newman MG. Executive function and other cognitive deficits are distal risk factors of generalized anxiety disorder 9 years later. Psychol Med. 2018;48(12):2045–53.
18. Cabrera I, Brugos D, Montorio I. Attentional biases in older adults with generalized anxiety disorder. J Anxiety Disord. 2020;71:102207.
19. Price RB, Eldreth DA, Mohlman J. Deficient prefrontal attentional control in late-life generalized anxiety disorder: an fMRI investigation. Transl Psychiatry. 2011;1(10):e46.
20. Mohlman J, Price RB, Vietri J. Attentional bias in older adults: effects of generalized anxiety disorder and cognitive behavior therapy. J Anxiety Disord. 2013;27(6):585–91.
21. Butters MA, Bhalla RK, Andreescu C, et al. Changes in neuropsychological functioning following treatment for late-life generalised anxiety disorder. Br J Psychiatry. 2011;199(3):211–8.
22. Caudle DD, Senior AC, Wetherell JL, et al. Cognitive errors, symptom severity, and response to cognitive behavior therapy in older adults with generalized anxiety disorder. Am J Geriatr Psychiatry. 2007;15(8):680–9.
23. Santabárbara J, Lipnicki DM, Olaya B, et al. Does anxiety increase the risk of all-cause dementia? An

updated meta-analysis of prospective cohort studies. J Clin Med. 2020;9(6):1791.

24. Karim HT, Ly M, Yu G, et al. Aging faster: worry and rumination in late life are associated with greater brain age. Neurobiol Aging. 2021;101:13–21.

25. Butnoriene J, Bunevicius A, Saudargiene A, et al. Metabolic syndrome, major depression, generalized anxiety disorder, and ten-year all-cause and cardiovascular mortality in middle aged and elderly patients. Int J Cardiol. 2015;190:360–6.

26. Tully PJ, Cosh SM, Baune BT. A review of the affects of worry and generalized anxiety disorder upon cardiovascular health and coronary heart disease. Psychol Health Med. 2013;18(6):627–44.

27. Nitschke JB, Sarinopoulos I, Oathes DJ, et al. Anticipatory activation in the amygdala and anterior cingulate in generalized anxiety disorder and prediction of treatment response. Am J Psychiatry. 2009;166(3):302–10.

28. Etkin A, Prater KE, Schatzberg AF, Menon V, Greicius MD. Disrupted amygdalar subregion functional connectivity and evidence of a compensatory network in generalized anxiety disorder. Arch Gen Psychiatry. 2009;66(12):1361–72.

29. Mohlman J, Price RB, Eldreth DA, Chazin D, Glover DM, Kates WR. The relation of worry to prefrontal cortex volume in older adults with and without generalized anxiety disorder. Psychiatry Res. 2009;173(2):121–7.

30. Karim H, Tudorascu DL, Aizenstein H, Walker S, Good R, Andreescu C. Emotion reactivity and cerebrovascular burden in late-life GAD: a neuroimaging study. Am J Geriatr Psychiatry. 2016;24(11):1040–50.

31. Andreescu C, Sheu LK, Tudorascu D, et al. Altered cerebral blood flow patterns associated with pathologic worry in the elderly. Depress Anxiety. 2011;28(3):202–9.

32. Andreescu C, Sheu LK, Tudorascu D, et al. Emotion reactivity and regulation in late-life generalized anxiety disorder: functional connectivity at baseline and post-treatment. Am J Geriatr Psychiatry. 2015;23(2):200–14.

33. Mantella RC, Butters MA, Amico JA, et al. Salivary cortisol is associated with diagnosis and severity of late-life generalized anxiety disorder. Psychoneuroendocrinology. 2008;33(6):773–81.

34. Lenze EJ, Mantella RC, Shi P, et al. Elevated cortisol in older adults with generalized anxiety disorder is reduced by treatment: a placebo-controlled evaluation of escitalopram. Am J Geriatr Psychiatry. 2011;19(5):482–90.

35. Rosnick CB, Wetherell JL, White KS, Andreescu C, Dison D, Lenze EJ. Cognitive-behavioral therapy augmentation of SSRI reduces cortisol levels in older adults with generalized anxiety disorder: a randomized clinical trial. J Consult Clin Psychol. 2016;84(4):345–52.

36. Calleo J, Sanley MA, Greisinger A, et al. Generalized anxiety disorder in older medical patients: diagnostic recognition, mental health management and service utilization. J Clin Psychol Med Settings. 2009;16(2):178–85.

37. Aggarwal R, Kunik M, Asghar-Ali A. Anxiety in later life. Focus (Am Psychiatr Publ). 2017;15(2):157–61.

38. Borkovec TD, Alcaine OM, Behar E. Avoidance theory of worry and generalized anxiety disorder. In: Generalized anxiety disorder: advances in research and practice. New York, NY: The Guilford Press; 2004. p. 77–108.

39. Roemer L, Salters K, Raffa SD, Orsillo SM. Fear and avoidance of internal experiences in GAD: preliminary tests of a conceptual model. Cogn Ther Res. 2005;29:71–88.

40. Mennin DS, Heimberg RG, Turk CL, Fresco DM. Applying an emotion regulation framework to integrative approaches to generalized anxiety disorder. Clin Psychol Sci Pract. 2002;9(1):85–90.

41. Koerner N, Dugas MJ. A cognitive model of generalized anxiety disorder: the role of intolerance of uncertainty. In: Davey GCL, Wells A, editors. Worry and its psychological disorders: theory, assessment and treatment. West Sussex: Wiley; 2006. p. 201–16.

42. Wells A. Meta-cognition and worry: a cognitive model of generalized anxiety disorder. Behav Cogn Psychother. 1995;23(3):301–20.

43. Garrido MM, Kane RL, Kaas M, Kane RA. Use of mental health care by community-dwelling older adults. J Am Geriatr Soc. 2011;59(1):50–6.

44. Wetherell JL, Petkus AJ, McChesney K, et al. Older adults are less accurate than younger adults at identifying symptoms of anxiety and depression. J Nerv Ment Dis. 2009;197(8):623–6.

45. Spitzer RL, Kroenke K, Williams JB, Lowe B. A brief measure for assessing generalized anxiety disorder: the GAD-7. Arch Intern Med. 2006;166(10):1092–7.

46. Wild B, Eckl A, Herzog W, et al. Assessing generalized anxiety disorder in elderly people using the GAD-7 and GAD-2 scales: results of a validation study. Am J Geriatr Psychiatry. 2014;22(10):1029–38.

47. Pachana NA, Byrne GJ, Siddle H, Koloski N, Harley E, Arnold E. Development and validation of the geriatric anxiety inventory. Int Psychogeriatr. 2007;19(1):103–14.

48. Byrne GJ, Pachana NA. Development and validation of a short form of the Geriatric Anxiety Inventory—the GAI-SF. Int Psychogeriatr. 2011;23(1):125–31.

49. Meyer TJ, Miller ML, Metzger RL, Borkovec TD. Development and validation of the Penn State worry questionnaire. Behav Res Ther. 1990;28(6):487–95.

50. Stanley MA, Novy DM, Bourland SL, Beck JG, Averill PM. Assessing older adults with generalized

anxiety: a replication and extension. Behav Res Ther. 2001;39(2):221–35.

51. Kilbourne AM, Beck K, Spaeth-Rublee B, et al. Measuring and improving the quality of mental health care: a global perspective. World Psychiatry. 2018;17(1):30–8.

52. Pinquart M, Duberstein PR. Treatment of anxiety disorders in older adults: a meta-analytic comparison of behavioral and pharmacological interventions. Am J Geriatr Psychiatry. 2007;15(8):639–51.

53. Cohen J. Statistical power analysis for the behavioral sciences. Hillsdale, NJ: Lawrence Erlbaum; 1988.

54. Thorp SR, Ayers CR, Nuevo R, Stoddard JA, Sorrell JT, Wetherell JL. Meta-analysis comparing different behavioral treatments for late-life anxiety. Am J Geriatr Psychiatry. 2009;17(2):105–15.

55. Hall J, Kellett S, Berrios R, Bains MK, Scott S. Efficacy of cognitive behavioral therapy for generalized anxiety disorder in older adults: systematic review, meta-Analysis, and meta-regression. Am J Geriatr Psychiatry. 2016;24(11):1063–73.

56. Nordhus IH, Pallesen S. Psychological treatment of late-life anxiety: an empirical review. J Consult Clin Psychol. 2003;71(4):643–51.

57. Stanley MA, Wilson NL, Novy DM, et al. Cognitive behavior therapy for generalized anxiety disorder among older adults in primary care: a randomized clinical trial. JAMA. 2009;301(14):1460–7.

58. Brenes GA, Danhauer SC, Lyles MF, Hogan PE, Miller ME. Telephone-delivered cognitive behavioral therapy and telephone-delivered nondirective supportive therapy for rural older adults with generalized anxiety disorder: a randomized clinical trial. JAMA Psychiatry. 2015;72(10):1012–20.

59. Hobbs MJ, Mahoney AEJ, Andrews G. Integrating iCBT for generalized anxiety disorder into routine clinical care: treatment effects across the adult lifespan. J Anxiety Disord. 2017;51:47–54.

60. Wetherell JL, Gatz M, Craske MG. Treatment of generalized anxiety disorder in older adults. J Consult Clin Psychol. 2003;71(1):31–40.

61. Barrowclough C, King P, Colville J, Russell E, Burns A, Tarrier N. A randomized trial of the effectiveness of cognitive-behavioral therapy and supportive counseling for anxiety symptoms in older adults. J Consult Clin Psychol. 2001;69(5):756–62.

62. Mohlman J, Gorenstein EE, Kleber M, De Jesus M, Gorman JM, Papp LA. Standard and enhanced cognitive-behavior therapy for late-life generalized anxiety disorder: two pilot investigations. Am J Geriatr Psychiatry. 2003;11(1):24–32.

63. Krasucki C, Howard R, Mann A. Anxiety and its treatment in the elderly. Int Psychogeriatr. 1999;11(1):25–45.

64. Balasubramaniam M, Joshi P, Alag P, et al. Antidepressants for anxiety disorders in late-life: a systematic review. Ann Clin Psychiatry. 2019;31(4):277–91.

65. Gupta A, Bhattacharya G, Farheen SA, et al. Systematic review of benzodiazepines for anxiety disorders in late life. Ann Clin Psychiatry. 2020;32(2):114–27.

66. Goncalves DC, Byrne GJ. Interventions for generalized anxiety disorder in older adults: systematic review and meta-analysis. J Anxiety Disord. 2012;26(1):1–11.

67. Lenze EJ, Rollman BL, Shear MK, et al. Escitalopram for older adults with generalized anxiety disorder: a randomized controlled trial. JAMA. 2009;301(3):295–303.

68. Lenze EJ, Mulsant BH, Shear MK, et al. Efficacy and tolerability of citalopram in the treatment of late-life anxiety disorders: results from an 8-week randomized, placebo-controlled trial. Am J Psychiatry. 2005;162(1):146–50.

69. Schuurmans J, Comijs H, Emmelkamp PM, et al. A randomized, controlled trial of the effectiveness of cognitive-behavioral therapy and sertraline versus a waitlist control group for anxiety disorders in older adults. Am J Geriatr Psychiatry. 2006;14(3):255–63.

70. Mokhber N, Azarpazhooh MR, Khajehdaluee M, Velayati A, Hopwood M. Randomized, single-blind, trial of sertraline and buspirone for treatment of elderly patients with generalized anxiety disorder. Psychiatry Clin Neurosci. 2010;64(2):128–33.

71. Katz IR, Reynolds CF 3rd, Alexopoulos GS, Hackett D. Venlafaxine ER as a treatment for generalized anxiety disorder in older adults: pooled analysis of five randomized placebo-controlled clinical trials. J Am Geriatr Soc. 2002;50(1):18–25.

72. Davidson J, Allgulander C, Pollack MH, et al. Efficacy and tolerability of duloxetine in elderly patients with generalized anxiety disorder: a pooled analysis of four randomized, double-blind, placebo-controlled studies. Hum Psychopharmacol. 2008;23(6):519–26.

73. Alexopoulos GS, Katz IR, Reynolds CF 3rd, Carpenter D, Docherty JP, Ross RW. Pharmacotherapy of depression in older patients: a summary of the expert consensus guidelines. J Psychiatr Pract. 2001;7(6):361–76.

74. McClelland J, Mathys M. Evaluation of QTc prolongation and dosage effect with citalopram. Ment Health Clin. 2016;6(4):165–70.

75. Kimura M, Tateno A, Robinson RG. Treatment of poststroke generalized anxiety disorder comorbid with poststroke depression: merged analysis of nortriptyline trials. Am J Geriatr Psychiatry. 2003;11(3):320–7.

76. Strawn JR, Geracioti L, Rajdev N, Clemenza K, Levine A. Pharmacotherapy for generalized anxiety disorder in adult and pediatric patients: an evidence-

based treatment review. Expert Opin Pharmacother. 2018;19(10):1057–70.

77. Koepke HH, Gold RL, Linden ME, Lion JR, Rickels K. Multicenter controlled study of oxazepam in anxious elderly outpatients. Psychosomatics. 1982;23(6):641–5.

78. Cohn JB. Double-blind safety and efficacy comparison of alprazolam and placebo in the treatment of anxiety in geriatric patients. Curr Ther Res. 1984;35:100–12.

79. Markota M, Rummans TA, Bostwick JM, Lapid MI. Benzodiazepine use in older adults: dangers, management, and alternative therapies. Mayo Clin Proc. 2016;91(11):1632–9.

80. Majercsik E, Haller J. Interactions between anxiety, social support, health status and buspirone efficacy in elderly patients. Prog Neuro-Psychopharmacol Biol Psychiatry. 2004;28(7):1161–9.

81. Sramek JJ, Hong WW, Hamid S, Nape B, Cutler NR. Meta-analysis of the safety and tolerability of two dose regimens of buspirone in patients with persistent anxiety. Depress Anxiety. 1999;9(3):131–4.

82. Montgomery S, Chatamra K, Pauer L, Whalen E, Baldinetti F. Efficacy and safety of pregabalin in elderly people with generalised anxiety disorder. Br J Psychiatry. 2008;193(5):389–94.

83. Wetherell JL, Petkus AJ, White KS, et al. Antidepressant medication augmented with cognitive-behavioral therapy for generalized anxiety disorder in older adults. Am J Psychiatry. 2013;170(7):782–9.

Panic Disorder

22

Siddharth Khasnavis and Ali Abbas Asghar-Ali

Epidemiology

Several studies have investigated the prevalence of panic disorder in older adults. A broad survey of community dwelling adults in the United States revealed a lifetime prevalence of 3.72% and 12-month prevalence of 1.17% among those 55 years and older. Those with panic disorder within the prior year were more likely to be female, report recent stressful life events, and have utilized emergency services [1]. A survey of Canadian adults 55 years and older suggested a 12-month prevalence of 0.82% with lifetime occurrence of 2.45%. Twelve-month prevalence decreased with age in this report from 1.3% (55 years old–64 years old) to 0.32% (65 years old–74 years old) and 0.50% (75 years and older) [2]. Similar findings were noted in a European sample of over 4000 adults comparing prevalence of panic disorder across all age-groups. While lifetime prevalence was highest in the 40–49 years age-group (3.3%), it steadily declined thereafter to the lowest of 0.5% in adults older than 80 years [3]. A review of multiple community surveys gathered from 1970s onwards, suggested a 1-month prevalence of panic disorder among those 65 years and older to be 0.2% for women and 0.0% for men [4]. Notably, the annual incidence of panic disorder in older individuals in this review was 0.04% suggesting that most cases reflected chronic, rather than a new onset, condition. Although in one community survey, 23% of individuals self-reported that symptoms related to panic disorder started after age 55 years, this did not sufficiently deter from the perspective that the prevalence of panic disorder decreases with age and most presentations among older adults represent a continuation of panic symptoms from earlier in life. Only one study has contrasted with this understanding and suggested that prevalence may be higher when examined in an outpatient geriatric psychiatry service as opposed to within the community [5]. However, this observation has not been replicated in literature and can also be impacted by selection bias.

The reason for the decline in the prevalence of panic disorder with age has been a subject of debate. Changes in neurotransmitter systems, psychological resiliency, cultural shifts, or evolving social interaction with age have been put forth as potential explanations [6].

S. Khasnavis (✉)
Department of Psychiatry, Yale University School of Medicine, New Haven, CT, USA
e-mail: Siddharth.Khasnavis@yale.edu

A. A. Asghar-Ali
Department of Psychiatry, Baylor College of Medicine, Houston, TX, USA
e-mail: asgharal@bcm.edu

Risk Factors

Epidemiological studies have interrogated risk factors and comorbidities in relation to panic disorder among older adults. Community surveys found that female gender, major depressive disorder, alcohol use disorder, stressful life events, and physical limitations or low quality of life were more frequently associated with panic disorder. The effect of marital status is less clear across studies. Similarly, while early childhood trauma or neglect increased the risk of panic disorder in young adulthood, this did not influence late onset panic disorder [7]. A comparison of early versus late onset panic disorder within Netherlands (with late onset defined as >48 years age) similarly noted that individuals with late onset panic disorder were less likely to report childhood trauma or separately, agoraphobia with their condition [8]. The combined influence of gender and alcohol use disorder was highlighted in a survey of over 18,000 community dwelling adults. Specifically, women with an alcohol use disorder had a higher prevalence of panic disorder than men with an alcohol use disorder [9]. In a smaller evaluation of 13 individuals with onset of panic disorder after 60 years, nearly half reported stressful life events and more than half reported concurrent depression and concurrent history of cardiovascular disease [10].

Assessment

Panic disorder is experienced as recurrent paroxysmal attacks driven by intense physical sensations or fear-based cognitions. The former may include palpitations, sweating, chest pain, or nausea while examples of the latter include fear of losing control or fear of dying. At least 4 or more symptoms must be present to characterize a panic attack. Subsequently, worry about recurrent attacks or maladaptive behaviors must be present for at least 1 month to meet the Diagnostic and Statistical Manual for Mental Disorders, Fifth Edition, Text Revision (DSM-5 TR) criteria for panic disorder. Lastly, the condition can be defined with concurrent agoraphobia, reflected by a marked worry about being in specific situations outside of the home [11, 12].

The DSM-5 TR framework is applicable across the lifespan, however, understanding specific characteristics of late life panic disorder can aid in the evaluation of older adults. Several studies have reported on features of panic disorder in older adults. For instance, a study of 70 adults aged 60 years and older identified 19 who experienced panic attacks though did not meet criteria for panic disorder. Dyspnea was reported as the most severe symptom during attacks, along with palpitations and difficulty with concentration. Fear of dying was rated lower in comparison [13]. Individuals experiencing panic attacks scored higher on the Anxiety Sensitivity Index (ASI) and most reported they had thought about seeking treatment, but not seriously. Similarly, a survey of 80 individuals over 60 years age revealed that individuals with panic disorder scored higher on measures of sympathetic arousal, somatization, and alcohol use disorder. In comparison, patients with generalized anxiety disorder scored higher on measures of depression and hostility [14]. A common understanding borne out of these studies is that older adults are often less likely to seek care for panic disorder and are more likely to present with physical, rather than, cognitive symptoms. Also, older adults may report either fewer or lower intensity of symptoms related to panic attacks than younger individuals [15].

The evaluation of panic disorder in older adults should mirror other psychiatric conditions within this age-group. A thorough psychiatric history forms the foundation, and specific inquiry about panic symptoms should be incorporated given older adults are less likely to seek care for this condition. Practitioners should be particularly vigilant around descriptions of sudden onset symptomatology with significant somatic basis. More so than other psychiatric conditions, medical conditions such as cardiac arrhythmia, hyperthyroidism, hypercalcemia, seizure, or hypoglycemic episodes can lead to, or mimic, panic attacks [16, 17]. Routine investigations may thus include vital signs, laboratory work-up that includes a metabolic panel, complete blood count, thyroid function tests, serum calcium, fasting glucose or hemoglobin A1c, and an electrocardiogram (ECG) [17]. Lastly, use, misuse or withdrawal from prescribed drugs or illicit substances can present as panic attacks. Thus, gathering a history about medication doses and changes in addition to substance use coupled with a urine toxicology screening will render a more comprehensive evaluation. Screening for co-morbid psychiatric conditions is crucial since panic disorder can be accompanied by major depressive disorder, generalized anxiety, and agoraphobia. Additional behavioral conditions which can be mis-represented as panic attacks may include re-experiencing of trauma in posttraumatic stress disorder (PTSD) or agitation seen with major neurocognitive disorder accompanied with behavioral symptoms.

Treatment

Strategies for treating panic disorder in older adults largely rely on data from studies and clinical practice within younger individuals. Where panic symptoms may be secondary to or exacerbated by a physical condition (i.e., hyperthyroidism, cardiac arrythmia), this should be addressed first. Attention must also be paid to substance use, especially the use of stimulating agent or withdrawal from substances such as alcohol or benzodiazepines. Attention to psychosocial factors such as social isolation, financial stress, food insecurity, or housing instability can be additionally helpful, considering that older individuals with psychiatric illness can be more vulnerable to such issues or limited in their ability to cope with them. Addressing social consequences or contributors will help augment psychotherapeutic and pharmacotherapeutic interventions. Pharmacological and psychotherapeutic tools for treating panic disorder are summarized in Table 22.1. The following sections review these in further detail.

Table 22.1 Treatment strategies for panic disorder in older individuals

Treatment	Tips about use
Selective serotonin reuptake inhibitor (SSRI)[a]	• Sertraline, fluoxetine, and paroxetine are approved by the FDA for treatment of panic disorder in adults • Citalopram and escitalopram have been examined in older individuals and may be considered for off-label use
Serotonin–norepinephrine reuptake inhibitor (SNRI)[a]	• Venlafaxine is FDA approved for use in panic disorder • Duloxetine may be considered for off-label use based on evidence supporting its use in adults
Tricyclic antidepressant (TCA)[a]	• Imipramine, desipramine, and clomipramine have evidence for use in adults with panic disorder • Studies are limited in older adults, and use is limited by tolerability and adverse effects[b]
Benzodiazepine (BZD)[a]	• Consider where immediate relief is required, when use is limited to short periods and when antidepressants are not tolerated or efficacious • Use is limited by greater propensity for adverse effects such as drowsiness, confusion, and falls in older adults • If used, lorazepam may be better tolerated in older adults
Cognitive behavioral therapy (CBT)	• Can be used as monotherapy or in combination with pharmacotherapy
Unified protocol	• Transdiagnostic approach as an alternative to disease specific manualized psychotherapy. See Ref. [32]
Relaxation and mindfulness-based interventions	• Beneficial for reducing anxiety symptoms in older adults • Have not been specifically examined in the treatment of panic disorder in older adults

[a]Can be used as monotherapy or combined with psychotherapy
[b]Hypotension, cardiac conduction abnormalities, anticholinergic and antihistaminic side effects

Pharmacotherapy

Serotonin reuptake inhibitors (SSRIs), serotonin–norepinephrine reuptake inhibitors (SNRIs), tricyclic antidepressants (TCAs), and benzodiazepines (BZDs) have all shown benefit in treating panic disorder. Meanwhile, antipsychotics, mood stabilizers, and buspirone monotherapy have not shown a benefit for this condition. Historically, SSRIs have been recommended ahead of other medication classes in treatment guidelines due to a lower risk of adverse effects. This view was additionally reinforced in a recent meta-analysis of randomized controlled trials in which sertraline and escitalopram most favorably balanced remission against adverse effects [18]. The authors observed that literature was comparably weighted in examining the benefits of SSRIs and benzodiazepines against a placebo, although studies on SSRIs delivered slightly more confidence when assessing remission rates. Other medication classes such as SNRIs and TCAs have received less attention in randomized trials and elicited lower confidence.

A handful of studies have specifically evaluated pharmacotherapy in older adults with panic disorder. In a study of 40 older adults, both citalopram and escitalopram led to reductions in weekly panic attacks by over 70% [19]. Moreover, escitalopram led to an earlier response with improvement noted within 2 weeks of initiating treatment. A double-blind cross over study separately corroborated the benefit of citalopram in older adults with panic disorder [20]. Likewise, sertraline has also been effective in treating this condition later in life, albeit in a small open label trial [21]. In another instance, the utility of paroxetine was highlighted in a Danish study of 120 adults (ages 21–69 years). Here, the mean number of panic attacks decreased by nearly 76% over 3 weeks with use of paroxetine, although, 77% of patients reported at least one adverse effect, with dizziness being the most common complaint [22]. Among TCAs, imipramine was

examined in older adults and showed a trend toward improvement, but it did not reach statistical significance [23].

The use of any pharmacotherapeutic agent should be pursued cautiously in older adults. This includes keeping in mind the pharmacokinetic and pharmacodynamic changes and closer monitoring for drug–drug interactions, polypharmacy, and fall risk. Older adults frequently manage a longer list of medications such that both medication burden and potential for medication error can influence the decision to pursue pharmacotherapy or choice of a particular agent. It is advisable to employ lower starting doses and titrate more gradually than in younger individuals to reduce emergence of adverse effects. With use of SSRIs, one should be cognizant of an increased risk of gastrointestinal bleeding and hyponatremia [24, 25]. QTc prolongation is a risk experienced with use of citalopram and escitalopram more than other SSRIs [26]. This risk can be mitigated in individuals by reviewing cardiovascular and medication history in advance and by avoiding supratherapeutic doses. Likewise, paroxetine, despite its noted benefit in this condition, should be used cautiously due to its greater anticholinergic side effects relative to other SSRIs. Compared to all SSRIs, TCAs present even greater risks in older adults including anticholinergic side effects, orthostatic hypotension, and cardiac arrhythmias, which limit their usage [27]. Recommendations around the use of benzodiazepines, on the other hand, are less clear. Across randomized controlled trials, BZDs were estimated to have remission rates comparable to TCAs in the treatment of panic disorder, however, their potential to cause drowsiness, falls, and confusion makes BZDs inappropriate for first line use [18]. Instead, they can be reserved for short-term use in more severe circumstances in which SSRIs have not reached their effect or are still being titrated. In such instances, lorazepam is commonly recommended in older individuals due to a safer mechanism of elimination compared to other BZDs [17].

Psychotherapy

Psychotherapies can also play a valuable role in the treatment of panic disorder. Among psychotherapies, cognitive behavioral therapy (CBT) remains superior to supportive and psychodynamic approaches to treatment of panic disorder [12]. In one trial involving both younger and older (greater than 60 years) patients, manualized therapy showed comparable reductions in avoidance behaviors and agoraphobic cognitions to paroxetine. Moreover, the effect on reducing avoidance was higher in older individuals [28]. Shorter duration of illness or older age of symptom onset was related to better outcomes with delivery of CBT. A separate report also across age-groups showed that cluster B personality features led to worse outcomes for avoidance behaviors after CBT; however, older adults with panic disorder demonstrated fewer cluster B symptoms than their younger counterparts [29]. Furthermore, a study involving 49 older adults compared CBT, paroxetine and watchful waiting, to find that standardized measures of agoraphobic cognitions and phobic avoidance improved similarly with both CBT and paroxetine [30]. A later analysis of the same cohort revealed that shorter duration of illness and late onset of panic disorder were associated with better outcomes with CBT over paroxetine [31]. Considering that panic disorder can be accompanied by other anxiety spectrum disorders, a novel approach is the use of a Unified Protocol (UP) in place of cognitive behavioral therapies developed around individual diagnoses. Barlow et al., described such an approach applied to 223 patients who were randomized to UP, disease specific therapy, or a waitlist [32]. The cohort included patients with generalized anxiety, social anxiety, obsessive compulsive disorder, and a subgroup of 59 patients with panic disorder. The UP focused on developing emotional awareness and understanding reactions as a core strategy. It was shown to be equivalent across diagnoses compared to condition specific protocols. Additional psychotherapies that have been considered in this age-group include relaxation-based therapy. Gould et al., tested video-based relaxation training in a sample of 40 adults over 60 years age who were randomized to either intervention or a wait list [33]. The cohort included patients with a spectrum of anxiety disorders. Across the entire cohort, treatment led to a reduction in the severity of anxiety as measured by the Geriatric Anxiety Scale (GAS). However, panic disorder was not adequately represented in this population to allow specific conclusions about the effect on relaxation training on this condition. A review of mindfulness-based therapy leads to similar findings. While shown in limited studies to be helpful with reducing geriatric anxiety symptoms, impact in panic disorder specifically is not demarcated in literature [34].

The key takeaway from these studies is that while the data are limited, many of the treatments shown to be beneficial among younger adults with panic disorder have shown efficacy in older individuals. An assessment of risks, benefits, and patient collaboration is even more necessary in older adults when considering their vulnerability to medication-related adverse effects compared to younger individuals. When available, and in line with patient preferences, psychotherapy is an effective strategy for treatment of panic disorder which also avoids medication related concerns. When disease severity and patient preference does lead to pharmacotherapy, SSRIs remain first line due to their lowest risk of adverse effects relative to other medication classes.

Conclusions

Panic disorder is an uncommon diagnosis in older adults and decreases in prevalence with age due to factors that not clearly understood. Thus, most cases of late life panic disorder reflect a continuation of chronic rather than new onset illness. Older adults are less likely to report panic attacks, less likely to seek care, and more likely to present their experience as physical complaints to medical providers. When assessing panic disorder, one should review psychiatric history thoroughly while also being attentive to medical comorbidities, medication use, and substance use which can all exacerbate or mimic panic attacks. Treatment of panic disorder in older adults can mirror strategies used in younger individuals, albeit with greater consideration given to medication interactions, adverse effects, and dosing strategies. Both manualized psychotherapy and pharmacotherapy primarily driven by SSRIs provide effective tools for treatment of this condition in older individuals.

References

1. Chou K-L. Panic disorder in older adults: evidence from the National Epidemiologic Survey on alcohol and related conditions. Int J Geriatr Psychiatry. 2010;25(8):822–32.
2. Corna LM, Cairney J, Herrmann N, Veldhuizen S, McCabe L, Streiner D. Panic disorder in later life: results from a National Survey of Canadians. Int Psychogeriatr. 2007;19(6):1084–96.
3. Olaya B, Moneta MV, Miret M, Ayuso-Mateos JL, Haro JM. Epidemiology of panic attacks, panic disorder and the moderating role of age: results from a population-based study. J Affect Disord. 2018;241:627–33.
4. Flint JA. Epidemiology and comorbidity of anxiety disorders in the elderly. Am J Psychiatry. 1994;151(5):640–9.
5. Raj BA, Corvea MH, Dagon EM. The clinical characteristics of panic disorder in the elderly: a retrospective study. J Clin Psychiatry. 1993;54(4):150–5.
6. Alastair FJ, Joan CM, Peter RV. Why is panic disorder less frequent in late life. Am J Geriatr Psychiatr. 1996;4(2):96–109.
7. Friedman S, Smith L, Fogel D, Paradis C, Viswanathan R, Ackerman R, et al. The incidence and influence of early traumatic life events in patients with panic disorder: a comparison with other psychiatric outpatients. J Anxiety Disord. 2002;16:259e72.
8. Tibi L, van Oppen P, Aderka IM, van Balkom AJLM, Batelaan NM, Spinhoven P, Penninx BW, Anholt GE. Examining determinants of early and late age at onset in panic disorder: an admixture analysis. J Psychiatr Res. 2013;47(12):1870–5.
9. Krystal JH, Leaf PJ, Bruce ML, Charney DS. Effects of age and alcoholism on the prevalence of panic disorder. Acta Psychiatr Scand. 1992;85(1):77–82.
10. Rakshanda H, Pollard AC. Late-life-onset panic disorder: clinical and demographic characteristics of a patient sample. J Geriatr Psychiatry Neurol. 1994;7(2):84–8.
11. American Psychiatric Association. Diagnostic and statistical manual of mental disorders. 5th ed; 2013. https://doi.org/10.1176/appi.books.9780890425596.
12. APA. Practice guidelines for the treatment of patients with panic disorder. 2nd ed; 2009.
13. Deer TM, Calamari JE. Panic symptomatology and anxiety sensitivity in older adults. J Behav Ther Exp Psychiatry. 1998;29(4):303–16.
14. Mohlman J, de Jesus M, Gorenstein EE, Kleber M, Gorman JM, Papp LA. Distinguishing generalized anxiety disorder, panic disorder, and mixed anxiety states in older treatment-seeking adults. J Anxiety Disord. 2004;18(3):275–90.
15. Katerndahl DA, Talamantes M. A comparison of persons with early-versus late-onset panic attacks. J Clin Psychiatry. 2000;61(6):422–7.
16. Te A, Tzong-Yow W, Chen Y-L, Pei D, Liu S-H, Yi-Ching S, Hsu C-H. Supraventricular Bigeminy in the elderly may mimic panic disorder deterioration. Psychogeriatrics. 2020;20(5):787–9.
17. Flint AJ, Gagnon N. Diagnosis and management of panic disorder in older patients. Drugs Aging. 2003;20(12):881–91.
18. Chawla N, Anothaisintawee T, Charoenrungrueangchai K, Thaipisuttikul P, McKay GJ, Attia J, Thakkinstian A. Drug treatment for panic disorder with or without agoraphobia: systematic review and network meta-analysis of randomised controlled trials. BMJ. 2022;376:e066084.
19. Rampello L, Alvano A, Raffaele R, Malaguarnera M, Vecchio I. New possibilities of treatment for panic attacks in elderly patients: escitalopram versus citalopram. J Clin Psychopharmacol. 2006;26(1):67–70.
20. Raffaele R, Vecchio I, Malaguarnera M, Rampello L, Ruggieri M, Nicoletti F. Therapy of panic attacks in the elderly. Arch Gerontol Geriatr Suppl. 2002;8:295–301.
21. Sheikh JI, Lauderdale SA, Cassidy EL. Efficacy of sertraline for panic disorder in older adults: a preliminary open-label trial. Am J Geriatr Psychiatry. 2004;12(2):230.
22. Oehrberg S, Christiansen PE, Behnke K, Borup AL, Severin B, Soegaard J, Calberg H, Judge R, Ohrstrom JK, Manniche PM. Paroxetine in the treatment of panic disorder. A randomised, double-blind, placebo-controlled study. Br J Psychiatry. 1995;167(3):374–9.
23. Sheikh JI, Swales PJ. Treatment of panic disorder in older adults: a pilot study comparison of alprazolam, imipramine, and placebo. Int J Psychiatry Med. 1999;29(1):107–17.
24. de Abajo FJ, Rodríguez LA, Montero D. Association between selective serotonin reuptake inhibitors and upper gastrointestinal bleeding: population based case-control study. BMJ. 1999;319(7217):1106–9.
25. Leth-Møller KB, Hansen AH, Torstensson M, Andersen SE, Ødum L, Gislasson G, Torp-Pedersen C, Holm EA. Antidepressants and the risk of hyponatremia: a Danish register-based population study. BMJ Open. 2016;6(5):e011200.
26. Castro VM, Clements CC, Murphy SN, Gainer VS, Fava M, Weilburg JB, et al. QT interval and antidepressant use: a cross sectional study of electronic health records. BMJ. 2013;346:f288.

27. Sultana J, Spina E, Trifirò G. Antidepressant use in the elderly: the role of pharmacodynamics and pharmacokinetics in drug safety. Exp Opin Drug Metab Toxicol. 2015;11(6):883–92.

28. Hendriks G-J, Kampman M, Keijsers GPJ, Hoogduin CAL, Oude Voshaar RC. Cognitive-behavioral therapy for panic disorder with agoraphobia in older people: a comparison with younger patients. Depress Anxiety. 2014;31(8):669–77.

29. Gulpers B, Voshaar RO, Kampman M, Verhey F, Alphen SVAN, Hendriks G-J. The impact of personality pathology on treatment outcome in late-life panic disorder. J Psychiatr Pract. 2020;26(3):164–74.

30. Hendriks G-J, Keijsers GPJ, Kampman M, Oude Voshaar RC, Verbraak MJPM, Broekman TG, Hoogduin CAL. A randomized controlled study of paroxetine and cognitive-Behavioural therapy for late-life panic disorder. Acta Psychiatr Scand. 2010;122(1):11–9.

31. Hendriks G-J, Keijsers GPJ, Kampman M, Hoogduin CAL, Oude Voshaar RC. Predictors of outcome of pharmacological and psychological treatment of late-life panic disorder with agoraphobia: predictors of outcome in late-life PD. Int J Geriatr Psychiatry. 2012;27(2):146–50.

32. Barlow DH, Farchione TJ, Bullis JR, Gallagher MW, Murray-Latin H, Sauer-Zavala S, Bentley KH, Thompson-Hollands J, Conklin LR, Boswell JF, Ametaj A, Carl JR, Boettcher HT, Cassiello-Robbins C. The unified protocol for transdiagnostic treatment of emotional disorders compared with diagnosis-specific protocols for anxiety disorders: a randomized clinical trial. JAMA Psychiatry. 2017;74(9):875–84.

33. Gould CE, Kok BC, Ma VK, Wetherell JL, Sudheimer K, Beaudreau SA. Video-delivered relaxation intervention reduces late-life anxiety: a pilot randomized controlled trial. Am J Geriatr Psychiatry. 2019;27(5):514–25.

34. Hazlett-Stevens H, Singer J, Chong A. Mindfulness-based stress reduction and mindfulness-based cognitive therapy with older adults: a qualitative review of randomized controlled outcome research. Clin Gerontol. 2019;42(4):347–58.

Siddharth Khasnavis and Ali Abbas Asghar-Ali

Epidemiology

OCD is less prevalent among older adults in comparison to younger individuals and relative to late life mood or anxiety disorders. The lifetime prevalence of OCD is reported to exceed 1.5% collectively across age-groups, but only up to 0.8% in adults over 60 years [1]. In a sample of adults over 60 years old in the United Kingdom, the 1-month prevalence of OCD was 0.2% among individuals between 60 and 74 years age. Obsessive compulsive symptoms, not meeting full diagnostic criteria, were more prevalent and associated with lower educational levels and lower quality of life [2]. A 2009 survey of Canadian adults 65 years and older recorded a 12-month prevalence of 1.5%. OCD was associated with lower educational level and being married, but not related to gender. Eighty percent of the people who were surveyed reported symptom onset before 60 years old and at a median age of 28.5 years, underscoring that a minority of individuals experience new onset OCD in older age [3]. OCD often co-occurred with depressive

symptoms and generalized anxiety disorder in this cohort. Likewise, in a Swedish cohort of 1018 individuals interviewed by trained staff, 2.9% met criteria for OCD over the prior month [4]. Nearly 20% with OCD also met criteria for major depressive disorder (MDD). In this study, OCD was found to be more prevalent in women than men over 70 years in age. Overall, what is evident from the range of studies is that a clear age cutoff for late-onset OCD has not been established. In some instances, the onset may be at the age of 30 years, whereas other studies have noted the age of onset as high as 60 years.

Epidemiological surveys have also attempted to better characterize late life OCD. Dell'Osso and colleagues compared the history of OCD among individuals who were below the age of 65 years with those over age 65 years. Across the sample, the mean age of onset was 19.2 years ± 9.9 years; although, in individuals over 65 years, mean age of onset was delayed by 10 years when compared to patients younger than 65 years. Older individuals were also less likely to have utilized cognitive behavioral therapy over their lifetime. At the same time, no significant differences were observed with regard to psychotropic medication exposure, suicide attempts, hospitalization history, or psychiatric and medical comorbidities [1]. A longitudinal follow-up study of individuals with OCD for up to 40 years showed that nearly 50% of them had an illness lasting over 30 years [5]. While most individuals

S. Khasnavis (✉)
Department of Psychiatry, Yale University School of
Medicine, New Haven, CT, USA
e-mail: Siddharth.Khasnavis@yale.edu

A. A. Asghar-Ali
Department of Psychiatry, Baylor College of
Medicine, Houston, TX, USA
e-mail: asgharal@bcm.edu

© The Author(s), under exclusive license to Springer Nature Switzerland AG 2024
R. R. Tampi, D. J. Tampi (eds.), *Treatment of Psychiatric Disorders Among Older Adults*,
https://doi.org/10.1007/978-3-031-55711-8_23

showed improvements in ratings of clinical severity or global function over time, only 20% showed complete recovery [5]. Furthermore, in most individuals, OCD symptoms qualitatively evolved with age. An example included a woman with fear of blushing during her adolescence which changed to obsessive thoughts about being slandered when she was in her 40 s. An additional study of late onset OCD, defined by the authors as emergence after age 30 years, showed that individuals with later onset were less likely to focus on contamination, somatic, or religious obsessions [6]. Overall, these studies further highlight that most late life OCD begins relatively early in life and the content or focus of obsessions and compulsions can change over time.

Risk Factors

There are few studies which have examined the predictors for late life OCD, whether presenting as a continuation of earlier illness, relapse, or new onset condition. Lower educational level has been a factor shown in several epidemiological surveys. In one report, older individuals with OCD were also more likely to demonstrate lower verbal IQ estimates and lower verbal fluency scores [2]. Late onset OCD defined as occurring after age 40 years was associated with female gender in one report [7]. In the same study, any traumatic event occurring after 40 years in age and a longer period of subclinical symptoms were also associated with higher likelihood of late onset OCD.

OCD occurring in older adults, particularly as a new onset illness, can be associated with underlying neurological illness. Case reports document OCD in association with Huntington's disease, frontotemporal dementia, dementia with Lewy bodies (DLB), Parkinson's disease, and cerebellar lesions [8–12]. Similarly, dopaminergic agents used to treat Parkinson's disease can also precipitate compulsive behaviors which resemble those in OCD [13].

Assessment

Evaluation of older adults with OCD should follow strategies used in younger individuals. Consider a structured interview using the Diagnostic and Statistical Manual for Mental Disorder, Fifth Edition, Text Revision (DSM-5 TR) criteria to ensure that both recurrent intrusive thoughts (obsessions) and repetitive behaviors or mental activities (compulsions) are assessed. Inquire about the level of distress associated with obsessions and how the individual has adapted to these experiences. Any functional impairment caused by compulsive behaviors should be similarly captured. Additionally, screen for suicidality given elevated risk in individuals with OCD and potential for self-harm to become a focus of intrusive obsessions [14]. Lastly, while patients often recognize their symptoms as ego-dystonic, this insight should not be assumed for all cases and instead explored.

While OCD may be comorbid with other psychiatric illnesses, it also shares symptoms with other psychiatric illnesses. Thus, there is a need for careful assessment of symptomatology to both understand it fully and appreciate the context. For instance, repetitive negative thoughts in a person with MDD may be ruminations or perhaps compulsive thoughts as part of co-occurring OCD [15]. Likewise, individuals with anxiety may report worrying which is subjectively intrusive. However, these intrusive cognitions are more likely connected to real life circumstances and congruent with the individual's values. Similarly, in posttraumatic stress disorder, individuals experience flashbacks and negative cognitions which have an intrusive quality and need to be differentiated from OCD [16].

As previously mentioned, a variety of neurological conditions can be accompanied by compulsive behaviors. In patients with new onset OCD in older age, there should be a higher index of suspicion and subsequently attention to a review of systems, examination and if possible, collateral from a family member or close acquaintance. Thus, in addition to a thorough history, routine investigations should include a brief cognitive screening, laboratory work-up that includes a complete blood count, metabolic panel, thyroid function tests, fasting glucose measurement, urine tox screen, and an electrocardiogram (ECG).

An understanding of the characteristics of late life OCD can aid in the diagnosis of this condition while psychometric instruments can provide further confidence. Regarding the former, at least one report comparing adults 60 years and older with younger individuals with OCD noted a greater tendency to engage in hand washing and fear of having sinned among older individuals [17]. On the other hand, older individuals had fewer concerns about symmetry or counting rituals compared to younger counterparts. Calamari et al., separately found that among older adults who were evaluated using the Obsessive Compulsive Inventory Revised (OCI-R), women scored higher on subscales for hoarding while men were higher on neutralizing subscales [18]. This study separately noted that the OCI-R as a self-reported instrument robustly correlated with OCD symptoms captured in interviews and maintained internal consistency when administered serially to individuals. The Yale Brown Obsessive Compulsive Scale (Y-BOCS) is a clinician administered scale which is also reliable for assessing OCD among older individuals.

Treatment

As with other conditions that have low prevalence in older adults, there are no randomized controlled trials focused on this age-group to guide optimal treatment for OCD [19]. Rather, evidence from the general adult population needs to be extrapolated to formulate treatment in older individuals. A multimodal approach utilizing pharmacotherapy and psychotherapy will be beneficial in most individuals [19]. Pharmacologic and psychotherapeutic tools for treating OCD are summarized in Table 23.1 and reviewed in subsequent sections. It should be noted that treatment

of comorbid psychiatric conditions and substance use is also vital. Furthermore, psychosocial interventions should be considered as OCD can disrupt routine functions and social connections in older adults [3]. Peer support, socialization, and case management can all be helpful to improve global function and facilitate holistic care.

In the general adult population, selective serotonin reuptake inhibitors (SSRIs), serotonin-norepinephrine reuptake inhibitors (SNRIs), tricyclic antidepressants (TCAs), and monoamine oxidase inhibitors (MAOIs) have all been utilized in the treatment of OCD, though, only clomipramine, sertraline, fluvoxamine, fluoxetine, and paroxetine have carried Food and Drug Administration (FDA) approval for treatment of OCD [20]. Not all classes of medications have equal efficacy. Historically, clomipramine was cited for its superiority over other agents; however, direct comparisons to SSRIs have showed only a small added benefit at the cost of more side effects compared to SSRIs [20]. Considering the weight of evidence and their better tolerance, SSRIs therefore serve as first-line treatment for OCD with higher doses and longer duration of treatment often needed for effect, relative to management of MDD [21]. Clomipramine is subsequently considered a second-line strategy. Among SNRIs, venlafaxine has shown benefit but with less evidence to support its use ahead of SSRIs [20]. Meanwhile, there is a paucity of trials to support monotherapy with duloxetine in OCD. In treatment refractory cases, antipsychotics are now considered an additional tool for off-label use—with risperidone and aripiprazole typically first line due to favorable tolerance over other antipsychotics [22]. In older adults, these present added risks and require more judicious use [23].

Pharmacotherapy in older adults should employ the same principles applied to treating other psychiatric disorders in this age-group [23]. This includes starting medications at a lower dose and escalating gradually to reduce the potential for adverse effects. One should also be attentive to drug–drug interactions, polypharmacy risk, and impact on medical comorbidities.

Table 23.1 Treatment strategies for OCD and hoarding disorder in older individuals

Treatment	Tips about use
OCD	
Cognitive behavioral therapy (ERP)[a]	• First-line monotherapy or in combination with pharmacotherapy
Selective serotonin reuptake inhibitor (SSRI)	• First-line monotherapy or in combination with ERP[a] • Sertraline, fluvoxamine, fluoxetine, and paroxetine are FDA approved for treatment of OCD • Citalopram and escitalopram may be used off-label
Clomipramine	• Second-line option or augmentation with SSRI • FDA approved for treatment of OCD in adults • Tolerability and adverse effects[b] limit use as a first-line option
Antipsychotics	• Consider as augmentation in moderate to severe cases • Third-line option when clomipramine is not tolerated, safe, or beneficial • Second-generation antipsychotics preferred in older individuals
Repetitive transcranial magnetic stimulation (rTMS)[c]	• FDA approved for treatment refractory OCD
Deep brain stimulation (DBS)[c]	• FDA approved for treatment refractory OCD
Electroconvulsive therapy (ECT)[c]	• Off-label use in treatment refractory OCD
Hoarding disorder	
Cognitive behavioral therapy (CBT)	• *CREST* protocol as one example of manualized therapy for hoarding disorder. See Ref. [57]
Psychotropics	• No agents specifically approved for hoarding disorder • Consider in the treatment of psychiatric comorbidities • SSRIs most relevant for comorbid OCD, anxiety, or depression

[a] Exposure and response prevention
[b] Hypotension, cardiac conduction abnormalities, anticholinergic and antihistaminic side effects
[c] Data for treatment of OCD in older individuals is very limited. Consider on a case-by-case basis with support of an interprofessional team

Case reports on pharmacotherapy in older adults hint that as with younger individuals, higher doses of medications may also be necessary for effect [24, 25]. Thus, medication side effects pose a particular challenge in the treatment of OCD, given treatment often relies on higher doses than typically used in mood and anxiety spectrum disorders [20, 21].

Review of treatment literature (primarily case reports) involving older adults suggests benefit from fluvoxamine, paroxetine, citalopram, sertraline, and venlafaxine [24]. Additionally, Austin et al. reported several cases which showed utility for clomipramine dosed up to 150 mg daily or fluoxetine in a 40–60 mg dose range [25]. Tranylcypromine and imipramine were likewise reported to be beneficial in earlier case reports when TCAs were more commonly used in treatment of OCD [26].

While numerous options exist, as in younger individuals with OCD, SSRIs should be utilized first as other classes of medications, especially TCAs can cause significant side effects such as anticholinergic effects. SSRIs are noted to have a response rate of 30–60% which can be enhanced by combining with psychotherapy [27]. SSRIs do carry an increased risk of gastrointestinal bleeding and hyponatremia which can be more concerning among older patients and should be monitored. Venlafaxine and clomipramine provide second-line options where SSRIs are insufficient [28]. Antipsychotics should ideally be avoided in older individuals but may be needed for augmentation in treatment refractory OCD [29]. There is at least one case report documenting the use of aripiprazole for treatment of self-harming obsessions in an older adult [27].

Psychotherapy

Cognitive behavioral therapy (CBT) is a crucial element of treatment for OCD in the general adult population, both alone and in combination with medications [19, 29]. Exposure and response prevention (ERP), the specific subtype of CBT recommended for OCD, involves graduated exposure to stimuli that provoke greater anxiety while preventing the individual from engaging in a compulsive ritual which relieves the anxiety [29]. For instance, in the treatment of contamination fears and repetitive hand washing, an individual may transition from touching a doorknob to picking an item out of the trash can while withholding hand washing for a specified duration of time. CBT has been shown to be beneficial among older adults in multiple case reports that outline the treatment of reassurance seeking behavior, contamination-related obsessions with compulsive handwashing, repetitive checking, sexual or religious obsessions, and intrusive thoughts about self-harm [27, 30–32]. Cognitive behavioral therapy was examined as an in-home strategy to treat an 86-year-old Veteran with obsessions about accidental harm and repetitive checking behaviors [33]. In response to treatment, the veteran reported a 50% reduction in subjective distress when not engaging in checking behavior. An important theme in this and other reports on the use of CBT in older individuals is the value of adapting the treatment protocol. Strategies include the addition of relaxation training, slowing of the protocol, simplification to accommodate for cognitive decline, and the addition of behavioral activation to treat concurrent depressive illnesses [32–34].

Other Treatments

While medications and psychotherapy are the primary tools for treating OCD, additional interventions have been explored in the general population. Deep brain stimulation (DBS) and repetitive transcranial magnetic stimulation (rTMS), for instance, are both approved by the FDA for treatment refractory OCD [35]. Transcranial direct current stimulation (tDCS) has also shown promise in refractory cases, though, does not have FDA approval [35]. Routine use of these modalities is limited by several barriers including availability of specialists and insurance approval [35]. Some interventional techniques have been documented for severe and refractory OCD in older adults. Casey et al. reported the off-label use of electroconvulsive therapy (ECT) in an 84-year-old woman with contamination fears, obsessions with bowel function, and cleaning/hand washing behaviors who previously did not respond to TCAs [36]. In this case, ECT was also continued in a maintenance phase due to initial benefit and later recurrence of symptoms. Cingulotomy was utilized for refractory OCD in another series of 33 cases of which 9 were older adults and up to 30% saw benefit from surgery [37]. Despite its approval for the treatment of OCD, data on the use of DBS in older individuals is lacking. A meta-analysis of randomized controlled trials involving this intervention did not yield studies which recruited geriatric patients [38]. The routine use of these modalities in the treatment of OCD among older adults ultimately requires data from many more controlled studies.

Treatment Summary

When weighing risks and benefits of OCD treatment in older adults, SSRIs and psychotherapy are supported by the greatest evidence for efficacy, safety, and access. Clomipramine and venlafaxine serve as second-line options. Although not FDA approved, antipsychotic medications are often used as augmentation agents before considering alternative neuromodulation interventions. With antipsychotic use, low starting doses and gradual titration are key to minimizing adverse effects. In the realm of neuromodulation, treatment strategy may be dictated by availability of specialized care. Where rTMS is available, it can offer a safer alternative to antipsychotic augmentation in older adults. A tool such as DBS, despite FDA approval, is likely to be employed last and in the most severe and refractory cases, given the need for interdisciplinary collaboration and separately, a higher risk of adverse outcomes from surgery in older individuals.

Hoarding Disorder

Hoarding disorder was included as a new diagnosis in the DSM-5. Historically seen as a condition secondary to OCD or OCPD (obsessive compulsive personality disorder), diagnostic separation was supported by findings that up to 80% of individuals with hoarding behavior do not have clinically impactful obsessive or compulsive symptoms [39]. Hoarding disorder is characterized by a reluctance to discard possessions which results in cluttering of one's personal space and significant distress or functional impairment [40]. Hoarding is discussed here for its historical affiliation with OCD, being shown to occur in up to 30% of individuals with OCD across studies [40]. The conditions can be seen as having shared cognitive and behavioral patterns. In hoarding, akin to obsessions and compulsions in OCD, individuals may have a fear of an adverse outcome if they are to discard certain possessions and thus develop a tendency to accumulate and retain belongings.

Epidemiology of Hoarding Disorder

Discrepancies in how hoarding was defined or assessed historically limited estimation of the prevalence of this disorder. To capture this more reliably, in-home interviews were utilized in a United Kingdom population of over 1600 adults from ages 16 years to 90 years [41]. After initially screening positive for hoarding behavior, 99 of 191 individuals completed detailed interviews and only 19 met the criteria for a hoarding disorder. The point prevalence of hoarding was estimated at 1.5% in this population. Comparisons within the population revealed that those with hoarding disorder confirmed on interviews were more likely to be older, financially stressed and widowed or divorced. This group was also more likely to report health issues as a barrier to daily functions. Compared directly against those who screened negative for hoarding disorder at the onset of the interview, those with hoarding disorder also reported psychological symptoms such as fatigue, depression, a history of PTSD, and

personality disorder more frequently. In another study involving a cohort of community dwelling adults of 34–94 years age from Baltimore, MD, point prevalence of pathological hoarding was measured at 5.3% (prior to establishment of DSM-5 criteria) [40]. Here, hoarding was more common within the 55–94 years age-group, and associated with lower household income, presence of specific personality traits (i.e., paranoid, schizotypal, obsessive compulsive), and childhood adversity such as excess physical discipline.

There have been additional efforts to characterize hoarding disorder in older adults. Ayers and colleagues conducted a survey of 18 adults over 60 years old, finding that all participants reported onset of illness prior to age 20 years [42]. They also noted that hoarding severity increased over lifetime and was most frequently comorbid with MDD, persistent depressive disorder, and OCD. In a separate study, the authors reported on cognitive function among individuals 58 years and older who did not have comorbid psychiatric disorders, including a neurocognitive disorder [43]. Individuals with hoarding disorder performed worse on subdomains of executive function including working memory, set shifting, inhibition, and flexibility of thought processes. Across similar works, it was shown that hoarding severity predicted greater disability with daily functions and was also associated with a higher number of medical conditions among older adults (most frequently cardiovascular) [44, 45]. Hoarding also increased health risks such as falls and poor hygiene and environmental risks such as fires among a cohort of adults older than 55 years when compared to an age matched control group [46].

Assessment of Hoarding Disorder

The assessment of hoarding is now aided by the established DSM-5 criteria. The condition is defined by a difficulty discarding possessions, irrespective of their value, and fueled by a perceived need to save the items. Attempts to discard possessions lead to distress and ultimately further accumulation of items. The clutter and congestion generated by this accumulation contribute to deterioration of living spaces and significant functional impairment [47].

When interviewing individuals with suspected pathological hoarding, it is important to screen for comorbidities. As outlined in population surveys, hoarding can co-occur with MDD, anxiety disorders, OCD, and PTSD [40, 42, 43]. Differentiation is aided by the observation that in contrast with OCD, individuals who hoard express fewer obsession and compulsions [48]. Similarly, in contrast with other psychiatric comorbidities, a person who hoards may not be distressed by their behavior or the dysfunction in their environment. Along with psychiatric conditions, medical comorbidities should also be reviewed given the association between hoarding severity and burden of medical issues. In older adults, hoarding may be a manifestation of a neuropsychiatric condition, e.g., an acquired brain injury, behavioral variant frontotemporal dementia, Parkinson's disease or dopamine agonist treatment, intellectual disability, or psychotic disorder [49]. Identifying an underlying neuropsychiatric cause for hording behavior can provide a distinct target for treatment and potentially also improve hoarding behaviors. Furthermore, intrinsic to hoarding disorder is a deterioration of living space and associated health risks. Thus, efforts should be made toward assessing the safety and livability of the home environment, especially given the increased risk of falls and other accidental injuries which may result from clutter [46]. Ideally a home visit would be performed to assess safety. Alternatively, images or collateral information may also provide insight into living conditions.

There have also been attempts to utilize psychometric instruments to support the evaluation for hoarding disorder. Examples include the Savings Inventory-Revised (SI-R), Clutter Image Rating scale (CIR), and Hoarding Disorder Dimensional scale (HD-D). In a broad review of hoarding-related psychometric scales, the SI-R was found to be the most consistent for tracking severity of hoarding disorder [50]. A dedicated review of the CIR among older adults showed significant correlation with the SI-R [51]. The CIR provides a means for assessing hoarding severity in the individual's home environment. The scale prompts rating of pictorial depictions of clutter of increasing severity (range of 1–9) in 3 separate rooms (living room, kitchen, and bedroom). A score of 4 or higher involving any one room is a suggested trigger for obtaining help, as it can reflect clinically significant interruption of routine functions [52].

Treatment of Hoarding Disorder

There is no proven role for pharmacologic agents in the treatment of hoarding disorder [53]. Nonetheless, medications can be considered for any comorbid psychiatric condition present alongside hoarding disorder. For treatment of hoarding itself, structured psychotherapies can be considered first-line treatment based on available outcome studies [53]. Manualized cognitive behavioral therapy for hoarding has been tested in individual format, web-based delivery and adapted to group settings with reported benefit on both observed and self-reported measures [54, 55]. An extended 15-month trial on web-based group treatment for hoarding, for instance, showed modest improvements on the CIR and CIR subscales [55]. In later works, the combination of cognitive rehabilitation (i.e., organization skills) and exposure-based treatment has shown improvements when measured by the SI-R, CIR, and the clinician global improvement ratings [56]. Published under the acronym CREST (cognitive rehabilitation and exposure/sorting therapy), this protocol was tested in a randomized clinical trial involving 58 adults divided into intervention or case management arms [57]. Participants of CREST showed a 38% reduction in symptoms on the SI-R compared to 25% for those who received case management. Similarly, exposure and response prevention (ERP), a validated psychotherapy for treating OCD, has been adapted to hoarding behaviors [54]. ERP can be used to target both the failure to discard belongings and compulsion to acquire and save items. Akin to OCD treatment, a patient could rank their distress related to discarding specific items and proceed to remove them based on the hierarchy. Outside the home environment, this may be conducted as an imaginal exposure. A host of studies have examined the use of ERP in which hoarding was occurring in the context of OCD. While ERP benefitted OCD symptoms typically assessed using the Y-BOCS, individuals with OCD that included hoarding behaviors showed lower response rates and higher treatment dropouts when compared to individuals with OCD without hoarding behaviors [54].

Amid the successes of psychotherapies for hoarding disorders, application in real world settings can face challenges such as treatment availability, treatment retention, and individuals' ability to participate because of cognitive decline. Donaldson et al., for instance, described a strategy to gradually increase participation in an older adult with neurocognitive decline and allow the individual to hand over hoarded items more easily [58]. Other authors have focused on treatment retention and in a study of 29 adults from age 52 years to 85 years, showed that those who did not complete behavioral therapy were more likely to report a lack of social support [59]. Likewise, higher levels of boredom and lower levels of self-control measured via subscales on the SI-R were associated with worse treatment outcomes. The authors posited that addressing these variables could improve retention in, and benefit from, treatment. Alongside this effort, there have been trials of community-based interventions for hoarding disorder. The previously noted CREST protocol was implemented as a multidisciplinary intervention that included psychotherapy, peer support, case management, and even post-treatment groups, and showed benefit in reducing hoarding severity and clutter among low-income older adults [60]. Overall, these studies highlight that as with the treatment of OCD, psychosocial interventions can be important adjuncts in the treatment of hoarding disorder in older adults.

Lastly it is valuable to review the safety and livability of the home environment, as these can be directly compromised by clutter and neglect of the personal space [46]. Risks may include falls, fire hazards, lack of access in an emergency, and direct risk to the individual based on the type of items being hoarded (i.e., spoiled foods, chemicals). Hoarding can potentially trigger complaints from neighbors, landlords, or local governing bodies, putting already vulnerable individuals at risk of eviction or legal repercussions. Assessing for these issues and using any available resources to manage them will facilitate well rounded care of older individuals with hoarding disorder. Table 23.1 lists the treatment strategies for OCD and hoarding disorder in older individuals.

Conclusions

OCD is among the less prevalent diagnoses among older adults, with most cases representing chronic, rather than new onset illness. New onset OCD is particularly uncommon after age 50 and warrants closer inspection for neurological disease, substance abuse, medical illness, or another psychiatric condition. Structured assessment of OCD can be supported with the clinician rated Y-BOCS or self-reported OCI-R scales. Both cognitive behavioral therapy and SSRIs serve as either first-line monotherapies or parallel interventions for treatment of OCD in older adults. Second-line options can include clomipramine and venlafaxine, with antipsychotics available for careful augmentation in refractory cases. Unlike OCD, hoarding disorder appears to increase in prevalence with age. Historically understood as being secondary to OCD, it is now recognized as an independent condition and known to co-occur with numerous psychiatric and neurological conditions. Hoarding can be associated with social isolation and reduced function among older through disruption of the living space, neglect of self-care, or falls and accidental injury. Thus far, only cognitive behavioral therapies have shown promise for treatment of this condition, and further study is needed to identify pharmacologic and integrated techniques to treat hoarding disorder. Ultimately, this is an area in which clinicians can have significant impact through timely assessment and collaboration with other providers and community supports.

References

1. Dell'Osso B, Benatti B, Rodriguez CI, Arici C, Palazzo C, Altamura AC, Hollander E, et al. Obsessive-compulsive disorder in the elderly: a report from the International College of Obsessive-Compulsive Spectrum Disorders (ICOCS). Eur Psychiatry. 2017;45:36–40.
2. Aykan RL, Stewart R. Obsessive and compulsive symptoms in a national sample of older people: prevalence, comorbidity, and associations with cognitive function. Am J Geriatr Psychiatry. 2013;21(3):263–71.
3. Grenier S, Préville M, Boyer R, O'Connor K. Prevalence and correlates of obsessive–compulsive disorder among older adults living in the community. J Anxiety Disord. 2009;23(7):858–65.
4. Klenfeldt IF, Karlsson B, Sigström R, Bäckman K, Waern M, Östling S, Gustafson D, Skoog I. Prevalence of obsessive-compulsive disorder in relation to depression and cognition in an elderly population. Am J Geriatr Psychiatry. 2014;22(3):301–8.
5. Skoog G, Skoog I. A 40-year follow-up of patients with obsessive-compulsive disorder. Arch Gen Psychiatry. 1999;56:121–7.
6. Grant JE, Mancebo MC, Pinto A, et al. Late-onset obsessive compulsive disorder: clinical characteristics and psychiatric comorbidity. Psychiatry Res. 2007;152(1):21–7.
7. Frydman I, et al. Late onset obsessive-compulsive disorder: risk factors and correlates. J Psychiatr Res. 2014;49:68–74.
8. Scicutella A. Late-life obsessive-compulsive disorder and Huntington's disease. J Neuropsychiatry Clin Neurosci. 2000;12(2):288–9.
9. Dondé C, Lepetit A, Dorey J-M, Herrmann M. Late-life atypical reactivation of obsessive-compulsive disorder associated with frontotemporal dementia. Rev Neurol. 2019;175(3):205–6.
10. Frileux S, Millet B, Fossati P. Late-onset OCD as a potential harbinger of dementia with Lewy bodies: a report of two cases. Front Psych. 2020;11:554.
11. Tonna M, Ottoni R, Ossola P, De Panfilis C, Marchesi C. Late-onset obsessive-compulsive disorder associated with left cerebellar lesion. Cerebellum. 2014;13(4):531–5.
12. Monaco L, Rita M, Di Stasio E, Zuccalà G, Petracca M, Genovese D, Fusco D, Silveri MC, et al. Prevalence of obsessive-compulsive symptoms in elderly Parkinson disease patients: a case-control study. Am J Geriatr Psychiatry. 2020;28(2):167–75.
13. Kelley BJ, Duker AP, Chiu P. Dopamine agonists and pathologic behaviors. Parkinson's Dis. 2012;2012:603631.
14. Albert U, De Ronchi D, Maina G, Pompili M. Suicide risk in obsessive-compulsive disorder and exploration of risk factors: a systematic review. Curr Neuropharmacol. 2019;17(8):681–96.
15. Cervin M. Obsessive-compulsive disorder: diagnosis, clinical features, nosology, and epidemiology. Psychiatr Clin North Am. 2023;46(1):1–16.
16. Dykshoorn KL. Trauma-related obsessive-compulsive disorder: a review. Health Psychol Behav Med. 2014;2(1):517–28.
17. Kohn R, Westlake RJ, Rasmussen SA, Marsland RT, Norman WH. Clinical features of obsessive-compulsive disorder in elderly patients. Am J Geriatr Psychiatry. 1997;5(3):211–5.
18. Calamari JE, Woodard JL, Armstrong KM, Molino A, Pontarelli NK, Socha J, Longley SL. Assessing older adults' obsessive-compulsive disorder symptoms: psychometric characteristics of the obsessive compulsive inventory-revised. J Obsessive Compuls Rel Dis. 2014;3(2):124–31.
19. Jenike MA. Geriatric obsessive-compulsive disorder. J Geriatr Psychiatry Neurol. 1991;4(1):34–9.
20. Reddy YCJ, Arumugham SS. Are current pharmacotherapeutic strategies effective in treating OCD? Expert Opin Pharmacother. 2020;21(8):853–6.
21. American Psychiatric Association. Practice guideline for the treatment of patients with obsessive-compulsive disorder. Arlington, VA: American Psychiatric Association; 2007. http://www.psych.org/psych_pract/treatg/pg/prac_guide.cfm
22. Thamby A, Jaisoorya TS. Antipsychotic augmentation in the treatment of obsessive-compulsive disorder. Indian J Psychiatry. 2019;61(Suppl 1):S51–7.
23. Kratz T, Diefenbacher A. Psychopharmacological treatment in older people: avoiding drug interactions and polypharmacy. Dtsch Arztebl Int. 2019;116(29–30):508–18.
24. Fernandes CP, Vilaverde D, Freitas D, Pereira F, Morgado P. Very late onset of obsessive-compulsive disorder: case report and review of published cases in those more than 60 years old. J Nerv Ment Dis. 2021;209(3):208–11.
25. Austin LS, Zealberg JJ, Bruce R, Lydiard. Three cases of pharmacotherapy of obsessive-compulsive disorder in the elderly. J Nerv Ment Dis. 1991;179(10):634–5.
26. Calamari JE, Faber SD, Hitsman BL, Poppe CJ. Treatment of obsessive compulsive disorder in the elderly: a review and case example. J Behav Ther Exp Psychiatry. 1994;25(2):95–104.
27. Lozano-Vicario L, Fernández-Sotos P, Lozoya-Moreno S, Del Yerro-Álvarez MJ. Late onset obsessive-compulsive disorder (OCD): a case report. Actas Espanolas De Psiquiatria. 2020;48(1):36–46.
28. Pittenger C, Bloch MH. Pharmacological treatment of obsessive-compulsive disorder. Psychiatr Clin North Am. 2014;37(3):375–91.
29. Jazi AN, Asghar-Ali AA. Obsessive-compulsive disorder in older adults: a comprehensive literature review. J Psychiatr Pract. 2020;26(3):175–84.
30. Halldorsson B, Salkovskis PM. Treatment of obsessive compulsive disorder and excessive reassurance seeking in an older adult: a single case quasi-experimental design. Behav Cogn Psychother. 2017;45(6):616–28.

31. Hirsh A, O'Brien K, Geffken GR, Adkins J, Goodman WK, Storch EA. Cognitive–behavioral treatment for obsessive-compulsive disorder in an elderly male with concurrent medical constraints. Am J Geriatr Psychiatry. 2006;14(4):380–1.

32. Jones MK, Wootton BM, Vaccaro LD. The efficacy of exposure and response prevention for geriatric obsessive compulsive disorder: a clinical case illustration. Case Rep Psychiatry. 2012;2012:1–5.

33. Lee LO, Rouse S, Mlinac ME. Home-based assessment and treatment of obsessive-compulsive disorder symptoms to reduce unnecessary emergency room usage in an older adult. J Cogn Psychother. 2019;33(1):82–94.

34. Noel NR, Seibell PJ, Nadeau JM, Storch EA. Treating just-right symptoms in geriatric obsessive-compulsive disorder. Indian J Psychiatry. 2016;58(4):481.

35. Kammen A, Cavaleri J, Lam J, Frank AC, Mason X, Choi W, Penn M, Brasfield K, Van Noppen B, Murray SB, Lee DJ. Neuromodulation of OCD: a review of invasive and non-invasive methods. Front Neurol. 2022;13:909264.

36. Casey DA, Davis MH. Obsessive-compulsive Disorder responsive to electroconvulsive therapy in an elderly woman. South Med J. 1994;87(8):862–4.

37. Jenike MA, Baer L, Ballantine HT, et al. Cingulotomy for refractory obsessive compulsive disorder: a long-term follow-up of 33 patients. Arch Gen Psychiatry. 1991;48(6):548–55.

38. Gadot R, Najera R, Hirani S, Anand A, Storch E, Goodman WK, Shofty B, Sheth SA. Efficacy of deep brain stimulation for treatment-resistant obsessive-compulsive disorder: systematic review and meta-analysis. J Neurol Neurosurg Psychiatry. 2022;93:1166–73.

39. Cath DC, Nizar K, Boomsma D, Mathews CA. Age-specific prevalence of hoarding and obsessive compulsive disorder: a population-based study. Am J Geriatr Psychiatry. 2017;25(3):245–55.

40. Samuels JF, Bienvenu OJ, Grados MA, Cullen B, Riddle MA, Liang KY, Eaton WW, Nestadt G. Prevalence and correlates of hoarding behavior in a community-based sample. Behav Res Ther. 2008;46(7):836–44.

41. Nordsletten AE, Reichenberg A, Hatch SL, Fernández de la Cruz L, Pertusa A, Hotopf M, Mataix-Cols D. Epidemiology of hoarding disorder. Br J Psychiatry. 2013;203(6):445–52.

42. Ayers CR, Saxena S, Golshan S, Wetherell JL. Age at onset and clinical features of late life compulsive hoarding. Int J Geriatr Psychiatry. 2010;25(2):142–9.

43. Ayers CR, Wetherell JL, Schiehser D, Almklov E, Golshan S, Saxena S. Executive functioning in older adults with hoarding disorder. Int J Geriatr Psychiatry. 2013;28(11):1175–81.

44. Ayers CR, Ly P, Howard I, Mayes T, Porter B, Iqbal Y. Hoarding severity predicts functional disability in late-life hoarding disorder patients. Int J Geriatr Psychiatry. 2014;29(7):741–6.

45. Ayers CR, Iqbal Y, Strickland K. Medical conditions in geriatric hoarding disorder patients. Aging Ment Health. 2014;18(2):148–51.

46. Diefenbach GJ, DiMauro J, Frost R, Steketee G, Tolin DF. Characteristics of hoarding in older adults. Am J Geriatr Psychiatry. 2013;21(10):1043–7.

47. American Psychiatric Association. Diagnostic and statistical manual of mental disorders. 5th ed; 2013. https://doi.org/10.1176/appi.books.9780890425596.

48. Neziroglu F, Weissman S, Allen J, McKay D. Compulsive hoarders: how do they differ from individuals with obsessive compulsive disorder? Psychiatry Res. 2012;200(1):35–40.

49. Gleason A, Perkes D, Wand AP. Managing hoarding and squalor. Aust Prescr. 2021;44(3):79–84.

50. Ong CW, Krafft J, Levin ME, Twohig MP. A systematic review and psychometric evaluation of self-report measures for hoarding disorder. J Affect Disord. 2021;290:136–48.

51. Dozier ME, Ayers CR. Validation of the clutter image rating in older adults with hoarding disorder. Int Psychogeriatr. 2015;27(5):769–76.

52. International OCD Foundation. Do I Have Hoarding Disorder? Retrieved January 3, 2023. https://hoarding.iocdf.org/about-hoarding/do-i-have-hoarding-disorder/

53. Ayers CR, Najmi S, Mayes TL, Dozier ME. Hoarding disorder in older adulthood. Am J Geriatr Psychiatry. 2015;23(4):416–22.

54. Williams M, Viscusi JA. Hoarding disorder and a systematic review of treatment with cognitive behavioral therapy. Cogn Behav Ther. 2016;45(2):93–110.

55. Muroff J, Steketee G, Himle J, Frost R. Delivery of internet treatment for compulsive hoarding (D.I.T.C.H.). Behav Res Ther. 2010;48(1):79–85.

56. Ayers CR, Saxena S, Espejo E, Twamley EW, Granholm E, Wetherell JL. Novel treatment for geriatric hoarding disorder: an open trial of cognitive rehabilitation paired with behavior therapy. Am J Geriatr Psychiatry. 2014;22(3):248–52.

57. Ayers CR, Dozier ME, Twamley EW, Saxena S, Granholm E, Mayes TL, Wetherell JL. Cognitive rehabilitation and exposure/sorting therapy (CREST) for hoarding disorder in older adults: a randomized clinical trial. J Clin Psychiatry. 2018;79(2):85.

58. Donaldson JM, Trahan MA, Kahng S. An evaluation of procedures to increase cooperation related to hoarding in an older adult with dementia. J Appl Behav Anal. 2014;47(2):410–4.

59. Weiss ER, Landers A, Todman M, Roane DM. Treatment outcomes in older adults with hoarding disorder: the impact of self-control, boredom and social support. Australas J Ageing. 2020;39(4):375–80.

60. Pittman JOE, Davidson EJ, Dozier ME, Blanco BH, Baer KA, Twamley EW, Mayes TL, Sommerfeld DH, Lagare T, Ayers CR. Implementation and evaluation of a community-based treatment for late-life hoarding. Int Psychogeriatr. 2021;33(9):977–86.

Part VII

Trauma and Stress Related Disorders

Posttraumatic Stress Disorder

Demetrius Woodard and Seetha Chandrasekhara

Introduction

Posttraumatic Stress Disorder (PTSD) is a condition that occurs in a person after exposure to an extreme stressor or traumatic event. Individuals may exhibit three distinct types of symptoms consisting of re-experiencing of the event, avoidance of reminders of the event, and hyperarousal for at least 1 month [1]. While traumatic events occur in many individuals, higher rates of PTSD have been documented in first responders to disasters and mass trauma, socially disadvantaged persons, younger persons, women, and military personnel. Research also shows a difference in probability that PTSD will develop based on sex and type of trauma (sexual assault, physical assault, and accidents) [2]. While the lifetime prevalence of PTSD in the United States of America was measured to be 6.1%, this figure spans all age-groups [3]. It is estimated that approximately 4.5% of older adults are diagnosed with PTSD, a rate lower in comparison to middle-aged and young adults [4]. Although not specific to older adults, studies have demonstrated that women are twice as likely to develop PTSD compared to men [5]. In the United States, the National Comorbidity Study estimated the lifetime prevalence in women as 9.7% and in men as 3.4% [6]. The development of PTSD in men and women differs between the type of trauma exposure with women being exposed to more sexual trauma [7]. There may also be more negative support systems and negative cognitions reported by women when compared to men [8, 9]. The Diagnostic and Statistical Manual of Mental Disorders Fifth Edition (DSM5) criteria for PTSD is listed in Table 24.1.

There are proposed factors for the above finding relative to other age-groups: less research, stigma, individuals' reluctance to admit PTSD symptoms, healthcare providers unsure of formal assessment and treatment of trauma in an older population, and higher occurrences of comorbid cognitive and sensory decline [1, 2]. Research also proposes that survivor bias could play a part in this difference as those with PTSD may be less likely to survive into late adulthood. It is important to note that PTSD was not introduced into diagnostic nomenclature until the 1980s, thus there could be members in the older adult cohort who experienced traumatic events and PTSD before it was formally recognized in literature [3].

D. Woodard
Department of Psychiatry, University of Pennsylvania Health System, Philadelphia, PA, USA
e-mail: demetrius.woodard@pennmedicine.upenn.edu

S. Chandrasekhara (✉)
Department of Psychiatry, Lewis Katz School of Medicine at Temple University,
Philadelphia, PA, USA
e-mail: tuc32963@temple.edu

© The Author(s), under exclusive license to Springer Nature Switzerland AG 2024
R. R. Tampi, D. J. Tampi (eds.), *Treatment of Psychiatric Disorders Among Older Adults*,
https://doi.org/10.1007/978-3-031-55711-8_24

Table 24.1 Criteria for post-traumatic stress disorder

Exposed to actual (or threatened) death, serious injury, or sexual violence in at least one of the below ways:
  – Direct experience
  – Witnessing traumatic event in person (occurring to others)
  – Learning event happened to close family or friend
  – Direct repeated exposure or repeated extreme details of traumatic event
  – Does not include exposure through electronic media (e.g., movies, television) unless related to work

At least one of the following intrusion symptoms occurring after traumatic event:
  – Recurrent and intrusive memories of traumatic event leading to distress
  – Recurrent dreams related to traumatic event causing distress
  – Dissociative reactions
  – Prolonged or intense psychological distress to cues that remind the individual of the event
  – Intense physiological reactions to cues that remind the individual of the event

At least one of the avoidance symptoms occurring after the traumatic event:
  – Avoiding distressing memories, thoughts, or feelings of event
  – Avoiding external reminders of event to prevent distress

At least two negative changes in cognitive and mood following traumatic event:
  – Unable to remember important detail of event
  – Exaggerated or continued negative beliefs or expectations about oneself, others, or environment
  – Blaming oneself for event due to distorted cognition
  – Negative emotional state
  – Decreased interest in activities
  – Feelings of detachment
  – Unable to experience positive emotions

At least two alterations in arousal/reactivity following traumatic event:
  – Irritability and anger
  – Reckless behavior
  – Hypervigilance
  – Heightened startle response
  – Difficulty with concentration
  – Disturbance of sleep

Symptoms persist longer than at least 1 month
Significant distress or functional impairment occurs
Not due to another medical condition or physiological response to a substance

[a] Specify—with dissociative symptoms (presence of derealization or depersonalization), with delayed expression (criteria not met until at least after 6 months of event)

In more than 50% of cases, PTSD co-occurs with mood, anxiety, or substance use disorders [3]. It is associated with serious disability, medical illness, and premature death [2]. Across the United States, research shows that older adults with chronic PTSD were three times more likely to have any disability, including mobility, self-care, and cognition, when compared to those with no PTSD [10]. In 2004, Schnurr and Green proposed a trauma model that postulates negative health consequences of traumatic exposure is conceptualized as a result of a significant distress reaction [11]. This aforementioned model suggests that PTSD affects physical health via biological, psychological, behavioral, and attentional changes.

Research shows that natural disasters also play a major part on the mental health of older adults and the development of PTSD. A meta-analysis performed by Parker et al. found that older adults were 2.11 times more likely to experience PTSD symptoms and 1.73 more likely to develop adjustment disorder when exposed to natural disasters and when compared with younger adults [12]. Some proposed factors that lead to this difference in mental health effects include lower ability to seek assistance after a natural disaster with increase in resulting morbidity and mortality, and a tendency of older adults to have a greater sense of loss after natural disasters. Researchers also proposed that the exposure hypothesis plays a part in older adults' varying psychological responses to natural disasters. The exposure hypothesis suggests that older adults are at a greater risk for worse mental health outcomes due to (1) reluctance to evaluate, (2) lower likelihood of receiving advanced warning in a timely manner, (3) disruption to accustomed way of life, and (4) a sense of deprivation resulting from their personal, physical, and social losses post disaster [12].

The COVID-19 pandemic affected many populations, particularly those with comorbidities like older adults [13]. A comprehensive review by Chamaa et al. suggested that older adults experienced increased psychological stress and fear relative to other age-groups due to increased risk of severe illness and symptoms, hospitalization, and intensive care (PTSD in the COVID-19 era) [14]. The incidence of COVID-19-associated PTSD in the older adult population is seen in many nations across the world. For example, researchers in Spain, France, and China found that 6.81%, 9.9%, and 26.8% (respectively) of people from the older age-group suffered from PTSD during the COVID-19 pandemic in 2021 [13–15].

Risk Factors Including Neurobiology

Since there are several forms of trauma, the intensity of the trauma and individual susceptibility interact to influence the likelihood of PTSD [1]. Factors associated with increased susceptibility include female sex, childhood trauma, fewer years of schooling, prior mental disorders, exposure to four or more traumatic events, and a history of exposure to interpersonal violence [2]. Interestingly, exposure to multiple traumatic events tends to exert a greater negative impact on the severity of posttraumatic outcomes when compared to a single, discrete traumatic experience [16]. Unfortunately, there is still not much research on cumulative trauma exposure in the older adult population and if it follows the same dose-response pattern seen in other age-groups. Research in younger populations has been extrapolated for consideration in this chapter due to the limited number of studies specifically evaluating older adults.

Current research suggests that there are several biologic risk factors that correlate to PTSD to date including genes, epigenetic regulation, neuroendocrine factors, inflammatory markers, autonomic-risk and resilience, and sleep disturbances [2]. It is currently believed that functional neural systems involved in fear learning, threat detection, emotional regulation, and contextual processing play a major role in the pathophysiology of PTSD [17]. Although research has been conducted to determine the neurobiological etiology of PTSD, multiple systems have been impli-

cated including serotonin, noradrenergic, glutamatergic, GABA, oxycontin, and cannabinoids [18].

Adverse childhood events (ACEs) such as sexual abuse, domestic violence, community violence, and emotional and physical abuse have been shown to be associated with adulthood PTSD, in a dose-response effect pattern [18]. Along with the aforementioned ACEs, witnessing domestic violence and incarceration of a parent increased odds for development of PTSD in both men and women older than 50 years in age [19]. There is much research on the effects of ACEs on young adult mood disorders; however, many researchers do not follow the research participants long enough to see the effects in older age (>50 years). However, it is important to note older adults who experienced their most distressing traumatic event during childhood exhibited more severe symptoms of PTSD and lower subjective happiness when compared with older adults who experienced their most distressing trauma after the transition to adulthood [20].

Evidence also shows that experiencing discrimination and prejudice has devastating effects on the recipient's physical and mental health. For example, studies displayed racial discrimination was a stronger predictor of trauma-related symptoms when compared to general life stress in a sample of Black and Asian college students [21]. Interestingly, vicarious trauma such as a Black American watching a video of a police killing a Black citizen also has a profound effect on one's mental health within the first 1–2 months of exposure to video [22]. This is important due to the increasing prevalence of social media usage and exposure to trauma provoking material to users of all age-groups. While it is now known that racial discrimination is a form of trauma for the recipient, PTSD due to racial trauma, is likely to be under-recognized due to (1) a lack of awareness among clinicians, (2) discomfort surrounding conversations about race in therapeutic settings, and (3) a lack of validated measures for its assessment [23].

While most studies focus on the effect of direct trauma, there is not much current literature on the effect of generational racial discrimination. Similar to racial discrimination, individuals who identify as lesbian, gay, bisexual, transgender, or queer (LGBTQ) experience trauma at higher rates than the general population and tend to have a higher prevalence of PTSD symptoms [24, 25]. There is still a lot of research that must be done to examine the relationship between sexual orientation disparities in PTSD treatment and possible elevated risk of exposure to violence and other traumatic events in the minority sexual orientation.

It is important for healthcare providers to be aware of the different forms of social determinants of health that can affect the mental well-being of older adults. These social determinants include demographic (age, race, gender), economic, environmental, and cultural/social factors impacting the health of older adults [26]. The health provider must establish rapport and a clear understanding of the social determinants that older adults encounter in order to provide the best care possible.

Assessment

When working with individuals with PTSD, it is vital that the healthcare provider obtains a thorough medical, psychiatric, family, military, social, and personal history [11]. The older adult should be asked specific questions pertaining to the traumatic event(s). There is often initial reluctance for older adults to disclose this information, so sensitivity is critical. Studies show that a PTSD diagnosis is linked to increased suicide risk in both military and civilian in the older adult demographic (>50 years old) [27]. Thus, it is important to assess for any prior/current suicidal ideation, suicidal attempts, and access to firearms. It is well established that veterans are at an increased risk for PTSD and substance use disorder when compared to the general population [28]. Even if an individual lacks military history, the healthcare provider should obtain a detailed substance use history.

The Clinician-Administered PTSD Scale (CAPS-5) is considered by many to be the gold standard in PTSD assessment. CAPS-5 is a 30-item questionnaire that corresponds to the Diagnostic and Statistical Manual fifth Edition (DSM5) diagnosis for PTSD [29]. It can be used to make a current diagnosis of PTSD, a lifetime diagnosis as well as assess symptoms over the past week. CAPS-5 also assesses the dissociative subtype of PTSD; either depersonalization or derealization. While research shows that the CAPS-5 diagnostic interview model is reliable, consistent, and valid, it is important to note that many of these studies focused on male veteran populations and did not focus on difference in gender, sex, or type of trauma experience [30].

There is also a self-reported PTSD checklist (PCL-5) available for PTSD assessment. PCL-5 is a 20 item self-reported questionnaire that is typically used for screening individuals for PTSD, making a provisional diagnosis and monitoring symptoms during or after treatment [31]. Current studies have shown the PCL-5 to be a consistent, reliable, and valid assessment tool in PTSD diagnosis as well [32]. While the PCL-5 can be used to make a provisional diagnosis, the gold standard for diagnosing PTSD is a clinical interview using a structured assessment model such as CAPS-5.

Treatments

There are many studies that have researched the efficacy of non-pharmacological and pharmacological strategies in the treatment of PTSD in adults [33]. For most adults with a PTSD diagnosis, non-pharmacologic treatment such as psychotherapy is the first-line option for treatment [34]. However, pharmacological treatments such as SSRIs can be used as an alternative first line or adjunct treatment if there are comorbid conditions present, such as depression.

Similar to clinician tendency to overlook the symptoms of PTSD in older adults, this population also experiences a disparity in treatment, as well. In a United States national investigation pertaining to mental health treatment for newly diagnosed PTSD in older veterans, Smith, et al. note that among veterans who received treatment, increased age was associated with decreased odds of receiving both psychotherapy and pharmacotherapy, decreased number of psychotherapy visits, and increased waiting times [35].

Non-pharmacological

The recommended first-line intervention for PTSD in adults is trauma-focused therapies including cognitive behavioral therapy (CBT), exposure therapy, and eye movement desensitization and reprocessing (EMDR) [34, 35]. Generally, trauma-focused CBT revolves around the therapist working with the individual to first identify maladaptive beliefs and then, focus on symptom reduction via thought exercises such as coping skills management and stress management [36]. In a systematic review, Hoffman, et al. reviewed 193 randomized controlled trials and discovered that cognitive processing therapy, a specific protocol of CBT, led to a reduction in PTSD symptoms (measured by the clinician-administered PTSD scale) when compared to the control sample of participants and results were sustained at 3- and 6-month intervals (standardized mean difference −1.35, 95% CI −1.77 to −0.94). Furthermore, more participants in this study who underwent cognitive processing therapy no longer met criteria for PTSD in comparison to the control group (risk difference 0.44, 95% CI 0.26–0.62) [37].

While cognitive processing therapy can be conducted in an individual or group setting, studies show that individual therapy leads to more effective results. Resick, et al. randomly assigned 268 military personnel (244 men [91.0%]; 24 women [9.0%]; mean [SD] age, 33.2 [7.4] years) with diagnosed PTSD to either group or individual cognitive processing therapy for a 6-week period [38]. The investigators found that participants in the individual cognitive processing therapy group displayed greater improvement in PTSD severity (mean [SE] difference on the PSS-I, −3.7 [1.4]; Cohen $d = 0.6$; $P = 0.006$).

The process of emotionally processing trauma through exposure is also a common therapy utilized in PTSD treatment [39]. While there are many forms of exposure therapy, prolonged exposure and written exposure are two of the most studied forms for PTSD treatment [39, 40]. While prolonged exposure therapy focuses on breathing retraining and gradual reintroducing exposure to a traumatic trigger over typically 12 sessions [39], written exposure focuses more on writing about the traumatic experience and discussing the thoughts and emotions that it evokes [40]. In a systematic review on psychotherapy for PTSD in older adults, Dinnen, et al. found that all the case studies and treatment outcome studies utilizing exposure therapy (e.g., imaginal exposure only; in vivo exposure only; full, manualized PE) reported at least some effectiveness in ameliorating symptoms related to trauma [41]. In a meta-analysis of seven trials including over 380 individuals with diagnosed PTSD, Cusack et al. found that exposure therapy leads to a marked improvement in PTSD symptoms when compared to a waitlist control group (standardized mean difference −1.27, 95% CI −1.54 to −1.0) [42]. Furthermore, this meta-analysis found that in 3 trials that included 197 individuals, 66% more individuals with exposure therapy did not meet criteria for PTSD versus waitlist control group (Number Needed to Treat (NNT) = 2).

Interestingly, prolonged exposure therapy has been found to be effective in populations exposed to multiple traumas when compared to a group who received present-centered therapy. In a randomized trial, Schnurr, et al. compared the effect of PTSD symptom reduction between prolonged exposure and present-centered therapy in a sample of 277 women with chronic PTSD with a mix of traumatic events (including sexual assault and military combat) [43]. The experimental group receiving prolonged exposure therapy displayed a larger reduction in PTSD symptoms (25 versus 17 points on the CAPS).

EMDR, a type of psychotherapy that combines elements of CBT and exposure therapy with instructed saccadic eye movements during exposure, is also an effective treatment for PTSD [44]. In contrast to other treatments that focus on changing emotions related to a traumatic event, EMDR focuses on the actual memory with the goal of changing the way the memory is stored in the brain. Typically, EMDR involves the individual conjuring up thoughts about the traumatic scene while the therapist moves 1–2 fingers across the person's visual field while the individual tracks the finger(s) until their anxiety decreases. The therapist then instructs the individual to generate an adaptive thought that is less distressing. Adaptive thinking involves recognizing unexpected situations and having the ability to consider multiple responses and decide on the most appropriate solution. Along with saccadic eye movements, the therapist may accelerate the learning process via introducing additional stimulation such as tapping or tones (bilateral stimulation) [44]. Chen, et al. performed a meta-analysis of 26 clinical studies to investigate the effects of EMDR on PTSD symptom reduction. This study revealed that EMDR significantly reduced PTSD symptoms ($g = -0.662$; 95% confidence interval (CI): -0.887 to -0.436) [45].

While current research focuses on the efficacy of the aforementioned therapies vs no therapeutic intervention, there is a scarcity of current literature comparing the efficacy of the therapies to each other. The aforementioned systemic review by Hoffman, et al. determined that high strength of evidence (SOE) supports efficacy of CBT-exposure and CBT-mixed treatment and moderate SOE supports efficacy of cognitive processing therapy and EMDR [37]. Therefore, choosing the best therapy depends on the individual's preference, the presentation, and the therapist's recommendation. Current research shows that physical activity decreased PTSD and depressive symptoms in participants with PTSD when compared to a control group of no physical activity [46]. While there is not much new data correlating physical activity and PTSD, it is important to consider it as a usual adjunct when combined with psychotherapy and medication.

The above studies were conducted with predominantly young adults, but Chen's meta-analysis age range went up to age 64 years [45]. When utilizing these therapies in older adults, there are special considerations to consider, especially related to cognitive or physical impairments. If there are noted issues with concentration, memory, and/or attention, a comprehensive cognitive evaluation should be performed [47].

Responses to questions may be more body-focused leading to more initial presentations to primary care clinics [47]. Adapting the therapeutic techniques may be necessary to accommodate individuals with specific needs or to adjust to sensory, physical, or cognitive impairments [48]. Caregivers should also be involved in the process to help reinforce concepts learned during therapy [48].

Pharmacological

Selective Serotonin Reuptake Inhibitor (SSRI)

Efficacy

SSRIs such as escitalopram, fluoxetine, paroxetine, and sertraline continue to be the first-line pharmacological treatment available for PTSD in adults. Williams, et al. in their meta-analysis found beneficial effect for SSRIs compared with placebo (risk ratio (RR) 0.66, 95% confidence interval (CI) 0.59–0.74; 8 studies, 1078 participants), which improved PTSD symptoms in 58% of SSRI participants compared with 35% of placebo participants, based on moderate-certainty evidence [49]. A meta-analysis performed by Hoskins, et al. also found that SSRI drugs were significantly superior to placebo on either clinician- and self-rated PTSD symptom severity combined (paroxetine) or clinician-rated PTSD symptom severity alone (fluoxetine) [50].

While there are not many studies that focus on SSRI efficacy specifically in the older adult population, the aforementioned systematic review from Dinnen, et al. determined evidence-based interventions validated in younger and middle-aged populations, such as SSRIs, appear acceptable and efficacious with older adults [51].

Adverse Effects

Serotonin receptors have many functions in the body including, but not limited to, mood, sleep, appetite, sexual function, and nausea. Generally, medications within the SSRI class exhibit side effects such as sexual dysfunction, sleep disturbances, weight changes, anxiety, dizziness, xerostomia, headache, and gastrointestinal distress [41, 52]. Studies also show SSRIs, particularly citalopram, may lead to QT interval prolongation in a dose-dependent pattern which can lead to a fatal arrhythmia, torsade de pointes [53]. It important for older adults taking SSRIs to be aware of using of other medications that increases serotonin including monoamine oxidase inhibitor, SSRIs, and tricyclic antidepressants as the increase in the number of serotonergic agents can increase the risk of developing serotonin syndrome [54].

Withdrawal

Williams et al. performed a meta-analysis examining the outcome of treatment withdrawal from SSRIs in the PTSD population [49]. There was evidence of a harm for the individual SSRI agents compared with placebo (RR 1.41, 95% CI 1.07–1.87; 14 studies, 2399 participants), particularly the SSRI paroxetine group when compared to the placebo group (RR 1.55, 95% CI 1.05–2.29; 5 studies, 1101 participants).

Serotonin and Norepinephrine Reuptake Inhibitors (SNRIs)

Venlafaxine

Compared to SSRIs, there are fewer studies on SNRIs effect on PTSD, particularly in the older adult population. In a 6-month, double-blind, placebo-controlled trial, Davidson, et al. randomly assigned 329 adults with PTSD to receive venlafaxine ER or placebo for 24 weeks. In this study, participants receiving venlafaxine ER were more likely to experience remission of PTSD symptoms compared with individuals receiving placebo (50.9 vs. 37.5%, $p = 0.01$) [50].

Noradrenergic and Specific Serotonergic Antidepressant

Mirtazapine

The Williams et al. meta-analysis reviewed 54 randomized controlled trials and found evidence of beneficial effect for mirtazapine (RR 0.45, 95% CI 0.22–0.94; 1 study, 26 participants) in 65% of people on mirtazapine when compared with 22% of placebo participants [49].

Tricyclic Antidepressants (C)

The aforementioned meta-analysis from Williams et al. also found evidence of beneficial effect for amitriptyline (RR 0.60, 95% CI 0.38–0.96) in 50% of amitriptyline participants compared with 17% of placebo participants, which improved PTSD symptoms [50]. However, it is important to note that TCAs are typically avoided in the older adult population due to adverse effects such as postural hypotension, which can contribute to falls and fractures, cardiac conduction abnormalities, and anticholinergic effect (delirium, urinary retention, dry mouth, and constipation) [52–55]. In a meta-analysis of cohort and case-control studies, Wu et al. found TCA use was associated with significantly increased fracture risk (relative risk [RR], 1.45; 95% confidence interval [CI], 1.31–1.60; $p < 0.001$) [56].

Alpha-Adrenergic Receptor Blockers

There is unclear evidence on the efficacy of alpha-adrenergic receptor blockers such as prazosin for the treatment of PTSD. A 15-week trial of prazosin led to decreased traumatic nightmares and hyperarousal symptoms with associated increased sleep quality and global function in a simple population of veterans with PTSD symptoms who returned from combat deployments to Iraq and Afghanistan [57]. However, prazosin did not show any effect on symptoms such as re-experiencing/intrusion and avoidance when compared to placebo groups. Some common side effects of prazosin such as hypotension, syncope, headaches, and drowsiness can occur more often in the older adult population due to possible drug interactions such as concurrent anti-hypertensive medications.

Antipsychotics

There are mixed results pertaining to the efficacy of using second-generation antipsychotics (SGA) in the treatment of PTSD in the older adult population. Villarreal et al. performed a clinical trial to examine the effect of quetiapine in a sample of 80 military veterans with documented PTSD symptoms [58]. Their study displayed reductions in CAPS total, re-experiencing, and hyperarousal scores when compared to the placebo. However, a larger trial involving over 200 United States military veterans displayed no reduction in PTSD symptoms after 6 months of risperidone [59]. Participants in this study also experienced typical side effects from SGA usage such as metabolic effects (weight gain), fatigue, somnolence, and hypersalivation.

Ketamine

While research pertaining to the benefits of ketamine in PTSD is still in the formative stages, there are promising results from early studies. In a clinical trial in 2018, 6 infusions of ketamine over 12 days led to rapid improvement in depressive and PTSD symptoms in a study population with comorbid treatment-resistant depression and chronic PTSD [60]. In 2019, Bryant et al. examined the effects of repeated IV ketamine in treatment-resistant depression in the older adult population (participants aged from 65 to 82 years). With a sample size of six, one participant failed to respond to the initial acute treatment phase, and four participants responded to the acute infusion phase, but did not sustain a response after eight maintenance infusions [61]. It is important to note that this is a novel treatment for treatment-resis-

tant depression and more research is needed to obtain a view of this treatment's efficacy, especially in older adults diagnosed with PTSD.

Due to the novelty of the treatment, there is not much research on the long-term side effects of ketamine in the older adult population. While individuals who chronically use recreational ketamine experience side effects such as neurological (cortical atrophy), urinary (dysuria, nocturia), cardiovascular (tachycardia, hypertension), and hepatotoxicity, it is important to note that it is unclear if these side effect occur in individuals receiving ketamine infusions for PTSD or depression [62].

Medication Dosages and Levels

For PTSD management, paroxetine typically has a starting dose of 20 mg (but could start at a lower dose of 5–10 mg) and a therapeutic dose of 20–60 mg. Sertraline typically starts at 50 mg (but could start at a lower dose of 12.5–25 mg) and a therapeutic dose of 50–250 mg. Fluvoxamine typically starts at 50 mg (but could start at a lower dose of 25 mg) and a therapeutic dose of 100–300 mg. Fluoxetine typically starts at 20 mg (but could start at a lower dose of 5–10 mg) and a therapeutic dose of 20–60 mg. Citalopram typically starts at 20 mg (but could start at a lower dose of 10 mg) and a therapeutic dose of 20–40 mg. Escitalopram typically starts at 10 mg (also the lowest starting dose) and a therapeutic dose of 20–40 mg. Finally, venlafaxine typically starts at 37.5 mg (also the lowest starting dose) and a therapeutic dose of 37.5–300 mg. Table 24.2 lists the starting doses, maximum doses and therapeutic ranges for medications used to treat PTSD.

Table 24.2 Medications for PTSD in older adults

Name	Indication	Starting dose (mg)	Maximum dose (mg)	Therapeutic range (mg)
Paroxetine	FDA approved	5	60	20–60
Sertraline	FDA approved	12.5	250	50–250
Fluvoxamine	Off-label	25	300	100–300
Fluoxetine	FDA approved	5	60	20–60
Citalopram	Off-label	10	40[a]	20–40
Escitalopram	Off-label	10	40[a]	20–40
Venlafaxine	FDA-conditional	37.5	300[a]	37.5–300

FDA Food and Drug Administration
[a] Above FDA-approved maximum dose for older adults

Evidence-based Treatment Algorithm

Treatment for PTSD should be initiated as soon as the diagnosis is made, to avoid any complications from the delay in treatment. The first-line for PTSD is trauma-focused psychotherapy rather than medications. If an individual does not respond to psychotherapy, pharmacologic management with an SSRI is the preferred alternative first-line (especially if the individual has comorbid mood disorders). If an individual does not respond to two or three different SSRIs/SNRIs, these medications can be switched to an SGA (especially if psychotic symptoms are present). In people with sleep disturbances such as nightmares, prazosin can be used as an adjunct medication with the previously established SSRIs. A proposed management algorithm is outlined in Fig. 24.1.

While there are many guidelines and treatment algorithms, the Veteran's Administration/Department of Defense (VA/DOD) Clinical Practice Guideline for the Management of Posttraumatic Stress Disorder and Acute Stress Disorder (VA) guideline is commonly used in the United States to determine PTSD management [63]. In a systematic review, Martin et al. examined the quality of 14 different PTSD treatment guidelines and found that while no guideline was perfect, the VA received some of the highest scores (along with guidelines published by American Psychiatric Association (APA) and World Health Organization (WHO)) [64].

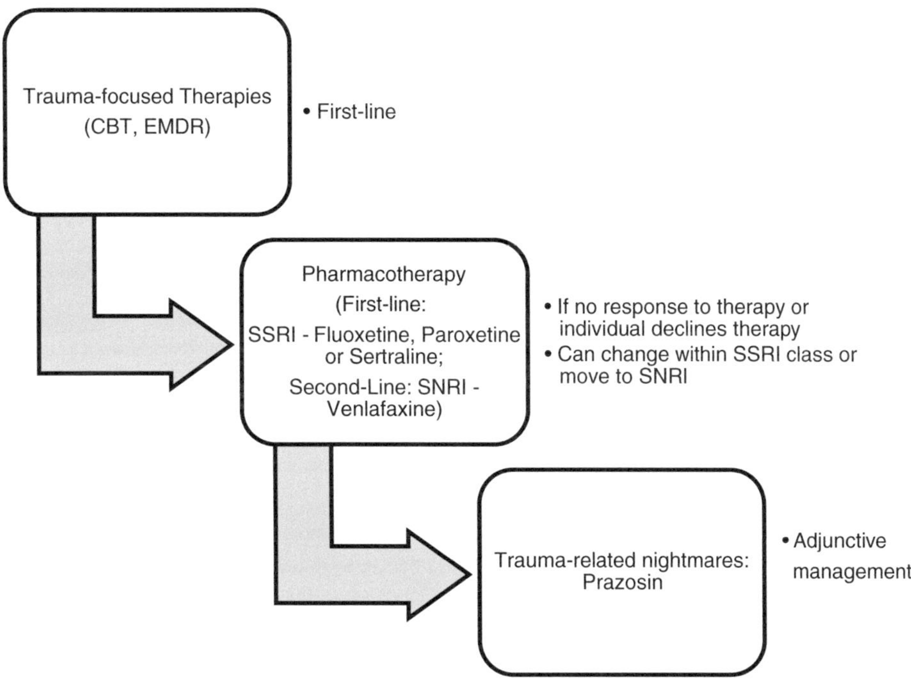

Fig. 24.1 Management algorithm. *CBT* cognitive behavioral therapy, *EMDR* eye movement desensitization reprocessing, *SNRI* serotonin and norepinephrine reuptake inhibitors

Conclusions

Posttraumatic stress disorder is a disorder that occurs following a singular or multiple distressing traumatic events and is often chronic in nature. While these traumatic events can occur either in childhood or adulthood, research points to childhood trauma leading to more severe PTSD symptoms later in life. Much of the research pertaining to PTSD in older adults revolves around the experience of military veterans and lacks a great deal of research examining the effects of other etiologies of trauma (abuse, social determinants of health, discrimination). There are many PTSD treatment guidelines that hold therapy modalities such as CBT, exposure therapy, and EMDR as first-line treatment. If therapy does not alleviate the PTSD symptoms, a SSRI can be added as a first-line alternative. PTSD is an under-researched disorder especially pertaining to the older adult demographic. This scarcity of literature makes proper care difficult for older adults with the disorder. Future research in PTSD in the older adult population should focus more on identification/assessment in populations with different traumatic experiences and treatment with novel management options such as ketamine.

References

1. Yehuda R. Post-traumatic stress disorder. N Engl J Med. 2002;346(2):108–14. https://doi.org/10.1056/nejmra012941.
2. Shalev A, Liberzon I, Marmar C. Post-traumatic stress disorder. N Engl J Med. 2017;376(25):2459–69. https://doi.org/10.1056/NEJMra1612499.
3. Goldstein R, et al. The epidemiology of DSM-5 posttraumatic stress disorder in the United States: results from the National Epidemiologic Survey on alcohol and related conditions-III. Soc Psychiatry Psychiatr Epidemiol. 2016;51(8):1137–48. https://doi.org/10.1007/s00127-016-1208-5.
4. Cook JM, McCarthy E, Thorp SR. Older adults with PTSD: brief state of research and evidence-based psychotherapy case illustration. Am J Geriatr Psychiatry. 2017;25(5):522–30. https://doi.org/10.1016/j.jagp.2016.12.016.
5. Christiansen DM, Elklit A. Sex differences in PTSD. In: Lazinica A, Ovuga E, editors. Posttraumatic stress disorder in a global context. Rijeka: InTech Open Access Book; 2012. p. 113–42.
6. Wang PS, et al. Twelve-month use of mental health services in the United States: results from the National Comorbidity Survey Replication. Arch Gen Psychiatry. 2006;62(6):629–40.
7. Tolin DF, Foa EB. Sex differences in trauma and posttraumatic stress disorder: a quantitative review of 25 years of research. Psychol Trauma Theory Res Pract Policy. 2008;3785 https://doi.org/10.1037/1942-9681.S.1.37.
8. Andrews B, Brewin CR, Rose S. Gender, social support and PTSD in victims of violent crime. J Trauma Stress. 2003;16:421–7. https://doi.org/10.1023/A:1024478305142.
9. Tolin DF, Foa EB. Gender and PTSD: a cognitive model. In: Kimerling R, Ouimette P, Wolfe J, editors. Gender and PTSD. New York, NY: The Guilford Press; 2003. p. 66–97.
10. Byers AL, et al. Chronicity of posttraumatic stress disorder and risk of disability in older persons. JAMA Psychiatry. 2014;71(5):540. https://doi.org/10.1001/jamapsychiatry.2014.5.
11. Schnurr PP. Physical Health and health services utilization. APA Handbook of Trauma. Psychology: Foundations in Knowledge (Vol. 1). 2014; 349–370. https://doi.org/10.1037/0000019-018.
12. Parker G, et al. Mental health implications for older adults after natural disasters—a systematic review and meta-analysis. Int Psychogeriatr. 2015;28(1):11–20. https://doi.org/10.1017/s1041610215001210.
13. González-Sanguino C, et al. Mental health consequences during the initial stage of the 2020 coronavirus pandemic (COVID-19) in Spain. Brain Behav Immun. 2020;87:172–6. https://doi.org/10.1016/j.bbi.2020.05.040.
14. Chamaa F, et al. PTSD in the COVID-19 era. Curr Neuropharmacol. 2021;19(12):2164–79. https://doi.org/10.2174/1570159X19666210113152954.
15. Cai X, et al. Psychological distress and its correlates among COVID-19 survivors during early convalescence across age groups. Am J Geriatr Psychiatry. 2020;28(10):1030–9. https://doi.org/10.1016/j.jagp.2020.07.003.
16. Ogle CM, Rubin DC, Siegler IC. Cumulative exposure to traumatic events in older adults. Aging Ment Health. 2013;18(3):316–25. https://doi.org/10.1080/13607863.2013.832730.
17. Kelmendi B, et al. PTSD: from neurobiology to pharmacological treatments. Eur J Psychotraumatol. 2016;7(1):31858. https://doi.org/10.3402/ejpt.v7.31858.
18. Chang X, et al. Associations between adverse childhood experiences and health outcomes in adults aged 18–59 years. PLoS One. 2019;14(2):e0211850. https://doi.org/10.1371/journal.pone.0211850.
19. Choi NG, et al. Association of Adverse childhood experiences with lifetime mental and substance use disorders among men and women aged 50+ years.

Int Psychogeriatr. 2016;29(3):359–72. https://doi.org/10.1017/s1041610216001800.

20. Ogle CM. The impact of the developmental timing of trauma exposure on PTSD symptoms and psychosocial functioning among older adults. Dev Psychol. 2013;49:2191–200. https://doi.org/10.1037/a0031985.supp.

21. Pieterse AL, et al. An exploratory examination of the associations among racial and ethnic discrimination, racial climate, and trauma-related symptoms in a college student population. J Couns Psychol. 2010;57(3):255–63. https://doi.org/10.1037/a0020040.

22. Bor J, et al. Police killings and their spillover effects on the mental health of black Americans: a population-based, quasi-experimental study. Lancet. 2018;392(10144):302–10. https://doi.org/10.1016/s0140-6736(18)31130-9.

23. Williams MT, et al. Assessing racial trauma within a DSM–5 framework: the UConn racial/ethnic stress and trauma survey. Pract Innov. 2018;3(4):242–60. https://doi.org/10.1037/pri0000076.

24. Seelman KL, Woodford MR, Nicolazzo Z. Victimization and microaggressions targeting LGBTQ college students: gender identity as a moderator of psychological distress. Microaggressions and Social Work Research, Practice and Education; 2020. p. 113–26. https://doi.org/10.4324/9780429460531-8.

25. Roberts AL, et al. Pervasive trauma exposure among us sexual orientation adults linked to posttraumatic stress disorder risk. Comprehen Psychiatry. 2010;6(51):e8–9. https://doi.org/10.1016/j.comppsych.2010.06.039.

26. Davison KM, et al. Post-traumatic stress disorder (PTSD) in mid-age and older adults differs by immigrant status and ethnicity, nutrition, and other determinants of health in the Canadian longitudinal study on aging (CLSA). Soc Psychiatry Psychiatr Epidemiol. 2021;56:963–80. https://doi.org/10.1007/s00127-020-02003-7.

27. Conejero I, et al. Suicide in older adults: current perspectives. Clin Interv Aging. 2018;13:691–9. https://doi.org/10.2147/cia.s130670.

28. Gros DF, et al. Relations among social support, PTSD symptoms, and substance use in veterans. Psychol Addict Behav. 2018;30(7):764–70. https://doi.org/10.1037/adb0000205.

29. Weathers FW et al. The Clinician-Administered PTSD Scale for DSM-5 (CAPS-5). 2013. [Assessment]. www.ptsd.va.gov.

30. Weathers FW, et al. The clinician-administered PTSD scale for DSM–5 (CAPS-5): development and initial psychometric evaluation in military veterans. Psychol Assess. 2018;30(3):383–95. https://doi.org/10.1037/pas0000486.

31. Weathers FW et al. The PTSD checklist for DSM-5 (PCL-5). 2013.

32. Forkus SR, et al. The posttraumatic stress disorder (PTSD) checklist for DSM–5: a systematic review of existing psychometric evidence. Clin Psychol Sci Pract. 2022;30:110–21. https://doi.org/10.1037/cps0000111.

33. Reisman M. PTSD treatment for veterans: what's working, what's new, and what's next. P T. 2016;41(10):623–7, 632-634

34. Watkins LE, Sprang KR, Rothbaum BO. Treating PTSD: a review of evidence-based psychotherapy interventions. Front Behav Neurosci. 2018;12:258. https://doi.org/10.3389/fnbeh.2018.00258.

35. Smith NB, et al. Mental health treatment for older veterans newly diagnosed with PTSD: a national investigation. Am J Geriatr Psychiatry. 2016;24(3):201–12. https://doi.org/10.1016/j.jagp.2015.02.001.

36. Beck JS. Cognitive behavior therapy: basics and beyond. 2nd ed. New York, NY: Guilford Press; 2011. p. 391.

37. Forman-Hoffman V, et al. Psychological and pharmacological treatments for adults with posttraumatic stress disorder: A systematic review update. Comparat Effect Rev. 2018;207 https://doi.org/10.23970/ahrqepccer207.

38. Resick PA, et al. Effect of group vs individual cognitive processing therapy in active-duty military seeking treatment for posttraumatic stress disorder. JAMA Psychiatry. 2017;74(1):28. https://doi.org/10.1001/jamapsychiatry.2016.2729.

39. Foa EB, Hembree E, Rothbaum BO. Prolonged exposure therapy for PTSD: emotional processing of traumatic experiences, therapist guide. New York, NY: Oxford University Press; 2007.

40. Sloan DM, Marx BP. Written exposure therapy for PTSD: a brief treatment approach for mental health professionals. American Psychological Press; 2019.

41. Dinnen S, Simiola V, Cook JM. Post-traumatic stress disorder in older adults: a systematic review of the psychotherapy treatment literature. Aging Ment Health. 2014;19(2):144–50. https://doi.org/10.1080/13607863.2014.920299.

42. Cusack K, et al. Psychological treatments for adults with posttraumatic stress disorder: a systematic review and meta-analysis. Clin Psychol Rev. 2016;43:128–41. https://doi.org/10.1016/j.cpr.2015.10.003.

43. Schnurr PP, et al. Cognitive behavioral therapy for posttraumatic stress disorder in women. JAMA. 2007;297(8):820. https://doi.org/10.1001/jama.297.8.820.

44. Shapiro F. Eye movement desensitization and reprocessing (EMDR) therapy: basic principles, protocols and procedures. 3rd ed. New York, NY: Guilford Press; 2017.

45. Chen Y-R, et al. Efficacy of eye-movement desensitization and reprocessing for patients with posttraumatic-stress disorder: A meta-analysis of randomized controlled trials. PLoS One. 2014;9(8):e103676. https://doi.org/10.1371/journal.pone.0103676.

46. Rosenbaum S, et al. Physical activity in the treatment of post-traumatic stress disorder: a systematic review and meta-analysis. Psychiatry Res. 2015;230(2):130–6. https://doi.org/10.1016/j.psychres.2015.10.017.

47. Aldwin CM, et al. Age differences in stress, coping, and appraisal: findings from the normative aging study. J Gerontol B Psychol Sci Soc Sci. 1996;51B:179–88.

48. Cook JM, et al. Symptom differences between older depressed primary care patients with and without history of trauma. Int J Psychiatry Med. 2001;31:401–14. https://doi.org/10.2190/61me-f2m0-3ph5-g59e.

49. Williams T, et al. Pharmacotherapy for post-traumatic stress disorder (PTSD). Cochrane Database Syst Rev. 2022;3:CD002795. https://doi.org/10.1002/14651858.cd002795.pub3.

50. Davidson J, et al. Treatment of posttraumatic stress disorder with venlafaxine extended release. Arch Gen Psychiatry. 2006;63(10):1158–65. https://doi.org/10.1001/archpsyc.63.10.1158.

51. Hoskins M, et al. Pharmacotherapy for post-traumatic stress disorder: systematic review and meta-analysis. Br J Psychiatry. 2015;206(2):93–100. https://doi.org/10.1192/bjp.bp.114.148551.

52. Chu A, Wadhwa R. Selective serotonin reuptake inhibitors—Statpearls—NCBI bookshelf. A Retrieved December 19, 2022, from https://www.ncbi.nlm.nih.gov/books/NBK554406/

53. Beach SR, et al. Meta-analysis of selective serotonin reuptake inhibitor–associated QTC prolongation. J Clin Psychiatry. 2014;75(05):e441–9. https://doi.org/10.4088/jcp.13r08672.

54. Scotton WJ, et al. Serotonin syndrome: pathophysiology, clinical features, management, and potential future directions. Int J Tryptophan Res. 2019;12:117864691987392. https://doi.org/10.1177/1178646919873925.

55. Wiese B. Geriatric depression: the use of antidepressants in the elderly. BC Medical Journal. 2011;53(7).

56. Wu Q, et al. Tricyclic antidepressant use and risk of fractures: a meta-analysis of cohort and case-control studies. J Bone Miner Res. 2013;28(4):753–63. https://doi.org/10.1002/jbmr.1813.

57. Raskind MA, et al. A trial of prazosin for combat trauma PTSD with nightmares in active-duty soldiers returned from Iraq and Afghanistan. Am J Psychiatry. 2013;170(9):1003–10. https://doi.org/10.1176/appi.ajp.2013.12081133.

58. Villarreal G, et al. Efficacy of quetiapine monotherapy in posttraumatic stress disorder: a randomized, placebo-controlled trial. Am J Psychiatry. 2016;173(12):1205–12. https://doi.org/10.1176/appi.ajp.2016.15070967.

59. Krystal JH. Adjunctive risperidone treatment for antidepressant-resistant symptoms of chronic military service–related PTSD. JAMA. 2011;306(5):493. https://doi.org/10.1001/jama.2011.1080.

60. Albott CS, et al. Efficacy, safety, and durability of repeated ketamine infusions for comorbid posttraumatic stress disorder and treatment-resistant depression. J Clin Psychiatry. 2018;79(3):17m11634. https://doi.org/10.4088/jcp.17m11634.

61. Bryant KA, et al. Effects of repeated intravenous ketamine in treatment-resistant geriatric depression. J Clin Psychopharmacol. 2019;39(2):158–61. https://doi.org/10.1097/jcp.0000000000001006.

62. da Frota Ribeiro CM, Riva-Posse P. Use of ketamine in elderly patients with treatment-resistant depression. Curr Psychiatry Rep. 2017;19(12):107. https://doi.org/10.1007/s11920-017-0855-x.

63. Veterans Affairs. 2017 clinical practice guideline for the management of PTSD. (2019, April 1). Retrieved December 19, 2022, from https://www.ptsd.va.gov/professional/treat/txessentials/cpg_ptsd_management.asp

64. Martin A, et al. Treatment guidelines for PTSD: a systematic review. J Clin Med. 2021;10(18):4175. https://doi.org/10.3390/jcm10184175.

Index

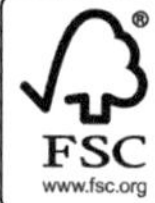

MIX
Papier aus verantwortungsvollen Quellen
Paper from responsible sources
FSC® C105338

If you have any concerns about our products,
you can contact us on
ProductSafety@springernature.com

In case Publisher is established outside the EU,
the EU authorized representative is:
Springer Nature Customer Service Center GmbH
Europaplatz 3, 69115 Heidelberg, Germany

Printed by Libri Plureos GmbH
in Hamburg, Germany